Oxford Textbook of

Movement Disorders

Oxford Textbook of

Movement Disorders

Edited by
David J. Burn
Institute for Ageing and Health
Newcastle University, UK

Series Editor
Christopher Kennard

OXFORD
UNIVERSITY PRESS

OXFORD
UNIVERSITY PRESS

Great Clarendon Street, Oxford, OX2 6DP,
United Kingdom

Oxford University Press is a department of the University of Oxford.
It furthers the University's objective of excellence in research, scholarship,
and education by publishing worldwide. Oxford is a registered trade mark of
Oxford University Press in the UK and in certain other countries

First Edition published in 2013

Impression: 1

British Library Cataloguing in Publication Data
Data available

ISBN 978–0–19–960953–6

Printed in China by
C&C Offset Printing Co. Ltd

Contents

List of Contributors

Lillian Acevedo Neurology Service, Hospital Clínic de Barcelona, Universitat de Barcelona (UB), Institut d'Investigacions Biomèdiques August Pi i Sunyer (IDIBAPS), Barcelona, Spain

Alberto Albanese Istituto Neurologico Carlo Besta, Milan, and Istituto di Neurologia, Università Cattolica del Sacro Cuore, Milan, Italy

Melissa J. Armstrong Department of Neurology, University of Maryland School of Medicine, Baltimore, MD, USA

Erika F. Augustine Department of Neurology, University of Rochester, School of Medicine and Dentistry, Rochester, NY, USA

Oliver Bandmann Department of Neuroscience, Sheffield Institute of Translational Neuroscience, University of Sheffield, Sheffield, UK

Roger A. Barker Department of Neurology and John van Geest Centre for Brain Repair, Addenbrooke's NHS Trust, Cambridge, UK

K.P. Bhatia National Hospital for Neurology and Neurosurgery, London, UK

José Brás Department of Molecular Neuroscience, Institute of Neurology, University College London, UK

S. Bressman Department of Neurology, Albert Einstein College of Medicine, New York, USA

David J. Brooks Imperial College London, UK

David J. Burn Institute for Ageing and Health, Newcastle University, Newcastle upon Tyne, UK

Francisco Cardoso Internal Medicine Department, Federal University of Minas Gerais, Belo Horizonte, MG, Brazil

Heidi Cartwright Neuroscience Research Australia and the University of New South Wales, Sydney, Australia

Leslie J. Cloud Virginia Commonwealth University, VCU Parkinson's Disease Research Center, Richmond, VA, USA

Carla Cordivari The National Hospital for Neurology and Neurosurgery and Institute of Neurology, University College Hospitals, London, UK

Marina A.J. de Koning-Tijssen Department of Neurology, University Medical Centre Groningen, University of Groningen, Groningen, The Netherlands

Günther Deuschl Department of Neurology, Christian-Albrechts-Universtität Kiel, Kiel, Germany

Mark J. Edwards Sobell Department of Motor Neuroscience and Movement Disorders, UCL Institute of Neurology, London, UK

Antonio A. Elia Istituto Neurologico Carlo Besta, Milan, Italy

Susan H. Fox Movement Disorder Clinic, Toronto Western Hospital, University Health Network and Division of Neurology, University of Toronto, Canada

Carles Gaig Neurology Service, Hospital Clínic de Barcelona, Universitat de Barcelona (UB), Institut d'Investigacions Biomèdiques August Pi i Sunyer (IDIBAPS), Barcelona, Spain

David Gallagher Department of Clinical Neurosciences, Institute of Neurology, University College London, UK

Glenda M. Halliday Neuroscience Research Australia and the University of New South Wales, Sydney, Australia

John Hardy Department of Molecular Neuroscience, Institute of Neurology, University College London, UK

Joseph Jankovic Parkinson Disease Center and Movement Disorders Clinic, Department of Neurology, Baylor College of Medicine, Houston, TX, USA

Christine Klein Department of Neurology, University of Lübeck, Lübeck, Germany

George Koutsis Department of Molecular Neuroscience, UCL Institute of Neurology, London, UK, and Department of Neurology, University of Athens Medical School, Athens, Greece

Florian Krismer Division of Neurobiology, Department of Neurology, Medical University, Innsbruck, Austria

Anthony Lang Movement Disorder Clinic, Toronto Western Hospital, University Health Network and Division of Neurology, University of Toronto, Canada

A.W. Lemstra Department of Neurology/Alzheimer Centre, VU Medical Centre, Amsterdam, The Netherlands

Shyamal H. Mehta Movement Disorders Program, Georgia's Health Sciences University, Augusta, GA, USA

Jonathan W. Mink Department of Neurology, University of Rochester, School of Medicine and Dentistry, Rochester, NY, USA

John C. Morgan Movement Disorders Program, Georgia's Health Sciences University, Augusta, GA, USA

Isabel Pareés Sobell Department of Motor Neuroscience and Movement Disorders, UCL Institute of Neurology, London, UK

Steffen Paschen Department of Neurology, University of Kiel, Kiel, Germany

Julie Phukan Department of Clinical Neurosciences, UCL Institute of Neurology, London, UK

Werner Poewe Department of Neurology, Medical University, Innsbruck, Austria

Josef Priller Department of Neuropsychiatry, Charité–Universitätsmedizin Berlin, Berlin, Germany

Paul J. Reading The James Cook University Hospital, Middlesbrough, UK

Anthony H.V. Schapira Department of Clinical Neurosciences, Institute of Neurology, University College London, UK

Susanne A. Schneider Department of Neurology, University of Kiel, Kiel, Germany

H. Seelaar Department of Neurology, Erasmus MC-University Medical Center Rotterdam, Rotterdam, the Netherlands

Kapil D. Sethi Movement Disorders Program, Georgia's Health Sciences University, Augusta, GA, USA

Binit Shah Movement Disorder Clinic, Toronto Western Hospital, University Health Network and Division of Neurology, University of Toronto, Canada

Sabine Spielberger Department of Neurology, Medical University, Innsbruck, Austria

M. Stamelou National Hospital for Neurology and Neurosurgery, London, UK

Gerald Stern Department of Clinical Neurology, University College Hospitals, London, UK

Sarah J. Tabrizi UCL Institute of Neurology and National Hospital for Neurology and Neurosurgery, London, UK

Rachel Tan Neuroscience Research Australia and the University of New South Wales, Sydney, Australia

Eduardo Tolosa Neurology Service, Hospital Clínic de Barcelona, Universitat de Barcelona (UB), Institut d'Investigacions Biomèdiques August Pi i Sunyer (IDIBAPS), Barcelona, Spain

J.C. van Swieten Department of Neurology, Erasmus MC-University Medical Center Rotterdam, Rotterdam, the Netherlands

Richard Walsh Movement Disorder Clinic, Toronto Western Hospital, University Health Network and Division of Neurology, University of Toronto, Canada

Thomas Warner Reta Lila Weston Institute of Neurological Studies, UCL Institute of Neurology, London, UK

William Weiner (deceased) Department of Neurology, University of Maryland School of Medicine, Baltimore, MD, USA

Gregor K. Wenning Division of Neurobiology, Department of Neurology, Medical University, Innsbruck, Austria

Thomas Wichmann Emory University, Atlanta, GA, USA

Edward J. Wild UCL Institute of Neurology and National Hospital for Neurology and Neurosurgery, London, UK

David R. Williams Van Cleef Roet Centre for Nervous Diseases, Monash University, Melbourne, Australia

Nicholas W. Wood Department of Molecular Neuroscience, UCL Institute of Neurology and UCL Genetics Institute, London, UK

List of Abbreviations

^{18}FDG	^{18}F-2-fluoro-2-deoxyglucose
^{123}I-FP-CIT	^{123}I-N-ω-fluoropropyl-2β-carbomethoxy-3β-(4-iodophenyl)nortropan
^{123}I-IBZM	^{123}I-iodobenzamine
^{123}IPT	[^{123}I]*N*-3-iodopro-pene-2-yl-2β-carbomethoxy-3β-4-chlorophenyl tropane
3-HK	3-hydroxykynurenine
5-HTP	5- hydroxytryptophan
6-OHDA	6-hydroxydopamine
AASLD	American Association for the Study of Liver Diseases
ABL	abetalipoproteinaemia
ACA	anterior cingulate area
ACD	alcoholic cerebellar degeneration
ACE	angiotensin-converting enzyme
ACTH	adrenocorticotrophic hormone
AD	Alzheimer's disease
ADC	AIDS dementia complex
ADCA	autosomal dominant cerebellar ataxia
ADEM	acute disseminated encephalomyelitis
ADHD	attention deficit–hyperactivity disorder
ADL	activities of daily living
ADNFLE	autosomal dominant nocturnal frontal lobe epilepsy
AED	antiepileptic drug
AFP	anterior forebrain pathway, alpha-fetoprotein
AGD	argyrophilic grain disease
AHD	acquired hepatocerebral degeneration
ALD	adrenoleucodystrophy
ALMA	alternating leg muscle activation
ALS	amyotrophic lateral sclerosis
AMRFS	action myoclonus renal failure syndrome
ANAB	antineuronal antibodies
AOA	ataxia with oculomotor apraxia
APD	atypical parkinsonian disorder, adult-onset primary dystonia
ARCA	autosomal recessive cerebellar ataxia
ARF	acute rheumatic fever
ARSACS	autosomal recessive spastic ataxia of Charlevoix-Saguenay
ASO	anti-streptolysin
ATA	ataxia telangiectasia
AVED	ataxia with vitamin E deficiency
BAC	bacterial artificial chromosome
BAL	British anti-lewisite
bd	twice daily
BDNF	brain-derived neurotrophic factor
BFC	benign familial chorea
bid	twice daily
BoNT	botulinum toxin
bp	base pair(s)
BP	*Bereitschaftspotential*
bvFTD	behavioural variant of frontotemporal dementia
CANVAS	cerebellar ataxia with neuropathy and bilateral vestibular areflexia syndrome
CBD	corticobasal degeneration
CBIT	comprehensive behavioural intervention for tics
CBS	corticobasal syndrome
cCT	cranial computed tomography
CFT	2-β-carbomethoxy-3-β-(4-fluorophenyl)tropane
CI	confidence interval
CJD	Creutzfeldt–Jakob disease
CM	centromedian nucleus of the thalamus
CMA	cingulate motor area
COMT	catechol-*O*-methyltransferase
CPAP	continuous positive airway pressure
CPG	central pattern generator
CR	controlled release
CRB	CREB-binding protein
C-reflex	cortical reflex
CSE	choreoathetosis/spasticity
CSF	cerebrospinal fluid
CSTC	cortico-striatal-thalamo-cortical
CT	computed tomography
CTX	cerebrotendinous xanthomatosis
CZi	caudal zona incerta

DA	dopamine agonist
DAT	dopamine transporter
DBA	dopamine-receptor blocking agent
DBS	deep brain stimulation
DDS	dopamine dysregulation syndrome
DIM	drug-induced myoclonus
DIP	drug-induced parkinsonism
DLB	dementia with Lewy bodies
DLPFC	dorsolateral prefrontal cortex
DM1	myotonic dystrophy type 1
DRB	dopamine-receptor-blocking drug
DRD	dopa-responsive dystonia
DRPLA	dentatorubral-pallidoluysian atrophy
DSM-IV	Diagnostic and Statistical Manual of Mental Disorders IV
DT	dystonic tremor
DTBZ	dihydrotetrabenazine
DTI	diffusion tensor imaging
DWI	diffusion-weighted imaging
EA	episodic ataxia
EBM	evidence based medicine
ECD	ethylene cysteinate dimer
EDS	excessive daytime sleepiness
EEG	electroencephalography, electroencephalographic, electroencephalogram
EFM	excessive fragmentary myoclonus
EFNS	European Federation of Neurological Societies
EKD	episodic kinesigenic dyskinesia
EMG	electromyography, electromyographic, electromyogram
EPaT	essential palatal tremor
EPS	extrapyramidal side effects
EPT	enhanced physiological tremor, exaggerated physiological tremor
ER	extended release
ET	essential tremor
FAB	Frontal Assessment Battery
FAHN	fatty acid hydroxylase-associated neurodegeneration
FAPED	familial acanthocytosis with paroxysmal exertion-induced dyskinesias and epilepsy
FCMTE	familial cortical myoclonic tremor and epilepsy
FDA	US Food and Drug Administration
FEF	frontal eye field
FHM	familial hemiplegic migraine
FIRDA	frontal intermittent rhythmic delta activity
fMRI	functional MRI
FoG	freezing of gait
FRDA	Friedreich's ataxia
FTD	frontotemporal dementia
FTDP-17	frontotemporal dementia with parkinsonism linked to chromosome 17
FTLD	frontotemporal lobe degeneration
FXTAS	fragile X-associated tremor–ataxia syndrome
GABA	gamma-aminobutyric acid
GABHS	group A beta-haemolytic streptococcus
GAD	glutamic acid decarboxylase
GBA	glucocerebrosidase
GCI	(oligodendro-)glial cytoplasmic inclusion
GDNF	glial-derived neurotrophic factor
GEPD	generalized epilepsy and paroxysmal dyskinesia
GI	gastrointestinal
GP	globus pallidus
GPe	external pallidal segment, globus pallidus externus
GPi	internal pallidal segment, globus pallidus internus
GSS	Gerstmann–Sträussler–Scheinker disease
gSSEP	giant somatosensory evoked potentials
GWAS	genome-wide association studies
HB–HC	hemiballism–hemichorea
HD	Huntington's disease
HDAC	histone deacetylase
HDL	Huntington's disease-like
HFT	hypnagogic foot tremor
HIV	human immunodeficiency virus
HMSN	hereditary motor and sensory neuropathy
HPRT	hypoxanthine-guanine phosphoribosyltransferase
ICCA	infantile familial convulsions and paroxysmal choreoathetosis
ICD	impulse control disorder
IL	interleukin
ILOCA	idiopathic late-onset cerebellar ataxia
INAD	infantile neuroaxonal dystrophy
iPS	induced pluripotent stem
iRBD	idiopathic REM sleep behaviour disorder
iRLS	idiopathic restless legs syndrome
ITD	idiopathic torsion dystonia
IVIG	intravenous immunoglobulin
KFR	Kayser–Fleischer ring
KMO	kynurenine 3-mono-oxygenase
LB	Lewy body
LDR	long-duration response
LN	Lewy neurite
LOFC	lateral orbitofrontal cortex
LSVT	Lee Silverman Voice Treatment
L-threo-DOPS	L-threo-dihydroxy-phenylserine
M1	primary motor cortex
MAO-B	monoamine oxidase type B
MAOI	monoamine oxidase inhibitor
MCA	Montreal Cognitive Assessment
MCI	mild cognitive impairment
MD	mediodorsal nucleus of the thalamus, myoclonus–dystonia
MDS	Movement Disorder Society
MEG	magnetoencephalography
MERRF	myoclonus epilepsy with ragged red fibres
MFS	Miller Fisher syndrome
MIBG	meta-iodobenzyl guanidine
MID	mitochondrial disorder
MIRAS	mitochondrial recessive ataxia syndrome
MLD	metachromatic leucodystrophy
MMSE	Mini Mental State Examination
MoCA	Montreal Cognitive Assessment
MOFC	medial orbitofrontal cortex
MP	^{11}C-methylphenidate
MPTP	1-methyl-4-phenyl-1,2,3-tetrahydropyridine
MRI	magnetic resonance imaging
MS	multiple sclerosis
MSA	multiple system atrophy

MSLT	Multiple Sleep Latency Test
MSN	medium spiny striatal projection neuron
MSS	Marinesco-Sjögren syndrome
MT	microtubule
NBIA	neurodegeneration with brain iron accumulation
NCC	nested case–control, neurocysticercosis
NCE	neuroacanthocytosis
NCI	neuronal cytoplasmic inclusion
NCL	neuronal ceroid lipofuscinosis
NCS	nerve conduction studies
NFLE	nocturnal frontal lobe epilepsy
NICE	National Institute for Health and Clinical Excellence
NIH	National Institutes of Health
NII	neuronal intranuclear inclusion
NINDS–SPSP	National Institute of Neurological Disorders and Stroke and Society for Progressive Supranuclear Palsy
NMDA	*N*-methyl-D-aspartate
NMS	neuroleptic malignant syndrome
NOS	not otherwise specified
NPC	Niemann–Pick disease type C
NPS	neuropsychiatric symptoms
OCB	oligoclonal band
OCD	obsessive–compulsive disorder
ODD	oppositional–defiant disorder
OH	orthostatic hypotension
OMD	oromandibular dystonia
OR	odds ratio
OrgT	organic tremor
OSA	obstructive sleep apnoea
OT	orthostatic tremor
PAGF	pure akinesia and gait freezing
PANDAS	paediatric autoimmune neuropsychiatric disorders associated with streptococcal infections
PAPS	primary antiphospholipid antibody syndrome
PATX	periodic ataxia
PCD	paraneoplastic cerebellar degeneration
PCR	polymerase chain reaction
PD	Parkinson's disease
PDD	Parkinson's disease dementia, pervasive developmental delay
PDRP	PD-related profile
PED	paroxysmal exercise-induced dyskinesia
PEG	percutaneous endoscopic gastrostomy
PET	positron emission tomography
Pf	parafascicular nucleus of the thalamus
PFS	Parkinson's Fatigue Scale
PHM	post-hypoxic myoclonus
PKAN	panthothenate kinase-associated neurodegeneration
PKD	paroxysmal kinesigenic dyskinesia
PLAN	*PLA2G6*-associated neurodegeneration
PLM	periodic limb movement
PLMD	periodic limb movement disorder
PMC	premotor cortex
PMD	psychogenic movement disorder
PME	progressive myoclonic epilepsy
PML	progressive multifocal leucoencephalopathy
PNFA	progressive non-fluent aphasia
PNKD	paroxysmal non-kinesigenic dyskinesia
PP	psychogenic parkinsonism
PPA	primary progressive aphasia
PPMS	primary progressive multiple sclerosis
PPN	pedunculopontine nucleus
PR	prolonged release
PSD	periodic sharp discharge, postsynaptic density
PSM	propriospinal myoclonus
PSP	progressive supranuclear palsy
PsyT	psychogenic tremor
PT	psychogenic tremor
PWT	primary writing tremor
QoL	quality of life
RBD	REM sleep behaviour disorder
RCT	randomized controlled trial
RD	Refsum's disease
RDP	rapid-onset dystonia–parkinsonism
REM	rapid eye movement
r-HGH	recombinant human growth hormone
RLS	restless legs syndrome
RMD	rhythmic movement disorder
ROI	region of interest
ROS	reactive oxygen species
RR	relative risk
RS	Richardson's syndrome
rTMS	repetitive transcranial magnetic stimulation
SANDO	sensory ataxic neuropathy, dysarthria, and ophthalmoparesis
SB	sleep bruxism
SBS	sequencing by synthesis
s.c.	subcutaneous
SC	Sydenham's chorea
SCA	spinocerebellar ataxia
sCJD	sporadic Creutzfeldt–Jakob disease
SCLC	small-cell lung cancer
SCM	sternocleidomastoid
SD	spasmodic dysphonia, Sydenham's disease
SDR	short-duration response
SEF	supplementary eye field
SEP	somatosensory evoked potential
SLE	systemic lupus erythematosus
SMA	supplementary motor area
SN	substantia nigra
SNc	substantia nigra pars compacta
SNP	single nucleotide polymorphism
SNr	substantia nigra pars reticulata
SNRI	serotonin–noradrenaline reuptake inhibitor
SOT	standard of truth
SPECT	single photon emission computed tomography
SPS	stiff person syndrome
SPT	symptomatic palatal tremor
SR	sepiapterin reductase
SREAT	steroid-responsive encephalopathy associated with autoimmune thyroiditis
SSEP	somatosensory evoked potential
SSPE	subacute sclerosing panencephalitis
SSRI	selective serotonin-reuptake inhibitor
STN	subthalamic nucleus

SWEDDs	scans without evidence of dopaminergic deficit
TA	tardive akathisia
TBZ	tetrabenzine
TCS	transcranial sonography
TD	tardive dyskinesia
tds	three times daily
TDt	tardive dystonia
TENS	transcutaneous electrical nerve stimulation
TH	tyrosine hydroxylase
TIC	Tourette Syndrome International Database Consortium
tid	three times daily
TMS	transcranial magnetic stimulation
TRIG	Tremor Investigation Group
TS	Tourette's syndrome
TST	task-specific tremor, triple stimulation test
UBS	ubiquitin proteasome system
UHDRS	Unified Huntington's Disease Rating Scale
UMSARS	Unified MSA Rating Scale
UPDRS	Unified Parkinson's Disease Rating Scale
UPS	ubiquitin–proteasome system
UPSIT	University of Pennsylvania Smell Identification Test
USCRS	UFMG Sydenham's Chorea Rating Scale
VA	ventral anterior nucleus of the thalamus
VGKC	voltage-gated potassium channel
VH	visual hallucination
Vim	ventrointermedius nucleus of the thalamus
VL	ventrolateral nucleus of the thalamus
VMAT2	vesicle monoamine transporter density
VPSG	polysomnography with audiovisual recording
VTA	ventral tegmental area
VWMD	vanishing white matter disease
WD	Wilson disease, Whipple's disease

CHAPTER 1

Overview and Historical Perspective

Gerald Stern

'A divine old age had slackened his mouth. He cast his spittle upon the ground and spat it out'.

Egyptian papyrus of 19th Dynasty *c.*1350–1200, describing an elderly king.

Ancient history

While early descriptions were inextricably influenced by mythology, magic, religion, superstition, traditional philosophies, and interpretations by shamans, obvious disorders of movement should have attracted 'clinical' attention. Interpretation of texts, such as the above, continue to remain uncertain. Certain early observations were remarkably sophisticated. In the Holy City of Varanasi (formerly Benares), within the Hindu University of India, original Sanskrit texts and incunabula reveal the contributions of Ayurvedic medicine (5000–3000 BC).

Diseases were then categorized into three bioentities: *vata* (psychomotor or life force), *pitta* (metabolic), and *kapha* (growth). Imbalance of *vata* gave rise to neurological disorders, which were further divided into *kampa* (tremor), *stambha* (stiffness), and *vishada* (depression). These could be compounded. Thus, *kamparata* indicated shaking palsy. Among the prescribed traditional medications were *atmaghupta* seed (*Mucuna pruriens*), containing levodopa, and extracts of three plants—*aswaghanda* root (*Withania somnifera*), *bala* (*Sida cordifolia*), and *paraseekayavanee* (*Hyoscyamus reticulatus*)—all solanaceous alkaloids similar to *Atropa belladona* (1). The latter were not introduced into European medicine until the nineteenth century, when they were used by a pupil of Charcot for the symptomatic treatment of Parkinson's disease. *Chandra*, the moon plant (*Rauwolfia serpentina*), long used as a sedative for recurring mania attributed to movements of the moon (lunacy), was rediscovered by Nathaniel Kline when serving in India during the Second World War. He introduced it to America—the first effective medication for chronic schizophrenia. It was soon discovered that sustained administration caused drug-induced parkinsonism and facilitated the recognition of dopamine as a neurotransmitter (2). Early Mesopotamian literature from the first half of the second millennium, which resisted translation of cuneiform scripts on clay tablets until the twentieth century, was often precise and sophisticated (3). It includes a compelling early description and prognosis of Parkinson's disease (4): 'If his head trembles, his neck and spine are bent, but he cannot stick out his tongue, his saliva flows from his mouth, his hands legs and feet all tremble at once and when he walks, he falls forwards, he will not get well'.

In the world's oldest continuous civilization, the present People's Republic of China, there is evidence stemming back to the second millennium BC indicating that Chinese society had its medicine men comparable to the shamans of North Asian tribal societies (5). However, in 1963 Keele observed '... it would seem probable that the first civilised people to free themselves from purely magico-religious concepts of disease were the ancient Chinese ...' (6). As in Europe, early observers often had difficulty in separating symptoms (*hou*), signs, syndromes, diseases (*chi*), causes, and treatments. Catalogues of diseases became compendious. Thus in 992, the massive Imperial Grace Formulary (*T'ai-ping sheng hui fang*) provided prescriptions for roughly a thousand distinct disorders (7).

Some traditional concepts may appear alien to contemporary eyes. For example, the notion of health (*ch'i*) was construed as a balance between two fundamental forces, the '*yin*' and the '*yang*' (8), yet there are implied notions, which ring familiar to present neurologists. In the earlier classics, excessive undisciplined emotions were recognized causes of disease (psychosomatics?). The conditions of health were partly inborn (genomics?), and partly due to food and drink (epigenetics *cum* nutrigenics?). Certain neurological diseases were described in meticulous detail; the clinical features and grim prognosis of rabies were set out in 556 BC '... when a mad dog bites someone, the patient becomes manic ... but if he remains well for 100 days he will remain safe ...' (5). During the Ming period (1368–1644), there are at least six separate descriptions of conditions resembling the shaking palsy (9). With respect to other neurodegenerations, in this vast ancient country where strongly held traditional values embraced profound family concern for the elderly, disabilities such as ageing may have been simply regarded as a fact of life demanding respect and support.

Claudius Galen (129–216), a Greek polymath from Pergamon, dominated Western medical science for over a thousand years until many of his opinions were refuted by Maimonides, Versalius, and William Harvey. Galen dissected many animals, published nearly 500 treatises, and wrote extensively on trauma and the nervous system (no doubt influenced by his experience as physician to the Roman School of Gladiators). He wrote in Greek but many of his works, translated later into Arabic (10), clearly document his extensive clinical experience and his insistence on a rational approach to medicine. Constantine reintroduced Greek medicine to Europe by patronage of translations of Aristotle, Hippocrates, and Galen into Latin. From these sources, classical notions of movement disorders are clearly documented. Galen recognized involuntary tremor (*voluntariae functionis laesio est impotentis*), tremor associated with stiffness (*quomodo a rigore differat*), and the influence of temperature (*affetus frigidus est*). Amongst several listed causes, he distinguished those related to poor nutrition (*causa alimenti indigentia*), those occurring in the mentally retarded (*est musculoram facultatis imbecillitus*), ocular tremor (*tremorum musculorum oculi*), and those related to psychiatric states including depression (*tremores convus superveniens mente ob melancholium*), and clearly separated the shaking of epilepsy (*tremors convulsivos*).

The early scientific enlightenment

In Europe, medieval physicians and anatomists rediscovered their heritage, albeit without the original Greek texts and usually through intermediate Syriac manuscripts. In the absence of drawings and diagrams, translational errors may well have occurred. In the *Anathomia of Mundius* (1538), the authorized textbook of medicine, there is a strange and fascinating confusion of Greek, Roman, Arabic, and medieval concepts (11). Mundinius states:

> At the base of the lateral ventricles lies a red sanguinous substance called vermis ... because it looks like an earthworm and because it moves like it. Namely it can contract ... and block the communication from one ventricle to another [ancient and medieval natural philosophy located phantasy in the anterior ventricle, imagination into the medial ventricle, and memory into the posterior ventricle] ... if then, the individual wishes to suspend cogitation, he elongates his worms and this prevents phantasy, memory and imagination from uniting and forming the 'common sense'...

Avicenna, the Arabic translator of Galen, had proposed 'vermis', whereas Galen speaks of choroid plexus and never vermis. Mundinius describes the wall of the lateral ventricle, to which the vermis is attached, as 'haunches'. Galen, who had a sound knowledge of the ventricles of the brain and adjacent structures, probably because he was familiar with the writings of Herophilus who had performed human necropsies in the School of Anatomy at Alexandria (circa 300 BC), referred to the basal ganglia as 'gluteal parts' or 'thighs'. Frederick Lewy (whose name is given to the Lewy body), a superb classical scholar as well as a seminal neuropathologist, was puzzled and shrewdly wrote, 'It may be luring to speculate whether the Greek *skelos* (thigh) may have been read as *skolex* (worm) by the Syriac expositor who preceded the Arabic translator Avicenna' (10). It was Thomas Willis who was responsible for much of the present nomenclature of the basal ganglia. In his *Cerebri Anatome* (1664), aided by the magnificent illustrations of Christopher Wren, Willis brought welcome clarity (12):

> ...In the foremost part of the brainstem, two prominent lentiform bodies... which are characterised by up-and-downward radiating medullating fibres, producing a striped appearance on their cut surface (corpus striatum)... Corpus striatum sive-medullae oblongatae apices sunt duo prominentiae lentiformis.

Willis authoritatively introduced the terms lenticular and striatum, using the terms synonymously when describing this structure as 'dissimilar to any other part of the brain' and quotes a sentence from Hainan's Arabic text of Galen concerning the glutea, so identifying striatum with glutea (12). Willis was also the first to clearly distinguish the striped anterior protruberance from the posterior non-striated lobe, which he called 'thalamus opticus', illustrating another probable misnomer. 'Thalamus' means a room or cavity and had been used by Galen for the chambers of the heart. He described the recess of the inferior horn of the lateral ventricle at its upward end as *thalame*, a loophole, which receives the 'spirit' by way of the hollow optic nerves. Hainan aptly depicts this region as a 'sleeping tent' (*hadjala*). Willis or his interpreters seem to have been more impressed by 'sleeping' than a 'tent' and thought of a bed rather than a bedroom.

As the detailed anatomy of the central nervous system was advancing, new findings continued to be described in classical languages. Just as traditionally, 'chorea' was derived from the Greek word for dance. In plays of ancient Greece, the chorus commented on the dramatic action utilizing dance, gesture, and mimicry. In many plays the chorus expressed to the audience what the actors could not say or provided insights and explanations, so the full repertoire of gestures was employed. Similarly, during the eighteenth and nineteenth centuries, knowledge of Greek or Latin was employed to describe new anatomical details.

The substantia innominata (1869) was the unnamed substance of Theodore Meynert (13). Déjèrine attributed to Burdach (1882) the name globus pallidum. Thomas von Sommering (1788), in his doctoral thesis 'De basi encephali et originibus nervorum', drew particular attention to the difference in appearance between the ashen or grey matter (substantiae cinereae) of the cortex and the brainstem: 'The mass is tinged a dark colour which in adults resembles neither the whiteness of the medulla nor the cinereal parts of the brain, but is, so to speak, midway between the cinereal and the medullary parts of the brain'. Later, the described a particular aggregation of dark substance within the cerebral peduncles. Sommering was familiar with the intimate relationship of the pigmented substance to the emerging third nerve fibres and noted that pigmentation was less distinct in the brains of newborn children and fetuses.

Alexander Munro (1783), the great Scottish anatomist did not seem to be aware of Sommering's priority: 'Nay in the middle substance of the brain and cerebellum, halfway between the surfaces of these and their ventricles and even within the crura cerebri... I have found a great quantity of ciniterous matter'. Blocq and Marinesco (1893) and Trétiakoff were amongst the first to relate 'Sömmering's substance, tache noire or locus niger crurum cerebri', now accepted as the substantia nigra, to disordered movement (14, 15).

The subthalamic nucleus also enjoyed a number of synonyms, including corps de Forel, discus lentiformis by Meynert, and nucleus amygdaliformis by Stilling, but most authors associated it with the name of Luys. Luys clearly showed this nucleus in his fine woodcut illustrated textbook (1876). He modestly, but erroneously, called the nucleus *bandelette accessoire de l'olive superiore* (16). The mysterious 'nucleus accumbens' simply means the nucleus leaning against the septum. Meanwhile, the era of classical neuropathology was accelerating, but not without controversy. In 1942, Lewy (10) observed the confusing apparent incompatibility between the autopsy findings of those who had suffered unequivocal movement disorders without gross demonstrable pathological changes, and frequent incidental findings in those who had shown no clinical evidence of disease. To some extent this was historically artefactual, as even by 1911, when light microscopy became routine, staining techniques were limited to the Weigert method. It was not until the Nissl stain became routine that microscopic details began to elucidate clinico-pathological links.

Pathological changes were found in conditions such as chorea (Alzheimer) (19) and Parkinson's disease (Lewy) (18), which appeared normal to the naked eye. Similarly, clinical distinctions were becoming more precise. Thomas Sydenham (1726) described 'Chorea St Viti', infectious chorea minor, and differentiated this from chorea major or 'dancing hysteria' (19). A non-infectious chronic hereditary form of chorea was reported by Dr Charles Walters when he wrote to Dunglison, his professor of medicine, on 5 May 1841. This was published the following year in the latter's *Practice of Medicine*. He wrote:

> ... somewhat common ... known among the common people as the 'magrums'... essentially spasmodic action of all or almost all the voluntary muscles... the disease is markedly hereditary... very rarely, it takes its appearance before adult life... it never ceases...in all cases it gradually induces a state of more or less perfect dementia...

Other reports followed: Gorman (1846) from Pennsylvania, Lyons from New York (1863), and finally on 15 February 1872 George Huntington read his famous paper summarizing his grandfather's (Dr Abel Huntington), his father's, and his own combined experience, stating: 'A form of this disease exists as far as I know almost exclusively in Long Island... the hereditary chorea' (20).

In 1961, MacDonald Critchley (21) elegantly set out the historical and geographical features of the illness, and how the largest of the American family groups could be traced back to East Anglia and the year 1630. Three young men left their native Suffolk village of Bures St Mary to settle in the American Colonies. There was intriguing evidence that they left because of their psychopathic behaviour. No fewer than seven of their daughters or granddaughters were regarded as witches. The fifth generation of the Bures family showed unequivocal evidence of Huntington's disease and Mary Bures' descendants constituted the largest family group in New England. The Peck family group was another, and originated when intermarriage took place with an affected member of the Wells family. The first member of this family originally dwelt 10 miles away from Bures (19).

Athetosis was first described by William Hammond (1869), Surgeon General of the United States Army. He proposed the name from the Greek indicating loss of stability. Hammond predicted (1871) that 'The phenomena indicated the implication of intracranial ganglia... one possible seat is the corpus striatum' (22) but he had to wait for 20 years until Gowers described a scar in the left optic thalamus in a patient with choreo-athetotic movement in the rigid left arm (22). Finally, Westphal (1883) reported 'A case of a disease of the central nervous system without anatomical changes, under the picture of a cerebrospinal grey degeneration' (24). In 1911, Alzheimer (17) showed that the illness was associated with giant multilobular glia nuclei '... all over the nervous system although the corpus striatum, optic thalamus, hypothalamus, pons and dentate nuclei were the parts most severely diseased'. In the following year Kinnier Wilson (25) described 'hepatolenticular degeneration'. This seems an appropriate historical time to end the classical period of 'diseases of the basal ganglia'.

Present challenges

In the following chapters, distinguished authorities provide comprehensive accounts of developments and advances in our understanding of movement disorders. Perhaps a further and final historical point may be made. On 28 April 1953 two young men rushed across the narrow road from the Cavendish Laboratories, Cambridge, England and entered the Eagle pub. One announced to the startled drinkers, 'We have just discovered the secret of life'. Apparently the crowd was not impressed. Francis Crick and his American colleague James Watson, without doing any experiments themselves but using paper cut-outs and metal rods and screws, had won the race to discover the structure of the double helix. Competitors had included Linus Pauling, a twice-honoured Nobel Prize Laureate. Two months later their historic paper was published: 'Molecular structure of nucleic acids. A structure for deoxyribose nucleic acid'. This contained an equally famous throw-away line: 'It has not escaped our notice that the specific pairing we have postulated immediately suggests a possible copying mechanism for the genetic material' (26).

The molecular revolution had begun. Since then, we have witnessed a tsunami of data. So far, apart from a few Mendelian single-gene neurodegenerative disorders such as Huntington's disease, tuberous sclerosis, spinal muscular atrophy, and myotonic dystrophies, the gap between genotype and phenotype remains vast and largely incomprehensible to clinicians. It seems that a quantum leap or paradigm shift is now required for us to evolve from traditional disease definitions and embrace the concept that all disease manifestations must be understood in complex molecular terms (27). Definitions such as 'the emergent properties of molecular networks as opposed to the core biological processes driven by responses to changes in a small number of genes' do not yet come easily to clinicians.

Perhaps a few final Cassandra comments and questions might be permitted? New, increasingly subtle clinico-pathological correlations at a classical and molecular level will continue to be discovered and rare new mutations and phenotypes will be charted, but there remains an urgent need to explain basic mechanisms. Not only why and when does a pathological process commence, but why are the majority spared? The enigma of selective system vulnerability has to be solved. The interval between the trigger or triggers to disadvantageous genetic processes and the appearance of demonstrable pathological events and—even longer—before subtle clinical events can be recognized will need to be elucidated. What factors accelerate the disease for an unfortunate minority and what permits others to run a more benign course? What determines vulnerability for some and protection for others? Only then will effective neuroprotection and treatments become a reality and replace symptomatic relief. Hopefully movement disorders will then enter their final historical phase.

References

1. Vaidya AB. Treatment of Parkinson's disease with cowhage plant—*Mucuna pruriens. Neurology (India)* 1987; 26: 171–6.
2. Carlsson A, Lindqvist M, Magnusson T. 3,4-Dihydroxyphenylalanine and 5-hydroxytryptophan as reserpine antagonists. *Nature* 1957; 180: 1200.
3. Reiner E. *Shurku collection of Sumerian and Arcadian incarnations.* Graz: Archiv für Orientschung Beheft, 1958.

4. Scurlock JA, Anderson BR. *Diagnosis in Assyrian and Babylonian medicine*. Chicago, IL: University of Illinois Press, 2005.
5. Sivin N. Medicine in Chinese culture. In: J. Needham (ed.) *Science and Civilisation in China*, pp. 38–94. Cambridge: Cambridge University Press, 2008.
6. Keele KD. *The evolution of clinical methods in medicine. Fitzpatrick Lectures, Royal College of Physicians. 1960–1*. London: Pitman, 1963.
7. Wang Huai-yin. *Thai phing sheng hui fang* (*Encyclopedia grace formulary of the Thai-phing-hsing-kuo Era, Sung*), 982.
8. Sivin N. *Traditional medicine in contemporary China*, pp. 106–9. Ann Arbor, MI: Centre for Chinese Studies, University of Michigan, 1987.
9. Moffett J. Personal communication. Needham Research Institute, Cambridge, 2001.
10. Lewy FH (1942). The diseases of the basal ganglia. *Res Publ Assoc Res Nerv Ment Dis* 1942; 21: 1–20.
11. Mundinus. *Anathomia Mundini per carpum castigata et postmodus cum apostillis ornate et noviter*, pp. 61–73. Venice: Bernadinus, 1538.
12. Willis T. *Cerebri anatome cui accessit nervorum descriptio et usus*. London: Roycroft, 1664.
13. Meynert T. Über die geweblichen Veraenderungen in den Centralorganen des Nervensystems bei einem Fall von Choreanminor. *Allg Wiener med Zeitg* 1868; 13: 67–76.
14. Stern G. The effects of lesions in the substantia nigra. *Brain* 1996; 89: 449–78.
15. Stern G. The language of the basal ganglia. *J Neural Transm (Suppl)* 1997; 51: 1–8.
16. Luys J. *Le cerveau et ses fonctions*. Paris: Librairie Germer Baillière, 1876.
17. Alzheimer A. Über die anatomische grundlage der Huntingtonschen Chorea und die choreatische Bewegungen uberhaupt. *Neurol Zbl* 1911; 30: 891.
18. Lewy FH. Die pathologische Anatomie der Paralysis agitans. *Lewandowsky's Handb* 1912; 3: 920.
19. Sydenham T (1726). Schedula monitoria de nova febris igressu. *Opera universa*, p. 526. Lugduni Batavorum apud Kerchem.
20. Huntington G. On chorea. *Med Surg Reporter* 1872; 26: 317.
21. Critchley M. *The black hole and other essays*, pp. 210–19. London: Pitman Medical, 1961.
22. Hammond WA. *A treatise on the diseases of the nervous system*, pp. 322, 654. New York: Appleton, 1871.
23. Gowers WR. On athetosis and posthemiplegic disorders of movement. *Med-chir Trans* 1876; 59: 271.
24. Westphal C. Über eine der Bilde der cerebrospinalen grauen Degeneration ähIichen Erkrankung des centralen Nervensystem ohne anatomischen Befund, etc. *Arch Psychiatr Nervenk*; 14: 87.
25. Wilson SAK. Progessive lenticular degeneration. *Brain* 1912; 34: 295.
26. Watson JD, Crick FHC. Molecular structure of nucleic acids. A structure for deoxyribose nucleic acid. *Nature* 1953; 171: 737.
27. Bell J (2010) Redefining disease. *Clin Med* 2010; 10: 584–94.

CHAPTER 2

Approach to History Taking and Examination of the Movement Disorder Patient

David J. Burn

Introduction

The characteristic feature of all movement disorders is an abnormality of the form and velocity of movements of the body. This rather vague definition disguises the sometimes bewildering spectrum of abnormal movements, their distribution, temporal evolution, underlying cause, and range of functional impacts. One of the reasons that many neurologists (including myself) are drawn into this subspecialty is that it remains very clinically based. Thus, an appreciation of the pattern of abnormal movements, enabling their phenomenology to be determined, is essential before embarking upon the correct diagnostic pathway. Failure to take this critical first step and to adopt a 'scattergun' approach to investigations is likely to be both time-consuming and costly.

The term 'movement disorder' has become synonymous with basal ganglia disease and extrapyramidal features. While it is true that many movement disorders arise from pathology within the basal ganglia, disorders such as myoclonus may arise from other neural structures, including the spinal cord. Moreover, the correlation between lesions within the basal ganglia and the occurrence and nature of any movement disorder produced is not always a close one. Given the extensive cerebral cortical connectivity of basal ganglia structures, it is unsurprising that movement disorders are also frequently associated with cognitive and neuropsychiatric problems. Indeed, these problems may precede and/or overshadow the abnormal movements.

The range of different movement disorders and their causes are discussed in the ensuing chapters of this book. This brief introduction to the topic will deal primarily with classification and broad issues relating to the approach to a patient with a suspected movement disorder.

Classification and definitions

Movement disorders can be categorized into akinetic–rigid and hyperkinetic; in other words, patients who either move too little or those who move too much. This simplistic approach is confounded where there are mixed signs. Someone with Parkinson's disease, for example, may be regarded as having an akinetic–rigid syndrome, but may also have prominent tremor. In such situations, it is best to categorize by the dominant movement disorder.

Akinetic–rigid disorders

The terms akinesia, bradykinesia, or hypokinesia are all used in the literature, sometimes with confusing results. Strictly speaking akinesia implies 'lack of movement'. Since very few patients are completely unable to move, it may not be the most appropriate term for this group of disorders, but its use has become embedded in movement disorder folklore. Bradykinesia means 'slow movement', whilst hypokinesia refers to poverty of movement, or movements that are smaller in amplitude than that intended. Akinesia has also been used as an umbrella term for bradykinesia, hypokinesia, and, most importantly, the progressive fatiguing and decrementing of repetitive movements such as finger or foot tapping. The latter more than anything captures the essence of 'parkinsonism', or an akinetic–rigid syndrome. Eliciting this in practice is not always easy and may require many repetitions to observe (>50 on occasion), whilst significant tremor may confound the interpretation. It is important not to perform the finger taps in tandem with the patient, since they may take visual cue from the examiner and appear spuriously better than they are with self-generated movements. Slowness of movement may sometimes be observed in pyramidal and cerebellar disturbances, underlining the importance of documenting fatigue and decrement as being specific to an extrapyramidal disorder.

Hyperkinetic disorders

In general, recognition and diagnosis of this group of disorders is more challenging than the akinetic–rigid syndromes. Some reviews have subclassified these movements into jerky and non-jerky syndromes (1). The former comprises myoclonus, chorea, and tics, whilst non-jerky hyperkinetic disorders include tremor and dystonia (2). The division is somewhat arbitrary, and confusion may occur where the movement disorder is mixed, as in so-called 'dystonic tics' for example.

Myoclonic movements are sudden, brief, shock-like involuntary movements which we all experience on occasion when falling off to sleep. Negative myoclonus occurs due to brief loss or inhibition of muscle tone. In the arms this may be due to asterixis, associated with hepatic or uraemic encephalopathy or carbon dioxide retention, whilst in the legs it may produce a 'bouncing gait' in the context of the post-anoxic Lance–Adams syndrome. Myoclonus may be described in terms of its distribution (focal, multifocal, segmental or generalized), aetiology (physiological, essential, epileptic or symptomatic), neurophysiology (cortical, subcortical, spinal and peripheral), and also by its triggers (spontaneous, action, stimulus-sensitive). Palatal myoclonus has been reclassified as a tremor disorder.

The *auditory startle response* is a polysynaptic reflex originating in the caudal brainstem which comprises a rapid eye blink followed by facial grimacing, flexion of the head, trunk, elbows, hips and knees, and raising of the shoulders in response to a sudden unexpected noise. Abnormal excessive startle may occur in hyperekplexia, as a manifestation of epilepsy, and various regional disorders of uncertain aetiology (latah reaction, miryachit, and the jumping Frenchmen of Maine). In a severe genetically determined form of startle disease (major hyperekplexia, associated with a mutation in the alpha-1 subunit of the glycine receptor) the motor response may be associated with transient generalized muscle stiffness and falls, with rapid recovery.

Chorea (from the Greek 'to dance') refers to quick, irregular, semi-purposive, and predominantly distal involuntary movements which can impart a 'fidgety' look to the patient. The involuntary movements may sometimes be subtle, and deciding whether the person is restless within the bounds of normality or whether they have chorea can be difficult. Occasionally the patient may 'convert' the choreiform movement into a voluntary action (for example, a movement of the forearm may be converted into drawing the arm up to check the time on a wrist-watch). Subjects with chorea also have motor impersistence, and this may manifest in some wonderfully descriptive signs such as the 'milk-maid grip' (inability to exert constant pressure whilst gently gripping two of the examiner's fingers) and 'trombone tongue' (rapid partial protrusion and retraction of the tongue when asked to keep it protruded).

Ballism is generally considered as part of the choreic spectrum. Initially the mainly proximal, large-amplitude, violent 'flinging' movements bear little resemblance to chorea, and may be associated with exhaustion as well as injury (to both patient and others). They are usually unilateral and result following vascular insult to the subthalamic nucleus, or immediately surrounding structures. As time passes, however, the ballistic movements subside into a choreiform phenotype. Bilateral ballism is rare and is often caused by metabolic abnormalities such as hyperglycaemia.

Tics are abrupt, jerky, non-rhythmic movements (motor tics) or sounds (vocal tics) that are temporarily suppressible by will power. These movements are preceded by a feeling of discomfort or an urge that is temporarily relieved by the tic. The distribution of tics is classically in the head and neck region, and the arms. A tic may be simple (for example, winking, wrinkling of the nose) or complex (for example, copying the movements or gestures of others—echopraxia—or touching objects). An ability to voluntarily suppress the tic is a key feature of this movement disorder, even though the suppression is associated with a build up of 'inner tension'.

Stereotypies are purposeless voluntary movements carried out in a repetitive fashion, often for long periods of time, and at the expense of all other activities. In contrast with tics, they are less paroxysmal, and may involve whole areas of the body. Hand wringing, typical of Rett syndrome, is an example of a stereotypy. Head banging and body rocking, seen in mental retardation of different aetiologies, are other commonly encountered examples of stereotypies.

History taking

The value of a careful history and examination can never be underestimated, even if the diagnosis may seem apparent from the moment the patient first walks into the clinic room. Regarding the history, one of my previous teachers in London used to say: 'If you have ten minutes with the patient, then spend nine taking the history'. This is sound advice, yet commonly overlooked in a busy clinic.

- *History of presenting complaint:* It may be difficult to date the precise onset of a movement disorder, but some idea of duration is important. Collateral history from a spouse or family member can be helpful here. Was the onset acute or gradual? It can also be helpful to ascertain where the problem began, and the nature of its spread. It can sometimes be useful to determine exacerbating and ameliorating factors, although most movement disorders are made worse by anxiety. Beware of the person with parkinsonism who uses a proxy symptom such as weakness or clumsiness; most patients do not complain of bradykinesia! Occasionally the person may not know why they are in clinic or why they were sent along; in my experience this has usually been the patient with chorea who is untroubled and largely unaware of their movement disorder. Always try to relate the symptoms to functional impact: what does it mean to the person in their everyday life? This will also have a bearing upon treatment decisions. I usually ask a few screening cognitive and neuropsychiatric questions at this point, if they have not already been covered, along with sleep pattern and possible parasomnias. Having a spouse or care-giver available at this point is particularly helpful. For example, the patient may be unaware or deny that they have been low in mood, irascible, or more apathetic. Collateral history can provide useful examples of cognitive impairment, such as inadvertently leaving gas or water on, getting lost in previously familiar surroundings, and so on. A bed-partner can describe better than anyone the likely occurrence of REM sleep behaviour disorder, and may even admit to moving into the spare bedroom in order to get a better night's sleep!
- *Past medical history:* Omit this at your peril, since systemic disorders can manifest as a movement disorder and the temporal association may not always be obvious. Examples include previous infections, stroke, and connective tissue disease. I would also include mental illness here, as this may signpost the need for a more detailed drug history, or provide clues to the diagnosis via a prodromal psychiatric disorder (e.g. neuroacanthocytosis, Huntington's).
- *Drug history:* Always consider drugs, both past and present, as a potential cause for the movement disorder. Tardive dyskinesias (commonly stereotypic movements, often orofacial in distribution, although a wide spectrum of drug-induced movement disorders has been described) may develop after relatively short exposure to the offending agent, but can persist for years.

A full list of medications previously taken by the patient should be obtained from the primary care practitioner if necessary. A high index of suspicion is required. While dopamine receptor blocking agents are well known to cause drug-induced parkinsonism and other tardive syndromes, agents such as valproate, amiodarone, and cinnarizine are less widely recognized to induce drug-induced movement disorders. If relevant, enquire about a history of drug abuse/'recreational' drug use.

- *Family history:* Drawing out the family pedigree can be helpful and avoids confusion at a later date. False-negative family histories may have several reasons, not least premature death of one or both parents (the cause of which may, in itself, be a clue). Non-paternity, adoption, and consanguinity may all be relevant, but questioning in such areas needs to be sensitively handled, and possibly best deferred to more expert genetic counselling.
- *Social history:* Smoking may be relevant if a paraneoplastic movement disorder is being considered (3), while the ability of alcohol to suppress tremor, dystonia, and other movements should always be established. The amount of alcohol necessary to have a beneficial effect should also be recorded, since most movement disorders will be suppressed after 10 pints of beer! It is also important to establish the home circumstances (stairs to negotiate, access to the property, etc.), and whether the person is dependent upon social services for their care. Where necessary, consider previous travel abroad and sexual history.
- *Systematic enquiry:* A full enquiry is time-consuming, but with practice questions can be targeted to clues obtained in the history. Sleep pattern may be relevant here, if it has not already been determined, along with olfactory and autonomic symptoms.

Examination

It is often helpful to call the patient in rather than relying upon a nurse to do this, since it affords the opportunity to watch the person walk in a larger area, turn, and encounter 'obstacles' such as doorways. More formal assessment of gait should include the 'pull test' and rotation of the trunk to ascertain axial rigidity. The inability of a patient to tandem walk for ten steps has been reported to differentiate patients with atypical parkinsonism from those with Parkinson's disease, although this finding needs to be independently replicated (1).

Observation during history taking allows the examiner to ascertain the nature of the movement disorder at rest, and its extent. It may also highlight inconsistencies and distractibility in the movement disorder, and reveal excessive sighing (characteristic of multiple system atrophy (MSA)) or other abnormal respiratory patterns. A brief cognitive assessment may be required, and is most easily performed with pen and paper testing, using a simple scale such as the Montreal Cognitive Assessment (MCA) (4) or the Mini-Mental State Examination (MMSE) (5). The latter is insensitive to executive dysfunction, so if this is suspected the MMSE should be supplemented with the Frontal Assessment Battery (FAB) (6), or components of this battery, such as a go–no go task, verbal fluency, or Luria test. Allowance may need to be made for abnormal movement interfering with drawing in these tests, but some indication of global cognitive function can be obtained fairly easily in most people. Observing the person write can be informative and may reveal, for example, dystonic posturing, corrugation on attempting to draw an Archimedes spiral, or micrographia. 'Fast micrographia' is said to be suggestive of pallidal lesions (7).

Thereafter, the neurological examination should be rigorous and systematic. Watch the eyes whilst the person is holding a target to ascertain whether they remain still, or describe abnormal movements, such as small side-to-side movements. These movements, described after their electro-oculographic appearance, are called macrosaccadic square-wave jerks. They are particularly frequent in progressive supranuclear palsy (PSP). Abnormal eye movements may also be helpful diagnostically, particularly saccadic movements in a person presenting with an akinetic–rigid syndrome (8). A normal saccadic eye movement is so fast that the examiner should only be able to see the pupil at the beginning and the end of the movement. In PSP the vertical and then horizontal saccadic eye movements are slowed to the point where the excursion of the pupil is clearly visible throughout the movement. In corticobasal degeneration there is typically a latent period between being given the command to look to one side and the eye movement itself (increased saccadic latency), although saccadic speed is near normal when it occurs. In Huntington's disease, early and consistent findings are an inability to suppress reflexive glances to novel visual stimuli which appear suddenly, and delayed initiation of voluntary saccades.

Eyelid dysfunction, such as reduced blink frequency, blepharoclonus, or apraxia of eyelid opening should be noted. In the upper limbs, subtle changes in extrapyramidal tone may be exaggerated by reinforcement or synkinesis—that is, asking the person to do something with the opposite arm, such as pretending to paint a wall. Tremor may be revealed by requesting the patient to perform serial seven subtractions from 100 with the arms resting comfortably on their lap in a semi-prone position. Eliciting progressive decrement of repetitive movements to determine bradykinesia has been described above.

Examination of cerebellar function may be difficult in the presence of involuntary movements and/or bradykinesia, but should still be documented. There may have already been clues from listening to the patient's speech (slurred dysarthria) or examining slow-pursuit eye movements (jerky slow pursuit and/or gaze-evoked nystagmus). Subtle heel–toe ataxia of gait may be observed in the patient with long-standing essential tremor, while ataxia may be noted in MSA, over and above parkinsonian features.

Reflexes are often unremarkable in many movement disorders, although it is not uncommon to elicit slightly brisker reflexes on the more affected side in early Parkinson's disease. There may be generalized hyper-reflexia in patients with MSA and PSP, while in neuroacanthocytosis ankle jerks are classically absent.

Asking the person to bring a video of their movement disorder can be helpful if it is intermittent. Alternatively, if no problem is apparent, consider whether the disorder is task specific (for example, a task-specific dystonia). In this situation, the patient may need to bring in a relevant piece of equipment, such as their guitar or a golf club, to demonstrate the problem!

Diagnostic formulation

As recommended in a recent review (1), addressing the following four questions consecutively is a helpful discipline in order to arrive at the correct diagnosis.

1. *Which types of movement disorder are present?* On a surprising number of occasions the movement disorder is not 'pure' and several phenomena may be present in the same patient. Examples include MSA (bradykinesia, ataxia, tremor, polyminimyoclonus), Huntington's disease (chorea, dystonia, bradykinesia), and tardive movement disorders related to dopamine receptor blocking drugs.
2. *What is the dominant movement disorder type?* Having identified the different components, it is important to ascertain the dominant movement type, since this will critically steer the differential diagnosis and investigational pathway. This may become more difficult in advanced disease states, where the initial characteristic movement disorder becomes masked by drug treatments, supervening progression, or secondary complications. Examples include florid levodopa-induced dyskinesias in Parkinson's, or an akinetic–rigid patient with advanced Huntington's disease. In such situations collateral history, old video footage, obtaining 'foreign' medical records, or repeated examinations to capture variability in the condition may all play a part in clarifying the situation.
3. *What are the associated features?* The presence of additional 'general medical' and/or neurological features on examination can provide further clues to the diagnosis, guiding the differential diagnosis of the dominant movement disorder. Illustrative examples would be corneal Kayser–Fleischer rings associated with Wilson disease, dysgraphaesthesia associated with corticobasal degeneration or hypothyroidism, and pulmonary abnormalities associated with some types of benign hereditary chorea.
4. *What is the differential diagnosis?* Having followed the above three steps it should be possible to draw up a differential diagnosis, using the history to contextualize the signs. In some cases the differential may be exceedingly short, and a specific diagnosis made rapidly or a diagnostic test requested. But in other situations it is excellent practice to list possible diagnoses, starting with the most likely first, since it is this list which will guide the first wave of investigations.

Ancillary investigations

It is beyond the scope of this chapter to comprehensively discuss ancillary investigations and studies that may be performed in different movement disorders. This will be covered under the relevant conditions. But some general principles are worth highlighting. In some situations no specific additional tests may be required to make a diagnosis. Parkinson's disease is regarded by many as one such example. The diagnosis is primarily clinical and while some diagnostic guidelines recommend brain imaging (e.g. computed tomography (CT) or magnetic resonance imaging (MRI)), this approach is not universally adopted. Where diagnostic doubt exists in a patient presenting with a 'monosymptomatic upper limb tremor', and it can be difficult to discriminate a tremor-dominant form of Parkinson's from dystonic tremor, then ^{123}I-N-ω-fluoropropyl-2β-carbomethoxy-3β-(4-iodophenyl) nortropan (^{123}I-FP-CIT) single photon emission computed tomography (SPECT) can be very useful. This ligand, which is now available in many countries, reflects the integrity of the nigrostriatal dopaminergic terminals, since it binds avidly to the presynaptic dopamine transporter. Therefore ^{123}I-FP-CIT SPECT is normal in subjects with dystonic or essential tremor and abnormal in people with Parkinson's disease. Even where the clinical signs are unilateral, SPECT images not uncommonly show bilateral abnormality, with reduced tracer binding in both putamens. In patients in whom there was diagnostic uncertainty between degenerative parkinsonism and non-degenerative tremor disorders, baseline imaging with ^{123}I-FP-CIT SPECT has shown 78% sensitivity and 97% specificity with reference to the 'gold standard' of clinical diagnosis at 3 years, compared with 93% and 46%, respectively, for baseline clinical diagnosis (9).

Establishing the phenomenology of the movement disorder is essential in order to guide which line of more complex investigations should be initiated. This avoids a potentially fruitless and expensive 'scattergun' approach. Often, the presence of additional clinical signs may allow the investigations requested to be refined even further.

Do not overlook simple tests, such as a full blood count, urea and electrolytes, liver function tests, thyroid function tests, blood glucose, or chest X-ray. The results from such a screen may yield important diagnostic clues, saving time and money in the long run (and also potential embarrassment!).

There should be a low threshold to undertake serum caeruloplasmin estimation, since Wilson disease may present with protean movement disorders and is eminently treatable. At a cut-off of 0.2g/L, serum caeruloplasmin is a simple screening test, although not very sensitive, since 5–20% of homozygous carriers will have normal results. Thus, while an abnormal result should prompt further screening (for example, ophthalmological assessment and urinary copper excretion), a normal serum caeruloplasmin level does not fully exclude Wilson disease.

In the absence of a clear clinical diagnosis, supported or not by a single definitive diagnostic test, a staged approach to investigation is recommended. Thus starting with relatively sensitive but non-specific tests such as simple blood tests and an MRI brain scan can give useful signposts towards the next stage of more specific imaging or genetic studies, for example. Finally, tissue may be required for diagnostic evaluation in some situations.

Management considerations

Some key general points that are worth remembering in clinic are illustrated in Box 2.1. Giving the diagnosis is done in a notoriously variable way and can have longer-term impact if done badly. For example, one international study suggested that satisfaction with the explanation of the condition of Parkinson's disease at diagnosis was a major determinant of subsequent quality of life (10).

Adherence to therapy is always likely to be greater when the patient is fully engaged in management decisions and understands the reason behind what is being recommended. For example, although it was long held that people with Parkinson's disease were conscientious about taking their medications regularly, a European study using electronic pill boxes has shown that, in a sample of 112 patients, whilst total median adherence (doses taken/doses prescribed) was 97.7%, timing adherence (doses taken at correct time intervals) was only 24.4% (11). If a patient has difficulty in accepting a diagnosis, or becomes upset by the explanation given, it may be useful to defer treatment discussions until they have had a chance to assimilate the situation better. Sometimes disability may be so minimal that no treatment is indicated, but this

Box 2.1 Key points in making management decisions

- Treat disability or poor quality of life, *not* recorded impairments.
- Remove potentially exacerbating/causative drugs whenever possible.
- Consider underlying depression when there seems to be a marked mismatch between impairment and reported disability.
- Patients do not always volunteer neuropsychiatric features like visual hallucinations. Ask!
- Members of the multidisciplinary team generally prefer an early referral.
- Never forget the need for genetic counselling and implications for other family members.
- If a psychogenic movement disorder is suspected the patient may be best managed by a formal admission and a staged multidisciplinary approach.

will also depend hugely upon patient expectations, their social situation, and comorbidities, *inter alia*. Until disease-modifying treatments are available for neurodegenerative movement disorders, at which time early diagnosis will assume huge importance, drug treatment is currently symptomatic. Therefore a balance needs to be struck between size of therapeutic effect, potential side effects (including long-term considerations such as propensity of an agent to cause problems such as dyskinesias) and, not infrequently, cost-effectiveness.

If there is a significant mismatch between reported disability (severe) and signs (mild), sometimes coupled with a history of apparent intolerance of medications, always consider an underlying affective disorder. Depression is an extremely common accompaniment of many movement disorders, and may indeed be integral to several, yet it is commonly under-diagnosed and under-treated.

Early referral to a multidisciplinary team is generally preferred, although the availability of specialist speech and language therapists, physiotherapists, occupational therapists, etc. is highly variable, even within some countries. Unfortunately, the evidence base for allied health professional interventions in this context is very weak, although this trend may gradually be reversing (12–14).

Management may sometimes involve *stopping* medication as much as *starting* new treatments if a drug-induced movement disorder is suspected. Re-scheduling a review after an appropriate interval to observe the effects of drug cessation can be very rewarding, particularly in the case of drug-induced parkinsonism. Unfortunately, as a rule tardive hyperkinetic disorders are more persistent.

Conclusion

The approach to history taking and examination of the movement disorder patient remains an art, and one that should be cultivated in training programmes and clinical meetings. Over-reliance upon unfocused investigations is a slippery slope which runs the risk of producing false-positive outcomes, prolonged diagnostic pathways, and increased financial pressures on health-care providers. This chapter has attempted to give an overview of several salient features in the clinical consultation, together with some general investigation and management principles. More specific details of individual conditions will be covered in subsequent chapters.

References

1. Abdo WF, van de Warrenburg BPC, Burn DJ, Quinn NP, Bloem BR. The clinical approach to movement disorders. *Nat Rev Neurol* 2010; 6: 29–37.
2. Robottom BJ, Factor SA, Weiner WJ. Movement disorders emergencies. Part 2: Hyperkinetic disorders. *Arch Neurol* 2011; 68: 719–24.
3. Grant R, Graus F. Paraneoplastic movement disorders. *Mov Disord* 2009; 24: 1715–24.
4. Chou KL, Amick MM, Brandt J, et al. A recommended scale for cognitive screening in clinical trials of Parkinson's disease. *Mov Disord* 2010; 25: 2501–7.
5. Folstein MF, Folstein SE, McHugh PR. 'Mini-Mental State'. A practical method for grading the cognitive state of patients for the clinician. *J Psychiatr Res* 1975; 12: 189–98.
6. Dubois B, Slachevsky A, Litvan I, Pillon B. The FAB: a frontal assessment battery. *Neurology* 2000; 55: 1621–6.
7. Kuoppamäki M, Rothwell JC, Brown RG, Quinn NP, Bhatia KP, Jahanshahi M. Parkinsonism following bilateral lesions of the globus pallidus: performance on a variety of motor tasks shows similarities with Parkinson's disease. *J Neurol Neurosurg Psychiatry* 2005; 76: 482–90.
8. Leigh RJ, Riley DE. Eye movements in parkinsonism: it's saccadic speed that counts. *Neurology* 2000: 54; 1018–19.
9. Cummings JL, Henchclife C, Schaier S, Simuni T, Waxman A, Kemp P. The role of dopaminergic imaging in patients with symptoms of dopaminergic system neurodegeneration. *Brain* 2011; 134: 3146–66.
10. Global Parkinson's Disease Survey Steering Committee. Factors impacting on quality of life in Parkinson's disease: results from an international study. *Mov Disord* 2002; 17: 60–7.
11. Grosset D, Antonini A, Canesi M, et al. Adherence to antiparkinson medication in a multicenter European study. *Mov Disord* 2009; 24: 826–32.
12. Nieuwboer A, Kwakkel G, Rochester L, et al. Cueing training in the home improves gait-related mobility in Parkinson's disease: the RESCUE trial. *J Neurol Neurosurg Psychiatry* 2007; 78: 134–40.
13. Clarke CE, Furmston A, Morgan E, et al. Pilot randomised controlled trial of occupational therapy to optimise independence in Parkinson's disease: the PD OT trial. *J Neurol Neurosurg Psychiatry* 2009; 80: 976–8.
14. Munneke M, Nijkrake MJ, Keus SH, et al. Efficacy of community-based physiotherapy networks for patients with Parkinson's disease: a cluster-randomised trial. *Lancet Neurol* 2010; 9: 46–54.

CHAPTER 3

Neuroanatomy for the Movement Disorder Specialist

Glenda M. Halliday, Rachel Tan, and Heidi Cartwright

General introduction

Normal motor control is a learned skill requiring the maturation of both the musculoskeletal system and the nervous system. Large parts of the brain are involved in coordinating and generating movements both directly and indirectly. Except for the muscles that activate the eye, which are innervated from midbrain nuclei, all the voluntary muscles of the body are directly innervated by motor neurons in the spinal cord and hindbrain.

The motor neuron

The motor neurons that directly innervate skeletal muscle constitute the final common pathway by which the nervous system controls movement and are often referred to as α-motor neurons (Fig. 3.1). In addition to α-motor neurons which innervate extrafusal muscle fibres, the ventral horn of the spinal cord and cranial nerve motor nuclei also contain γ-motor neurons (Fig. 3.1). These neurons innervate the polar, contractile elements of intrafusal muscle fibres, maintaining the sensitivity of the stretch reflex (the γ-reflex loop, Fig. 3.1). Both α- and γ-motor neurons are under the influence of descending pathways from the brain (Fig. 3.1).

Conscious control of the motor neuron

Descending neural drive from motor cortical centres generate volitional movements through the corticospinal and corticobulbar outputs, as well as corticoreticulospinal tracts (1). The important role of motor cortical outputs has been recognized since the nineteenth and twentieth centuries when stimulation of the motor cortex was found to elicit movements, and sectioning of the corticospinal tract and lesions in this system were found to impair volitional movement, causing paralysis and weaknesses. Axons from the corticospinal tract synapse directly onto motor neurons (termed corticomotoneuronal connections (Fig. 3.1)) and also onto interneurons within the spinal cord. The corticospinal tract itself contains the bulk of direct corticofugal outputs destined to recruit spinal motor neurons (1).

Motor cortices

Pyramidal neurons in the somatomotor cortices send corticospinal and corticobulbar axons through the corticospinal tract. These cortices comprise the primary motor cortex, ventral and dorsal premotor areas (both subfields of area 6), supplementary motor areas and (rostral, dorsal, and ventral) cingulate motor areas (Fig. 3.2). The precise borders of these cortices have been disputed, partly because it is difficult to depict the areas precisely on maps of the cortical surface which cannot reveal the borders in the depths of sulci (for a review, see (2)).

The primary motor cortex corresponds to cytoarchitectonic area 4 of Brodmann's classification of the human brain (3, 4). As well as its own local circuitry, it contains a topographically organized motor output to the bulbar muscles as well as the trunk and extremities. The ventral premotor cortex corresponds to the lower part of Brodmann's area 6 and can be functionally subdivided into two or three regions (for a review of the different terminologies and the possible function of these non-primary motor cortical areas, see (5)). The ventral premotor areas are likely to be involved in the transformation of information about peripersonal space and visual space into motor commands for movements, particularly of the upper limb. The dorsal premotor cortex corresponds to the superior part of area 6 which also can be subdivided on functional grounds (F2 and F7). The precise role of F2 is debated, but it is involved in reaching and visual signalling. The F7 area is involved in eye movement control, and perhaps also in stimulus–response associations for movements (6).

The mesial part of area 6 was once considered to be a single area, the supplementary motor area (7). It is now subdivided into the supplementary motor area (SMA) proper, or F3, and the pre-supplementary motor area (pre-SMA), or F6. The SMA

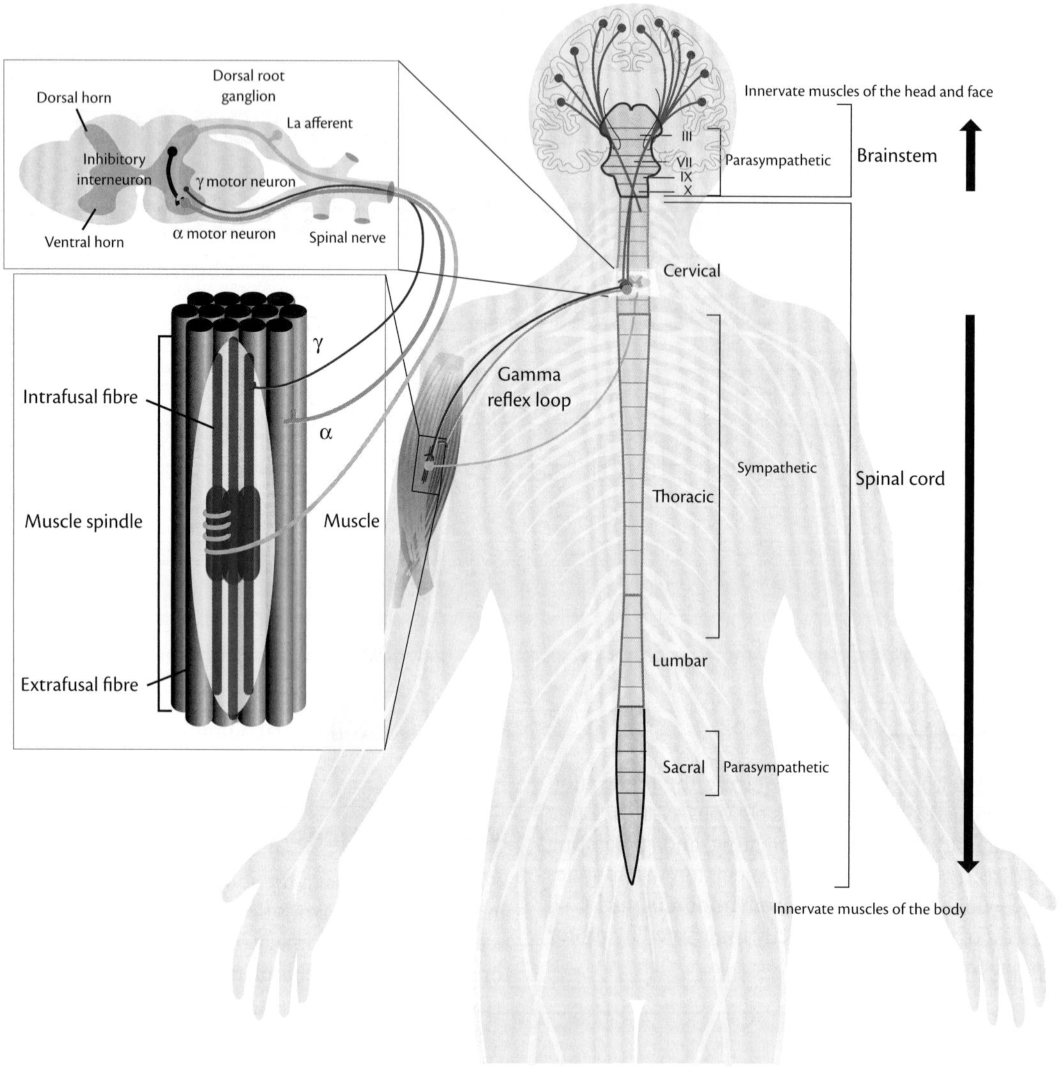

Fig. 3.1 Illustration of main motor pathways involved in the volitional control of movement. The two major efferent pathways under corticomotor control are the α-motor neurons (light green) and the much smaller γ-motor neurons (dark green), located within the ventral horn of the spinal cord. The α-motor neurons innervate the extrafusal muscle fibres causing the muscle to contract. The γ-motor neurons attach to the intrafusal fibres found within the muscle spindle and provide stretch sensitivity via the Ia afferent fibres (grey) which activate the α-motor neurons (gamma reflex loop). This loop helps regulate the muscle length and tone and is important for reflexes. The Ia afferent, along with corticospinal projections, also excites associated interneurons (black) which regulate the reflex by inhibiting the α-motor neurons.

proper is involved in preparation and selection of movements, and perhaps in the initial learning of motor sequences (8), while the pre-SMA can modify these movements based on cognitive, sensory, and motivational signals. Finally, there are motor cortical areas within the cingulate sulcus (Brodmann areas 23 and 24), termed the rostral, dorsal, and ventral cingulate motor areas. The motor function of these non-primary motor cortical areas has been obtained using a mixture of methods, including electrical stimulation and neurophysiological mapping, neuroanatomical tracing, and functional neuroimaging in primates. Not only do they contain some somatotopic organization (e.g. face, arm, and leg separations) but also they have some direct projections of varying strength to the primary motor cortex and also to the brainstem and spinal cord (1, 9, 10). They provide the interface between sensorimotor, limbic, and executive systems, modifying movement in response to pain, attentional, and arousal states.

Primary motor cortex

The primary motor cortex is unusual in that it has a low density of neurons, lacking an obvious layer IV and containing giant Betz cells, giving it the greatest cortical thickness (~3.8 mm), with the adjacent sensory cortex being thinnest (~1.8 mm) (2). Presumably this allows substantial synaptic integration for flexible selection of motor outputs. Pyramidal cells with output to subcortical and cortical regions are distributed throughout layers II–VI, with the majority in layers III and V (Fig. 3.3). Layer V has a low density of neuronal packing and ~15% of cells have corticospinal axons. Such projections make up about 30% of the descending corticospinal tract. The projecting axons are largely myelinated with a range of conduction velocities.

The intrinsic connectivity of the primary motor cortex, as in most of the cortex, is arranged radially in columns (Fig. 3.3). Intrinsic non-pyramidal neurons (including stellate and basket cells) have radially oriented dendrites and make largely local

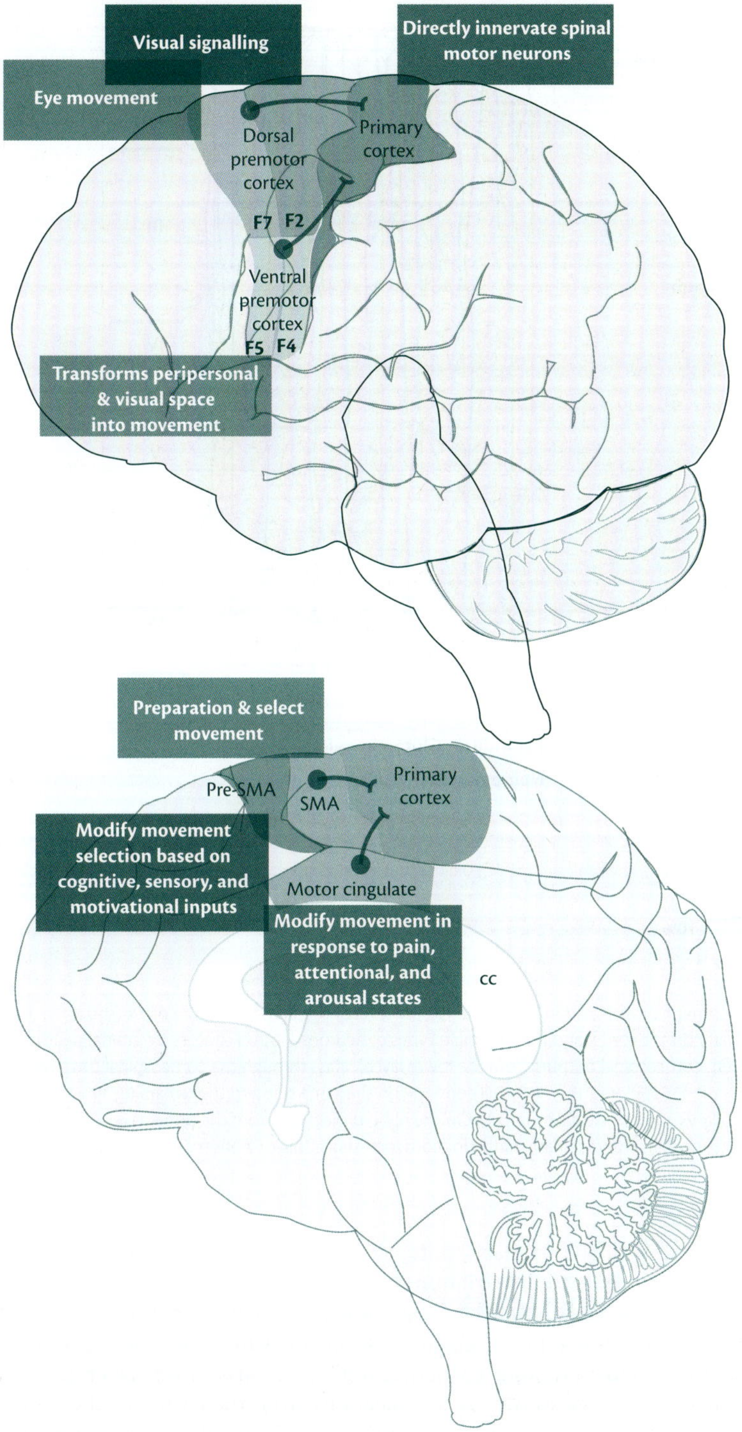

Fig. 3.2 Cortical regions involved in motor control and their functions. Corticocortical excitatory projections to the primary motor cortex are indicated in green. SMA, supplementary motor cortex; cc, corpus callosum.

connections (Fig. 3.3). Basket cells exert GABAergic inhibition of pyramidal cell output, part of a recurrent laterally spreading inhibitory circuit (11). About a third of local pairs of primary cortical cells show evidence of correlated drive during tasks, indicating they receive common inputs (12, 13).

Cortical and thalamic input to motor cortices

Various neuroanatomical techniques and electrophysiological mapping have shown that many cortical areas project directly to the primary motor cortex (5). These include the premotor areas, supplementary motor areas, and cingulate motor areas (Fig. 3.2). Some degree of somatotopic organization is maintained in these projections to the primary motor cortex. Sensory information from parietal areas also projects either directly or indirectly through the sensory cortex to the motor cortex (14). Corticocortical projection neurons are usually derived from the small supragranular pyramidal neurons and provide excitatory drive to supragranular neurons in nearby cortical regions. Within the cortical columns, these

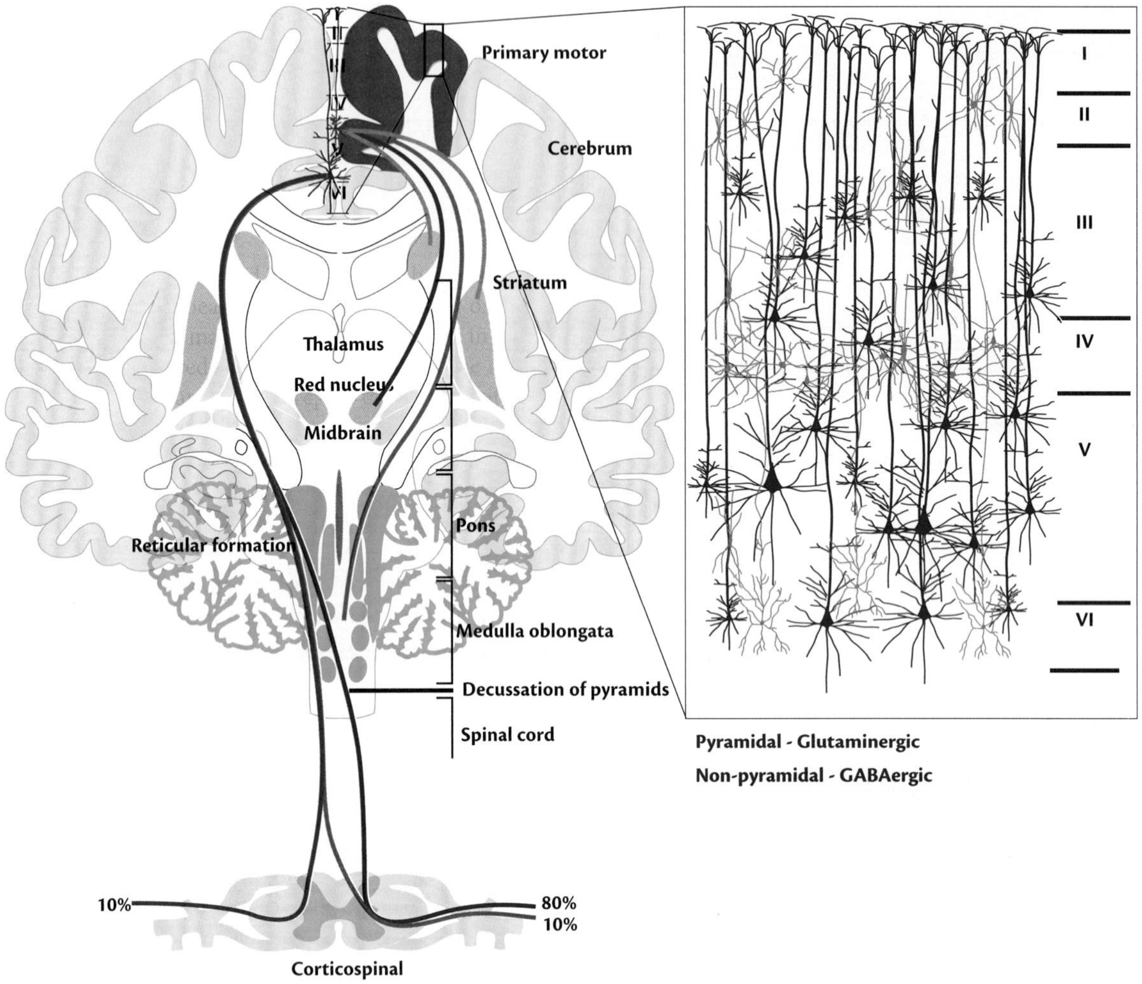

Fig. 3.3 Diagram of the main descending pathways from the primary motor cortex. Coronal section of the brain at the level of the primary motor cortex (shown in dark green). The box enlargement shows the layered configuration of the primary motor cortex and the two main types of neurons—the excitatory pyramidal neurons (dark green) and the regulating inhibitory interneurons (light green). On the left, corticospinal outputs from the lower layer V pass through the corticospinal tract. Most corticospinal fibres cross over to the contralateral side at the pyramidal decussation (80%). A further 10% will continue on the same side and the remaining 10% will cross over at the level they exit. All three pathways will synapse with the medullary motor nuclei (see Fig. 3.1). On the right, projections from the upper layer V and layer III pyramidal neurons terminate subcortically in the striatum (corticostriatal), red nucleus (rubrospinal), midbrain (corticomesencephalic), pons (corticopontine), and medullary reticular formation (corticoreticular).

supragranular neurons provide strong excitatory drive to the large layer V pyramidal output neurons, thus reinforcing the thalamic input to these neurons.

A number of thalamic nuclei assist in determining cortical activity by facilitating information transfer from one cortical region to another through a feedforward mechanism (15). In particular, the ventral anterior thalamus feeds forward executive information to premotor cortices (under basal ganglia influence), the ventrolateral anterior thalamus feeds forward premotor information to the primary motor cortex (under basal ganglia and cerebellar influence), and the ventrolateral posterior thalamus provides feedback from the primary motor cortex (under cerebellar influence). These reciprocal and non-reciprocal corticothalamocortical connections form cohesive integrated circuits for the control of movement (15).

Corticospinal outputs and their origin

In addition to major corticofugal outputs to the medullary motor nuclei and the spinal cord from the lower part of layer V in the primary motor cortex, the upper part of layer V has outputs to the striatum, red nucleus, pons, and reticular formation (Fig. 3.3). The focal outputs to the principal relay nuclei of the thalamus originate in layer VI, while corticocortical, corticostriate, and corticocallosal fibres arise from layer III (16, 17). The most direct projections from the cortex to the motor neuron arise largely from the caudal part of the primary motor cortex (9) (Fig. 3.2). These outputs diverge at the motor neuron level such that one corticospinal axon can supply more than one motor neuron pool monosynaptically, and it probably synapses on many motor neurons within each pool (18). The primary motor cortex is concerned not with contraction of single muscles, but with whole groups of functionally related muscles. It is concerned to bring them to action both in specific movements and when maintaining a more static posture (19). The divergence of primary motor cortical output and the presence of multiple motor cortical areas allows for parallel control of muscle activity.

Major regulators of the motor cortices

Two major subcortical systems are crucial for adequate volitional movement: the cerebellum and basal ganglia systems. Both systems comprise a large number of integrated regions (see below) which impact on the motor system at the level of the thalamus and brainstem. The thalamus contains aspiny excitatory glutamatergic neurons which conduct short-latency excitatory responses after appropriate cortical excitation, and thalamic regions participating in motor control include specific ventral, posterior, and intralaminar nuclei (20), regions with direct input from motor cortices. Reciprocal and non-reciprocal excitatory input to the thalamus (Fig. 3.4) allows the synchronization of thalamocortical oscillations and information flow across functionally related cortical fields (21). Cortical regions associated with executive function (such as dorsolateral prefrontal cortex) have non-reciprocal connections to thalamic regions projecting to premotor cortices (ventral anterior thalamus), while premotor cortices have non-reciprocal connections with thalamic regions projecting to primary motor cortex (ventrolateral thalamus) (15) (Fig. 3.4). These interconnections between the cortex and thalamus largely determine cortical activity, facilitating information transfer from one cortical region to another through a feedforward mechanism (Fig. 3.4). The output nuclei of the basal ganglia inhibit thalamocortical activity in the ventral anterior, anterior ventrolateral, and caudal intralaminar nuclei (15), while the output nuclei of the cerebellum excite thalamocortical activity in the ventrolateral posterior and ventrointermedial nuclei.

Just as lesion and stimulation studies show the importance of motor cortical outputs, comparable approaches to the study of these major subcortical systems have revealed that they profoundly gate and modify movements. Depending on the location of lesions or stimulation, there can be extreme poverty of all movements, abnormal postures, and uncontrollable rhythmic motor outputs (22). Our understanding of how these regions integrate motor information is largely based on knowledge of their relationship to the corticospinal system, giving three types of subcortical regions to consider—those receiving direct information from and influencing motor cortical regions, those with projections to motor regions, and those regions performing internal monitoring and regulation.

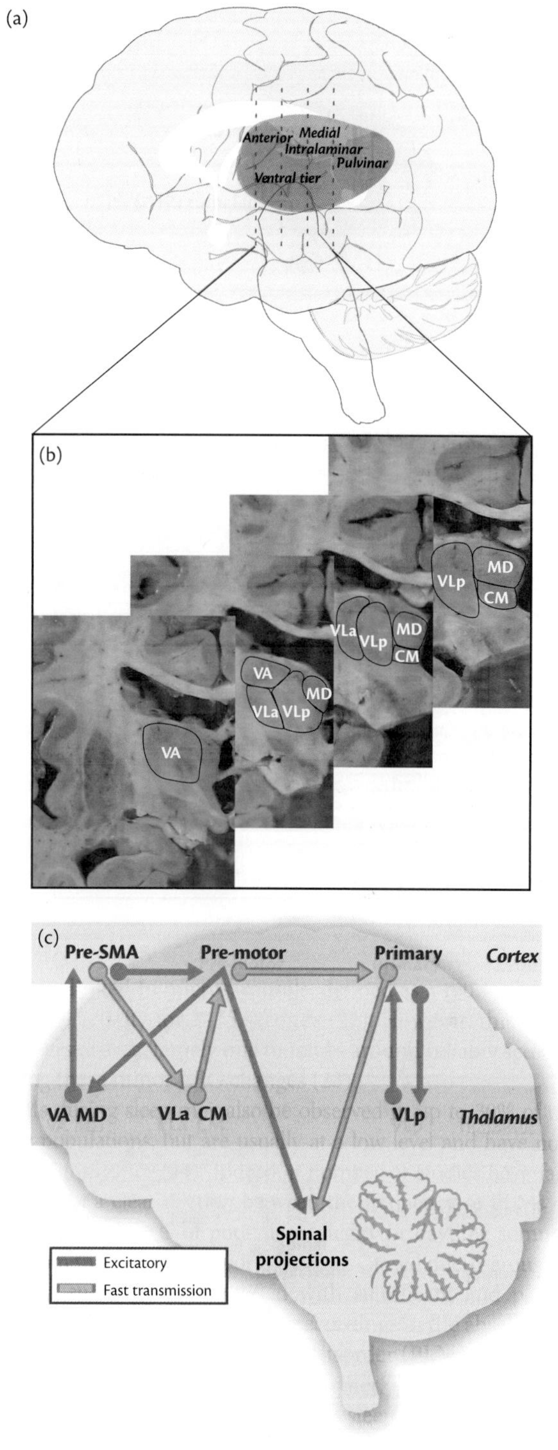

Fig. 3.4 Thalamic motor areas and their involvement in motor control. (a) Position of the thalamus in the brain showing the major anatomical subdivisions. (b) Human coronal sections through the motor regions of the thalamus. (c) Diagram showing the main corticothalamic-cortical pathways involved in movement (see text). CM, central median; pre-SMA, pre-supplementary motor area; MD, medial dorsal thalamus; VA, ventral anterior thalamus; VLa, ventral lateral anterior thalamus; VLp, ventral lateral posterior thalamus.

The basal ganglia system

The basal ganglia comprise a number of anatomically integrated regions involved in motor control (21, 23). They also play important roles in emotional, motivational, associative, and cognitive functions. Basal ganglia regions include the caudate nucleus, putamen, internal and external segments of the globus pallidus, subthalamic nucleus, and substantia nigra. The basal ganglia directly inhibit ventral anterior regions of the thalamus to influence motor control (Fig. 3.5). Basal ganglia regions have complex anatomical interconnections that are not fully characterized electrophysiologically.

Basal ganglia regions receiving motor input

The largest subcortical region receiving input from both supragranular and infragranular regions of the motor cortices is the putamen (23). Together with the caudate nucleus, this striatal area receives information from all cortical regions. The putamen passes on processed information through both a direct activating pathway and an indirect inactivating pathway to the basal ganglia output nuclei, the internal globus pallidus, and the substantia nigra pars reticulata (23) (Fig. 3.5). These basal ganglia regions are small in

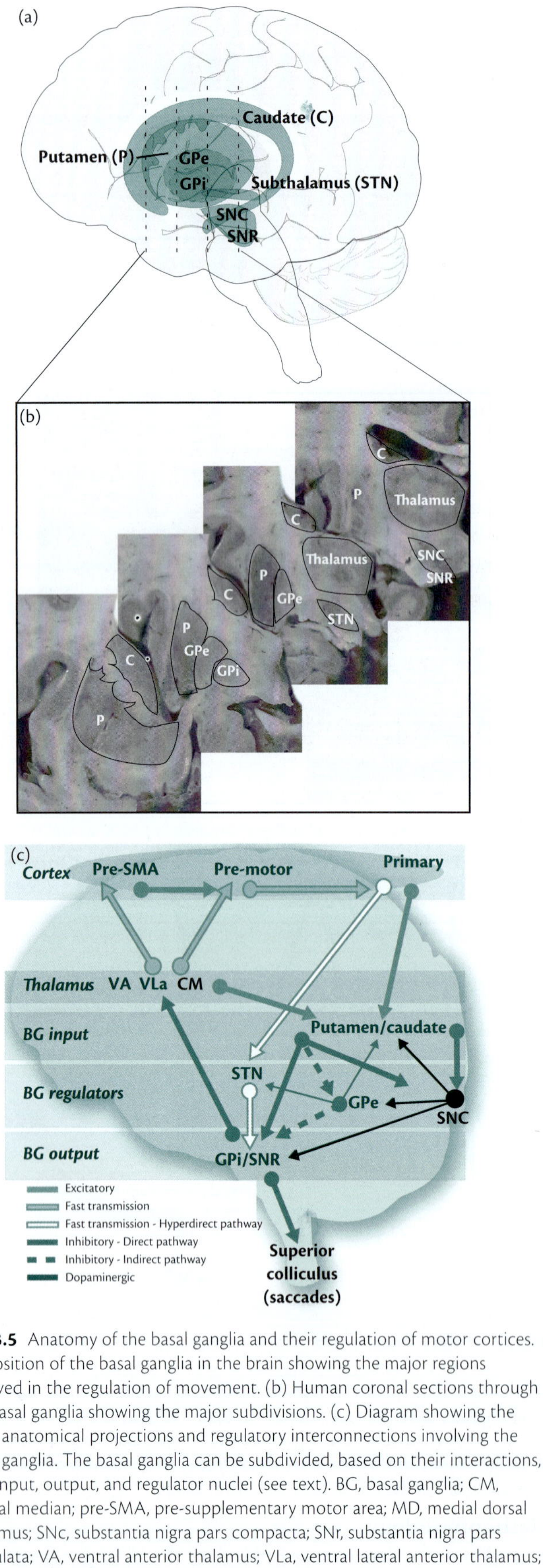

Fig. 3.5 Anatomy of the basal ganglia and their regulation of motor cortices. (a) Position of the basal ganglia in the brain showing the major regions involved in the regulation of movement. (b) Human coronal sections through the basal ganglia showing the major subdivisions. (c) Diagram showing the main anatomical projections and regulatory interconnections involving the basal ganglia. The basal ganglia can be subdivided, based on their interactions, into input, output, and regulator nuclei (see text). BG, basal ganglia; CM, central median; pre-SMA, pre-supplementary motor area; MD, medial dorsal thalamus; SNc, substantia nigra pars compacta; SNr, substantia nigra pars reticulata; VA, ventral anterior thalamus; VLa, ventral lateral anterior thalamus; VLp, ventral lateral posterior thalamus.

comparison with the striatum (100-fold fewer neurons) and contain large aspiny GABAergic inhibitory projection neurons.

Striatal neurons also receive excitatory thalamic input from the ventral anterior, ventrolateral, and caudal intralaminar nuclei and inhibitory input from the external globus pallidus, and are modulated by dopamine from the substantia nigra pars compacta and the mesencephalic tegmentum (23, 24) (Fig. 3.5). Overall, dopamine enhances activity in the direct pathway and decreases activity in the indirect pathway (25). The striatum contains mainly GABAergic spiny projection neurons and a small population of GABAergic and cholinergic interneurons (~3% of striatal neurons). Striatal spiny neurons project to the globus pallidus and substantia nigra, as well as giving rise to dense local arbours which contact other spiny neurons (23). They are usually silent and discharge only when cortical information is received. The GABAergic interneurons establish contacts with the dendritic shafts of neighbouring spiny neurons and form the structural basis for feedforward striatal surround inhibition. Striatal cholinergic interneurons, in contrast, are tonically active and play a major role in the learning of reward behaviour.

The smallest subcortical region receiving pyramidal input from layer V neurons of the motor cortices is the subthalamic nucleus (26). This is the only cortical input to this nucleus and this hyperdirect pathway conveys powerful excitatory effects from the motor cortices to the globus pallidus and substantia nigra pars reticulata, bypassing the striatum, with shorter conduction times compared with the direct striatal pathway (26) (Fig. 3.5). It also receives significant inhibitory input from the globus pallidus and striatum (27) (Fig. 3.5). The subthalamic nucleus contains aspiny excitatory glutamatergic neurons that conduct short-latency excitatory responses to the globus pallidus and substantia nigra after cortical excitation.

Internal regulators of the basal ganglia

There is significant internal modulation of the hyperdirect, direct, and indirect basal ganglia pathways. One of the basal ganglia regions most influencing striatal processing is the dopaminergic substantia nigra pars compacta, as discussed above, although pallidal and thalamic projections also significantly modify striatal output. The large tonically active aspiny dopaminergic neurons of the substantia nigra pars compacta receive input directly from striatal spiny projection neurons which modifies their firing rate and patterns (25) (Fig. 3.5). This reinforces wanted behaviours and suppresses those that are unwanted. These dopaminergic neurons also receive significant innervation from cortical, limbic, and brainstem regions and play a role in shifting attentional sets.

The basal ganglia region with the most internal connections is the external segment of the globus pallidus (23) (Fig. 3.5). These pallidal neurons receive most input from the striatum and the subthalamic nucleus, as well as a small dopaminergic projection from the substantia nigra (Fig. 3.5). Individual neurons in the external globus pallidus innervate the output nuclei as well as the subthalamic nucleus and the substantia nigra pars compacta (23) (Fig. 3.5). About 25% of them also innervate the striatal GABAergic spiny neurons. These neurons provide the anatomical substrate for the synaptic integration of functionally diverse cortical information within the basal ganglia and appear to work in parallel with the subthalamic nucleus and striatum to set up appropriate oscillatory activity within the basal ganglia (27). Therefore they are in a position to provide level-setting control of the activity through virtually the whole of the basal ganglia system.

The cerebellar system

The cerebellum plays an important role in motor control by modulating the primary motor cortex as well as spinally projecting brainstem regions to make movements integrated and seamless into a coordinated whole (28–31). The cerebellum directly excites the brainstem reticular formation, the red nucleus, and the ventrolateral thalamus to influence and regulate movements (Fig. 3.6). Similarly to the basal ganglia system, there are three types of subcortical regions to consider—those receiving direct information from and influencing motor cortical regions or spinal cord, those with projections to these motor regions, and those performing internal monitoring and regulation.

Regions receiving motor input

The cerebellum receives input from the motor cortices through neurons in the pontine nuclei (28–31). These neurons receive direct projections from the motor cortices through the corticopontine tract, and the pontine nuclei in turn project axons across the midline to the contralateral cerebellum via the middle cerebellar peduncles to form the pontocerebellar projection (Fig. 3.6). The cerebellum also receives input from Golgi tendon organs and muscle spindles, which carry information concerning muscle tension and limb position via spinocerebellar pathways, and afferents from the accessory cuneate nucleus (28–31) (Fig. 3.6). Both these relays enter the cerebellum via the inferior cerebellar peduncle. Lastly, the cerebellum receives input from other brainstem nuclei including, importantly, the inferior olive, which receives projections in turn from the spinal cord and from the red nucleus and motor cortex (32) (Fig. 3.6).

Based on the type of motor input, the cerebellum may be functionally divided into three regions: the spinocerebellum, the cerebrocerebellum, and the vestibulocerebellum (30). The spinocerebellum receives and compares motor commands with sensory information to adjust motor control and improve accuracy between intent and action. Spinocerebellar pathways in the inferior cerebellar peduncle synapse on neurons in the fastigial and interposed deep nuclei, as well as the cerebellar cortex. The vermis and intermediate hemispheres of the spinocerebellum project to the fastigial nucleus and the interposed nuclei, respectively. Purkinje cells of the vestibulocerebellum send their axons through the superior cerebral peduncle to the vestibular nuclei (30, 31). The vestibular nuclei play a role in coordinating head and eye movements via the medial vestibulospinal tract, as well as eye movement control via fibres in the medial longitudinal fasciculus to extraocular motor nuclei. The cerebrocerebellum receives input directly from the pontine nuclei through the middle cerebellar peduncle (30, 31).

Internal anatomy of the cerebellum

At the cellular level, the cerebellar cortex is uniformly organized and based on five types of neurons organized into three layers: the deep layer of granule cells, the intermediate layer of Purkinje cells, and the superficial layer of Golgi, stellate, and basket cells (28–31). Embedded within the white matter of the cerebellum are three pairs of deep nuclei (lateral, interposed, and medial), which are the final output centres for the cerebellum (28–31).

The deep nuclei are innervated by the inhibitory Purkinje cells of the cerebellar cortex (Fig. 3.6). Purkinje cells are the targets of climbing fibres originating from the inferior olivary nuclear complex and, to a lesser extent, mossy fibres from the pons, brainstem, and spinal cord relay nuclei (28–31). Although each Purkinje cell receives only a single climbing afferent, each climbing fibre makes multiple synapses with one Purkinje cell, forming one of the strongest excitatory connections in the central nervous system (32). Purkinje cells are in turn inhibited by the stellate cells and basket cells which receive their predominant input from the parallel fibres of granule cells (28–32). The granule cells are the only excitatory interneurons in the cerebellum and are the target of mossy fibres originating from the pontine other large pre-cerebellar nuclei. The axons of granule cells bifurcate to form parallel fibres which synapse on Purkinje cells and other cerebellar interneurons (28–31).

Excitatory cerebellar output (30, 31, 33–35)

The fastigial nucleus projects most of its axons through the inferior cerebellar peduncle to brainstem nuclei, generating the reticulospinal and vestibulospinal tracts. The vestibulospinal tract controls balance and postural tone. The interposed nuclei project through the superior cerebellar peduncle to the magnocellular component of the red nucleus and, via the ventrolateral nucleus of the thalamus, to motor cortices, influencing the rubrospinal and lateral corticospinal tracts. The cerebrocerebellar cortex sends efferent projections to neurons in the dentate nucleus which project to the ventrolateral thalamus which directly influences motor cortices. Axons from the dentate nucleus also project to the ipsilateral inferior olivary nucleus, the major source of input to the cerebellum, via the parvocellular division of the red nucleus.

Brainstem and spinal pattern generators for rhythmic movements

Rhythmic motor patterns (walking, scratching, breathing) are stereotyped and complex, but are subject to continuous voluntary control. Brown (36) was the first to recognize that the alternate flexion and extension of leg muscles in walking could be produced by rhythmic central circuits, now known as central pattern generators (CPGs). He demonstrated this in cats with a transected spinal cord, showing that they could generate sustained rhythmic output without requiring input from either supraspinal structures or sensory receptors (36). Further work has shown that rhythmic locomotion requires activation of both CPG regions and regions responsible for generating muscle tone (37). Both CPG regions for the coordination of rhythmic movements and regions responsible for muscle tone are located in the brainstem and spinal cord (Fig. 3.7), and are activated and modified by the integration of afferent inputs from brain regions involved in organizing motor and autonomic activities (38).

Muscles are in a constant state of partial contraction called muscle tone, which is a requirement for their use and necessary for postural stability during all movements. This is the only aspect of skeletal muscle activity that cannot be controlled voluntarily, even when a muscle is relaxed (37). Muscle tone is regulated by excitatory descending monoaminergic and other reticulospinal inputs to

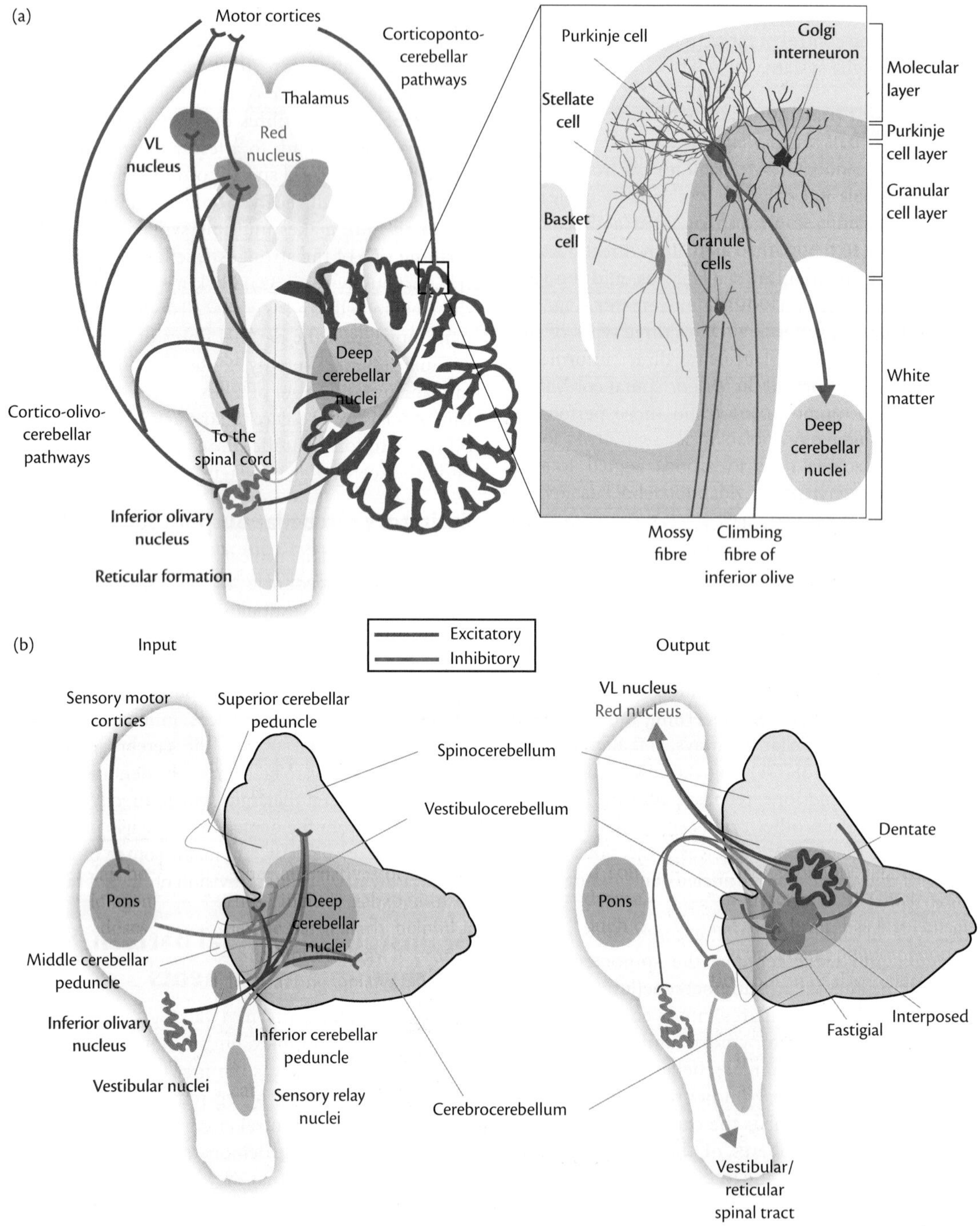

Fig. 3.6 Anatomy of the cerebellum and its involvement in motor control. (a) There are two main descending pathways from the motor cortex to the cerebellum: the corticopontocerebellar and the cortico-olivocerebellar pathways. Both pathways target the Purkinje cells of the cerebellar cortex (see inset) which then project through the deep cerebellar nuclei to the thalamus and red nucleus to regulate the motor cortices and spinal cord. Inset: Illustration of the three layers of the cerebellar cortex and the five types of neurons involved, including the major inhibitory output neuron, the Purkinje cell. (b) The cerebellar cortex can be divided into three functional regions based on their connectivity and function. The spinocerebellum is the cortical region located medially in the cerebellum (vermis and paravermis). Spinocerebellar Purkinje cells receive input from the pons, the inferior olive, and the sensory relay nuclei in the upper spinal cord and medulla oblongata. These Purkinje cells then project to the interposed deep cerebellar nuclei which regulate motor pathways via the red nucleus and thalamocortical systems. The cerebrocerebellum comprises the cortical regions located in the lateral cerebellar hemispheres. Cerebrocerebellar Purkinje cells receive input from the pons and inferior olive and then project to the dentate nuclei which directly influence the motor cortices via the ventrolateral (VL) nucleus as well as to the red nucleus. Inhibitory neurons in the dentate nuclei also project to the inferior olivary nucleus. The vestibulocerebellum is the cortical region located adjacent to the fourth ventricle (flocculonodular lobe). Vestibulocerebellar Purkinje cells receive input from the pons, the inferior olive, and the vestibular nuclei. These Purkinje cells project to the fastigial nuclei which relay back to the vestibular nuclei and reticular formation to influence reticulospinal and vestibulospinal pathways.

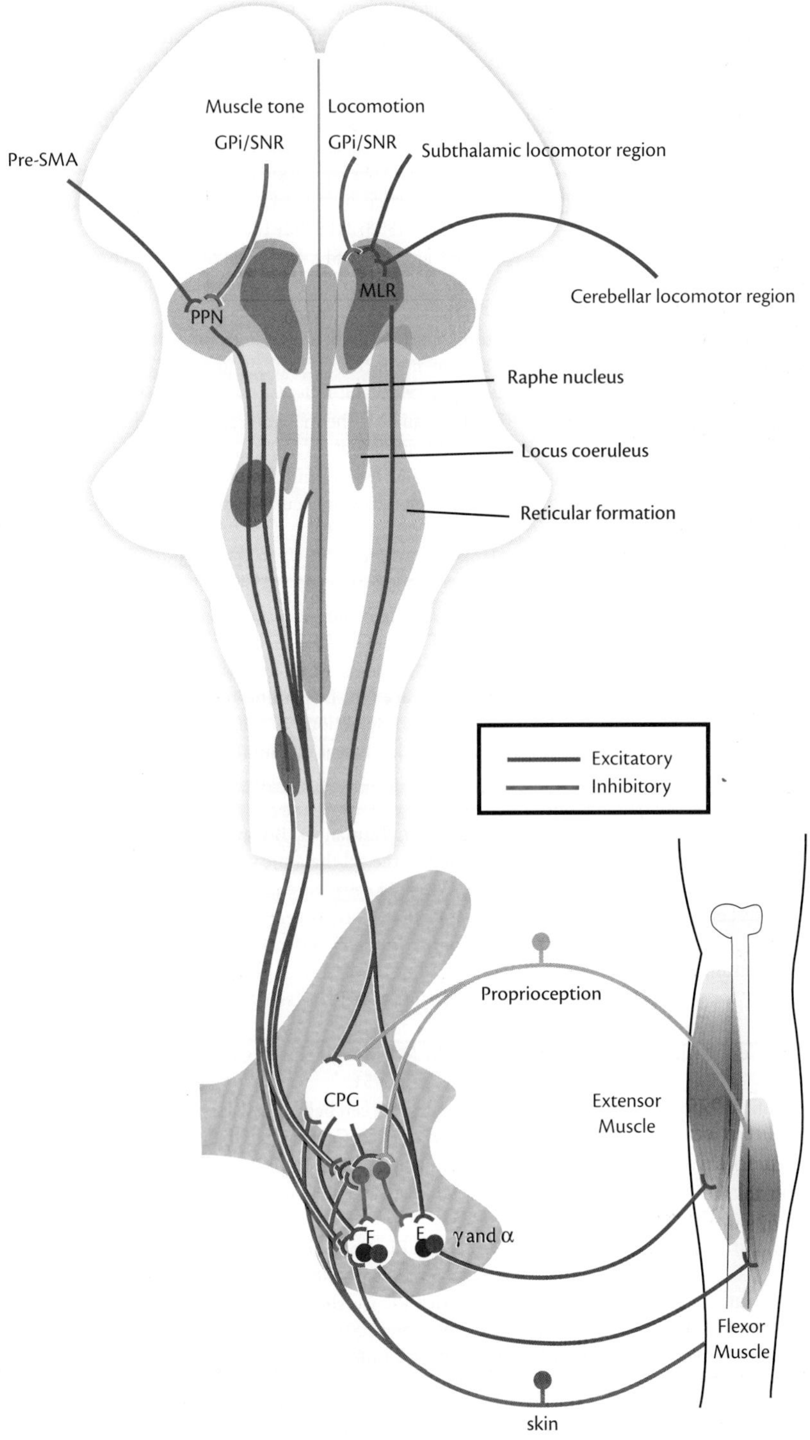

Fig. 3.7 Pathways involved in locomotor patterns and muscle tone. Locomotion (right): Subthalamic/cerebellar locomotor regions synapse on the mesencephalic locomotor region (MLR) in the pedunculopontine tegmental region, innervating the interneurons of the spinal central pattern generators (CPGs) either directly or through reticulospinal neurons. These pathways are regulated by the inhibitory inputs from the basal ganglia (GPi/SNR). Muscle tone (left): Monoaminergic locus coeruleus and raphe nuclei projections excite spinal motor neurons. Pontoreticular neurons excite inhibitory neurons in the medulla oblongata (reticulospinal neurons) and spinal cord (spinal interneurons), both of which inhibit spinal motor neurons. These two spinal projection systems have reciprocal inhibitory interactions. Cholinergic neurons in the pedunculopontine tegmental nucleus (PPN) receive direct input from the pre-SMA of the motor cortices as well as from the basal ganglia (GPi/SNR) to modulate muscle tone by directly exciting the pontine reticular formation. Inset: All three pathways are influenced by external stimuli from the skin and proprioceptive afferents. E, extensor motor neurons; F, flexor motor neurons; GPi, internal globus pallidus; SNR, substantia nigra pars reticulata.

motor spinal neurons (Fig. 3.7), and inhibited via cholinoceptive pontine reticular formation neurons which excite inhibitory neurons in the medulla oblongata (reticulospinal neurons) and spinal cord (spinal interneurons), both of which inhibit spinal motor neurons (Fig. 3.7). The excitatory and inhibitory muscle tone projections have reciprocal inhibitory interactions (37). Consequently, muscle tone is achieved by the counterbalance between these excitatory and inhibitory systems.

CPGs in the spinal cord are composed of interneuronal circuits that evoke rhythmic movements for basic, multi-joint, and multi-limb patterns (37). Spinal cord CPGs are activated by direct corticospinal input as well as by the mesencephalic locomotor region in the pedunculopontine region (directly and via medullary reticulospinal neurons) (Fig. 3.7). Sensory afferents from proprioceptive and skin receptors can activate and modify these patterns (37, 39), and reticulospinal and vestibulospinal inputs select and enhance the spinal repertoire by improving the control of muscle tone, varying the speed and quality of oscillatory patterns for locomotion (Fig. 3.7). The mesencephalic locomotor region and medullary reticular formation receive basal ganglia and cerebellar inputs, respectively, from the subthalamic and cerebellar locomotor regions (37) (Fig. 3.7). This complex coordination is necessary for humans to change patterns voluntarily during locomotion (e.g. when circumventing obstacles).

Conclusion

Movement is coordinated by a complex integrated network of brain regions. Of primary importance for voluntary purposeful movements is the motor neuron and its direct activation by the primary motor cortex. However, effective movement cannot be achieved without the integration of information from other motor cortices, the monitoring and modulation of this information flow through the thalamocortical circuits by both the basal ganglia and cerebellum, all on a background of appropriate muscle tone to enable the most time- and energy-effective inaction of the selected motion. For learned stereotyped movements some automation is achieved through brainstem and spinal central pattern generators. Disruption to different parts of this complex neural network produces very diverse movement disorders.

References

1. Dum RP, Strick PL. Motor areas in the frontal lobe of the primate. *Physiol Behav* 2002; 77: 677–82.
2. Zilles K. Architecture of the human cerebral cortrex: regional and laminar organization. In: G. Paxinos (ed.) *The Human Nervous System* (2nd edn), pp. 997–1055. New York: Academic Press, 2004.
3. Brodmann K. *Vergleichende lokalisationslehre der Grosshirnrinde*. Leipzig: Barth, 1909.
4. Geyer S, Ledberg A, Schleicher A, et al. Two different areas within the primary motor cortex of man. *Nature* 1996; 382: 805–7.
5. Matelli M, Luppino G, Geyer S, Zilles K. Motor cortex. In: G. Paxinos (ed.) *The Human Nervous System* (2nd edn), pp. 973–96. New York: Academic Press, 2004.
6. Passingham RE. *The frontal lobe and voluntary action*. Oxford: Oxford University Press, 1993.
7. Penfield W, Welch K. The supplementary motor area of the cerebral cortex; a clinical and experimental study. *AMA Arch Neurol Psychiatry* 1951; 66: 289–317.
8. Tanji J. New concepts of the supplementary motor area. *Curr Opin Neurobiol* 1996; 6: 782–7.
9. Lemon RN, Maier MA, Armand J, Kirkwood PA, Yang HW. Functional differences in corticospinal projections from macaque primary motor cortex and supplementary motor area. *Adv Exp Med Biol* 2002; 508: 425–34.
10. Miyachi S, Lu X, Inoue S, et al. Organization of multisynaptic inputs from prefrontal cortex to primary motor cortex as revealed by retrograde transneuronal transport of rabies virus. *J Neurosci* 2005; 25: 2547–56.
11. Hendry SH, Houser CR, Jones EG, Vaughn JE. Synaptic organization of immunocytochemically identified GABA neurons in the monkey sensory-motor cortex. *J Neurocytol* 1983; 12: 639–60.
12. Fetz EE, Shupe LE. Neural network models of the primate motor system. In: R. Eckmiller (ed.) *Advanced neural computers*, pp. 43–50. Amsterdam: Elsevier, 1991.
13. Baker SN, Olivier E, Lemon RN. An investigation of the intrinsic circuitry of the motor cortex of the monkey using intra-cortical microstimulation. *Exp Brain Res* 1998; 123: 397–411.
14. Jones EG. Ascending inputs to, and internal organization of, cortical motor areas. *Ciba Found Symp* 1987; 132: 21–39.
15. Haber S, McFarland NR. The place of the thalamus in frontal cortical-basal ganglia circuits. *Neuroscientist* 2001; 7: 315–24.
16. Jones EG, Wise SP. Size, laminar and columnar distribution of efferent cells in the sensory-motor cortex of monkeys. *J Comp Neurol* 1977; 175: 391–438.
17. Jones EG. Laminar distribution of cortical efferent cells. In: A. Peters, EG Jones (eds). *Cerebral cortex*. New York: Plenum Press; 1984.
18. Lemon RN, Baker SN, Davis JA, Kirkwood PA, Maier MA, Yang HS. The importance of the cortico-motoneuronal system for control of grasp. *Novartis Found Symp* 1998; 218: 202–18.
19. Kurtzer I, Herter TM, Scott SH. Random change in cortical load representation suggests distinct control of posture and movement. *Nat Neurosci* 2005; 8: 498–504.
20. Darian-Smith C, Darian-Smith I. Thalamic projections to areas 3a, 3b, and 4 in the sensorimotor cortex of the mature and infant macaque monkey. *J Comp Neurol* 1993; 335: 173–99.
21. Guillery RW, Sherman SM. The thalamus as a monitor of motor outputs. *Philos Trans R Soc Lond B Biol Sci* 2002; 357: 1809–21.
22. Vilensky JA, Gilman S. Integrating the work of D. Denny-Brown and some of his contemporaries into current studies of the primate motor cortex. *J Neurol Sci* 2001; 182: 83–7.
23. Bolam JP, Hanley JJ, Booth PA, Bevan MD. Synaptic organisation of the basal ganglia. *J Anat* 2000; 196: 527–42.
24. Smith Y, Raju DV, Pare JF, Sidibe M. The thalamostriatal system: a highly specific network of the basal ganglia circuitry. *Trends Neurosci* 2004; 27: 520–7.
25. Onn SP, West AR, Grace AA. Dopamine-mediated regulation of striatal neuronal and network interactions. *Trends Neurosci* 2000; 23: S48–56.
26. Hamani C, Saint-Cyr JA, Fraser J, Kaplitt M, Lozano AM. The subthalamic nucleus in the context of movement disorders. *Brain* 2004; 127: 4–20.
27. Bevan MD, Magill PJ, Terman D, Bolam JP, Wilson CJ. Move to the rhythm: oscillations in the subthalamic nucleus–external globus pallidus network. *Trends Neurosci* 2002; 25: 525–31.
28. Ramnani N. The primate cortico-cerebellar system: anatomy and function. *Nat Rev Neurosci* 2006; 7: 511–22.
29. Apps R, Garwicz M. Anatomical and physiological foundations of cerebellar information processing. *Nat Rev Neurosci* 2005; 6: 297–311.
30. Grimaldi G, Manto M. Topography of Cerebellar Deficits in Humans. *Cerebellum* 2012; 11: 336–51.
31. Manto M. The cerebellum, cerebellar disorders, and cerebellar research—two centuries of discoveries. *Cerebellum* 2008; 7: 505–16.
32. Ausim Azizi S. ... And the olive said to the cerebellum: organization and functional significance of the olivo-cerebellar system. *Neuroscientist* 2007; 13: 616–25.
33. Middleton FA, Strick PL. Cerebellar output: motor and cognitive channels. *Trends Cogn Sci* 1998; 2: 348–54.
34. Middleton FA, Strick PL. Cerebellar projections to the prefrontal cortex of the primate. *J Neurosci* 2001; 21: 700–12.
35. Dum RP, Strick PL. An unfolded map of the cerebellar dentate nucleus and its projections to the cerebral cortex. *J Neurophysiol* 2003; 89: 634–9.
36. Brown TG. On the nature of the fundamental activity of the nervous centres; together with an analysis of the conditioning of rhythmic activity in progression, and a theory of the evolution of function in the nervous system. *J Physiol* 1914; 48: 18–46.
37. Takakusaki K, Tomita N, Yano M. Substrates for normal gait and pathophysiology of gait disturbances with respect to the basal ganglia dysfunction. *J Neurol* 2008; 255 (Suppl 4): 19–29.
38. Grillner S, Wallen P. Central pattern generators for locomotion, with special reference to vertebrates. *Annu Rev Neurosci* 1985; 8: 233–61.
39. Jankowska E, Lundberg A, Stuart D. Propriospinal control of interneurons in spinal reflex pathways from tendon organs in the cat. *Brain Res* 1983; 261: 317–20.

CHAPTER 4

Functional Aspects of the Basal Ganglia

Thomas Wichmann

Introduction

Our understanding of basal ganglia function has changed substantially over recent decades. For many years these structures were mainly associated with the control of movement, as many movement disorders have been related to basal ganglia pathology. However, there is growing recognition that these structures are more broadly involved in the control and adaptation of behaviour. The relevant systems-level anatomy will be reviewed here, followed by a discussion of the proposed functions of these structures.

Overview of basal ganglia anatomy

General circuit anatomy

The basal ganglia are components of a system of segregated parallel circuits which originate from pre- and post-central portions of the cerebral cortex, traverse the basal ganglia and thalamus, and then return to the frontal area of origin (1–9). The circuits were designated 'motor', 'oculomotor', 'associative', and 'limbic' circuits (1), reflecting the functions of the cortical areas involved. As shown in Fig. 4.1, these circuits are functionally distinct although they are thought to utilize the same basic anatomical building blocks. Studies have shown that at least some of the larger circuits (e.g. the motor circuit) are comprised of parallel subcircuits (e.g. individual subcircuits for different parts of the body) (4, 10, 11).

An interesting long-standing debate concerns the question of the degree of functional convergence of these parallel basal ganglia–thalamocortical circuits or subcircuits (discussed in refs 12, 13). It is obvious that anatomical convergence must occur, as cortical projections outnumber the striatal neurons that receive such inputs, and striatal projecting neurons, in turn, outnumber the neurons in other portions of the basal ganglia. Moreover, the dendritic trees of many basal ganglia neurons are large and obviously receive inputs from multiple axons. However, studies have demonstrated little functional convergence in healthy animals (14–17), with individual neurons showing very high functional specificity. The functional separation between neighbouring subcircuits appears to break down in dopamine-depleted animals, with receptive fields of neurons in the basal ganglia and thalamus growing wider, although there are no obvious anatomical changes, such as altered synaptic densities or sizes of dendritic trees (e.g. 18–21). This suggests that circuit separation may be a functional process rather than being entirely structurally determined. It is tempting to speculate that the active segregation of parallel circuits is a dopamine-dependent basal ganglia process, but neither the involvement of dopamine nor the role of the basal ganglia in this process have been directly demonstrated.

The circuitry within the basal ganglia has also been studied. As shown in Fig. 4.2, the neuronal connections seem to form a complicated system of negative (and positive) feedback circuits. However, it is important to recognize that most of the connections are very specific within each of the brain structures involved. Therefore it is not known whether they truly form closed feedback loops or whether, instead, they serve to connect closely related neighbouring basal ganglia territories.

Figure 4.2 shows that the striatum (including the putamen and caudate nucleus) and the subthalamic nucleus (STN) function as input structures, receiving topographically organized projections from cortex, while the internal segment of the globus pallidus (GPi) and the substantia nigra pars reticulata (SNr) are the basal ganglia output structures, projecting to the thalamus and brainstem. The striatum is connected to the output structures via two different pathways, a monosynaptic GABAergic pathway (the so-called 'direct' pathway), and a polysynaptic connection ('indirect pathway'), consisting of a GABAergic projection from the striatum to the external pallidal segment (GPe), which then projects to the GPi and SNr either directly or via the intercalated STN.

The separation of the direct and indirect pathways has been intensively debated. Separation of these pathways was initially proposed on the basis of tract-tracing and immunohistochemical studies, showing that the indirect (striato-GPe) pathway originated from striatal neurons that express encephalin, while the direct (striato-GPi/SNr) pathway originated in striatal neurons

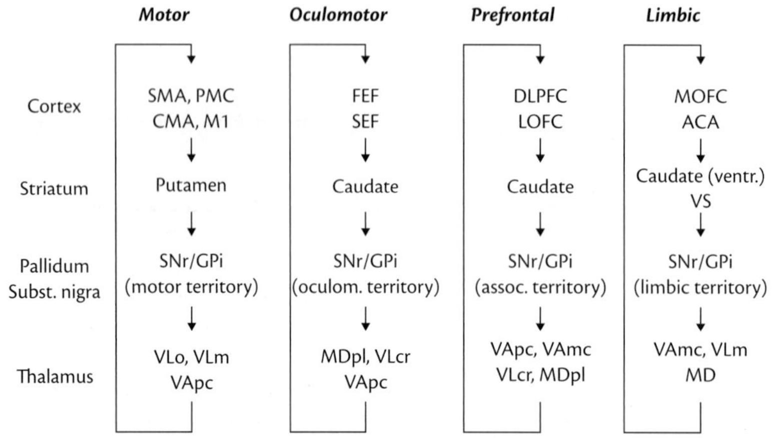

Fig. 4.1 Circuit anatomy of the cortex–basal ganglia–thalamocortical circuits. The basal ganglia are part of multiple segregated circuits that involve specific territories in the basal ganglia and associated areas of thalamus and cortex. ACA, anterior cingulate area; CMA, cingulate motor area; DLPFC, dorsolateral prefrontal cortex; FEF, frontal eye fields; LOFC, lateral orbitofrontal cortex; M1, primary motor cortex; MD, mediodorsal nucleus of the thalamus; MDpl, mediodorsal nucleus of thalamus, pars lateralis; MOFC, medial orbitofrontal cortex; PMC, pre-motor cortex; SMA, supplementary motor area; SEF, supplementary eye field; VApc, ventral anterior nucleus of thalamus, pars parvocellularis; VAmc, ventral anterior nucleus of thalamus, pars magnocellularis; VLm, ventrolateral nucleus of thalamus, pars medialis; VLo, ventrolateral nucleus of thalamus, pars oralis; VLcr, ventrolateral nucleus of thalamus, pars caudalis, rostral division. See text for other abbreviations. Reproduced, with permission, from Wichmann T, Delong MR. Deep brain stimulation for neurologic and neuropsychiatric disorders. *Neuron* 2006; 52: 197–204.

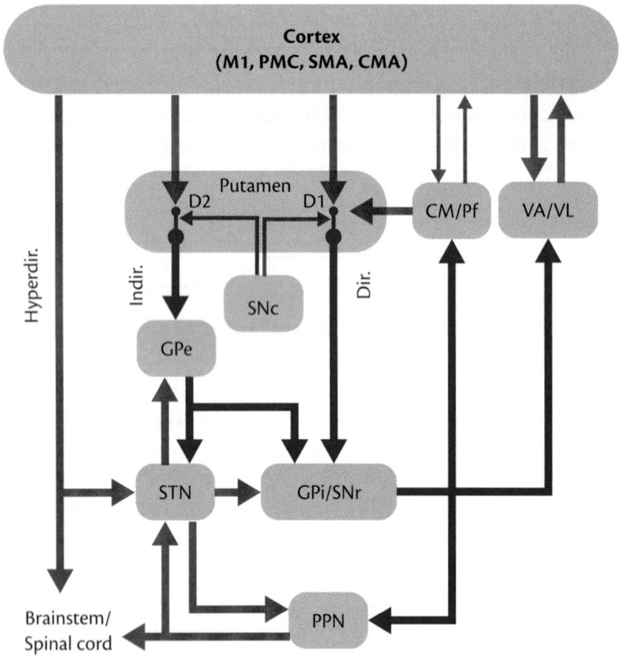

Fig. 4.2 Connections between basal ganglia nuclei, thalamus, and cortex, forming the 'motor circuit' of the basal ganglia. Green arrows indicate inhibitory connections; grey arrows indicate excitatory connections. Abbreviations: CM, centromedian nucleus of thalamus; CMA, cingulate motor area; Dir., direct pathway; D1, D2, dopamine receptor subtypes; Indir., indirect pathway; M1, primary motor cortex; Pf, parafascicular nucleus of the thalamus; PMC, pre-motor cortex; PPN, pedunculopontine nucleus; SMA, supplementary motor area. See text for other abbreviations. Reproduced, with permission, from Galvan A, Wichmann T. Pathophysiology of parkinsonism. *Clin Neurophysiol* 2008; 119: 1459–74.

expressing substance P (summarized in ref. 22). Furthermore, in histochemical studies and studies in transgenic mice, striatal direct-pathway neurons express dopamine D1 receptors while the indirect-pathway neurons express dopamine D2 receptors (23–25), with virtually no overlap between the two groups of striatal cells, although it was recently shown that the interpretation of studies in the transgenic animals may require some caution (26). However, the complete separation of direct and indirect pathways has not been confirmed by single-cell tracing studies in which many individual striatal neurons were, in fact, shown to project to both pallidal segments in monkeys, or, in rodents, to the GP (the rodent equivalent of GPe) and the SNr (27, 28). Determining the degree of separation between the direct and indirect pathways remains an important goal because some of the prominent models of basal ganglia function are built around the idea that the direct and indirect pathways operate relatively independently on basal ganglia output (see below). Such models would have to be substantially revised if collaterals of the same individual axons were found to be involved in both the direct and indirect pathways.

Besides participating in the indirect pathway of the basal ganglia, the STN also receives monosynaptic cortical inputs (29–31). The corticosubthalamic pathway has been called the 'hyperdirect' pathway, to emphasize that this pathway may provide the basal ganglia output nuclei with faster access to cortical information than is possible via the trans-striatal direct/indirect pathways (32–37).

The functionally relevant question of which types of cortical neurons provide input to the basal ganglia (and, thus, which type of information is being processed in these nuclei) remains open. In rodents, evidence has accumulated that direct-pathway neurons receive inputs from inter-hemispheric projecting cortical neurons, while the striatal neurons that give rise to the indirect pathway receive collaterals of the pyramidal tract (38). However, in electrophysiological studies in primates, neurons in cortex that gave rise to the pyramidal tract were found to differ substantially from those projecting to the striatum (39, 40). In partial agreement with these findings, single-cell tracing studies in monkeys showed two separate types of cortical neurons projecting to the striatum, including a smaller group with downstream projections and collaterals to striatal neurons, and a much larger group that sends terminations exclusively to the striatum (41).

The origin(s) of the corticosubthalamic pathway are also not clear. It appears that this pathway is separate from the corticostriatal pathway (41), and data in cats and rodents suggest that it may arise as axon collaterals of other corticofugal systems, such as the corticospinal tract (42–44), but this has not been confirmed in primates.

Basal ganglia outputs project to the thalamus in a topographically specific manner. In primates, movement-related output from the basal ganglia, mostly emanating from GPi, reaches the ventrolateral nucleus of the thalamus (VL), while non-motor output of the basal ganglia, emanating from the SNr, reaches the ventral anterior nucleus (VA). The basal ganglia–thalamocortical circuits are then at least partially closed by projections from the VL and VA nuclei to motor and non-motor areas, respectively, of the frontal cortex.

Additional basal ganglia output projections are directed at the brainstem, including prominent reciprocal connections to the pedunculopontine nucleus (PPN) (see discussion in ref. 45) and other brainstem areas, which may then give rise to descending projections, as well as reciprocal projections between the SNr/STN and the superior colliculus, known to be involved in the regulation of saccades and orienting movements (9, 46–52).

Interneurons and neuromodulators

Interneurons in the striatum are considered to be important to basal ganglia function. Interneurons constitute about 5% of all striatal neurons in rodents, but may account for a larger proportion of striatal cells in primates. Most interneuron classes are GABAergic (53–56). An important group of neurons within this category is the parvalbumin-positive 'fast-spiking' interneurons, which receive cortical input and provide significant GABAergic inhibition to neurons around them, including striatal output neurons (57). Non-GABAergic interneuron classes also exist, most notably the cholinergic interneurons. As discussed below, these neurons are active during reward learning and are strongly driven by thalamostriatal inputs.

Another important feature of basal ganglia function is that the activity of basal ganglia cells is subject to modulation by neuromodulators. Of these, the functions of dopamine are strongly emphasized in all of the proposed functions of the basal ganglia. Dopamine is released at both striatal and extrastriatal basal ganglia locations from terminals of the nigrostriatal projection (emanating from the SNc) and from projections from the ventral tegmental area (VTA). Judging by studies in dopamine-depleted animals and parkinsonian patients, the steady-state levels of dopamine strongly influence the overall activity and activity patterns in the basal ganglia. In addition, the studies by Schultz and other authors (58) have implicated the phasic release of dopamine, together with changes in acetylcholine levels (59), in regulating the strength of corticostriatal synapses, a function that may be highly important in the context of reward-based learning (see below). Dopaminergic inputs to the striatum may also have trophic functions, helping to maintain the morphology of dendritic spines. Consistent with this, it has been shown in (dopamine-depleted) patients with Parkinson's disease, and in rodent and monkey models of parkinsonism, that there is a substantial reduction in the size of dendritic trees, and other changes in dendritic spine morphology, in the parkinsonian state (60–66).

Thalamostriatal projections

While nuclei of the thalamus that receive basal ganglia output are often considered only as a relay between the basal ganglia and cortex, there is accumulating evidence that neurons in several thalamic nuclei also project back to the basal ganglia (67, 68). This is particularly true for the caudal intralaminar nuclei (the centromedian nucleus (CM) and the parafascicular nucleus (Pf)), which receive topographically organized input from the basal ganglia and send a massive projection back to the striatum (67, 69). In primates, the CM receives collaterals of the movement-related GPi projection to the VL, and projects to the 'motor' portion of the striatum (the putamen), while the Pf receives inputs from the non-motor output projections of the basal ganglia, and projects to non-motor portions of the striatum (the caudate nucleus). Although the CM and Pf inputs directly target the striatal projection neurons and cholinergic striatal interneurons (67, 70), the responses of striatal neurons to these inputs are not simply a reflection of the thalamic (glutamatergic) inputs, but also are strongly shaped by the intra-striatal circuitry, resulting in very complex response patterns (71, 72). In addition to feeding back basal ganglia output to the striatum, neurons in the CM also respond to salient stimuli in the environment, and may help to regulate reward-related activities (particularly those of the cholinergic neurons in the striatum) by favouring attention to relevant environmental stimuli (59, 73–77). The CM/Pf also sends projections to the STN (78–87), but the functions of these connections are not known.

Interactions between cerebellum and basal ganglia

For many years, researchers have seen the basal ganglia–thalamocortical and cerebello-thalamocortical systems as anatomically and functionally distinct systems. In recent years, this view has softened considerably, with the demonstration of anatomical connections between the two systems. A bisynaptic pathway linking the deep cerebellar nuclei to the striatum via the centrolateral nucleus of the thalamus was first demonstrated in mice (88), and later in primates (89). A connection between the STN and the cerebellar cortex was documented more recently (90). There is also evidence that the striatum receives inputs from portions of the ventral thalamus that are related to the cerebellum (discussed in ref. 67). Of course, further interactions between the cerebellar and basal ganglia circuits occur at the cortical level. The functional significance of the cortical and subcortical interplay between the two systems is not clear, but there is evidence from studies in rodent models and in patients that disturbances of these interactions may be relevant in the expression of some movement disorders, such as tremor and dystonia.

Basal ganglia functions

The rapidly advancing knowledge of basal ganglia anatomy, as well as clinical observations in people with basal ganglia diseases, has resulted in the formulation of concrete hypotheses about their involvement in movement-related functions. In contrast, despite solid anatomical evidence that large portions of the basal ganglia belong to non-motor circuits, little is known about the role that these structures play in non-motor functions. Therefore most of the following descriptions of basal ganglia functions focus on their possible motor functions, followed by only a very brief discussion of non-motor functions.

Inhibition of thalamocortical activities

Several of the major hypotheses regarding the function of the basal ganglia are built around the notion that the output from the basal ganglia inhibits thalamocortical activities, and therefore fundamentally serves to limit cortical activation (and movement). This concept makes sense from an anatomical point of view but, like any other hypothesis regarding the functions of these structures, the view that such inhibition is essential must be weighed against the fact that near-complete lesions of the basal ganglia output nuclei in animals and in patients with movement disorders have relatively few detrimental effects on behaviour (see below). This discrepancy can be interpreted either as evidence in favour of a view that the effects of basal ganglia on cortical functions are subtle, and therefore that their absence is hard to detect, or that the basal ganglia have effects on thalamocortical activity which are at least partially redundant, so that they can be compensated for. The latter view is also supported by the observation that altered firing rates and patterns in basal ganglia output, as have been documented in movement disorders such as Parkinson's disease (see review in ref. 91) and dystonia (e.g. 92), are seemingly far more disruptive to behaviour than the complete absence of basal ganglia output following therapeutic or experimental lesioning.

Action selection and scaling of movement

The interplay between direct and indirect basal ganglia pathways is central to several specific hypotheses regarding the motor functions of the basal ganglia, based on the notion that activation of the direct and indirect pathways have opposing effects on basal ganglia output. Specifically, it is thought that the direct pathway suppresses basal ganglia output by monosynaptic GABAergic inhibition, which may lead to disinhibition of thalamic and cortical activities, and, potentially, to facilitation of movement. In contrast, activation of striatal source neurons of the indirect pathway is expected to result in inhibition of GPe cells, which would lead to disinhibition of STN neurons, and thus increased drive of the basal ganglia output nuclei GPi and SNr. Increased basal ganglia output would eventually lead to greater inhibition of thalamocortical projections, and to a reduction of movement.

One hypothesis that makes use of this opposition between the direct and indirect pathways is the 'scaling' hypothesis. This states that the direct and indirect pathways interact to regulate the amplitude or speed of movement. In this model, activation of the direct pathway facilitates movement by disinhibition of thalamocortical neurons. The facilitated movement is then terminated (or its amplitude is limited) by the inhibitory actions of the indirect pathway, leading to increased basal ganglia output. Evidence for such a role of the basal ganglia comes from studies of the activity of pallidal neurons in monkeys trained to perform movements with different amplitudes (93). Another hypothesis is that the basal ganglia contribute to an 'action selection' mechanism by which activation of the direct pathway facilitates intended movements or motor programs, while unintended movements are suppressed by activation of the indirect and hyperdirect pathways, perhaps acting in a centre-surround fashion (e.g. 22, 32, 94, 95). This 'focusing' hypothesis relies on the possibility that direct- and indirect-pathway neurons in the striatum receive information about intended and unintended movements, respectively, or that the opposing activation patterns of the direct and indirect pathways are produced by specific inhibitory effects in the striatum—for instance, mediated by lateral inhibition of striatal output neurons through fast-spiking GABAergic interneurons (53, 57, 96, 97).

Both the scaling and action selection (focusing) hypotheses are complicated by the fact that the firing activity of basal ganglia neurons in relation to limb movement is too slow to allow for meaningful scaling or focusing. Even the fastest route by which the cerebral cortex would have access to the basal ganglia (i.e. the corticosubthalamic pathway (32)) would be active only after cortical selection of motor programs has occurred. Accordingly, phasic changes in neuronal activity in the STN and GPi in relation to the onset of limb movement occur relatively late with respect to ongoing movements, often after the start of EMG activity of related muscles (14, 93, 98–100). Additional uncertainty with regard to the scaling and focusing hypotheses arises from the fact that the input to the striatum does not appear to reflect 'motor programs' in a recognizable manner. Taken together, these findings make it unlikely that functions like scaling and focusing are primarily mediated by the basal ganglia. More likely, these functions rely heavily on cortical processing, even if the basal ganglia are also involved.

Response inhibition

The inhibition of ongoing motor programs is important under behavioural situations that require 'set'-shifting, or stop-signal inhibition. Under these conditions, ongoing movements or motor programs are inhibited or terminated in response to external cues (101, 102). It has been suspected for many years that the basal ganglia are part of a network that serves this inhibitory function (34, 103), and that dysfunction in this network may be important in the pathophysiology of a variety of disorders including, in particular, attention deficit hyperactivity disorder (ADHD) (104–109). Imaging and other studies have suggested that the response inhibition network includes not only the basal ganglia, but also several frontal and prefrontal regions (particularly the right inferior prefrontal cortex and the pre-supplementary motor area (pre-SMA)) (105, 110). Involvement of the basal ganglia in the response inhibitory network is supported by the observation that lesions in the basal ganglia produce deficits in response inhibition (as measured with stop-signal reaction time tasks) that are similar in extent to those produced by prefrontal cortical damage (111).

The STN may have a particularly prominent role in this inhibitory network, as it is anatomically positioned to drive inhibitory pallidal and nigral output, which may then act to inhibit thalamocortical transmission (32, 34, 94, 112–117). Consistent with such a role, studies of the effects of STN lesions in rats showed clear impairments of response inhibition in situations of behavioral conflict (118–120). The STN has also been shown to play a role in inhibiting automatic eye movements when switching to voluntary eye movements (121). Similar evidence is available with regard to a basal ganglia role in inhibiting limb movements (but see ref. 122).

Areas of the basal ganglia other than the STN may also be involved in response inhibition functions. For instance, lesions of the rodent striatum increase stop-signal reaction times (123, 124), and imaging and other studies have led to speculation that functional disturbances of associative portions of the striatum may play a role in the development of features of ADHD (e.g. 108, 125), which may be considered the result of failure of response inhibition.

Additional evidence for a role of the basal ganglia in response inhibition comes from studies of deep brain stimulation (DBS) and other functional neurosurgical interventions, which are frequently performed as treatment in patients with advanced movement disorders. STN-DBS treatment in patients with Parkinson's disease has been shown to interfere with response inhibition functions, as measured in cognitive and motor tasks (126–132). Most studies have shown STN-DBS to be related to impaired response inhibition, resulting, for instance, in a higher number of commission errors in Go–No Go tasks (131), but improvements in response inhibition have also been described (133). More recent research suggests that the effects of STN-DBS on response inhibition functions may, in fact, be specific to the location stimulated: stimulation of the dorsal (motor) portion of the STN was found to influence response inhibition in a Go–No Go task less than stimulation of the ventral (non-motor) portion of the nucleus (134).

Other movement-related functions

Procedural learning

One of the most active lines of research into basal ganglia functions addresses its role in procedural learning, i.e. the implicit acquisition of motor sequences and habits (e.g. 135–139). Large-scale regional shifts of basal ganglia activity have been observed when animals learn new tasks. The 'associative' caudate nucleus appears to be involved in early phases of learning, while the 'motor' putamen is more prominently engaged when animals execute previously learned movement sequences (140–149). Studies in rodents have shown that the activities of individual striatal neurons or neuron groups also change during learning. In many neurons, neuronal spiking activities gradually shift to emphasize the beginning and end of movement sequences (150–152), which is interpreted as evidence for shifts in the encoded information in these cells. However, it is unclear whether the shifts in the involvement of basal ganglia regions, or in the firing patterns of individual cells, originate in the basal ganglia, or whether they occur first in the cerebral cortex or thalamus, and are then only secondarily reflected at the basal ganglia level. Thus, it is perhaps more appropriate to see these changes as properties of the corticobasal ganglia–thalamocortical circuits rather than as properties of the basal ganglia per se (for discussion, see ref. 153). This broader view is also supported by experiments comparing sequence learning in normal monkeys and monkeys in which the internal pallidum was inactivated. These experiments failed to reveal any specific impairments of motor sequence learning in the lesioned animals (154, 155).

The learning of action sequences has also been extensively studied in the avian equivalent of the basal ganglia–thalamocortical circuitry, the so-called anterior forebrain pathway (AFP) (156). During a critical developmental period, young songbirds learn by imitating adult birds to produce the species-specific sounds they will use for communication and courtship. Interruption in the AFP, specifically in area X, homologous to the striatum and pallidum in mammals, interferes with the acquisition of songs during the critical period, or with the maintenance of learned songs thereafter (157–160).

Clinical support for the notion that the basal ganglia are essential to procedural learning comes from studies that have shown that procedural learning is disturbed in patients with basal ganglia pathologies (such as Parkinson's or Huntington's diseases), as opposed to the loss of explicit memory functions by patients with hippocampal pathologies (such as amnestic patients with Alzheimer's disease) (161–168). Specific disturbances in the control of habitual behaviours, but not goal-directed behaviours, were recently postulated to occur in patients with Parkinson's disease (169). This hypothesis is based on the observation that the dopamine loss in Parkinson's disease affects the putamen (associated with habitual behaviours) more than the caudate nucleus (more closely associated with goal-directed behaviours). Another clinical entity, obsessive compulsive disorder, has also been interpreted as a disorder of the procedural learning function of the basal ganglia (170). However, as in the experimental animal studies mentioned above, it cannot be said with certainty whether the learning impairments in these disorders are specific to the basal ganglia, as patients with disorders like Parkinson's or Huntington's diseases almost always also have substantial pathology outside the basal ganglia which may contribute to the deficits (171–177).

Reward learning

The basal ganglia were first identified as having a specific role in reward learning in studies of the response properties of dopaminergic neurons in the SNc. These neurons tend to fire in relation to (positive) prediction errors in rewarded tasks (178–184). This model was later extended into an 'actor–critique' model in which the dopamine signal to the striatum would serve as the 'critique' of the actions of the medium spiny neurons in a particular behavioural context, always acting to maximize the amount of reward to the animal.

Dopamine release from terminals of the nigrostriatal projection in reward-driven learning situations appears to be closely coordinated with the activity of cholinergic interneurons in the striatum, which are thought to signal salience, driven by their inputs from the intralaminar thalamic nuclei (59, 74–77, 185–190). It was shown that the arrival of reward information in the striatum triggers a pause in the firing of these 'tonically active' cholinergic interneurons which coincides with an increase in dopaminergic signalling (59, 186, 191, 192). Together with other intrastriatal mechanisms, specifically the endocannabinoid and adenosinergic systems (e.g. 193–198), dopamine release influences the synaptic strength of specific corticostriatal synapses that may be relevant to maximize behaviours that will produce reward.

In addition to the positive error prediction signals mentioned above, recent studies have suggested that negative prediction error signals may reach the basal ganglia from the lateral habenula. These signals influence SNc neuron activity, and thus may further modulate dopamine release in the striatum (199–204).

The concept that the basal ganglia are involved in reward learning has obvious clinical relevance. For instance, disorders of habit formation (such as addiction) have been linked to altered dopaminergic signalling in the striatum (136, 138, 147, 169), and disorders that are characterized by altered dopaminergic transmission, such as Parkinson's disease, may be associated with changes in reward learning (205, 206).

Control of bimanual movements

Because parkinsonian patients have significant problems with the performance of bimanual movements, especially anti-phase movements (207, 208), many studies have been designed to examine the role of the basal ganglia in these movements, using functional MRI (fMRI) and other functional tests. For example, it was shown that DBS of the STN reduces the impact of motivation on the performance of bimanual movements (209), and that changes in the activation patterns of the STN and GP may be involved in, or be reflective of, age-related declines in the performance of bimanual switching tasks (210). In a task involving temporally uncoupled bimanual finger movements, fMRI showed increased activation within right pre-motor and dorsolateral prefrontal, bilateral inferior parietal, basal ganglia, and cerebellar areas, identifying the basal ganglia as part of a larger bimanual movement circuitry (211) that is disturbed in Parkinson's disease (208). As with the role of the basal ganglia in learning, the basal ganglia are rarely seen to be active alone in tests of bimanual movements, so their function is very difficult to separate from that of associated cortical areas.

Non-motor functions

There is increasing discussion of the role of limbic portions of the basal ganglia in the control of motivation and mood, in addition to their role in cognition (as discussed earlier under response inhibition). There is also evidence that the basal ganglia and associated areas of the thalamus, particularly the CM–Pf complex, are involved in the regulation of pain-related behaviours, and potentially in the modulation of nociceptive information (212–214) and feeding behaviours (including responses to appetitive stimuli (215)). Like other basal ganglia areas, the STN may be involved in associative and limbic functions, as demonstrated by DBS surgery which may result in mood and cognition changes (216), and from animal studies in which STN interventions were shown to lead to changes in motivation and attention (120, 217–221). As with the potential motor functions of the basal ganglia, the non-motor functions of these structures cannot be considered apart from cortical and thalamic functions.

Conclusion

The fact that the basal ganglia are very closely linked to the thalamocortical operations in the form of modularly organized closed loops makes it virtually impossible to assign specific functions to these nuclei distinct from those of the other related brain regions. The behavioural and other roles of these structures are inextricably linked to anatomically associated areas of thalamus, cortex, and perhaps brainstem and cerebellum. All of these structures are simultaneously involved in behavioural control, and disease conditions in any of these brain areas will affect activity patterns in all of the related structures. Identifying the role of the basal ganglia is further complicated by the apparently substantial redundancy in these circuits, which accounts for the relative lack of functional deficits observed in animals and patients with basal ganglia lesions.

However, a few generalizations can be made. One is that, although the basal ganglia are important for the planning and on-line control of movement, as proposed by the focusing, scaling, and response inhibition models described above, it is probably too simple to conclude that this is their 'function', because lesions of the basal ganglia output nuclei have little or no effect on most movements in normal animals or humans (168). Indeed, patients undergoing pallidotomy, an obviously major interruption of the motor circuit, have no perceived complaints or clearly observable disturbances of voluntary movement, and experimental inactivation of the pallidum in monkeys results in slowing, but no obvious disinhibitory phenomena (154, 155).

Another general observation is that the basal ganglia appear to have a predominantly inhibitory role in the modulation of behaviour. By virtue of their tonic inhibitory output to the thalamus, they may serve to limit cortical activation. As mentioned before, this possibility has been examined in several different contexts, including action selection, the scaling of movement, the inhibition of behaviours under conflict situations, or the termination of motor programs that are already underway. A second major modulatory role of these structures arises from the fact that connections within the basal ganglia (and specifically in the striatum) are subject to considerable plasticity, allowing them to be 'tuned' to the actions of the modulatory network to permit behavioural responses that are likely to be rewarded, while suppressing others that would interfere, or to bundle sequences of movement into larger units. Basal ganglia inactivation has relatively few effects on behaviour, but disturbances of basal ganglia processing such as those seen in Parkinson's disease (reviewed in ref. 91) or dystonia result in major behavioural impairments, ranging from motor abnormalities such as akinesia (poverty of movement), bradykinesia (slowness of movement), or involuntary movements, to obsessive–compulsive symptoms or behavioural disinhibition.

It is worthwhile pointing out here some aspects of our models of basal ganglia function that may need revision. For instance, the basic assumption that basal ganglia output generally acts to inhibit thalamocortical and brainstem operations should be re-evaluated. Many studies have shown that the interactions between GABAergic and glutamatergic systems may result in a variety of discharge patterns (for instance, oscillatory phenomena or rebound bursts) which are not fully explained by simple inhibitory interactions, and are not well integrated into current models of basal ganglia activities.

It is also not clear to what extent the separation of neighbouring 'channels' within the basal ganglia is a by-product of the anatomical arrangement of these pathways, and to what extent it is an actively maintained condition. Another potentially undue bias is our almost exclusive focus on basal ganglia–thalamocortical circuits. As mentioned above, the basal ganglia have strong reciprocal interactions with brainstem areas such as the PPN, but little is known of the function(s) of these interactions.

Finally, it is obvious that our views of basal ganglia functions are strongly biased by the fact that movements are easier to examine than cognition or emotion. Given the anatomy of the basal ganglia–thalamocortical system, it is likely that some of the modulatory functions of the basal ganglia functions described above for behaviour also apply to non-motor domains, and there is growing recognition that the cognitive and emotional abnormalities in ADHD, obsessive–compulsive disorder, and other conditions involve the basal ganglia. The possibility that the basal ganglia may not only reflect primary cortical changes but also play a more active role in cognition and emotion has become apparent from changes in these domains observed with DBS surgery and other functional surgical interventions. While such changes are currently most often seen as unwanted side effects of DBS treatments for movement disorders, it may become possible to harness our understanding of non-motor functions in the future to treat conditions such as obsessive–compulsive disorder, ADHD, or even depression, with targeted neurosurgical interventions.

Acknowledgements

The preparation of this article was supported through grants from the NIH/NINDS (R01-NS054976, R01-NS071074 and P50-NS071669 (TW)), and by NIH/NCRR grant RR-000165 (Yerkes National Primate Centre).

References

1. Alexander GE, DeLong MR, Strick PL. Parallel organization of functionally segregated circuits linking basal ganglia and cortex. *Annu Rev Neurosci* 1986; 9: 357–81.
2. Joel D, Weiner I. The organization of the basal ganglia–thalamocortical circuits: open interconnected rather than closed segregated. *Neuroscience* 1994; 63: 363–79.
3. DeLong M, Wichmann T. Changing views of basal ganglia circuits and circuit disorders. *Clin EEG Neurosci* 2010; 41: 61–7.
4. Hoover JE, Strick PL. Multiple output channels in the basal ganglia. *Science* 1993; 259: 819–21.
5. Middleton FA, Strick PL. Basal ganglia and cerebellar loops: motor and cognitive circuits. *Brain Res Rev* 2000; 31: 236–50.
6. Kelly RM, Strick PL. Macro-architecture of basal ganglia loops with the cerebral cortex: use of rabies virus to reveal multisynaptic circuits. *Prog Brain Res* 2004; 143: 449–59.
7. Alexander GE, Crutcher MD. Functional architecture of basal ganglia circuits: neural substrates of parallel processing. *Trends Neurosci* 1990; 13: 266–71.
8. Alexander GE, Crutcher MD, DeLong MR. Basal ganglia–thalamocortical circuits: parallel substrates for motor, oculomotor, 'prefrontal' and 'limbic' functions. *Prog Brain Res* 1990; 85: 119–46.
9. McHaffie JG, Stanford TR, Stein BE, Coizet V, Redgrave P. Subcortical loops through the basal ganglia. *Trends Neurosci* 2005; 28: 401–7.
10. Turner RS, Grafton ST, Votaw JR, Delong MR, Hoffman JM. Motor subcircuits mediating the control of movement velocity: a PET study. *J Neurophysiol* 1998; 80: 2162–76.
11. Turner RS, Desmurget M, Grethe J, Crutcher MD, Grafton ST. Motor subcircuits mediating the control of movement extent and speed. *J Neurophysiol* 2003; 90: 3958–66.
12. Bar-Gad I, Heimer G, Ritov Y, Bergman H. Functional correlations between neighboring neurons in the primate globus pallidus are weak or nonexistent. *J Neurosci* 2003; 23: 4012–16.
13. Morris G, Nevet A, Bergman H. Anatomical funneling, sparse connectivity and redundancy reduction in the neural networks of the basal ganglia. *J Physio, Paris* 2003; 97: 581–9.
14. Wichmann T, Bergman H, DeLong MR. The primate subthalamic nucleus. I: Functional properties in intact animals. *J Neurophysiol* 1994; 72: 494–506.
15. Bergman H, Feingold A, Nini A, et al. Physiological aspects of information processing in the basal ganglia of normal and parkinsonian primates. *Trends Neurosci* 1998; 21: 32–8.
16. Raz A, Vaadia E, Bergman H. Firing patterns and correlations of spontaneous discharge of pallidal neurons in the normal and the tremulous 1-methyl-4-phenyl-1,2,3,6-tetrahydropyridine vervet model of parkinsonism. *J Neurosci* 2000; 20: 8559–71.
17. Jaeger D, Kita H, Wilson CJ. Surround inhibition among projection neurons is weak or nonexistent in the rat neostriatum. *J Neurophysiol* 1994; 72: 2555–8.
18. Pessiglione M, Guehl D, Rolland AS, et al. Thalamic neuronal activity in dopamine-depleted primates: evidence for a loss of functional segregation within basal ganglia circuits. *J Neurosci* 2005; 25: 1523–31.
19. Rothblat DS, Schneider JS. Alterations in pallidal neuronal responses to peripheral sensory and striatal stimulation in symptomatic and recovered parkinsonian cats. *Brain Res* 1995; 705(1–2): 1–14.
20. Schneider JS. Responses of striatal neurons to peripheral sensory stimulation in symptomatic MPTP-exposed cats. *Brain Res* 1991; 544: 297–302.
21. Leblois A, Meissner W, Bezard E, Bioulac B, Gross CE, Boraud T. Temporal and spatial alterations in GPi neuronal encoding might contribute to slow down movement in parkinsonian monkeys. *Brain Res* 2006; 24: 1201–8.
22. Albin RL, Young AB, Penney JB. The functional anatomy of basal ganglia disorders. *Trends Neurosci* 1989; 12: 366–75.
23. Day M, Wokosin D, Plotkin JL, Tian X, Surmeier DJ. Differential excitability and modulation of striatal medium spiny neuron dendrites. *J Neurosci* 2008; 28: 11603–14.
24. Kravitz AV, Freeze BS, Parker PR, et al. Regulation of parkinsonian motor behaviours by optogenetic control of basal ganglia circuitry. *Nature* 2010; 466: 622–6.
25. Gong S, Zheng C, Doughty ML, et al. A gene expression atlas of the central nervous system based on bacterial artificial chromosomes. *Nature* 2003; 425: 917–25.
26. Kramer PF, Christensen CH, Hazelwood LA, et al. Dopamine D2 receptor overexpression alters behavior and physiology in Drd2-EGFP mice. *J Neurosci* 2011; 31: 126–32.
27. Wu Y, Richard S, Parent A. The organization of the striatal output system: a single-cell juxtacellular labeling study in the rat. *Neurosci Res* 2000; 38: 49–62.
28. Parent A, Charara A, Pinault D. Single striatofugal axons arborizing in both pallidal segments and in the substantia nigra in primates. *Brain Res* 1995; 698: 280–4.
29. Afsharpour S. Topographical projections of the cerebral cortex to the subthalamic nucleus. *J Comp Neurol* 1985; 236(1): 14–28.
30. Nambu A, Tokuno H, Inase M, Takada M. Corticosubthalamic input zones from forelimb representations of the dorsal and ventral divisions of the premotor cortex in the macaque monkey: comparison with the input zones from the primary motor cortex and the supplementary motor area. *Neurosci Lett* 1997; 239(1): 13–16.
31. Hartmann-von Monakow K, Akert K, Kunzle H. Projections of the precentral motor cortex and other cortical areas of the frontal lobe to the subthalamic nucleus in the monkey. *Exp Brain Res* 1978; 33: 395–403.
32. Nambu A, Tokuno H, Takada M. Functional significance of the cortico-subthalamo-pallidal 'hyperdirect' pathway. *Neurosci Res* 2002; 43: 111–17.
33. Nambu A, Mori S, Stuart DG, Wiesendanger M. A new dynamic model of the cortico-basal ganglia loop. *Prog Brain Res* 2004; 461–6.
34. Aron AR, Poldrack RA. Cortical and subcortical contributions to stop signal response inhibition: role of the subthalamic nucleus. *J Neurosci* 2006; 26: 2424–33.
35. Leblois A, Boraud T, Meissner W, Bergman H, Hansel D. Competition between feedback loops underlies normal and pathological dynamics in the basal ganglia. *J Neurosci* 2006; 26: 3567–83.
36. Heida T, Marani E, Usunoff KG. The subthalamic nucleus. II: Modelling and simulation of activity. *Adv Anat Embryol Cell Biol* 2008; 199: 1–85, vii.
37. Marani E, Heida T, Lakke EA, Usunoff KG. The subthalamic nucleus. I: Development, cytology, topography and connections. *Adv Anat Embryol Cell Biol* 2008; 198: 1–113, vii.
38. Lei W, Jiao Y, Del Mar N, Reiner A. Evidence for differential cortical input to direct pathway versus indirect pathway striatal projection neurons in rats. *J Neurosci* 2004; 24: 8289–99.
39. Turner RS, DeLong MR. Corticostriatal activity in primary motor cortex of the macaque. *J Neurosci* 2000; 20: 7096–108.
40. Bauswein E, Fromm C, Preuss A. Corticostriatal cells in comparison with pyramidal tract neurons: contrasting properties in the behaving monkey. *Brain Res* 1989; 493: 198–203.
41. Parent M, Parent A. Single-axon tracing study of corticostriatal projections arising from primary motor cortex in primates. *J Comp Neurol* 2006; 496: 202–13.
42. Iwahori N. A Golgi study on the subthalamic nucleus of the cat. *J Comp Neurol* 1978; 182: 383–97.
43. Giuffrida R, Li Volsi G, Maugeri G, Perciavalle V. Influences of pyramidal tract on the subthalamic nucleus in the cat. *Neurosci Lett* 1985; 54: 231–5.
44. Kitai ST, Deniau JM. Cortical inputs to the subthalamus: intracellular analysis. *Brain Res* 1981; 214: 411–15.

45. Mena-Segovia J, Bolam JP, Magill PJ. Pedunculopontine nucleus and basal ganglia: distant relatives or part of the same family? *Trends Neurosci* 2004; 27: 585–8.
46. Coizet V, Graham JH, Moss J, et al. Short-latency visual input to the subthalamic nucleus is provided by the midbrain superior colliculus. *J Neurosci* 2009; 29: 5701–9.
47. Liu P, Basso MA. Substantia nigra stimulation influences monkey superior colliculus neuronal activity bilaterally. *J Neurophysiol* 2008; 100: 1098–112.
48. Kaneda K, Isa K, Yanagawa Y, Isa T. Nigral inhibition of GABAergic neurons in mouse superior colliculus. *J Neurosci* 2008; 28: 11071–8.
49. Hikosaka O. Basal ganglia mechanisms of reward-oriented eye movement. *Ann NY Acad Sci* 2007; 1104: 229–49.
50. Sato M, Hikosaka O. Role of primate substantia nigra pars reticulata in reward-oriented saccadic eye movement. *J Neurosci* 2002; 22: 2363–73.
51. Basso MA, Wurtz RH. Neuronal activity in substantia nigra pars reticulata during target selection. *J Neurosci* 2002; 22: 1883–94.
52. Hikosaka O, Takikawa Y, Kawagoe R. Role of the basal ganglia in the control of purposive saccadic eye movements. *Physiol Rev* 2000; 80(3): 953–78.
53. Chuhma N, Tanaka KF, Hen R, Rayport S. Functional connectome of the striatal medium spiny neuron. *J Neurosci* 2011; 31: 1183–92.
54. Tepper JM, Wilson CJ, Koos T. Feedforward and feedback inhibition in neostriatal GABAergic spiny neurons. *Brain Res Rev* 2008 Aug; 58(2): 272–81.
55. Wilson CJ. GABAergic inhibition in the neostriatum. *Prog Brain Res* 2007; 160: 91–110.
56. Tepper JM, Koos T, Wilson CJ. GABAergic microcircuits in the neostriatum. *Trends Neurosci* 2004; 27: 662–9.
57. Mallet N, Le Moine C, Charpier S, Gonon F. Feedforward inhibition of projection neurons by fast-spiking GABA interneurons in the rat striatum *in vivo*. *J Neurosci* 2005; 25: 3857–69.
58. Schultz W. Behavioral dopamine signals. *Trends Neurosci* 2007; 30: 203–10.
59. Cragg SJ. Meaningful silences: how dopamine listens to the ACh pause. *Trends Neurosci* 2006; 29: 125–31.
60. Villalba RM, Smith Y. Differential structural plasticity of corticostriatal and thalamostriatal axo-spinous synapses in MPTP-treated Parkinsonian monkeys. *J Comp Neurol* 2011; 519: 989–1005.
61. Villalba RM, Lee H, Smith Y. Dopaminergic denervation and spine loss in the striatum of MPTP-treated monkeys. *Exp Neurol* 2009; 215: 220–7.
62. Gerfen CR. Indirect-pathway neurons lose their spines in Parkinson disease. *Nat Neurosci* 2006; 9: 157–8.
63. Deutch AY. Striatal plasticity in parkinsonism: dystrophic changes in medium spiny neurons and progression in Parkinson's disease. *J Neural Transm Suppl* 2006; (70): 67–70.
64. Zaja-Milatovic S, Milatovic D, Schantz AM, et al. Dendritic degeneration in neostriatal medium spiny neurons in Parkinson disease. *Neurology* 2005; 64: 545–7.
65. Stephens B, Mueller AJ, Shering AF, et al. Evidence of a breakdown of corticostriatal connections in Parkinson's disease. *Neuroscience* 2005; 132: 741–54.
66. McNeill TH, Brown SA, Rafols JA, Shoulson I. Atrophy of medium spiny I striatal dendrites in advanced Parkinson's disease. *Brain Res* 1988; 455: 148–52.
67. Smith Y, Raju DV, Pare JF, Sidibe M. The thalamostriatal system: a highly specific network of the basal ganglia circuitry. *Trends Neurosci* 2004; 27: 520–7.
68. McFarland NR, Haber SN. Convergent inputs from thalamic motor nuclei and frontal cortical areas to the dorsal striatum in the primate. *J Neurosci* 2000; 20: 3798–813.
69. Haber SN, Calzavara R. The cortico-basal ganglia integrative network: the role of the thalamus. *Brain Res Bull* 2009; 78: 69–74.
70. Smith Y, Raju D, Nanda B, Pare JF, Galvan A, Wichmann T. The thalamostriatal systems: anatomical and functional organization in normal and parkinsonian states. *Brain Res Bull* 2009; 78: 60–8.
71. Nanda B, Galvan A, Smith Y, Wichmann T. Effects of stimulation of the centromedian nucleus of the thalamus on the activity of striatal cells in awake rhesus monkeys. *Eur J Neurosci* 2009; 29: 588–98.
72. Zackheim J, Abercrombie ED. Thalamic regulation of striatal acetylcholine efflux is both direct and indirect and qualitatively altered in the dopamine-depleted striatum. *Neuroscience* 2005; 131: 423–36.
73. Matsumoto N, Minamimoto T, Graybiel AM, Kimura M. Neurons in the thalamic CM–Pf complex supply striatal neurons with information about behaviorally significant sensory events. *J Neurophysiol* 2001; 85(2): 960–76.
74. Minamimoto T, Kimura M. Participation of the thalamic CM-Pf complex in attentional orienting. *J Neurophysiol* 2002; 87: 3090–101.
75. Minamimoto T, Hori Y, Kimura M. Complementary process to response bias in the centromedian nucleus of the thalamus. *Science* 2005; 308: 1798–1801.
76. Minamimoto T, Hori Y, Kimura M. Roles of the thalamic CM–PF complex–basal ganglia circuit in externally driven rebias of action. *Brain Res Bull* 2009; 78: 75–9.
77. Shimo Y, Hikosaka O. Role of tonically active neurons in primate caudate in reward-oriented saccadic eye movement. *J Neurosci* 2001; 21: 7804–14.
78. Sugimoto T, Hattori T. Confirmation of thalamosubthalamic projections by electron microscopic autoradiography. *Brain Res* 1983; 267: 335–9.
79. Royce GJ, Mourey RJ. Efferent connections of the centromedian and parafascicular thalamic nuclei: an autoradiographic investigation in the cat. *J Comp Neurol* 1985; 235: 277–300.
80. Carpenter MB, Jayaraman A. Subthalamic nucleus of the monkey: connections and immunocytochemical features of afferents. *J Hirnforsch* 1990; 31: 653–68.
81. Sadikot AF, Parent A, Francois C. Efferent connections of the centromedian and parafascicular thalamic nuclei in the squirrel monkey: a PHA-L study of subcortical projections. *J Comp Neurol* 1992; 315: 137–59.
82. Mouroux M, Feger J. Evidence that the parafascicular projection to the subthalamic nucleus is glutamatergic. *NeuroReport* 1993; 4: 613–15.
83. Feger J, Bevan M, Crossman AR. The projections from the parafascicular thalamic nucleus to the subthalamic nucleus and the striatum arise from separate neuronal populations: a comparison with the corticostriatal and corticosubthalamic efferents in a retrograde fluorescent double-labelling study. *Neuroscience* 1994; 60: 125–32.
84. Mouroux M, Hassani OK, Feger J. Electrophysiological study of the excitatory parafascicular projection to the subthalamic nucleus and evidence for ipsi- and contralateral controls. *Neuroscience* 1995; 67: 399–409.
85. Deschenes M, Bourassa J, Doan VD, Parent A. A single-cell study of the axonal projections arising from the posterior intralaminar thalamic nuclei in the rat. *Eur J Neurosci* 1996; 8: 329–43.
86. Lanciego JL, Gonzalo N, Castle M, Sanchez-Escobar C, Aymerich MS, Obeso JA. Thalamic innervation of striatal and subthalamic neurons projecting to the rat entopeduncular nucleus. *Eur J Neurosci* 2004; 19: 1267–77.
87. Tande D, Feger J, Hirsch EC, Francois C. Parafascicular nucleus projection to the extrastriatal basal ganglia in monkeys. *NeuroReport* 2006; 17: 277–80.
88. Ichinohe N, Mori F, Shoumura K. A di-synaptic projection from the lateral cerebellar nucleus to the laterodorsal part of the striatum via the central lateral nucleus of the thalamus in the rat. *Brain Res* 2000; 880: 191–7.
89. Hoshi E, Tremblay L, Feger J, Carras PL, Strick PL. The cerebellum communicates with the basal ganglia. *Nat Neurosci* 2005; 8: 1491–3.
90. Bostan AC, Dum RP, Strick PL. The basal ganglia communicate with the cerebellum. *Proc Natl Acad Sci USA* 2010; 107: 8452–6.
91. Galvan A, Wichmann T. Pathophysiology of parkinsonism. *Clin Neurophysiol* 2008; 119: 1459–74.

92. Schrock LE, Ostrem JL, Turner RS, Shimamoto SA, Starr PA. The subthalamic nucleus in primary dystonia: single-unit discharge characteristics. *J Neurophysiol* 2009; 102: 3740–52.
93. Georgopoulos AP, DeLong MR, Crutcher MD. Relations between parameters of step-tracking movements and single cell discharge in the globus pallidus and subthalamic nucleus of the behaving monkey. *J Neurosci* 1983; 3: 1586–98.
94. Mink JW. The basal ganglia: focused selection and inhibition of competing motor programs. *Prog Neurobiol* 1996; 50: 381–425.
95. Nambu A. Seven problems on the basal ganglia. *Curr Opin Neurobiol* 2008; 18: 595–604.
96. Kawaguchi Y, Aosaki T, Kubota Y. Cholinergic and GABAergic interneurons in the striatum. *Nihon Shinkei Seishin Yakurigaku Zasshi* 1997; 17: 87–90.
97. Mallet N, Ballion B, Le Moine C, Gonon F. Cortical inputs and GABA interneurons imbalance projection neurons in the striatum of parkinsonian rats. *J Neurosci* 2006; 26: 3875–84.
98. Mitchell SJ, Richardson RT, Baker FH, DeLong MR. The primate globus pallidus: neuronal activity related to direction of movement. *Exp Brain Res* 1987; 68: 491–505.
99. Anderson ME, Turner RS. A quantitative analysis of pallidal discharge during targeted reaching movement in the monkey. *Exp Brain Res* 1991; 86: 623–32.
100. Turner RS, Anderson ME. Pallidal discharge related to the kinematics of reaching movements in two dimensions. *J Neurophysiol* 1997; 77: 1051–74.
101. Verbruggen F, Logan GD. Models of response inhibition in the stop-signal and stop-change paradigms. *Neurosci Biobehav Rev* 2009; 33: 647–61.
102. Liddle EB, Scerif G, Hollis CP, et al. Looking before you leap: a theory of motivated control of action. *Cognition* 2009; 112: 141–58.
103. Band GP, van Boxtel GJ. Inhibitory motor control in stop paradigms: review and reinterpretation of neural mechanisms. *Acta Psychol (Amst)* 1999; 101: 179–211.
104. Aron AR, Poldrack RA. The cognitive neuroscience of response inhibition: relevance for genetic research in attention-deficit/hyperactivity disorder. *Biol Psychiatry* 2005; 57: 1285–92.
105. Dickstein SG, Bannon K, Castellanos FX, Milham MP. The neural correlates of attention deficit hyperactivity disorder: an ALE meta-analysis. *J Child Psychol Psychiatry* 2006; 47: 1051–62.
106. Robbins TW. Shifting and stopping: fronto-striatal substrates, neurochemical modulation and clinical implications. *Philos Trans R Soc Lond B Biol Sci* 2007; 362: 917–32.
107. Groman SM, James AS, Jentsch JD. Poor response inhibition: at the nexus between substance abuse and attention deficit/hyperactivity disorder. *Neurosci Biobehav Rev* 2009; 33: 690–8.
108. Casey BJ, Castellanos FX, Giedd JN, et al. Implication of right frontostriatal circuitry in response inhibition and attention-deficit/hyperactivity disorder. *J Am Acad Child Adolesc Psychiatry* 1997; 36: 374–83.
109. Armstrong IT, Munoz DP. Inhibitory control of eye movements during oculomotor countermanding in adults with attention-deficit hyperactivity disorder. *Exp Brain Res* 2003; 152: 444–52.
110. Aron AR, Behrens TE, Smith S, Frank MJ, Poldrack RA. Triangulating a cognitive control network using diffusion-weighted magnetic resonance imaging (MRI) and functional MRI. *J Neurosci* 2007; 27: 3743–52.
111. Rieger M, Gauggel S, Burmeister K. Inhibition of ongoing responses following frontal, nonfrontal, and basal ganglia lesions. *Neuropsychology* 2003; 17: 272–82.
112. Chambers CD, Garavan H, Bellgrove MA. Insights into the neural basis of response inhibition from cognitive and clinical neuroscience. *Neurosci Biobehav Rev* 2009; 33: 631–46.
113. Kuhn AA, Williams D, Kupsch A, et al. Event-related beta desynchronization in human subthalamic nucleus correlates with motor performance. *Brain* 2004; 127: 735–46.
114. Aron AR, Durston S, Eagle DM, Logan GD, Stinear CM, Stuphorn V. Converging evidence for a fronto-basal-ganglia network for inhibitory control of action and cognition. *J Neurosci* 2007; 27: 11860–4.
115. Eagle DM, Baunez C, Hutcheson DM, Lehmann O, Shah AP, Robbins TW. Stop-signal reaction-time task performance: role of prefrontal cortex and subthalamic nucleus. *Cereb Cortex* 2008; 18: 178–88.
116. Isoda M, Hikosaka O. Role for subthalamic nucleus neurons in switching from automatic to controlled eye movement. *J Neurosci* 2008; 28: 7209–18.
117. Eagle DM, Baunez C. Is there an inhibitory-response-control system in the rat? Evidence from anatomical and pharmacological studies of behavioral inhibition. *Neurosci Biobehav Rev* 2010; 34: 50–72.
118. Baunez C, Humby T, Eagle DM, Ryan LJ, Dunnett SB, Robbins TW. Effects of STN lesions on simple vs choice reaction time tasks in the rat: preserved motor readiness, but impaired response selection. *Eur J Neurosci* 2001; 13: 1609–16.
119. Baunez C, Nieoullon A, Amalric M. In a rat model of parkinsonism, lesions of the subthalamic nucleus reverse increases of reaction time but induce a dramatic premature responding deficit. *J Neurosci* 1995; 15: 6531–41.
120. Baunez C, Robbins TW. Bilateral lesions of the subthalamic nucleus induce multiple deficits in an attentional task in rats. *Eur J Neurosci* 1997; 9: 2086–99.
121. Hikosaka O, Isoda M. Brain mechanisms for switching from automatic to controlled eye movements. *Prog Brain Res* 2008; 171: 375–82.
122. Tunik E, Houk JC, Grafton ST. Basal ganglia contribution to the initiation of corrective submovements. *NeuroImage* 2009; 47: 1757–66.
123. Eagle DM, Robbins TW. Inhibitory control in rats performing a stop-signal reaction-time task: effects of lesions of the medial striatum and d-amphetamine. *Behav Neurosci* 2003; 117: 1302–17.
124. Dalley JW, Cardinal RN, Robbins TW. Prefrontal executive and cognitive functions in rodents: neural and neurochemical substrates. *Neurosci Biobehav Rev* 2004; 28: 771–84.
125. Booth JR, Burman DD, Meyer JR, et al. Larger deficits in brain networks for response inhibition than for visual selective attention in attention deficit hyperactivity disorder (ADHD). *J Child Psychol Psychiatry* 2005; 46: 94–111.
126. Jahanshahi M, Ardouin CM, Brown RG, et al. The impact of deep brain stimulation on executive function in Parkinson's disease. *Brain* 2000; 123: 1142–54.
127. Schroeder U, Kuehler A, Haslinger B, et al. Subthalamic nucleus stimulation affects striato-anterior cingulate cortex circuit in a response conflict task: a PET study. *Brain* 2002; 125: 1995–2004.
128. Witt K, Pulkowski U, Herzog J, et al. Deep brain stimulation of the subthalamic nucleus improves cognitive flexibility but impairs response inhibition in Parkinson disease. *Arch Neurol* 2004; 61: 697–700.
129. Ray NJ, Jenkinson N, Brittain J, et al. The role of the subthalamic nucleus in response inhibition: evidence from deep brain stimulation for Parkinson's disease. *Neuropsychologia* 2009; 47: 2828–34.
130. Hershey T, Revilla FJ, Wernle A, Gibson PS, Dowling JL, Perlmutter JS. Stimulation of STN impairs aspects of cognitive control in PD. *Neurology* 2004; 62: 1110–14.
131. Ballanger B, van Eimeren T, Moro E, et al. Stimulation of the subthalamic nucleus and impulsivity: release your horses. *Ann Neurol* 2009; 66: 817–24.
132. Frank MJ, Samanta J, Moustafa AA, Sherman SJ. Hold your horses: impulsivity, deep brain stimulation, and medication in parkinsonism. *Science* 2007; 318: 1309–12.
133. van den Wildenberg WP, van Boxtel GJ, van der Molen MW, Bosch DA, Speelman JD, Brunia CH. Stimulation of the subthalamic region facilitates the selection and inhibition of motor responses in Parkinson's disease. *J Cogn Neurosci* 2006 Apr; 18(4): 626–36.
134. Hershey T, Campbell MC, Videen TO, et al. Mapping Go–No-Go performance within the subthalamic nucleus region. *Brain* 2010; 133: 3625–34.

135. Yin HH, Mulcare SP, Hilario MR, et al. Dynamic reorganization of striatal circuits during the acquisition and consolidation of a skill. *Nat Neurosci* 2009; 12: 333–41.
136. Graybiel AM. Habits, rituals, and the evaluative brain. *Annu Rev Neurosci* 2008; 31: 359–87.
137. Graybiel AM. The basal ganglia: learning new tricks and loving it. *Curr Opin Neurobiol* 2005; 15: 638–44.
138. Pennartz CM, Berke JD, Graybiel AM, et al. Corticostriatal interactions during learning, memory processing, and decision making. *J Neurosci* 2009; 29: 12831–8.
139. Kubota Y, Liu J, Hu D, et al. Stable encoding of task structure coexists with flexible coding of task events in sensorimotor striatum. *J Neurophysiol* 2009; 102: 2142–60.
140. Miyachi S, Hikosaka O, Lu X. Differential activation of monkey striatal neurons in the early and late stages of procedural learning. *Exp Brain Res* 2002; 146: 122–6.
141. Nakahara H, Doya K, Hikosaka O. Parallel cortico-basal ganglia mechanisms for acquisition and execution of visuomotor sequences – a computational approach. *J Cogn Neurosci* 2001; 13: 626–47.
142. Rand MK, Hikosaka O, Miyachi S, et al. Characteristics of sequential movements during early learning period in monkeys. *Exp Brain Res* 2000; 131: 293–304.
143. Hikosaka O, Nakahara H, Rand MK, Sakai K, Lu X, Nakamura K, et al. Parallel neural networks for learning sequential procedures. *Trends Neurosci* 1999; 22: 464–71.
144. Hikosaka O, Miyashita K, Miyachi S, Sakai K, Lu X. Differential roles of the frontal cortex, basal ganglia, and cerebellum in visuomotor sequence learning. *Neurobiol Learn Mem* 1998; 70: 137–49.
145. Miyachi S, Hikosaka O, Miyashita K, Karadi Z, Rand MK. Differential roles of monkey striatum in learning of sequential hand movement. *Exp Brain Res* 1997; 115: 1–5.
146. Restivo L, Frankland PW. Shifting to automatic. *Front Integr Neurosci* 2010; 4: 1.
147. Ashby FG, Turner BO, Horvitz JC. Cortical and basal ganglia contributions to habit learning and automaticity. *Trends Cogn Sci* 2010; 14: 208–15.
148. Steele CJ, Penhune VB. Specific increases within global decreases: a functional magnetic resonance imaging investigation of five days of motor sequence learning. *J Neurosci* 2010; 30: 8332–41.
149. Swett BA, Contreras-Vidal JL, Birn R, Braun A. Neural substrates of graphomotor sequence learning: a combined FMRI and kinematic study. *J Neurophysiol* 2010; 103: 3366–77.
150. Jin X, Costa RM. Start/stop signals emerge in nigrostriatal circuits during sequence learning. *Nature* 2010; 466: 457–62.
151. Fujii N, Graybiel AM. Time-varying covariance of neural activities recorded in striatum and frontal cortex as monkeys perform sequential-saccade tasks. *Proc Natl Acad Sci USA* 2005; 102: 9032–7.
152. Jog MS, Kubota Y, Connolly CI, Hillegaart V, Graybiel AM. Building neural representations of habits. *Science* 1999; 286: 1745–9.
153. Haber SN, Knutson B. The reward circuit: linking primate anatomy and human imaging. *Neuropsychopharmacology* 2010; 35: 4–26.
154. Desmurget M, Turner RS. Motor sequences and the basal ganglia: kinematics, not habits. *J Neurosci* 2010; 30: 7685–90.
155. Wenger KK, Musch KL, Mink JW. Impaired reaching and grasping after focal inactivation of globus pallidus pars interna in the monkey. *J Neurophysiol* 1999; 82: 2049–60.
156. Reiner A, Yamamoto K, Karten HJ. Organization and evolution of the avian forebrain. *Anat Rec A Discov Mol Cell Evol Biol* 2005; 287: 1080–102.
157. Gale SD, Perkel DJ. Anatomy of a songbird basal ganglia circuit essential for vocal learning and plasticity. *J Chem Neuroanat* 2010; 39: 124–31.
158. Fee MS, Scharff C. The songbird as a model for the generation and learning of complex sequential behaviors. *ILAR J* 2010; 51: 362–77.
159. Kojima S, Doupe AJ. Activity propagation in an avian basal ganglia-thalamocortical circuit essential for vocal learning. *J Neurosci* 2009; 29: 4782–93.
160. Doupe AJ, Perkel DJ, Reiner A, Stern EA. Birdbrains could teach basal ganglia research a new song. *Trends Neurosci* 2005; 28: 353–63.
161. Knowlton BJ, Mangels JA, Squire LR. A neostriatal habit learning system in humans. *Science* 1996; 273: 1399–402.
162. Yin HH, Knowlton BJ. The role of the basal ganglia in habit formation. *Nat Rev Neurosci* 2006; 7: 464–76.
163. Moustafa AA, Gluck MA. Computational cognitive models of prefrontal–striatal–hippocampal interactions in Parkinson's disease and schizophrenia. *Neural Netw* 2011; 24: 575–91.
164. Doyon J. Motor sequence learning and movement disorders. *Curr Opin Neurol* 2008; 21: 478–83.
165. Ghilardi MF, Eidelberg D, Silvestri G, Ghez C. The differential effect of PD and normal aging on early explicit sequence learning. *Neurology* 2003; 60: 1313–19.
166. Nakamura T, Ghilardi MF, Mentis M, et al. Functional networks in motor sequence learning: abnormal topographies in Parkinson's disease. *Hum Brain Mapp* 2001; 12: 42–60.
167. Carbon M, Ghilardi MF, Feigin A, et al. Learning networks in health and Parkinson's disease: reproducibility and treatment effects. *Hum Brain Mapp* 2003; 19: 197–211.
168. Obeso JA, Jahanshahi M, Alvarez L, et al. What can man do without basal ganglia motor output? The effect of combined unilateral subthalamotomy and pallidotomy in a patient with Parkinson's disease. *Exp Neurol* 2009; 220: 283–92.
169. Redgrave P, Rodriguez M, Smith Y, et al. Goal-directed and habitual control in the basal ganglia: implications for Parkinson's disease. *Nat Rev Neurosci* 2010; 11: 760–72.
170. Graybiel AM, Rauch SL. Toward a neurobiology of obsessive–compulsive disorder. *Neuron* 2000; 28: 343–7.
171. Korczyn AD, Gurevich T. Parkinson's disease: before the motor symptoms and beyond. *J Neurol Sci* 2010; 289: 2–6.
172. Braak H, del Tredici K. Neuroanatomy and pathology of sporadic Parkinson's disease. *Adv Anat Embryol Cell Biol* 2009; 201: 1–119.
173. Braak H, Del Tredici K. Invited article: Nervous system pathology in sporadic Parkinson disease. *Neurology* 2008; 70: 1916–25.
174. Cummings DM, Milnerwood AJ, Dallerac GM, Vatsavayai SC, Hirst MC, Murphy KP. Abnormal cortical synaptic plasticity in a mouse model of Huntington's disease. *Brain Res Bull* 2007; 72: 103–7.
175. Cepeda C, Wu N, Andre VM, Cummings DM, Levine MS. The corticostriatal pathway in Huntington's disease. *Prog Neurobiol* 2007; 81: 253–71.
176. Paulsen JS, Magnotta VA, Mikos AE, et al. Brain structure in preclinical Huntington's disease. *Biol Psychiatry* 2006; 59: 57–63.
177. Kassubek J, Juengling FD, Ecker D, Landwehrmeyer GB. Thalamic atrophy in Huntington's disease co-varies with cognitive performance: a morphometric MRI analysis. *Cereb Cortex* 2005; 15: 846–53.
178. Fiorillo CD, Tobler PN, Schultz W. Discrete coding of reward probability and uncertainty by dopamine neurons. *Science* 2003; 299: 1898–902.
179. Waelti P, Dickinson A, Schultz W. Dopamine responses comply with basic assumptions of formal learning theory. *Nature* 2001; 412: 43–8.
180. Schultz W, Tremblay L, Hollerman JR. Reward processing in primate orbitofrontal cortex and basal ganglia. *Cerebr Cortex* 2000; 10: 272–84.
181. Schultz W, Dickinson A. Neuronal coding of prediction errors. *Annu Rev Neurosci* 2000; 23: 473–500.
182. Hollerman JR, Schultz W. Dopamine neurons report an error in the temporal prediction of reward during learning. *Nat Neurosci* 1998; 1: 304–9.
183. Schultz W, Dayan P, Montague PR. A neural substrate of prediction and reward. *Science* 1997; 275: 1593–9.
184. Mirenowicz J, Schultz W. Preferential activation of midbrain dopamine neurons by appetitive rather than aversive stimuli. *Nature* 1996; 379: 449–51.
185. Humphries MD, Gurney KN. The role of intra-thalamic and thalamocortical circuits in action selection. *Network* 2002; 13: 131–56.

186. Aosaki T, Miura M, Suzuki T, Nishimura K, Masuda M. Acetylcholine–dopamine balance hypothesis in the striatum: an update. *Geriatr Gerontol Int* 2010; 10 (Suppl 1): S148–57.
187. Aosaki T, Kimura M, Graybiel AM. Temporal and spatial characteristics of tonically active neurons of the primate's striatum. *J Neurophysiol* 1995; 73: 1234–52.
188. Hori Y, Minamimoto T, Kimura M. Neuronal encoding of reward value and direction of actions in the primate putamen. *J Neurophysiol* 2009; 102: 3530–43.
189. Samejima K, Ueda Y, Doya K, Kimura M. Representation of action-specific reward values in the striatum. *Science* 2005; 310: 1337–40.
190. Aosaki T, Tsubokawa H, Ishida A, Watanabe K, Graybiel AM, Kimura M. Responses of tonically active neurons in the primate's striatum undergo systematic changes during behavioral sensorimotor conditioning. *J Neurosci* 1994; 14: 3969–84.
191. Morris G, Arkadir D, Nevet A, Vaadia E, Bergman H. Coincident but distinct messages of midbrain dopamine and striatal tonically active neurons. *Neuron* 2004; 43: 133–43.
192. Ding JB, Guzman JN, Peterson JD, Goldberg JA, Surmeier DJ. Thalamic gating of corticostriatal signaling by cholinergic interneurons. *Neuron* 2010; 67: 294–307.
193. Ferre S, Lluis C, Justinova Z, et al. Adenosine–cannabinoid receptor interactions. Implications for striatal function. *Br J Pharmacol* 2010; 160: 443–53.
194. Kreitzer AC, Malenka RC. Endocannabinoid-mediated rescue of striatal LTD and motor deficits in Parkinson's disease models. *Nature* 2007; 445: 643–7.
195. Yin HH, Lovinger DM. Frequency-specific and D2 receptor-mediated inhibition of glutamate release by retrograde endocannabinoid signaling. *Proc Natl Acad Sci USA* 2006; 103: 8251–6.
196. Kreitzer AC, Malenka RC. Dopamine modulation of state-dependent endocannabinoid release and long-term depression in the striatum. *J Neurosci* 2005; 25: 10537–45.
197. Adermark L, Talani G, Lovinger DM. Endocannabinoid-dependent plasticity at GABAergic and glutamatergic synapses in the striatum is regulated by synaptic activity. *Eur J Neurosci* 2009; 29: 32–41.
198. Adermark L, Lovinger DM. Frequency-dependent inversion of net striatal output by endocannabinoid-dependent plasticity at different synaptic inputs. *J Neurosci* 2009; 29: 1375–80.
199. Matsumoto M, Hikosaka O. Representation of negative motivational value in the primate lateral habenula. *Nat Neurosci* 2009; 12: 77–84.
200. Wickens J. Toward an anatomy of disappointment: reward-related signals from the globus pallidus. *Neuron* 2008; 60: 530–1.
201. Matsumoto M, Hikosaka O. Negative motivational control of saccadic eye movement by the lateral habenula. *Prog Brain Res* 2008; 171: 399–402.
202. Hikosaka O, Sesack SR, Lecourtier L, Shepard PD. Habenula: crossroad between the basal ganglia and the limbic system. *J Neurosci* 2008; 28: 11825–9.
203. Matsumoto M, Hikosaka O. Lateral habenula as a source of negative reward signals in dopamine neurons. *Nature* 2007; 447: 1111–15.
204. Ji H, Shepard PD. Lateral habenula stimulation inhibits rat midbrain dopamine neurons through a GABA(A) receptor-mediated mechanism. *J Neurosci* 2007; 27: 6923–30.
205. Kunig G, Leenders KL, Martin-Solch C, Missimer J, Magyar S, Schultz W. Reduced reward processing in the brains of Parkinsonian patients. *NeuroReport* 2000; 11: 3681–7.
206. Voon V, Hassan K, Zurowski M, et al. Prevalence of repetitive and reward-seeking behaviors in Parkinson disease. *Neurology* 2006; 67: 1254–7.
207. Song YG, Yoo KS, Park KW, Park JH. Coordinative and limb-specific control of bimanual movements in patients with Parkinson's disease and cerebellar degeneration. *Neurosci Lett* 2010; 482: 146–50.
208. Wu T, Wang L, Hallett M, Li K, Chan P. Neural correlates of bimanual anti-phase and in-phase movements in Parkinson's disease. *Brain* 2010; 133: 2394–409.
209. Sauleau P, Eusebio A, Vandenberghe W, Nuttin B, Brown P. Deep brain stimulation modulates effects of motivation in Parkinson's disease. *NeuroReport* 2009; 20: 622–6.
210. Coxon JP, Goble DJ, van Impe A, de Vos J, Wenderoth N, Swinnen SP. Reduced basal ganglia function when elderly switch between coordinated movement patterns. *Cereb Cortex* 2010; 20: 2368–79.
211. Meister IG, Foltys H, Gallea C, Hallett M. How the brain handles temporally uncoupled bimanual movements. *Cereb Cortex* 2010; 20: 2996–3004.
212. Chudler EH, Dong WK. The role of the basal ganglia in nociception and pain. *Pain* 1995; 60: 3–38.
213. Weigel R, Krauss JK. Center median–parafascicular complex and pain control. Review from a neurosurgical perspective. *Stereotact Funct Neurosurg* 2004; 82: 115–26.
214. Harte SE, Spuz CA, Borszcz GS. Functional interaction between medial thalamus and rostral anterior cingulate cortex in the suppression of pain affect. *Neuroscience* 2011; 172: 460–73.
215. Ono T, Nishijo H, Nishino H. Functional role of the limbic system and basal ganglia in motivated behaviors. *J Neurol* 2000; 247 (Suppl 5): V23–32.
216. Temel Y, Blokland A, Steinbusch HW, Visser-Vandewalle V. The functional role of the subthalamic nucleus in cognitive and limbic circuits. *Prog Neurobiol* 2005; 76: 393–413.
217. Baunez C, Gubellini P. Effects of GPi and STN inactivation on physiological, motor, cognitive and motivational processes in animal models of Parkinson's disease. *Prog Brain Res* 2010; 183: 235–58.
218. Guigoni C, Li Q, Aubert I, et al. Involvement of sensorimotor, limbic, and associative basal ganglia domains in l-3,4-dihydroxyphenylalanine-induced dyskinesia. *J Neurosci* 2005; 25: 2102–7.
219. Darbaky Y, Baunez C, Arecchi P, Legallet E, Apicella P. Reward-related neuronal activity in the subthalamic nucleus of the monkey. *NeuroReport* 2005; 16: 1241–4.
220. Baunez C, Dias C, Cador M, Amalric M. The subthalamic nucleus exerts opposite control on cocaine and 'natural' rewards. *Nat Neurosci* 2005; 8: 484–9.
221. Baunez C, Amalric M, Robbins TW. Enhanced food-related motivation after bilateral lesions of the subthalamic nucleus. *J Neurosci* 2002; 22: 562–8.
222. Wichmann T, Delong MR. Deep brain stimulation for neurologic and neuropsychiatric disorders. *Neuron* 2006; 52: 197–204.

CHAPTER 5

Electrophysiological Approaches to the Movement Disorder Patient

Carla Cordivari

Introduction

Neurophysiological techniques are an objective way of investigating movement disorders and can support the clinical diagnosis as well as monitoring their severity and the effects of treatment. Over the past 25 years there have been enormous advances in our understanding of the pathophysiology of movement disorders, and this has been paralleled by the broadening range of investigative techniques available to clinicians. Many of these techniques, particularly transcranial magnetic stimulation (TMS), have been extremely useful in supporting clinical findings. However, the inter-individual variability in the responses, particularly for TMS, has resulted in difficulties in translating this method into a definite clinically applicable diagnostic use. As a result, many neurophysiological methods are still only used for research purposes.

In this chapter we will discuss the most common neurophysiological tests. These should always be interpreted in conjunction with clinical features. These techniques may disclose information that cannot be obtained by clinical observation alone.

Tremor

Tremor is the most common movement disorder and the most frequently evaluated by neurophysiological studies (1).

Tremor is a rhythmical oscillatory movement of a body part. It may be a symptom of many diseases affecting the nervous system, but may also occur in normal subjects as a manifestation of physiological tremor. More than with any other movement disorders, the neurophysiological findings of tremor cannot be evaluated in isolation, as a proper diagnosis often requires a close correlation with the clinical features. The conditions favouring tremor (rest, postural, action) and the presence of associated neurological signs provide important guidance in the electrophysiological diagnosis of tremor.

Neurophysiological tests using multichannel electromyographic (EMG) recording and accelerometer data identify the type of tremor on the basis of its frequency, pattern of muscle activation, duration, and amplitude of the muscle bursts (2).

Tremor can arise from different sources. It is possible to separate a central tremor from peripheral tremor by using an external loading of the limb (500–1000 g in the hand). External loading typically reduces the tremor frequency in peripheral tremor (physiological tremor, exaggerated physiological tremor (EPT), neuropathic tremor), but not in central tremor (Parkinson's disease (PD), essential tremor (ET), dystonic tremor (DT), cerebellar tremor). However, most pathological tremors are generated from a central oscillator and this test is not always necessary. The amplitude of the tremor is actually of very little diagnostic value, but can be useful for objectively monitoring the response to treatment.

The pattern of muscle activation between agonist and antagonist muscles (synchronous versus alternating) is not pathognomonic for a particular subtype of tremor. Both synchronous and alternating patterns of muscle activity can be seen in several tremor disorders. Furthermore, the pattern of muscle activity is often influenced by 'crosstalk' activity from agonist–antagonist muscles which further limits its diagnostic utility.

Tremor results in bursts of muscle activity, and the duration of the burst is directly related to the tremor frequency. Faster tremors, such as orthostatic tremor and tremor of cortical origin (rhythmic cortical myoclonus), produce shorter bursts of muscle activity.

For diagnostic purposes, the frequency of the tremor is the most useful piece of information that can be gained neurophysiologically. Tremor occurring at frequencies higher than 11 Hz is definitely pathological and usually represented by orthostatic tremor with a frequency of 13–18 Hz. Patients with orthostatic tremor present clinically with gait unsteadiness and a trembling sensation that occurs on standing. The clinical examination is unremarkable and tremor is frequently palpable but not seen because of the very high frequency. The pathognomonic neurophysiological feature is a 'coherent' tremor activity of the lower limbs at 13–18 Hz that is absent when lying or sitting (3). This tremor can be studied by simply positioning one surface electrode or accelerometer on the quadriceps or tibial muscles and recording the frequency of muscle bursts (see Fig. 5.1).

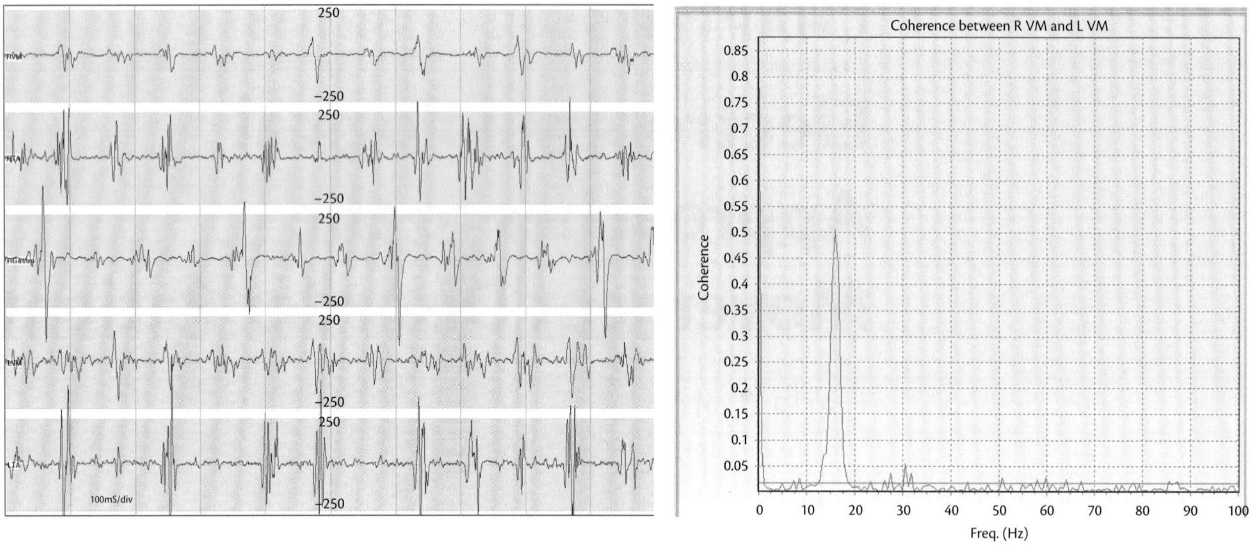

Fig. 5.1 13 Hz orthostatic tremor and right and left vastus medialis coherence at 13 Hz.

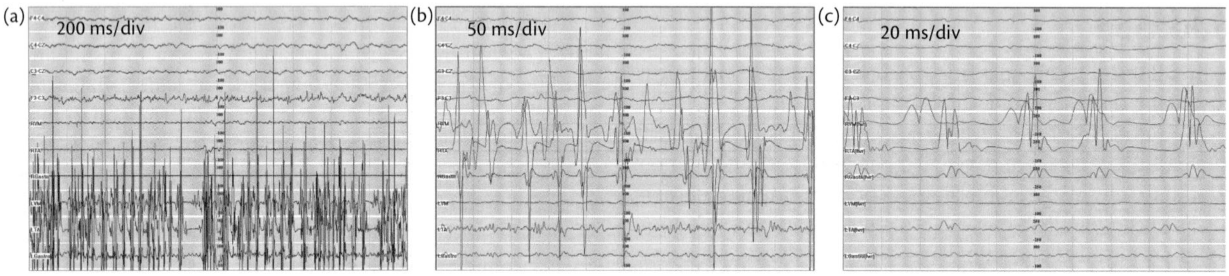

Fig. 5.2 (a) Negative myoclonus in ~20 Hz tremor. (b) Short duration muscle bursts of 30 ms. (c) Rostro-caudal progression.

Fast rhythmical cortical myoclonus can also produce a tremor in this or a higher frequency range. Cortical myoclonus may present with a fast and rhythmic activity resembling a tremor (4, 5). Hereditary forms have recently been identified, and individuals frequently present with cortical myoclonus and epilepsy (6–9). It is a postural 'tremor' with a jerky action. Surface EMG recording reveals a high frequency rhythmic activity up to 20 Hz with muscle bursts of very short duration (less than 50 ms). When such a high frequency is recorded a multichannel EMG recording may be necessary to show the characteristic pattern of muscle recruitment, with rostro-caudal progression reflecting propagation along the pyramidal pathway. Rhythmic cessation of muscle tone, which is characteristic of negative cortical myoclonus or asterixis, is also seen. The predominant involvement of distal muscles of the hands and face simply reflects the disproportionately large representation of these body parts within the sensorimotor cortex. Simultaneous EEG recording may be useful to detect cortical abnormalities such as spikes, polyspikes, or runs of rhythmic slow activity (10) (see Fig. 5.2).

Tremors occurring at frequencies lower than 4 Hz are rare and represent midbrain (rubral or Holmes) tremor, cerebellar tremor (2–4 Hz), and palatal tremor (1–3 Hz). They are easily distinguished on clinical grounds (11).

The pure rest tremor seen in some patients with *Parkinson's disease (PD)* is characteristically greater than 4 Hz, although the upper frequency limit of these tremors has not been firmly established. For those parkinsonian patients with a combination of rest and postural/kinetic tremors, the frequency of the latter may be similar to or more than 1.5 Hz higher than the rest tremor frequency.

Physiological and enhanced physiological tremors are characterized by relatively high frequencies (7–12 Hz). Physiological tremors are present in many normal individuals and generally have no clinical significance. The enhanced physiological tremor is mainly postural, with a high frequency between 7 and 12 Hz and relatively low amplitude. Typically, it is aggravated by drugs, alcohol withdrawal, and hyperthyroidism. It occurs also under conditions of stress, fatigue, anxiety, or hypoglycaemia (1).

In classic *essential tremor (ET)*, the rate of tremor may vary between 4 and 12 Hz, with older patients typically demonstrating tremor frequencies towards the lower range. In contrast, younger patients with mild ET tend to have tremor frequencies that extend into the 7–12 Hz range of physiological tremor. A kinetic component, when present, is generally at the same frequency. Functional disabilities include problems with handwriting, drinking, eating, dressing, and speaking. It is still debated whether ET can be defined as a 'bilateral, largely symmetrical postural or kinetic tremor involving hands and forearms that is visible and persistent'. It is also accepted that it can be unilateral at onset but will ultimately become bilateral in all sufferers (11).

Neuropathic tremor is relatively uncommon and generally consists of irregular postural or kinetic tremors of variable frequency ranging from 4 to 11 Hz. It occurs in the context of an established peripheral neuropathy (12).

Dystonic tremor is an irregular tremor (jerky tremor), usually below 7 Hz, which is associated with dystonic postures in the affected extremity or elsewhere. It is subject to position- and task-specific worsening, and increases with attempts to move the body part in the opposite direction to the dystonic pattern (11). This may be associated with head dystonia. Although classified separately, some tremors such as 'primary writing tremor' (frequency 5–7 Hz) and 'vocal tremor', which produces a quivering of the speech at a frequency of approximately 3–8 Hz, actually represent a form of dystonic tremor. Dystonic tremor is a mainly postural or action tremor but may also be present at rest and resemble PD (13).

Most pathological tremors occur at intermediate frequencies (4–9 Hz), and therefore it is not possible to distinguish those entities on the basis of the frequency of the tremor alone as in individual cases their frequencies often overlap. Additional tests and neurological findings are useful in classifying these tremors.

Recent studies with patients suspected to have tremulous dominant early PD but no evidence of nigrostriatal denervation on dopamine transporter scanning (scans without evidence of dopaminergic deficit (SWEDDs)), suggest that these subjects may in fact have dystonic tremor (13). It is very important to distinguish these two forms of tremor as the prognosis is different; SWEDDs are not likely to progress in severity or to develop long-term motor and non-motor complications, as seen in PD. Furthermore, a correct diagnosis will avoid inappropriate use of PD drug treatments (14).

In SWEDDs and patients with dystonic or essential tremor, no re-emerging tremor is seen as it occurs immediately after changing from rest to a position with the arm outstretched at shoulder level. In contrast, patients with PD with a postural tremor have a 're-emergent' postural tremor, starting on average after 3–4 s. SWEDDs and those with segmental dystonia exhibit an abnormally exaggerated response to the paired associative stimulation (PAS) protocol which involves repeated pairing of median nerve and motor cortical magnetic stimulation given at inter-stimulus intervals of 25 ms (14).

There are features that can help to distinguish between PD patients and SWEDDs which may be useful in clinical practice: lack of true bradykinesia, presence of dystonia, and head tremor favoured a diagnosis of SWEDDs, whereas re-emergent tremor, true fatiguing or decrement, good response to dopaminergic drugs, and presence of non-motor symptoms favour PD (13, 14).

Patients with essential tremor can easily be confused with a dystonic tremor when a minimal dystonic component is present; lack of an exaggerated response to the PAS protocol supports the diagnosis of essential tremor. However, the role of TMS in improving diagnostic accuracy has not been fully validated (15).

Psychogenic tremor

Psychogenic tremor (PsyT) is the most commonly reported psychogenic movement disorder. Neurophysiological studies are helpful in distinguishing between PsyT and organic tremor (OrgT).

Variation in the frequency of the tremor in response to weight loading can assist in differentiating PsyT from OrgT (16, 17). In the former, the frequency of tremor increases with weight load owing to an increase in coactivation to maintain the oscillation. With OrgT the frequency tends to remain the same in tremors of central origin or reduce in physiological tremor (15, 16). In PsyT, amplitude and frequency decrease during distraction (counting, tapping). Furthermore, tapping different frequencies with the unaffected hand 'entrains' the same frequency on the tremulous side. Ballistic movements performed on the contralateral limb can also significantly reduce the tremor amplitude or even produce a pause in the tremor (18–21). Increased coherence between limbs in bilateral tremor is also a pointer to a psychogenic aetiology. Muscle coactivation between agonist and antagonist muscles is often recorded (coactivation sign).

When the onset of tremor can be recorded, a tonic coactivation occurring in the antagonist muscles is seen 300 ms before the onset of the tremor burst in PsyT (16). A set of scoring criteria using the sum results from all these individual tests has recently been reported to be both sensitive and specific in the diagnosis of PysT (22).

Myoclonus

Myoclonus is an involuntary movement disorder which occurs in many different conditions with a wide variety of different aetiologies and neurophysiological phenomena, but with a common semiological element: sudden, brief, shock-like, involuntary movements caused by muscular contractions or inhibitions (23).

Muscle contraction produces positive myoclonus, and muscle inhibition causes negative myoclonus. It can be focal, multifocal, generalized, spontaneous, or reflex. It may occur at rest, when maintaining a posture, or during action. Myoclonus is classified according to its physiopathological basis as cortical, reticular, or spinal (10, 24).

Cortical myoclonus is characterized by jerks of short duration, involving many muscles and usually synchronously in agonists and antagonists. Myoclonus may be positive at rest or triggered by movements, or negative when the limbs are outstretched against gravity. Cortical myoclonus is most marked in the distal limb, and in focal forms is usually confined to this site. If widespread, myoclonus is multifocal, and in some cases there are additional bilateral or generalized jerks. It may affect speech and gait.

Reflex jerks may be elicited by touch and tap, or visual stimuli (reflex myoclonus). When there is sensitivity to auditory stimuli, this suggests a startle syndrome, although some patients may have a combination of cortical myoclonus and pathological startle. Multifocal jerks occurring with voluntary action are very suggestive of a cortical origin for the myoclonus. Jerks are usually arrhythmic but can also be rhythmic (cortical tremor) or periodic.

The myoclonus is usually due to a lesion of the sensorimotor cortex which results in an abnormal discharge that is conducted rapidly down the corticospinal pathways to produce abrupt excitation or inhibition of spinal motor neurons and cause brief contraction or inhibition of innervated muscles (jerk).

Positive myoclonus is represented by brief jerks of electromyographic (EMG) activity with a duration usually less than 70 ms, while negative myoclonus is produced by a sudden interruption of a tonic muscle contraction (between 50 and 400 ms). EMG recording from an extremity can also demonstrate spread of jerks (or periods of 'muscle silence') from the proximal to the distal muscle with a velocity corresponding to that of alpha motor fibres. For this reason muscle activity is recorded from several limb and cranial muscles using multichannel EMG (25).

The simultaneous recording of EMG and EEG allows analysis of the relationship between myoclonic and cortical events. Cortical activities are recorded by classical EEG using a 10–20 montage. In cortical myoclonus the EEG often shows multifocal or generalized spike and wave discharges, or multiple spike and wave discharges, which are usually time-locked to the muscle jerks. While the EEG may not show any time-locked abnormality in some cases, EEG back-averaging can disclose myoclonus-related EEG activity that may not be recognized on the conventional polygraph. This technique can determine the precise time interval from the EEG activity to the myoclonus. It also identifies the scalp distribution of the myoclonus-related EEG activity based on simultaneous multichannel recordings.

EEG–EMG back-averaging is performed by analysing the recording offline and placing a marker at the onset of each myoclonic jerk. Then the EEG is averaged around the marker, for example 200 ms before and 200 ms after (see Fig. 5.3).

Back-averaging analysis shows a positive–negative biphasic spike at the central electrode somatotopically representing the muscle from which the myoclonus is recorded. The initial positive precedes the onset of myoclonic EMG discharge in a hand muscle by approximately 20 ms. The more distal the muscle the myoclonus is recorded from, the longer is the EEG–EMG time interval. Myoclonus-related discharge spreads through the motor cortex within one hemisphere, and also transcallosally to the homologous area of the contralateral motor cortex (10–15 ms) (26). Unfortunately, EEG back-averaging analysis is limited by muscle activity artefacts on the scalp, and also in cases where the jerks are of high frequency or are infrequent.

In subjects in whom myoclonic EMG bursts are of small amplitude, or are repeated rhythmically at high frequency, frequency analysis has advantages over back-averaging. Frequency analysis of both EMG–EMG and EEG–EMG coherence can detect a pathologically exaggerated common drive in distal limb muscles, showing significant coherence in the physiological range (15–60 Hz) and also, in some cases, at much higher frequencies (27).

Another feature of cortical myoclonus is the enlarged somatosensory evoked potential (SEP) obtained by median nerve stimulation and recorded over the parietal cortex. These SEPs are obtained by averaging EEGs over several hundreds of peripheral nerve stimuli. The initial components, a post-central negative peak (N20) and a pre-central positive peak (P20), are not enhanced; however, the subsequent components (P25, P30, N35) are three to ten times larger than normal. It is generally agreed that 10 μV represents the threshold above which cortical responses are considered enlarged, yielding so-called giant SEPs. Giant SEPs are commonly found in patients with cortical myoclonus, in particular those with progressive myoclonic epilepsy, and are presumably related to a hyperexcitable sensorimotor cortex (25).

Not all patients with cortical myoclonus display giant SEPs. In this case it is useful to assess cortical excitability by studying the recovery cycle of SEPs (SEP-R) using paired-pulse stimuli. In normal subjects the second cortical SEP is attenuated at an inter-stimulus interval below 100 ms. The finding of SEPs that are larger after a paired-pulse stimulation than after a single stimulation is strongly suggestive of cortical hyperexcitability and thus, in the context of myoclonus, of a cortical origin (10).

Further supportive evidence for a cortical origin of the jerks can be obtained by also assessing the long-latency reflex (C-reflex) which can be simultaneously recorded with SEPs. The long-loop reflex (C-reflex) is obtained by sub-threshold motor stimulation of the median nerve at 2–3 Hz and is recorded from both thenar muscles. It has an ipsilateral latency of around 45 ms, and is 10–15 ms longer contralaterally because of the transcallosal transit time (26). Muscles should be recorded at rest and then during a weak tonic contraction.

The presence of a C-reflex at rest is always pathological and indicates cortical hyperexcitability. It should be noted that a C-reflex can be found during weak muscle activation even in healthy subjects. Recording the muscle activity during a weak contraction is useful for detecting any stimulus-related EMG silent periods which reflect an abnormal negative long latency (negative C-reflex).

It must be remembered that the presence of a C-reflex indicates only that the myoclonus is reflex and so sensitive to somatosensory stimuli. As reflex myoclonus can also be subcortical (i.e. reticular

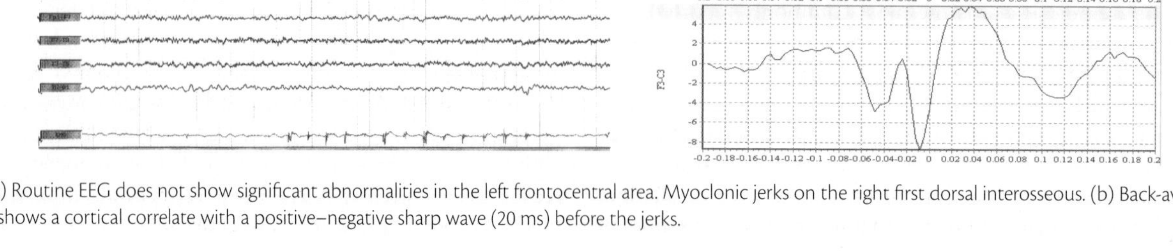

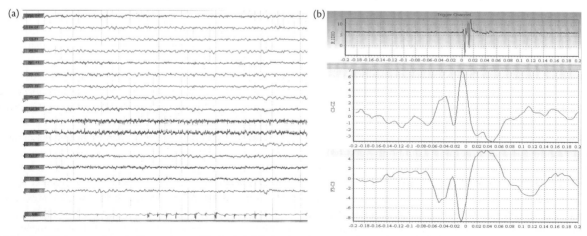

Fig. 5.3 (a) Routine EEG does not show significant abnormalities in the left frontocentral area. Myoclonic jerks on the right first dorsal interosseous. (b) Back-averaging of 50 jerks shows a cortical correlate with a positive–negative sharp wave (20 ms) before the jerks.

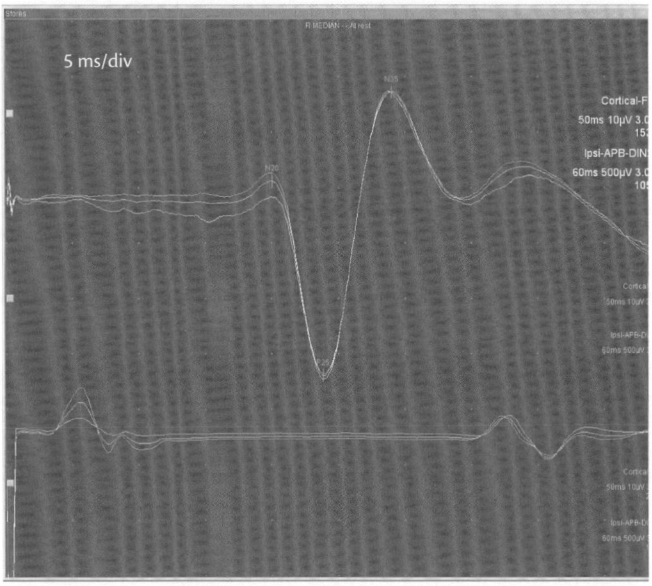

Fig. 5.4 Giant evoked potential with P25/N35 of 53 μV, C-reflex at latency of 40 ms.

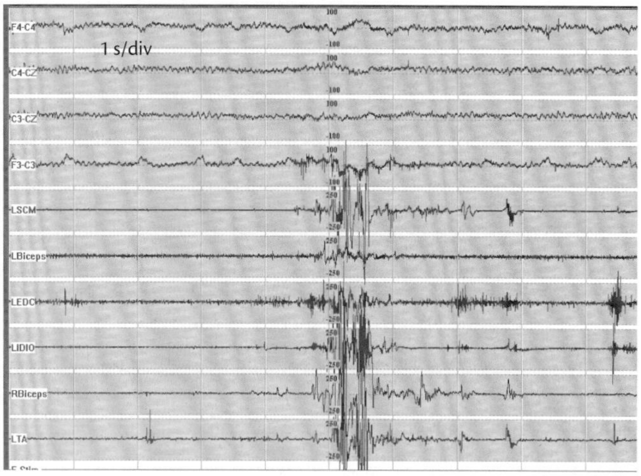

Fig. 5.5 Patient with myoclonus dystonia (ε-sarcoglycan gene).

reflex myoclonus), its presence does not definitely indicate a cortical origin for the myoclonus (see Fig. 5.4).

A C-reflex is frequently found in corticobasal degeneration (CBD), a disease in which SEPs are not enlarged and EEG back-averaging fails to reveal a pre-myoclonus spike (28).

In Creutzfeldt–Jakob disease (CJD), myoclonus is not stimulus-sensitive and occurs continuously and quasi-periodically in the resting condition every 600–1500 ms. There may be accompanying dystonic posturing. EMG bursts are similar to, or slightly longer than, those of classical cortical myoclonus. Periodic sharp discharges (PSDs) are usually associated with muscle jerks, but can occur independently. EEG spike wave and EMG activity correlate loosely. On back-averaging, the negative spike wave is much smaller than the PSD recorded with the raw EEG. The time interval between EEG and jerks is 50–85 ms (much longer than required for conduction through the pyramidal tract). Typical cortical reflex myoclonus may be seen in the late stages of the disease.

In subacute sclerosing panencephalitis (SSPE) sudden movements followed by a tonic phase ('hung-up jerks') can be related to periodic high amplitude EEG discharges occurring every 4–13 s.

Myoclonus dystonia is a movement disorder characterized by a combination of rapid brief muscle contraction (myoclonus) and/or sustained twisting and repetitive movements that result in an abnormal posture (dystonia). Myoclonic jerks typically affect the neck, trunk, and upper limbs, with less common involvement of the legs (29). About 50% of patients have additional focal or segmental dystonia, presenting as cervical dystonia or writer's cramp. Myoclonus dystonia is characterized by multifocal, focal, and generalized jerks of brief and long duration, and spasms. Often they are stimulus-sensitive and may present a startle response. No cortical origin has been found for the absence of enlarged SEPs and positive cortical event on EEG back-averaging (see Fig. 5.5).

Reticular myoclonus (brainstem myoclonus) is characterized by generalized jerks with prominent involvement of proximal and flexor muscles. Jerks may be spontaneous or stimulus-induced, particularly with respect to sound (30). The jerks originate from the brainstem reticular formation. The first muscle to be activated is the trapezius or sternocleidomastoid (SCM). Subsequently, there is spread to cranial and caudal muscles with different velocities of propagation but with a constant pattern of muscle activation. Myoclonic jerks may be associated with cortical spikes, but the lack of correlation between the two suggests that spikes are projected to, but do not originate in, the cortex. Evoked potentials are not increased in amplitude, but there may be an enhanced C-reflex.

The normal human startle response consists of a brief flexion response, most marked in the upper half of the body, elicited by unexpected auditory, and sometimes somaesthetic, visual or vestibular stimuli. The nucleus reticularis pontis caudalis seems to be particularly important. Conduction of efferent impulses both upwards and downwards from the generator, possibly in the medial reticular formation, is slow. The shortest latencies are 20–50 ms for the orbicularis oculi muscle, while in the quadriceps the latency of the responses reaches 100–150 ms. EMG responses in the intrinsic hand and foot muscles are particularly delayed. Auditory startle reflex EMG latencies are rather variable. The constant reflex EMG activity in orbicularis oculi is the most important event in the normal auditory startle reflex. Considering the auditory blink reflex in orbicularis oculi as separated from the startle response, the earliest muscle recorded is the SCM with a latency of <100ms. The activity then spreads up the brainstem from cranial nerve XI to cranial nerve V and down the spinal cord (reflex brainstem myoclonus). In physiological startle the stimulus-induced response tends to habituate, and disappears after four to six stimuli. Exaggerated startle responses are seen in hyperekplexia, neuropsychiatric startle syndrome, and stimulus-induced epilepsy or other movement disorders such as stiff person syndrome or tics (30) (see Fig. 5.6).

Two different patterns of *spinal myoclonus* are recognized: propriospinal myoclonus and segmental myoclonus. In the latter, myoclonus is limited to muscles innervated by one to two contiguous spinal segments. It is often caused by a structural lesion of the spinal cord, although in some cases no lesion is found. The myoclonus is often rhythmic and may persist during sleep. Stimulus sensitivity is unusual.

When segmental myoclonus is suspected a multichannel EMG recording should be performed in distant muscles belonging to the

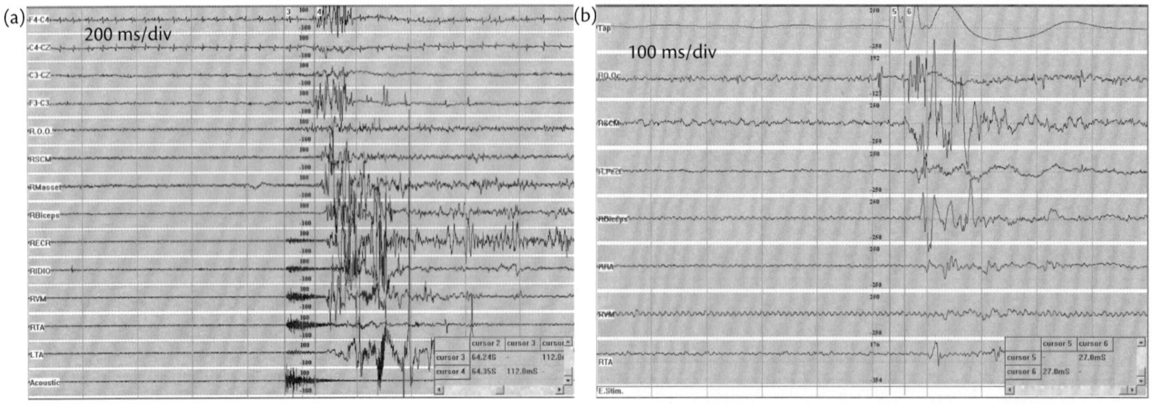

Fig. 5.6 (a) Acoustic stimulation. (b) Tapping on the nose.

same myotome, and it is useful to study at least two myotomes. The frequency of the jerks is highly variable, and EMG burst can have a duration of up to 1000 ms (31).

Propriospinal myoclonus is characterized by axial muscle contractions usually causing flexion of the trunk and typically induced by lying down. Rhythmicity is not common in propriospinal myoclonus, although 'runs' or clusters of jerks are seen. It is hypothesized that propriospinal myoclonus arises from a spinal myoclonic generator recruiting axial muscles up and down the spinal cord via long propriospinal pathways (31, 32). The propagation of the myoclonic discharge within the spinal cord can be studied by recording proximal upper limb, trunk (cervical, thoracic paraspinal, and rectus abdominis), and lower limb muscles.

Propriospinal myoclonus is characterized by arrhythmic sequences or runs of axial jerks producing flexion or extension of the trunk. Bursts of muscle activity vary from 50 ms to 4 s. EMG jerks arise from abdominal or cervical spinal segments and slowly spread rostrally and caudally at <10 m/s. Cranial muscles are not involved, with the exception of the neck. This form of myoclonus can be stimulus-sensitive (see Fig. 5.7).

Cervical trauma, albeit mild, is reported in some idiopathic cases, and some have viral myelitis. Most cases are labelled as idiopathic as no structural lesion is found. As the 'typical' clinical and electrophysiological features of propriospinal myoclonus can be voluntarily mimicked, and in some cases an immediate response to a placebo dose of botulinum toxin has been reported, a psychogenic aetiology should be considered in idiopathic cases (33, 34). Interestingly, however, ultrastructural lesions in the spinal tracts have recently been reported using diffusion tensor magnetic resonance imaging (35).

Psychogenic myoclonus

Jerking of the limbs that superficially resembles spinal segmental myoclonus may also be seen in patients where either the clinical course or investigations reveal the cause to be psychogenic (34, 36). In psychogenic movement disorders, multichannel surface EMG recording of the jerks may show an inconsistent pattern of muscle activation, variable intermuscular latencies, and distractibility.

A useful tool that can distinguish between organic and psychogenic jerks is the detection of a *Bereitschaftspotential* (BP) via jerk-locked back-averaging analysis (34, 36). The BP consists of an early (early BP) and a late (late BP) component, the former starting 2 s and the latter 400 ms before the jerk onset. Both the components have a cortical generator: the early BP originates from the supplementary motor area (SMA) and the late BP from the primary motor cortex (M1).

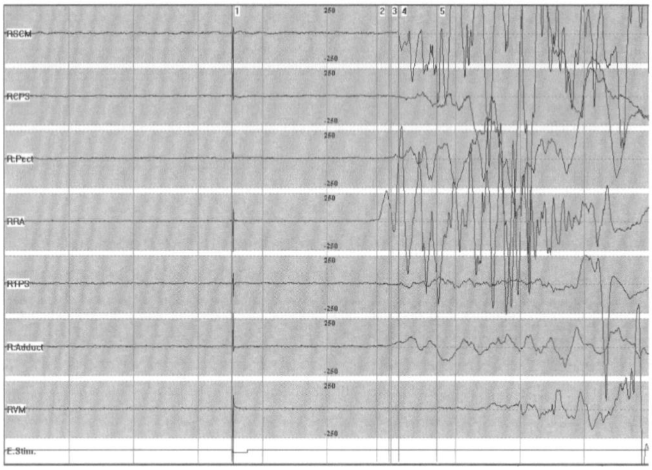

Fig. 5.7 Multichannel EMG recording in propriospinal myoclonus.

BPs can be recorded prior to self-paced voluntary movements. A 'typical' BP has never been recorded prior to proven organic myoclonus. Its presence in patients with jerks or other intermittent movements indicates that there is a (conscious or unconscious) volition component in the origin of these jerks.

The BP is obtained by back-averaging epochs of EEG preceding the muscle jerks. As this test requires a low/high-pass filter (0.05 Hz) the patient has to be very quiet between the jerks as the EEG recording is less stable and more sensitive to artefact. The eyes should be covered with cotton-wool pads to avoid blink artefact. This technique is not useful when the jerks are too frequent (with inter-jerk interval <2 s) or too few (poor signal-to-noise ratio requires at least 40 jerks). As this test involves the average of many jerks it is always possible that some organic jerks are averaged with jerks where a minor voluntary component is included. The converse situation may also occur (in particular in patients with axial jerks). Therefore a cautious interpretation of these features is necessary in such cases.

It is also important to note that healthy people do not have a pre-movement potential when jerks occur in response to external

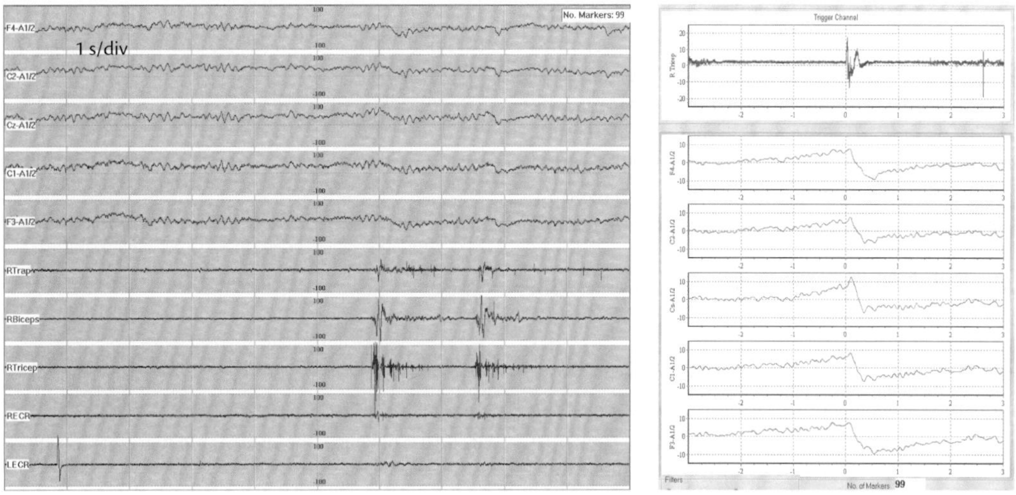

Fig. 5.8 Filters 0.05–10 Hz: amplitude axis in μV; 3 s pre- and post-trigger. Back-averaging for detection of BP.

stimuli, while patients with tics and myoclonus dystonia may have an abbreviated pre-movement potential (see Fig 5.8).

Dystonia

Dystonia is characterized by co-contraction of agonist and antagonist muscles and overflow of muscle contraction, which refers to activation of muscles not required to perform the desired action. This may be due to impaired inhibition at multiple levels in the central nervous system. In dystonia, there is reduced reciprocal inhibition in the spinal cord, abnormal inhibitory function localized in the brainstem (enhanced blink reflex), and reduced inhibition in the cortex, measured by transcranial magnetic stimulation (TMS) (37). TMS has provided useful information on pathophysiology of dystonia, but the technique is of limited help for diagnostic purposes in individual patients. The triple stimulation test (TST) has proved to be a useful screening tool in patients with prolonged central motor conduction times and mutations in the *PARK2* gene, particularly because such mutations are a relatively common cause of young-onset PD.

Patients with dystonia caused by mutations in *TOR1A* gene display abnormalities on some TMS measures (e.g. intra-cortical inhibition and silent period). Unaffected carriers of the mutation appear to have similar abnormalities and this may be used to identify asymptomatic carriers (15).

In patients with primary dystonia, including those with *DYT1* mutations, there is an enhanced response to non-invasive brain stimulation protocols which can induce plastic changes in the motor system. Thus, PAS and repetitive transcranial magnetic stimulation (rTMS) protocols all produce larger and more long-lasting effects in patients with dystonia compared with healthy controls. Interestingly, non-manifesting carriers of the *DYT1* mutation show a subnormal response to such protocols, indicating that abnormalities in the control of plastic changes in the brain may be a primary driving force behind the development of dystonia.

Video multichannel EMG recording for cervical dystonia is a useful tool to identify the dystonic neck muscles to be treated with botulinum toxin in cases where the clinical examination alone fails to determine which muscles contribute to the dystonic movement. Multichannel EMG recording of bilateral neck muscles (SCM, splenius capitus, levator scapulae, and trapezius) is useful to identify 'leading' overactive neck muscles which are active at the onset of dystonic spasms and those muscles that show paradoxical activity, leading to restriction of head movements. For this reason, patients need to be studied at rest and during rotation and tilt of the neck.

The selection of incorrect muscles for injection of botulinum toxin may explain why some patients have a suboptimal response (Fig. 5.9).

More sophisticated analyses of EMG discharges consider EMG–EMG coherence. This may disclose the character of the descending discharges responsible for the abnormal muscle activity in dystonia (38). An abnormal 4–7 Hz drive is seen in dystonic muscles in patients with the *DYT1* gene mutation, idiopathic torticollis, and myoclonus dystonia.

In the arms there is evidence of an abnormal corticomuscular drive in the 15–30 Hz band leading to co-contraction between antagonistic muscles, with the exception of writer's cramp where a discrete peak in EMG–EMG coherence may be seen at 11–12 Hz.

Psychogenic dystonia

A clinical distinction between organic and psychogenic dystonia can be extremely challenging. Most electrophysiological studies so far have focused on patients with a fixed dystonia syndrome

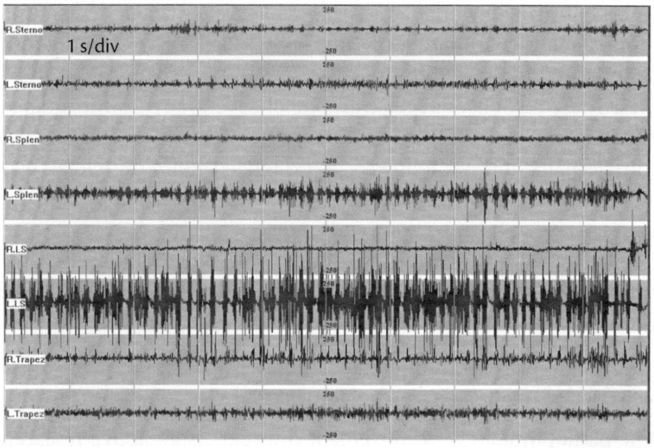

Fig. 5.9 Overactivity of left splenius capitus and levator scapulae at rest.

or psychogenic dystonia affecting limb, trunk, and neck muscles. While these patients show the same abnormalities of short- and long-interval intracortical inhibition, cortical silent period, and spinal reciprocal inhibition as patients with primary dystonia, the response to a plasticity protocol (paired associative stimulation) is abnormal only in primary dystonia. However, these similarities and differences between psychogenic and primary dystonia have only been reported at a group level, hence their usefulness as a discriminating tool for individuals remains to be proved.

An enhanced R2 blink reflex recovery curve in patients with blepharospasm is useful in distinguishing an organic from a psychogenic origin. In this protocol, surface EMG is recorded from the orbicularis oculi muscles. Electrical stimulation is applied to the supraorbital nerve in the supraorbital notch while the patient is at rest with eyes gently closed. Blink reflex in response to paired stimulation is assessed at interstimulus intervals of 200, 300, 500, and 1000 ms. R2 is usually completely abolished at interstimulus intervals <200 ms; it then slowly recovers, reaching about 40–50% at the 500 ms interval and 70–90% at the 1500 ms interval (39).

This test shows that the recovery curve is normal in patients with atypical (presumed psychogenic) blepharospasm, while in patients with organically determined blepharospasm the recovery of R2 response is in an interstimulus interval <200 ms. Patients with solely involuntary levator palpebrae inhibition exhibit a normal R2 recovery cycle.

Rigidity

Stiff person syndrome

This syndrome is characterized by axial rigidity at rest, involving mainly trunk and proximal lower limb muscles. Exteroceptive stimuli may evoke a sudden exacerbation of rigidity (reflex spasm) (40). A crucial finding is the presence of continuous motor unit activity in the paraspinal muscles that persists even when trying to relax. EMG electrical silence cannot be obtained. The rigidity and continuous motor unit activity lessen or even disappear during sleep and after spinal or general anaesthesia, indicating a central source (41).

Exteroceptive or cutaneomuscular reflexes are enhanced, habituate poorly, and spread as reflex spasms into muscles normally not involved in the reflex. These findings point to enhanced spinal interneuronal excitability due to defects within either spinal interneuronal networks at a segmental level or their descending control. Polysynaptic reflexes are characteristically exaggerated in both upper and lower limbs as well as the axial (paraspinal) muscles. These responses begin with one or several myoclonic jerks at short intervals (50–70 ms) that are synchronous in antagonistic muscle pairs and are followed by prolonged tonic muscle activation (observed clinically as spasm) (42). This pattern appears to be characteristic of stiff person syndrome.

Patients with stiff limb syndrome present continuous motor units at rest at least in one limb. Spasms tend to involve repetitive grouped discharges of motor units (see Fig. 5.10).

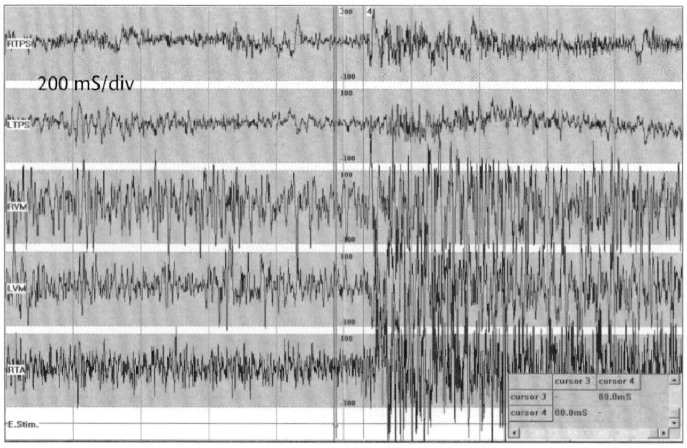

Fig. 5.10 Continuous motor activity in the legs and exteroceptive reflex.

Conclusion

The pathophysiology of movement disorders is an active research field. Neurophysiological diagnostic support is still limited in most of the tremors in the intermediate frequency range, as the clinical features often guide the interpretation of the neurophysiological findings. Studies involving a larger number of patients may help in validating the techniques. Unfortunately, many techniques are not widely available in the clinical setting and have limited clinical application as they are not particularly user-friendly (e.g. TMS and coherence studies). Dystonia of psychogenic origin and organic movement disorders continue to present diagnostic challenges which may be helped by further studies. In the field of myoclonus, neurophysiology provides better support even when the EEG fails to show abnormalities. In such cases, polygraphic recording is necessary to demonstrate the origin of the myoclonus. Startle responses may be a guide in the diagnosis of brainstem pathology and in exaggerated startle responses.

Acknowledgements

I would like to express special thanks to Mr Nathan Toms for the excellent technical support he has provided for many years.

References

1. Jankovic J, Fahn S. Physiologic and pathologic tremors. Diagnosis, mechanism, and management. *Ann Intern Med* 1980; 93: 460–5.
2. Deuschl G. Neurophysiological tests for the assessment of tremors. *Adv Neurol* 1999; 80: 57–65.
3. McManis PG, Sharbrough FW. Orthostatic tremor: clinical and electrophysiologic characteristics. *Muscle Nerve* 1993; 16: 1254–60.
4. Ikeda A, Kakigi R, Funai N, Neshige R, Kuroda Y, Shibasaki H. Cortical tremor: a variant of cortical reflex myoclonus. *Neurology* 1990; 40(10): 1561–65.
5. Toro C, Pascual-Leone A, Deuschl G, Tate E, Pranzatelli MR, Hallett M. Cortical tremor. A common manifestation of cortical myoclonus. *Neurology* 1993; 43: 2346–53.
6. Elia M, Musumeci SA, Ferri R, et al. Familial cortical tremor, epilepsy, and mental retardation: a distinct clinical entity? *Arch Neurol* 1998; 55: 1569–73.
7. Okuma Y, Shimo Y, Hatori K, Hattori T, Tanaka S, Mizuno Y. Familial cortical tremor with epilepsy. *Parkinsonism Relat Disord* 1997; 3: 83–7.
8. Striano P, Robbiano A, Zara F, Striano S. Familial cortical tremor and epilepsy: a well-defined syndrome with genetic heterogeneity waiting for nosological placement in the ILAE classification. *Epilepsy Behav* 2010; 19: 669.
9. van Rootselaar AF, van Schaik IN, van den Maagdenberg AM, Koelman JH, Callenbach PM, Tijssen MA. Familial cortical myoclonic tremor with epilepsy: a single syndromic classification for a group of pedigrees bearing common features. *Mov Disord* 2005; 20(6): 665–73.

10. Shibasaki H, Hallett M. Electrophysiological studies of myoclonus. *Muscle Nerve* 2005; 31(2): 157–74.
11. Deuschl G, Bain P, Brin M. Consensus statement of the Movement Disorder Society on Tremor. Ad Hoc Scientific Committee. *Mov Disord* 1998;13 (Suppl 3): 2–23.
12. Deuschl G, Bergman H. Pathophysiology of nonparkinsonian tremors. *Mov Disord* 2002; 17 (Suppl 3): S41–8.
13. Schneider SA, Edwards MJ, Mir P, et al. Patients with adult-onset dystonic tremor resembling parkinsonian tremor have scans without evidence of dopaminergic deficit (SWEDDs). *Mov Disord* 2007; 22: 2210–15.
14. Schwingenschuh P, Ruge D, Edwards MJ, et al. Distinguishing SWEDDs patients with asymmetric resting tremor from Parkinson's disease: a clinical and electrophysiological study. *Mov Disord* 2010; 25: 560–9.
15. Edwards MJ, Talelli P, Rothwell JC. Clinical applications of transcranial magnetic stimulation in patients with movement disorders. *Lancet Neurol* 2008; 7: 827–40.
16. Deuschl G, Koster B, Lucking CH, Scheidt C. Diagnostic and pathophysiological aspects of psychogenic tremors. *Mov Disord* 1998; 13: 294–302.
17. Zeuner KE, Shoge RO, Goldstein SR, Dambrosia JM, Hallett M. Accelerometry to distinguish psychogenic from essential or parkinsonian tremor. *Neurology* 2003; 61: 548–50.
18. Kumru H, Valls-Sole J, Valldeoriola F, Marti MJ, Sanegre MT, Tolosa E. Transient arrest of psychogenic tremor induced by contralateral ballistic movements. *Neurosci Lett* 2004; 370: 135–9.
19. McAuley J, Rothwell J. Identification of psychogenic, dystonic, and other organic tremors by a coherence entrainment test. *Mov Disord* 2004; 19: 253–67.
20. McAuley JH, Rothwell JC, Marsden CD, Findley LJ. Electrophysiological aids in distinguishing organic from psychogenic tremor. *Neurology* 1998; 50: 1882–4.
21. O'Suilleabhain PE, Matsumoto JY. Time-frequency analysis of tremors. *Brain* 1998; 121: 2127–34.
22. Schwingenschuh P, Katschnig P, Seiler S, et al. Moving toward 'laboratory-supported' criteria for psychogenic tremor. *Mov Disord* 2011; 26: 2509–15.
23. Caviness JN, Brown P. Myoclonus: current concepts and recent advances. *Lancet Neurol* 2004; 3: 598–607.
24. Shibasaki H. Neurophysiological classification of myoclonus. *Neurophysiol Clin* 2006; 36(5–6): 267–9.
25. Cassim F, Houdayer E. Neurophysiology of myoclonus. *Neurophysiol Clin* 2006; 36: 281–91.
26. Brown P, Day BL, Rothwell JC, Thompson PD, Marsden CD. Intrahemispheric and interhemispheric spread of cerebral cortical myoclonic activity and its relevance to epilepsy. *Brain* 1991; 114: 2333–51.
27. van Rootselaar AF, Maurits NM, Koelman JH, et al. Coherence analysis differentiates between cortical myoclonic tremor and essential tremor. *Mov Disord* 2006; 21: 215–22.
28. Thompson PD, Day BL, Rothwell JC, Brown P, Britton TC, Marsden CD. The myoclonus in corticobasal degeneration. Evidence for two forms of cortical reflex myoclonus. *Brain* 1994; 117: 1197–207.
29. Kinugawa K, Vidailhet M, Clot F, Apartis E, Grabli D, Roze E. Myoclonus dystonia: an update. *Mov Disord* 2009; 24: 479–89.
30. Brown P, Rothwell JC, Thompson PD, Britton TC, Day BL, Marsden CD. The hyperekplexias and their relationship to the normal startle reflex. *Brain* 1991; 114: 1903–28.
31. Brown P, Rothwell JC, Thompson PD, Marsden CD. Propriospinal myoclonus: evidence for spinal 'pattern' generators in humans. *Mov Disord* 1994; 9: 571–6.
32. Brown P, Thompson PD, Rothwell JC, Day BL, Marsden CD. Axial myoclonus of propriospinal origin. *Brain* 1991; 114: 197–214.
33. Kang SY, Sohn YH. Electromyography patterns of propriospinal myoclonus can be mimicked voluntarily. *Mov Disord* 2006; 21: 1241–4.
34. Esposito M, Edwards MJ, Bhatia KP, Brown P, Cordivari C. Idiopathic spinal myoclonus: a clinical and neurophysiological assessment of a movement disorder of uncertain origin. *Mov Disord* 2009; 24: 2344–9.
35. Roze E, Bounolleau P, Ducreux D, et al. Propriospinal myoclonus revisited: clinical, neurophysiologic, and neuroradiologic findings. *Neurology* 2009; 72: 1301–9.
36. van der Salm SM, Koelman JH, Henneke S, van Rootselaar AF, Tijssen MA. Axial jerks: a clinical spectrum ranging from propriospinal to psychogenic myoclonus. *J Neurol* 2010; 257: 1349–55.
37. Hallett M. Neurophysiology of dystonia: the role of inhibition. *Neurobiol Dis* 2011; 42: 177–84.
38. Grosse P, Edwards M, Tijssen MA, et al. Patterns of EMG–EMG coherence in limb dystonia. *Mov Disord* 2004; 19: 758–69.
39. Aramideh M, Ongerboer de Visser BW. Brainstem reflexes: electrodiagnostic techniques, physiology, normative data, and clinical applications. *Muscle Nerve* 2002; 26: 14–30.
40. Hadavi S, Noyce AJ, Leslie RD, Giovannoni G. Stiff person syndrome. *Pract Neurol* 2011; 11: 272–82.
41. Lorish TR, Thorsteinsson G, Howard FM Jr. Stiff-man syndrome updated. *Mayo Clin Proc* 1989; 64: 629–36.
42. Armon C, McEvoy KM, Westmoreland BF, McManis PG. Clinical neurophysiologic studies in stiff-man syndrome: use of simultaneous video-electroencephalographic-surface electromyographic recording. *Mayo Clin Proc* 1990; 65: 960–7.

CHAPTER 6

Movement Disorders: Structural and Functional Imaging

David J. Brooks

Structural imaging in Parkinsonian disorders

Parkinsonism (a combination of bradykinesia, rigidity, tremor) can result when the nigrostriatal dopaminergic projections or the outflow tracts from the striatum and pallidum are interrupted. In Parkinson's disease (PD) the neurons of the substantia nigra compacta (SNc) are targeted by Lewy body inclusions. In multiple system atrophy (MSA), an atypical form of degenerative parkinsonism associated with autonomic failure and ataxia, argyrophilic inclusions are additionally found in the striatum, while progressive supranuclear palsy (PSP) is associated with neurofibrillary tangles in the SNc, basal ganglia, and oculomotor nuclei.

Magnetic resonance imaging

Conventional magnetic resonance imaging (MRI) weighted to detect T_1- and T_2-relaxation times of water protons can sensitively exclude structural causes of parkinsonism, such as basal ganglia tumors, toxic necrosis such as after methcathinone (ephedrone) ingestion, small vessel ischaemic disease, and calcification, and can detect cortical atrophy and hydrocephalus (1). Volumetric MRI has so far failed to demonstrate a reduction in SNc volume in PD, probably because of the difficulty in defining the borders of this structure owing to its high iron content. Diffusion tensor imaging (DTI) uses field gradient sequences which allow MRI to detect the directionality (anisotropy) and amplitude of water movement along fibre tracts. In a recent series, DTI was reported to detect reduced anisotropy of SNc water diffusion in 100% of *de novo* PD cases, changes being greatest in the lateral nigra where pathology is known to be most severe (see Fig. 6.1) (2).

While the striatum is pathologically spared in PD, the putamen in patients with MSA shows reduced signal on T_2-weighted MRI when cell loss and iron deposition are present (Fig. 6.2a). This is often accompanied by a lateral rim of increased signal due to gliosis. If degeneration of the pons has occurred, the lateral as well as longitudinal pontine fibres become evident as high signal manifesting as the 'hot cross bun' sign (Fig. 6.2b) (3,4). In advanced MSA cerebellar and pontine atrophy becomes visually obvious, and increased signal can be detected in the middle cerebellar peduncles. PSP patients do not show the putamen signal changes characteristic of MSA but develop third-ventricular widening and midbrain atrophy—the humming bird sign on sagittal views. Superior cerebellar peduncle atrophy differentiates PSP patients from other parkinsonian conditions.

Corticobasal degeneration (CBD) is a tauopathy characterized by swollen achromatic neurons in the inferior parietal and premotor cortex, striatum, SNc, and dentate nuclei. MRI characteristically shows asymmetric hemispheric atrophy in established cases. While the above MRI changes can all be found in atypical parkinsonian syndromes, they are not sensitive markers of these disorders, being generally only seen in more advanced cases. Diffusion-weighted MRI provides a more sensitive modality for discriminating atypical from typical parkinsonian disorders. Most cases of probable MSA and PSP diagnosed on clinical criteria both show increased putamen water diffusivity, whereas this is absent in typical PD (5). However, MSA and PSP can be discriminated from each other by the presence of altered signal in the middle cerebellar peduncles in the former and the superior cerebellar peduncles in the latter (6).

Transcranial sonography

Transcranial sonography (TCS) reveals structural midbrain and striatal changes in parkinsonian disorders as hyperechogenic signals (Fig. 6.3). Over 90% of cases with clinically established PD show increased midbrain echogenicity with TCS, but this can also be seen in 10% of elderly normals and 15% of essential tremor cases, so the specificity of this finding is suboptimal (7). The intensity of midbrain hyperechogenicity detected with TCS does not correlate with disability in PD and remains static over five years despite clinical progression (8). It has been suggested that its presence is a marker of susceptibility to PD rather than a state marker, and may be reflecting the presence of midbrain iron deposition rather than dopamine cell loss. In support of this, abnormal nigral hyperechogenicity can be detected in subjects at risk for PD, such as carriers of alpha synuclein, *LRRK2*, *parkin*, and

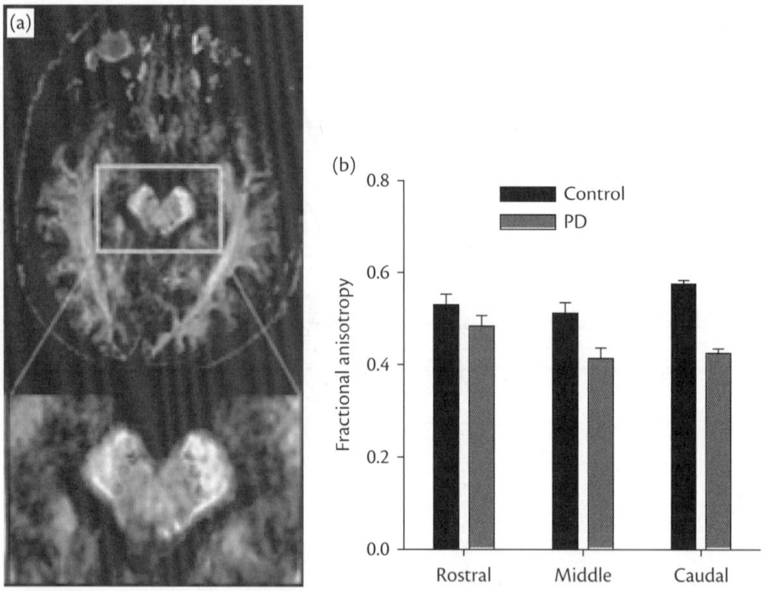

Fig. 6.1 Fractional anisotropy (FA) of the midbrain. Nigral FA is reduced in a rostral caudal gradient in PD. (Picture from Vaillancourt et al. 2009)

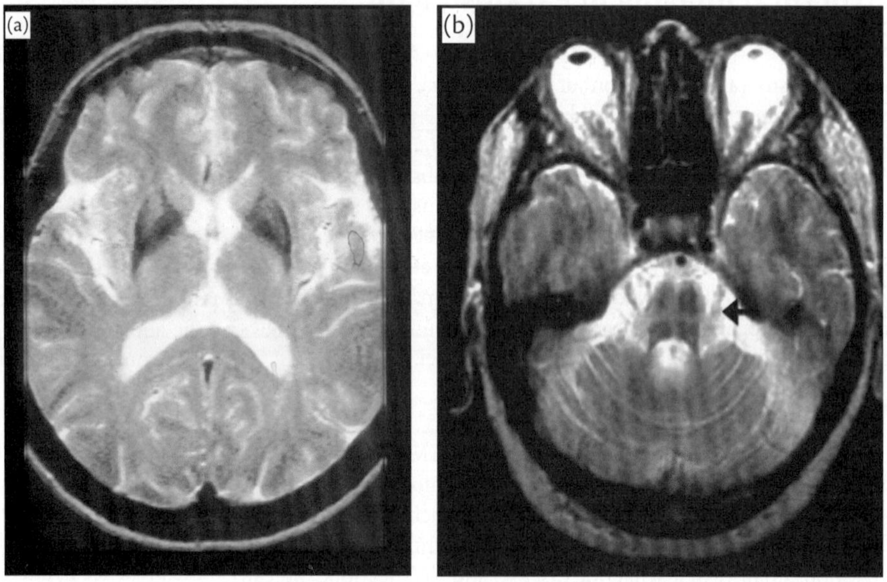

Fig. 6.2 T_2-weighted MRI showing (a) low lateral putamen signal at the same level as the pallidum in MSA and (b) the pontine 'hot cross bun sign' in MSA.

DJ1 gene mutations (9) or subjects with late-onset hyposmia (10). Nigral hyperechogenicity is not seen in atypical parkinsonian disorders despite the presence of dopamine cell loss at post-mortem. Hyperechogenic lentiform signals can be detected in MSA cases which, when combined with absent midbrain hyperechogenicity, can help discriminate them from PD (11).

Structural imaging in hyperkinetic disorders

Dystonia

The most common familial form of generalized dystonia is an autosomal dominant disorder associated with a *DYT1* gene mutation which has around 40% penetrance and is generally early onset starting in a lower limb. The *DYT1* mutation is a GAG deletion within the coding region of the gene on chromosome 9q34 which codes for torsin A, an ATP-binding protein of unknown function. A second generalized dystonia locus has been mapped to chromosome 8p (*DYT6*); affected individuals tend to have adult-onset dystonia presenting with craniocervical or focal symptoms.

Conventional MRI findings in idiopathic and genetic dystonias are normal, although acquired dystonia cases may show structural lesions in the lentiform nucleus or posterior thalamus (12). Wilson disease patients characteristically show cystic lesions in their basal ganglia. However, diffusion tensor imaging has revealed abnormal water diffusivity in the basal ganglia of cervical dystonia patients (13). As DTI detects the directionality of water flow, it allows bundles of nerve fibres to be delineated—a process known as tractography. In dystonia associated with *DYT1* gene mutations, abnormal

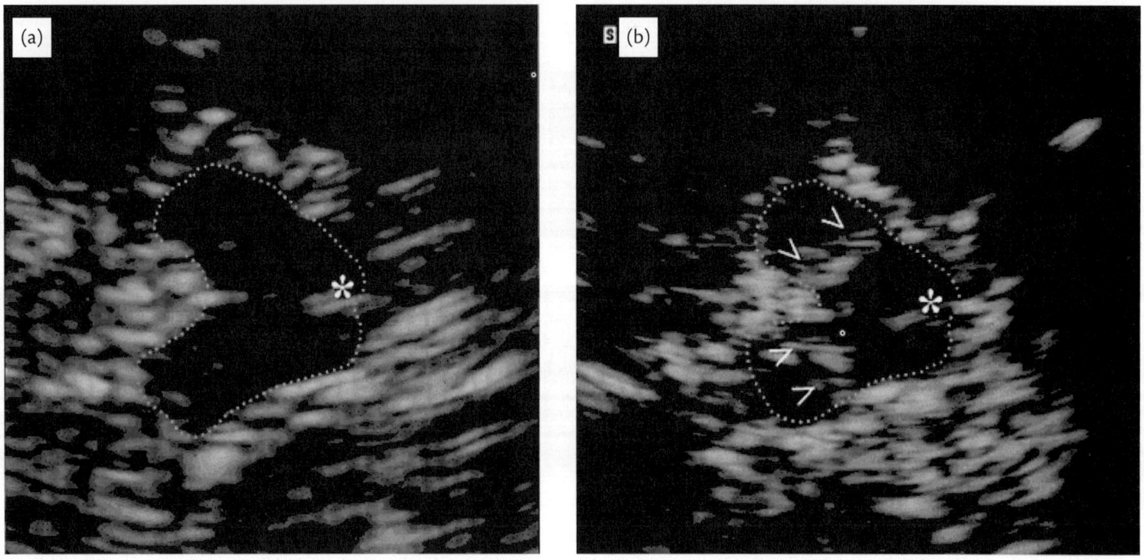

Fig. 6.3 Transcranial sonography showing hyperechogenicity from the lateral midbrain (substantia nigra) in PD. (Picture from Berg et al. 2001)

structural connectivity between the cerebellar nuclei and the thalamus and between frontal cortex and striatum can be demonstrated with tractography, although conventional MRI appears normal (14). These findings all support idiopathic and genetic dystonias arising from an abnormal structural development of subcortical–cortical connections.

Huntington's disease

Huntington's disease (HD) is an autosomal dominantly transmitted disorder associated with an excess of CAG triplet repeats (>38) in the *huntingtin* (*HTT*) gene on chromosome 4. The function of this gene is still uncertain, but the pathology of HD targets medium spiny projection neurons in the striatum, causing intranuclear and cytoplasmic inclusions to form. While altered striatal T_2-weighted MRI signal and caudate atrophy are only visually evident in cases of established HD (15), MR volumetry reveals subclinical caudate and putamen atrophy in pre-manifest gene carriers close to predicted symptom onset (16). Striatal atrophy becomes more marked as they become symptomatic and develop motor signs. Aylward and colleagues (17) were able to predict time of conversion from preclinical to clinical HD by measuring caudate volumes. These workers suggested that caudate volume may be a useful outcome measure for assessing treatment effectiveness in both pre-manifest and symptomatic subjects.

Functional imaging

The changes in regional cerebral function that characterize different movement disorders can be examined in two main ways: first, focal changes in resting levels of regional cerebral metabolism, blood flow, and neuroreceptor availability can be measured. Secondly, abnormal patterns of regional brain activation, evidenced as changes in blood flow or levels of neurotransmitter release, can be detected when patients with movement disorders perform motor and cognitive tasks or are exposed to drug challenges.

Parkinson's disease

The presynaptic dopaminergic system

Dopamine terminal function in PD can be examined *in vivo* in three main ways:

- terminal dopa decarboxylase activity can be measured with ^{18}F-dopa positron emission tomography (PET);
- the availability of dopamine transporters (DATs) can be assessed with ^{11}C-methylphenidate (MP) PET or tropane-based PET and single photon emission computed tomography (SPECT) markers such as ^{11}C-2-β-carbomethoxy-3-β-(4-fluorophenyl)tropane (^{11}C-CFT), ^{18}F-FP-CIT, ^{123}I-altropane, ^{123}I-β-CIT, and ^{123}I-FP-CIT;
- vesicle monoamine transporter density (VMAT2) can be studied with ^{11}C- or ^{18}F-dihydrotetrabenazine (DTBZ) PET (Fig. 6.4) (18).

In PD patients with early stage 1 disease affecting only one side bilaterally reduced putamen tracer uptake can be seen, activity being most depressed in the putamen contralateral to the clinically affected limbs. Head-of-caudate dopamine terminal function remains relatively preserved until later in the condition. Onset of symptoms has been estimated to occur after a 30–50% loss of putamen dopamine terminal function (19). Unlike nigral hyperechogenicity, reductions in putamen dopamine terminal function correlate well with severity of limb rigidity and bradykinesia although, interestingly, they correlate poorly with severity of tremor (20).

PET and SPECT can differentiate clinically probable PD from normal subjects or benign essential and dystonic tremor patients with a sensitivity and specificity of around 90% (21). An abnormal PET or SPECT scan provides support for a diagnosis of a dopamine-deficient parkinsonian syndrome and a rationale for treating with dopaminergic agents, while a normal scan effectively excludes this diagnosis.

Several studies have examined the utility of using DAT imaging to determine whether 'grey' parkinsonian cases are associated with

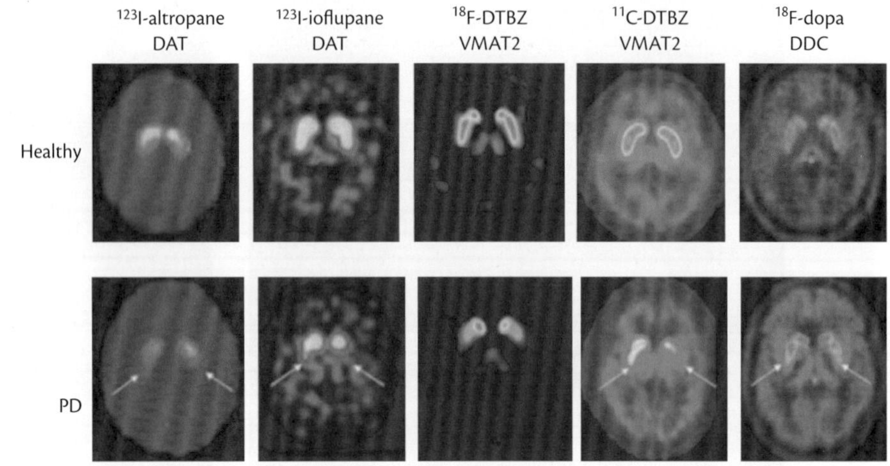

Fig. 6.4 SPECT and PET images of dopamine terminal function in normal subjects and early PD patients.

striatal dopamine deficiency. In the Query PD study the standard of truth (SOT) was the clinical impression of two movement disorder experts after 6 months of clinical follow-up (22). While referring clinicians showed 92% sensitivity for diagnosing dopamine-deficient parkinsonism, their baseline clinical specificity was poor (30%) compared with the SOT, while baseline imaging specificity with ^{123}I-β-CIT SPECT was 100%. These findings suggest that clinicians tend to overdiagnose PD when uncertain. The Clinically Uncertain Parkinsonian Syndromes (CUPS) trial was designed to establish whether knowledge of baseline striatal DAT binding influenced the diagnosis and subsequent management of patients with uncertain PD (23). When FP-CIT SPECT findings were revealed to clinicians, the diagnosis of dopamine-deficient parkinsonian syndrome was revised in 52% of the 118 cases and the management strategy changed in 72% of cases. A two-year follow-up found that 90% of subjects still retained the diagnosis assigned after baseline FP-CIT SPECT findings were released (24). The CUPS study supports the view that including a measure of striatal dopaminergic function in the work-up of uncertain parkinsonian cases influences their subsequent management.

There was no non-imaged control group as a comparator in the CUPS study, so the prevalence of change in management plan without SPECT was not determined. The PDT409 study, which had a similar design but included a control arm, has recently reported (25). There were around 130 possible PD cases in each arm, and patients were assessed at baseline and assigned a diagnosis and management plan. Twelve weeks after FP-CIT SPECT or no imaging they were re-assessed and their diagnosis and management reviewed. Forty-four per cent who had SPECT versus 12% who were not imaged had a change in their diagnosis after 12 weeks of follow-up, while 49% in the imaging arm versus 31% in the non-imaged arm had a change of management plan.

A common cause of confusion with PD is adult-onset dystonic tremor which can present as an asymmetric resting arm tremor with impaired arm swing and cogwheel rigidity, but without evidence of true akinesia (26). In these cases functional imaging should be considered to avoid inappropriate medication with dopaminergic agents. Other causes of confusion include drug-associated and psychogenic parkinsonism. Marshall and co-workers (27) presented eleven patients who initially fulfilled diagnostic criteria for PD and were treated with dopaminergic agents, but in whom emerging diagnostic doubts led to DAT imaging with FP-CIT SPECT. This was negative, and subsequent withdrawal of antiparkinsonian therapy was achieved without clinical deterioration, suggesting that dopaminergic imaging can be valuable where inappropriate use of antiparkinsonian medication is suspected.

Postsynaptic dopaminergic receptor binding

The striatum contains primarily dopamine D1 and D2 receptor subtypes which both play a role in modulating locomotor function. ^{123}I-iodobenzamine (^{123}I-IBZM) SPECT studies have reported normal levels of striatal D2 binding in untreated PD (Fig. 6.5) while ^{11}C-raclopride PET detects a 10–20% increase in putamen D2 availability (18). As ^{11}C-raclopride competes with endogenous dopamine for D2 binding, this raised receptor availability probably reflects dopamine depletion rather than an adaptive rise in receptor numbers. In chronically levodopa-exposed PD cases levels of putamen D2 binding normalize as synaptic levels of dopamine are restored.

Measuring striatal dopamine

As ^{11}C-raclopride competes with synaptic dopamine to bind to D2 receptors its uptake is sensitive to changes in synaptic levels of striatal dopamine. PET can be used to detect changes in dopamine induced by drugs or behaviour. Microdialysis studies in animals suggest that a 10% reduction in striatal ^{11}C-raclopride binding reflects a fivefold increase in synaptic dopamine levels (28). When

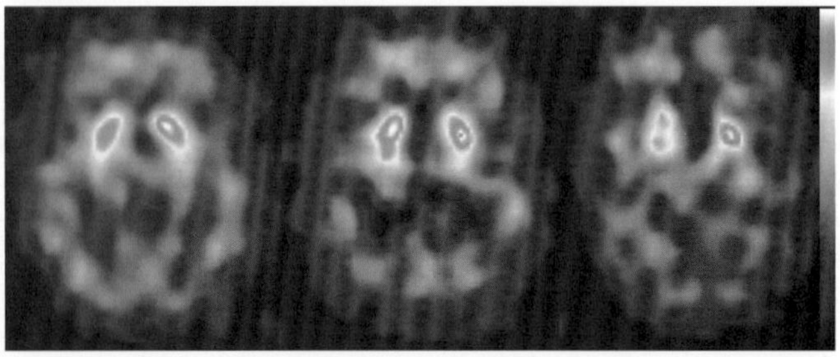

Fig. 6.5 ^{123}I-IBZM SPECT images of dopamine D2 receptor binding in a normal subject and in PD and MSA cases. Striatal D2 binding is reduced in the MSA case. (Picture courtesy of Dr G. Wenning)

PD patients take oral levodopa, transient rises in synaptic dopamine result. ^{11}C-raclopride PET has shown that improvement in disability after levodopa correlates with the estimated rises in putamen dopamine (29). Some PD patients compulsively take far larger doses of levodopa than are clinically required—this has been termed the dopamine dysregulation syndrome (DDS). Compared with PD patients who are not compulsively taking excess medication, DDS patients show enhanced levodopa-induced dopamine release in the ventral striatum (30). PD cases who develop impulse control disorders, such as compulsive gambling, when administered dopamine agonist therapy also release higher levels of ventral striatal dopamine when exposed to the relevant stimuli such as games of chance (31).

Detection of preclinical PD

It has been estimated from post-mortem studies that, for every patient who develops clinical PD, there are ten subclinical cases with incidental brainstem Lewy body disease in the community. The greatest risk factors for PD are age and a family history. Late-onset idiopathic hyposmia and REM sleep behaviour disorder (RBD) are also associated with later onset of Lewy body disorders. ^{18}F-dopa PET has detected subclinically reduced dopaminergic function in asymptomatic identical twins and relatives of idiopathic PD cases, and in *parkin* and *LRRK2* gene carriers (18). Reduced striatal DAT binding can be detected in around 10% of late-onset hyposmic subjects (32) and a majority of patients with idiopathic RBD (33).

Levodopa-induced dyskinesias

PD patients with early disease and sustained therapeutic responses to levodopa show a reduction in striatal ^{11}C-raclopride binding after oral levodopa that is maintained for several hours, compatible with a sustained increase in synaptic dopamine levels (34). In contrast, fluctuators show larger, but short-lived, falls in ^{11}C-raclopride uptake, implying that pulsatile swings in dopamine levels are occurring. As loss of dopamine terminals in PD becomes severe, the striatum fails to store dopamine and buffer synaptic levels when exogenous levodopa is taken. This is magnified by the relatively greater loss of dopamine transporters from terminals, the route for dopamine reuptake, compared with dopa decarboxylase activity (35). Pulsatile swings in synaptic dopamine levels will promote internalization of dopamine receptors which are then unavailable and so fluctuating treatment responses result. The severity of peak dose dyskinesias following oral levodopa administration to PD patients has been shown to correlate with the rises of synaptic dopamine induced, as reflected by levels of reductions in putaminal ^{11}C-raclopride binding (29).

The striatum contains high densities of adenosine A2A sites which are found on striatal neurons of the indirect pathway and regulate its activity. Uptake of ^{11}C-SCH442416, a marker of A2A binding, is normal in the striatum of non-dyskinetic subjects but is raised in dyskinetic cases (36). *N*-methyl-D-aspartate (NMDA) receptors are a subclass of glutamate receptors containing a voltage-gated ion channel which is opened during learning and memory tasks. ^{11}C-CNS5161 PET is a marker of NMDA ion channel activity, and recently this has been shown to be increased at the time PD patients are experiencing levodopa-induced dyskinesias (37). This could help to explain the beneficial mode of action of amantadine, an NMDA channel blocker.

Modifying progression of PD

As functional imaging can objectively follow loss of dopamine terminal function in PD, it provides a potential means of monitoring the efficacy of putative neuroprotective agents. In the REAL PET (^{18}F-dopa) and CALM PD (β-CIT SPECT) trials (38, 39), early PD patients were shown to lose dopamine terminal function a third more slowly if treated with a dopamine agonist as opposed to levodopa. The incidence of complications was also significantly reduced in the agonist cohorts, but improvements in disability were greater in the levodopa cohorts. The interpretation of these data has remained controversial because of the discordance between imaging and clinical outcomes. It is possible that levodopa acts directly to downregulate β-CIT and ^{18}F-dopa uptake, thus confounding the utility of these imaging biomarkers for assessing neuroprotective efficacy in the presence of dopaminergic agents. PET and SPECT have also been used as imaging biomarkers to examine the possible neuroprotective efficacy of riluzole and paliroden (^{18}F-dopa PET), TCH346, and CEP1347 (β-CIT SPECT)—these trials were all negative and CEP1347 treatment was shown to depress striatal β-CIT uptake (40).

Two major double-blind controlled trials on the efficacy of implantation of human fetal cells in PD have been sponsored by the National Institutes of Health (NIH) in the USA (41, 42). Despite both histological and ^{18}F-dopa PET evidence of graft function, neither of these controlled trials demonstrated clinical efficacy according to their primary endpoints. However, there were indications that younger, more severely affected patients benefited from intrastriatal implantation of human fetal dopamine cells. An issue raised by both these trials was the occurrence of problematic 'off' period dyskinesias in many implanted patients.

Glial-derived neurotrophic factor (GDNF) is a potent neurotrophic factor known to prevent the degeneration of dopamine neurons in rodent and primate models of PD where nigral degeneration is toxically induced with 6-hydroxydopamine (6-OHDA) or 1-methyl-4-phenyl-1,2,3,6-tetrahydropyridine MPTP. A small open trial showed the efficacy of intra-putaminal infusions of GDNF in five PD patients along with 16–26% increases in ^{18}F-dopa storage at the site of the catheter tip (43). However, a randomized placebo-controlled study in 36 cases failed to show a clinical benefit of this procedure although, again, consistent local increases in ^{18}F-dopa storage were seen (44). These restorative trials suggest that increasing dopamine storage capacity by implanting fetal cells, or via inducing terminal sprouting with trophic factors, is not enough to guarantee a therapeutic response unless appropriate connectivity is also established.

Non-motor complications of PD

A majority of PD patients experience depressive symptoms. It has been suggested that serotonergic loss might contribute to depression in PD; to date, however, the results from neuroimaging studies have not supported this view. PD patients with and without depression have shown similar median raphe uptake of ^{11}C-WAY 100635 binding, a marker of 5HT1A sites on serotonergic cell bodies (45). Midbrain uptake of ^{123}I-β-CIT reflects serotonin transporter availability and does not differ between PD patients with and without depression or correlate with Hamilton Depression Rating Scale scores (46). The PET tracer ^{11}C-RT132 binds with similar affinity to dopamine and noradrenaline transporters.

Remy and co-workers used ^{11}C-RT132 PET to assess PD patients with and without depression (47). The depressed PD patients had lower ^{11}C-RT132 binding in the locus coeruleus and areas of the limbic system than non-depressed PD patients. This finding suggests that loss of limbic dopamine and noradrenaline rather than serotonin may be most relevant to the pathogenesis of depression in patients with PD.

Eighty per cent of PD patients will develop dementia if they survive for 20 years with their illness. This can reflect both the presence of cortical Lewy body disease and the degeneration of dopaminergic and cholinergic projections to cortical areas. Cholinergic terminal function can be assessed with ^{11}C-NMP4A PET, a marker of acetylcholine sterase activity. Non-demented PD patients show focally reduced cholinergic function in parietal and occipital cortex. When dementia is present, PD cases manifest a global and more severe reduction of cortical ^{11}C-NMP4A binding (48). Cortical acetylcholinesterase activity correlates with MMSE scores and performance on executive tests such as card sorting and trail making in PD (49). These results suggest that progressive cognitive impairment in PD is in part a consequence of cholinergic deficit.

Levels of ^{18}F-2-fluoro-2-deoxyglucose (^{18}FDG) uptake reflect neuronal synaptic activity. In non-demented PD patients cortical FDG uptake is generally within normal limits, but covariance analysis reveals an abnormal profile of relatively increased lentiform nucleus and reduced frontoparietal metabolism (50). This has been labelled the PD-related profile (PDRP), and its degree of expression correlates with degree of motor disability. The PDRP normalizes after successful treatment with dopaminergic drugs or deep brain stimulation. Frankly demented PD patients show an Alzheimer's disease (AD) pattern of impaired brain glucose utilization, with the posterior cingulate, parietal, and temporal association areas being most affected (51). It remains unclear whether the pattern of glucose hypometabolism in demented PD patients reflects coincidental AD, cortical Lewy body disease, loss of cholinergic projections, or some other degenerative process. In cases proved to have cortical Lewy body disease there tends to be greater occipital cortex hypometabolism than in Alzheimer patients (52). The PET ligand ^{11}C-PIB, a neutral thioflavin-T analogue developed to image β-amyloid plaques in AD, has recently been employed to assess PD patients with dementia. Only a minority of these cases showed increased ^{11}C-PIB uptake, suggesting that amyloid pathology is not a major contributor to their cognitive problems (53).

Cardiac sympathetic function

^{123}I meta-iodobenzyl guanidine (^{123}I-MIBG) SPECT is a marker of adrenergic terminal function and can be used to study functional integrity of cardiac sympathetic innervation in PD. The mediastinal ^{123}I-MIBG signal is reduced in a majority of PD cases, even when no clinical evidence of autonomic failure is present. However, in stage 1 PD 50% of cases still show normal cardiac MIBG uptake, so this approach is not as sensitive a marker for PD as DAT imaging (54).

Atypical parkinsonian syndromes

Multiple system atrophy (MSA)

^{18}FDG PET studies in MSA show reduced levels of striatal, brainstem, and cerebellar glucose metabolism, in contrast to PD where these are preserved (55,56). The presynaptic dopaminergic system is impaired in a similar way to PD so that, while ^{18}F-dopa PET, VMAT2, and DAT imaging can separate PD and MSA from normal, they cannot reliably discriminate these two parkinsonian conditions (18).

Unlike PD, MSA is associated with loss of putamen dopamine D2 binding (Fig. 6.5), but this is mild and does not provide a sensitive discriminator of MSA from PD. In one series ^{123}I-IBZM SPECT detected reduced striatal D2 binding in only two-thirds of *de novo* parkinsonian patients who had a negative apomorphine response and were thought to have possible MSA (57).

^{123}I-MIBG SPECT, a marker of adrenergic terminal function, is normal in MSA as the autonomic dysfunction results from loss of pre- rather than post-synaptic innervation (58). This differentiates MSA from PD, where the sympathetic loss is postsynaptic, and provides another means of discriminating these two conditions (Fig. 6.6).

Progressive supranuclear palsy (PSP)

PSP is characterized pathologically by neuronal loss in the substantia nigra, pallidum, superior colliculi, brainstem nuclei, and peri-aqueductal grey matter, with intra-neuronal neurofibrillary tangle formation. FDG PET reveals depressed frontal cortex, basal ganglia, cerebellar, and thalamic glucose metabolism in PSP which correlates with disease duration and performance on psychometric tests of frontal function (18, 59). The presence of reduced striatal metabolism sensitively discriminates 90% of PSP cases from PD. However, as striatal hypometabolism is also a feature of MSA, FDG PET cannot reliably discriminate these atypical conditions.

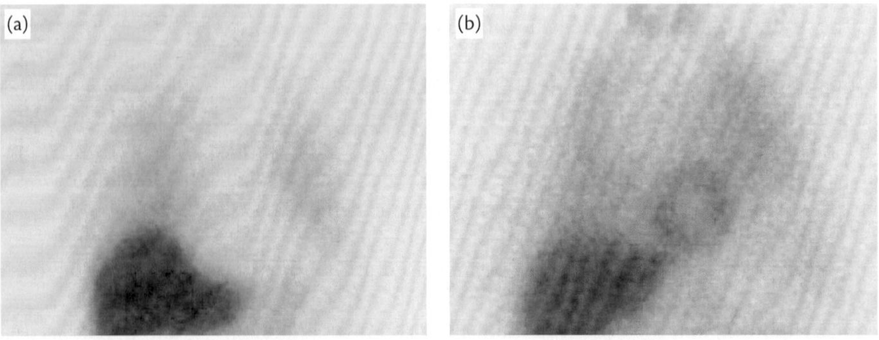

Fig. 6.6 ^{123}I-MIBG images of cardiac sympathetic function in (a) PD and (b) MSA. (Picture from S. Braune et al. *Neurology* 1999; 53: 1020–5)

The pathology of PSP uniformly targets nigrostriatal dopaminergic projections and so, in contrast to PD and MSA, putamen and caudate ^{18}F-dopa uptake and DAT binding are equivalently reduced, resulting in a uniform loss of striatal signal (60). Striatal D2 binding is reduced in a majority of PSP cases and this can be detected with ^{11}C-raclopride PET or IBZM SPECT (18).

Involuntary movement disorders

Huntington's disease (HD) and other choreas

HD is an autosomal dominantly transmitted disorder associated with an excess of CAG triplet repeats (>38) in the *huntingtin* (*HTT*) gene on chromosome 4. Other degenerative disorders associated with chorea include neuroacanthocytosis (NA), dentatorubral-pallidoluysian atrophy (DRPLA), and benign familial chorea (BFC). The inflammatory disorders systemic lupus erythematosus (SLE) and Sydenham's chorea are also associated with chorea, as is chronic neuroleptic exposure.

Clinically affected HD patients show severely reduced striatal levels of resting glucose metabolism as do NA, DRPLA, and some BFC patients (61–63). In contrast, striatal glucose metabolism is normal in inflammatory or tardive choreas. The medium spiny striatal neurons that degenerate in HD express D2 receptors. ^{11}C-raclopride PET studies show that striatal D2 binding is reduced by at least 30% when HD patients manifest symptoms (64, 65). Reduced striatal ^{11}C-raclopride binding is also seen in NA but, in contrast, normal striatal D2 binding is found in SLE and tardive choreas (66).

Around 50% of pre-manifesting adult HD gene carriers show reduced levels of striatal glucose metabolism and D2 binding, indicating that their disease is already active (67). The rate of progression of HD can be tracked using PET as a biomarker. Caudate glucose metabolism has been reported to decline by 3% per annum, while striatal D2 binding declines by 3–6%. These findings suggest that functional imaging could provide an objective means of following HD progression in the event of effective neuroprotective or restorative interventions being found.

Microglia constitute 10–20% of white cells in the brain and form its natural defence mechanism. They are normally in a resting state, but local injury causes them to activate and swell, expressing HLA antigens on the cell surface and releasing cytokines such as IL1 and TNFα. The mitochondria of activated microglia express the translocator protein (TSPO) which is a steroid transporter although it was previously known as the peripheral benzodiazepine site. ^{11}C-PK11195 is an isoquinoline which binds selectively to the TSPO and so provides an *in vivo* PET marker of microglial activation.

Post-mortem studies of HD brains have shown a significant accumulation of activated microglia in the basal ganglia and the frontal cortex. HD patients show significant increases in striatal ^{11}C-PK11195 binding (Fig. 6.7b) which correlate with clinical disease severity measured with the Unified Huntington's Disease Rating Scale (UHDRS), with striatal reductions in ^{11}C-raclopride binding, and with the size of the patients' CAG triplet expansion (68). Increased striatal and cortical ^{11}C-PK11195 binding can also be seen in many adult pre-manifest HD gene carriers, suggesting that microglial activation is an early event. Taken together, the findings from post-mortem and neuroimaging studies support the view that activated microglia contribute to the ongoing neuronal degeneration in HD.

Dystonia

FDG PET shows normal levels of resting glucose metabolism in *DYT1* carriers but covariance analysis reveals an abnormal resting metabolic profile where levels of lentiform nucleus glucose metabolism are relatively reduced and frontal metabolism is raised (14). This pattern is seen whether *DYT1* gene carriers are clinically affected or asymptomatic, and is a pattern that is almost the reverse of that reported for Parkinson's disease. A PET study of *DYT1* dystonic patients performed while they slept also showed this abnormal profile of resting glucose metabolism, confirming that it is not movement-related. A similar profile has been reported in *DYT6* dystonia and essential blepharospasm. These findings suggest that dysfunction of a common network involving the basal ganglia and frontal cortex may underlie all genetic dystonias.

^{18}F-dopa PET and ^{123}I-β-CIT SPECT studies have shown normal dopamine storage in the majority of idiopathic torsion

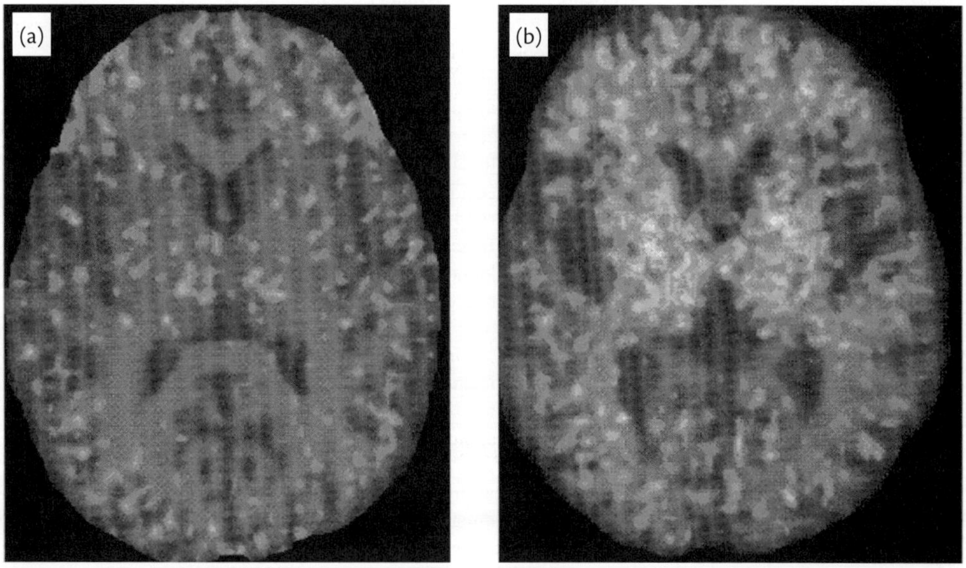

Fig. 6.7 ^{11}C-PK11195 PET scans of (a) a healthy subject and (b) HD gene carrier. Mild microglial activation is seen in the thalamus of the healthy control whereas significantly raised activation is evident in the frontal cortex and striata of the HD patient. (Picture courtesy of Dr Nicola Pavese)

dystonia (ITD) cases. In contrast, PET and SPECT have shown that striatal D2 binding is reduced (69, 70). This could conceivably lead to decreased activity of the indirect striatopallidal pathway which normally acts to inhibit unwanted movement or actions. Recently it has been reported uptake of ^{11}C-flumazenil, a marker of benzodiazepine receptor binding on the $GABA_A$ complex, is reduced in motor and pre-motor areas in a group of *DYT1* cases and cases with sporadic dystonia (71). Such a deficit in GABAergic function could result in a failure of normal cortical inhibitory circuits, also allowing involuntary muscle contractions to occur.

Dopa-responsive dystonia (DRD) and dystonia–parkinsonism

Dominantly inherited DRD is related to a mutation in the *DYT5* gene coding for GTP cyclohydrolase 1. This enzyme constitutes part of the tetrahydrobiopterin synthetic pathway, the co-factor for tyrosine hydroxylase. Patients are unable to manufacture levodopa, and hence dopamine, from endogenous tyrosine but can still convert exogenous levodopa to dopamine. DRD cases generally present in childhood with diurnally fluctuating dystonia and later develop background parkinsonism. Occasionally, the condition presents as pure parkinsonism in adulthood. ^{18}F-dopa PET and ^{123}I-β-CIT SPECT findings are normal in most DRD patients (72), thus distinguishing this condition from early-onset dystonia–parkinsonism where severely reduced putamen ^{18}F-dopa and ^{123}I-β-CIT uptake is found (73).

Conclusions

Structural imaging

- Structural changes in PD nigra can be detected with both transcranial sonography and diffusion tensor MRI.
- Midbrain hyperechogenicity reveals a susceptibility to PD rather than correlating with severity of disease.
- Atypical parkinsonian syndromes can be sensitively discriminated from typical PD by abnormal putamen signals detectable with both diffusion-weighted MRI and transcranial sonography.
- DTI can detect changes in structural connectivity in genetic dystonias, revealing abnormal cerebellar–thalamic and frontostriatal tractography.

Functional imaging

- PET and SPECT provide a sensitive and objective means of detecting dopamine terminal dysfunction in PD where clinical doubt exists, thus providing a rationale for a trial of dopaminergic medication.
- FDG PET can demonstrate striatal hypometabolism in suspected atypical PD variants, so discriminating them from PD.
- PET and SPECT can detect subclinical dopamine terminal dysfunction in subjects at risk for PD if present and detect reduced striatal D2 binding in pre-manifest HD gene carriers. This could help identify cases for neuroprotective approaches if a successful therapy is identified.
- Imaging potentially enables PD and HD progression to be objectively monitored and the efficacy of putative neuroprotective and restorative approaches to be evaluated. However, direct effects of any intervention on the imaging modality can be a confound.
- FDG PET reveals a common abnormal profile of resting glucose metabolism in the genetic dystonias.
- PET can detect striatal inflammation (microglial activation) in pre-manifesting HD gene carriers and this may act to drive neuronal loss.

References

1. Brooks DJ. Technology insight: imaging neurodegeneration in Parkinson's disease. *Nature Clin Pract Neurol* 2008; 4: 267–77.
2. Vaillancourt DE, Spraker MB, Prodoehl J, et al. High-resolution diffusion tensor imaging in the substantia nigra of de novo Parkinson disease. *Neurology* 2009; 72: 1378–84.
3. Schrag A, Good CD, Miszkiel K, et al. Differentiation of atypical parkinsonian syndromes with routine MRI. *Neurology* 2000; 54: 697–702.
4. Brooks DJ, Seppi K, for the Neuroimaging Working Group on MSA. Proposed neuroimaging criteria for the diagnosis of multiple system atrophy. *Mov Disord* 2009; 24: 949–64.
5. Seppi K, Schocke MF, Esterhammer R, et al. Diffusion-weighted imaging discriminates progressive supranuclear palsy from PD, but not from the parkinson variant of multiple system atrophy. *Neurology* 2003; 60: 922–7.
6. Nicoletti G, Lodi R, Condino F, et al. Apparent diffusion coefficient measurements of the middle cerebellar peduncle differentiate the Parkinson variant of MSA from Parkinson's disease and progressive supranuclear palsy. *Brain* 2006; 129: 2679–87.
7. Berg D, Siefker C, Becker G. Echogenicity of the substantia nigra in Parkinson's disease and its relation to clinical findings. *J Neurol* 2001; 248: 684–9.
8. Berg D, Merz B, Reiners K, Naumann M, Becker G. Five-year follow-up study of hyperechogenicity of the substantia nigra in Parkinson's disease. *Mov Disord* 2005; 20: 383–5.
9. Walter U, Klein C, Hilker R, et al. Brain parenchyma sonography detects preclinical parkinsonism. *Mov Disord* 2004; 19: 1445–9.
10. Sommer U, Hummel T, Cormann K, et al. Detection of presymptomatic Parkinson's disease: combining smell tests, transcranial sonography, and SPECT. *Mov Disord* 2004; 19: 1196–202.
11. Behnke S, Berg D, Naumann M, Becker G. Differentiation of Parkinson's disease and atypical parkinsonian syndromes by transcranial ultrasound. *J Neurol Neurosurg Psychiatry* 2005; 76: 423–5.
12. Bhatia KP, Marsden CD. The behavioural and motor consequences of focal lesions of the basal ganglia in man. *Brain* 1994; 117: 859–76.
13. Colosimo C, Pantano P, Calistri V, et al. Diffusion tensor imaging in primary cervical dystonia. *J Neurol Neurosurg Psychiatry* 2005; 76: 1591–3.
14. Carbon M, Eidelberg D. Abnormal structure–function relationships in hereditary dystonia. *Neuroscience* 2009; 1641: 220–9.
15. Savoiardo M, Strada L, Oliva D, Girotti F, Dincerti L. Abnormal MRI signal in the rigid form of Huntington's disease. *J Neurol Neurosurg Psychiatry* 1991; 54: 888–91.
16. Aylward EH, Codori AM, Barta PE, et al. Basal ganglia volume and proximity to onset in presymptomatic Huntington disease. *Arch Neurol* 1996; 53: 1293–6.
17. Aylward EH, Codori AM, Rosenblatt A, et al. Rate of caudate atrophy in presymptomatic and symptomatic stages of Huntington's disease. *Mov Disord* 2000; 15: 552–60.
18. Brooks DJ. Imaging approaches to Parkinson disease. *J Nucl Med* 2010; 51: 596–609.
19. Morrish PK, Rakshi JS, Sawle GV, Brooks DJ. Measuring the rate of progression and estimating the preclinical period of Parkinson's disease with [^{18}F]dopa PET. *J Neurol Neurosurg Psychiatry* 1998; 64: 314–19.

20. Vingerhoets FJG, Schulzer M, Calne DB, Snow BJ. Which clinical sign of Parkinson's disease best reflects the nigrostriatal lesion? *Ann Neurol* 1997; 41: 58–64.
21. Benamer TS, Patterson J, Grosset DG, et al. Accurate differentiation of parkinsonism and essential tremor using visual assessment of [123I]-FP-CIT imaging: the [123I]-FP-CIT Study Group. *Mov Disord* 2000; 15: 503–10.
22. Jennings DL, Seibyl JP, Oakes D, et al. ^{123}I beta-CIT and single-photon emission computed tomographic imaging vs clinical evaluation in Parkinsonian syndrome: unmasking an early diagnosis. *Arch Neurol* 2004; 61: 1224–9.
23. Catafau AM, Tolosa E. Impact of dopamine transporter SPECT using ^{123}I-ioflupane on diagnosis and management of patients with clinically uncertain parkinsonian syndromes. *Mov Disord* 2004; 19: 1175–82.
24. Tolosa E, Borght TV, Moreno E. Accuracy of DaTSCAN 123I-ioflupane SPECT in diagnosis of patients with clinically uncertain parkinsonism. 2: Year follow-up of an open-label study. *Mov Disord* 2007; 22: 2346–51.
25. Kupsch A, Bajaj N, Weiland F, et al. Changes in clinical management following DaTSCAN™ ioflupane imaging in patients with a clinically uncertain parkinsonian syndrome: interim report. *Neurology* 2011; 76: A276.
26. Schwingenschuh P, Ruge D, Edwards MJ, et al. Distinguishing SWEDDs patients with asymmetric resting tremor from Parkinson's disease: a clinical and electrophysiological study. *Mov Disord* 2010; 25: 560–9.
27. Marshall VL, Patterson J, Hadley DM, Grosset KA, Grosset DG. Successful antiparkinsonian medication withdrawal in patients with parkinsonism and normal FP-CIT SPECT. *Mov Disord* 2006; 21: 2247–50.
28. Laruelle M. Imaging synaptic neurotransmission with *in vivo* binding competition techniques: a critical review. *J Cereb Blood Flow Metab* 2000; 20: 423–51.
29. Pavese N, Evans AH, Tai YF, et al. Clinical correlates of levodopa-induced dopamine release in Parkinson disease: a PET study. *Neurology* 2006; 67: 1612–17.
30. Evans AH, Pavese N, Lawrence AD, et al. Compulsive drug use linked to sensitized ventral striatal dopamine transmission. *Ann Neurol* 2006; 59: 852–8.
31. Steeves TD, Miyasaki J, Zurowski M, et al. Increased striatal dopamine release in Parkinsonian patients with pathological gambling: a [^{11}C] raclopride PET study. *Brain* 2009; 132: 1376–85.
32. Ponsen MM, Stoffers D, Booij J, et al. Idiopathic hyposmia as a preclinical sign of Parkinson's disease. *Ann Neurol* 2004; 56: 173–81.
33. Eisensehr I, Linke R, Noachtar S, et al. Reduced striatal dopamine transporters in idiopathic rapid eye movement sleep behaviour disorder—comparison with Parkinson's disease and controls. *Brain* 2000; 123: 1155–60.
34. de la Fuente-Fernandez R, Lu JQ, Sossi V, et al. Biochemical variations in the synaptic level of dopamine precede motor fluctuations in Parkinson's disease: PET evidence of increased dopamine turnover. *Ann Neurol* 2001; 49: 298–303.
35. Troiano AR, de la Fuente-Fernandez R, Sossi V, et al. PET demonstrates reduced dopamine transporter expression in PD with dyskinesias. *Neurology* 2009; 72: 1211–16.
36. Ramlackhansingh AF, Bose SK, Ahmed I, et al. Adenosine A2A receptor availability in Parkinson's disease patients with and without levodopa induced dyskinesias studied with C-11 SCH442416 PET. *Neurology* 2010; 74: A588
37. Ahmed I, Bose SK, Pavese N, et al. Glutamate NMDA receptor dysregulation in Parkinson's disease with dyskinesias. *Brain* 2011; 134: 979–86.
38. Whone AL, Watts RL, Stoessl J, et al. Slower progression of PD with ropinirole versus L-dopa: the REAL-PET study. *Ann Neurol* 2003; 54: 93–101.
39. Parkinson Study Group. Dopamine transporter brain imaging to assess the effects of pramipexole vs levodopa on Parkinson disease progression. *JAMA* 2002; 287: 1653–61.
40. Parkinson Study Group. Mixed lineage kinase inhibitor CEP-1347 fails to delay disability in early Parkinson disease. *Neurology* 2007; 69: 1480–90.
41. Freed CR, Greene PE, Breeze RE, et al. Transplantation of embryonic dopamine neurons for severe Parkinson's disease. *N Engl J Med* 2001; 344: 710–19.
42. Olanow CW, Goetz CG, Kordower JH, et al. A double-blind controlled trial of bilateral fetal nigral transplantation in Parkinson's disease. *Ann Neurol* 2003; 54: 403–14.
43. Gill SS, Patel NK, Hotton GR, et al. Direct brain infusion of glial cell line-derived neurotrophic factor in Parkinson disease. *Nat Med* 2003; 9: 589–95.
44. Lang AE, Gill S, Patel NK, et al. Randomized controlled trial of intraputamenal glial cell line-derived neurotrophic factor infusion in Parkinson disease. *Ann Neurol* 2006; 59: 459–66.
45. Brooks DJ, Pavese N. Imaging non-motor aspects of Parkinson's disease. In: Chaudhuri KR, Tolosa E, Schapira A, Poewe W (eds) *Non-motor symptoms of Parkinson's disease*, pp. 59–72. Oxford, New York: Oxford University Press, 2009.
46. Kim SE, Choi JY, Choe YS, Choi Y, Lee WY. Serotonin transporters in the midbrain of Parkinson's disease patients: a study with 123I-beta-CIT SPECT. *J Nucl Med* 2003; 44: 870–6.
47. Remy P, Doder M, Lees AJ, Turjanski N, Brooks DJ. Depression in Parkinson's disease: loss of dopamine and noradrenaline innervation in the limbic system. *Brain* 2005; 128: 1314–22.
48. Hilker R, Thomas AV, Klein JC, et al. Dementia in Parkinson disease: functional imaging of cholinergic and dopaminergic pathways. *Neurology* 2005; 65: 1716–22.
49. Bohnen NI, Kaufer DI, Hendrickson R, et al. Cognitive correlates of cortical cholinergic denervation in Parkinson's disease and parkinsonian dementia. *J Neurol* 2006; 253: 242–7.
50. Eidelberg D. Metabolic brain networks in neurodegenerative disorders: a functional imaging approach. *Trends Neurosci* 2009; 32: 548–57.
51. Kuhl DE, Metter EJ, Benson DF. Similarities of cerebral glucose metabolism in Alzheimer's and Parkinsonian dementia. *J Cereb Blood Flow Metab* 1985; 5: S169–70.
52. Vander-Borght T, Minoshima S, Giordani B, et al. Cerebral metabolic differences in Parkinson's and Alzheimer's disease matched for dementia severity. *J Nucl Med* 1997; 38: 797–802.
53. Edison P, Rowe CC, Rinne JO, et al. Amyloid load in Parkinson's disease dementia and Lewy body dementia measured with [^{11}C]PIB positron emission tomography. *J Neurol Neurosurg Psychiatry* 2008; 79: 1331–8.
54. Nagayama H, Hamamoto M, Ueda M, Nagashima J, Katayama Y. Reliability of MIBG myocardial scintigraphy in the diagnosis of Parkinson's disease. *J Neurol Neurosurg Psychiatry* 2005; 76: 249–51.
55. Antonini A, Kazumata K, Feigin A, et al. Differential diagnosis of parkinsonism with [^{18}F]fluorodeoxyglucose and PET. *Mov Disord* 1998; 13: 268–74.
56. Spetsieris PG, Ma Y, Dhawan V, Eidelberg D. Differential diagnosis of parkinsonian syndromes using PCA-based functional imaging features. *NeuroImage* 2009; 45: 1241–52.
57. Schwarz J, Tatsch K, Gasser T, et al. 123I-IBZM binding compared with long-term clinical follow up in patients with *de novo* parkinsonism. *Mov Disord* 1998; 13: 16–19.
58. Druschky A, Hilz MJ, Platsch G, et al. Differentiation of Parkinson's disease and multiple system atrophy in early disease stages by means of I-123-MIBG-SPECT. *J Neurol Sci* 2000; 175: 3–12.
59. Eckert T, Barnes A, Dhawan V, et al. FDG PET in the differential diagnosis of parkinsonian disorders. *NeuroImage* 2005; 26: 912–21.
60. Burn DJ, Sawle GV, Brooks DJ. The differential diagnosis of Parkinson's disease, multiple system atrophy, and Steele–Richardson–Olszewski syndrome: discriminant analysis of striatal ^{18}F-dopa PET data. *J Neurol Neurosurg Psychiatry* 1994; 57: 278–84.
61. Kuwert T, Lange HW, Langen KJ, et al. Cortical and subcortical glucose consumption measured by PET in patients with Huntington's disease. *Brain* 1990; 113: 1405–23.

62. Dubinsky RM, Hallett M, Levey R, Di Chiro G. Regional brain glucose metabolism in neuroacanthocytosis. *Neurology* 1989; 39: 1253–5.
63. Hosokawa S, Ichiya Y, Kuwabara Y, et al. Positron emission tomography in cases of chorea with different underlying diseases. *J Neurol Neurosurg Psychiatry* 1987; 50: 1284–7.
64. Turjanski N, Weeks R, Dolan R, et al. Striatal D_1 and D_2 receptor binding in patients with Huntington's disease and other choreas: a PET study. *Brain* 1995; 118: 689–96.
65. Antonini A, Leenders KL, Eidelberg D. [C-11]Raclopride-PET studies of the Huntington's disease rate of progression: relevance of the trinucleotide repeat length. *Ann Neurol* 1998; 43: 253–5.
66. Andersson U, Eckernas SA, Hartvig P, et al. Striatal binding of 11C-NMSP studied with positron emission tomography in patients with persistent tardive dyskinesia: no evidence for altered dopamine receptor binding. *J Neural Transm* 1990; 79: 215–26.
67. Andrews TC, Weeks RA, Turjanski N, et al. Huntington's disease progression: PET and clinical observations. *Brain* 1999; 122: 2353–63.
68. Tai YF, Pavese N, Gerhard A, et al. Microglial activation in presymptomatic Huntington's disease gene carriers. *Brain* 2007; 130: 1759–66.
69. Naumann M, Pirker W, Reiners K, et al. Imaging the pre- and postsynaptic side of striatal dopaminergic synapses in idiopathic cervical dystonia: a SPECT study using [^{123}I]epidepride and [^{123}I]β-CIT. *Mov Disord* 1998; 13: 319–23.
70. Perlmutter JS, Stambuk MK, Markham J, et al. Decreased [F-18] spiperone binding in putamen in idiopathic focal dystonia. *J Neurosci* 1997; 17: 843–50.
71. Garibotto V, Romito LM, Elia AE, et al. *In vivo* evidence for GABAA receptor changes in the sensorimotor system in primary dystonia. *Mov Disord* 2011; 26: 852–7.
72. Snow BJ, Nygaard TG, Takahashi H, Calne DB. Positron emission tomography studies of dopa-responsive dystonia and early-onset idiopathic parkinsonism. *Ann Neurol* 1993; 34: 733–8.
73. Turjanski N, Bhatia K, Burn DJ, et al. Comparison of striatal ^{18}F-dopa uptake in adult-onset dystonia-parkinsonism, Parkinson's disease, and dopa-responsive dystonia. *Neurology* 1993; 43: 1563–8.

CHAPTER 7

Genetic Techniques, Impact and Diagnostic Issues in Movement Disorders

José Brás and John Hardy

Advances in the diagnosis of movement disorders

The last decade has seen remarkable progress in molecular genetics, which has allowed us to gain greater insight into the molecular events underlying inherited neurological diseases. For those diseases where a clear Mendelian pattern of inheritance is present, a majority of the common genes harbouring pathogenic mutations has been identified, allowing, in some cases, the correct reclassification of heterogeneous clinical syndromes, in addition to enabling novel diagnostic possibilities. It is expected that ultimately these findings will form the basis of new therapeutic and preventive approaches.

A major part of this revolution in the genetics of neurological disorders, and movement disorders in particular, comes from the understanding that, in many cases, a single gene, containing a single mutation and acting in a purely dominant or recessive mode, does not explain the genetic component of that particular disease. In these cases, common genetic variability may act as a risk for the development of the disease, but is not the single underlying cause.

Huntington's disease is the classic example of a purely genetic movement disorder (1). Here, the presence of an expanded version of the *huntingtin* gene invariably means the development of the disease, while its absence precludes it, simultaneously helping our understanding of the pathobiology of the disease and implying that routine molecular diagnostic tests can be provided by simple assays, usually based on the polymerase chain reaction (PCR). At the opposite end of the spectrum are diseases such as Parkinson's disease, where clear Mendelian inheritance represents a minority of cases, and several genes are known to contain pathogenic mutations (2–7). Depending on the size of these genes, this may render molecular diagnosis too costly or time-consuming; in addition, if some of these mutations are not simple sequence changes, and therefore sequencing the genes fails to detect them. Again, Parkinson's disease provides such an example: some mutations in the *PRKN* gene are heterozygous deletions of complete exons, which are undetectable by routine sequencing (8).

Notwithstanding the fact that only a small percentage of movement disorders can be effectively treated, molecular diagnosis remains a very important tool because it provides valuable information for the affected individual, allowing them to make informed life choices, including family planning.

Genetic knowledge of the aetiology of neurological diseases has been expanded based on recent advances in genomic technologies. These have allowed us to look at genetic variability linked to disease from a completely different perspective than was possible five to ten years ago. These advances have allowed us to move from studying one individual exon at a time, to being able to interrogate the entire genome of an individual in a single experiment. This clearly has the potential to impact on the diagnosis of these diseases and, in a way, revolutionize molecular diagnosis.

In this chapter we will discuss the applicability of these new technologies to diagnosis, consider their limitations and pitfalls, and look at the next wave of genomic technologies that are likely to turn the promise of personalized medicine into a reality.

Sanger sequencing: the cornerstone of diagnostic tests

The gold standard for genetic diagnosis is Sanger sequencing. Here, one is able to interrogate small fragments of DNA—typically <800 base pairs (bp)—for sequence changes. This method is based on a methodological approach taken by Fred Sanger and Alan Coulson in the late 1970s (9, 10), but greatly improved in speed and ease of use by the employment of automated DNA sequencing instruments. The principle of capillary sequencing is based on the incorporation of the four nucleotides, each carrying its own specific dye, enabling identification of the base present at any given position of the DNA sequence being analysed. Following PCR amplification of the locus of interest from genomic DNA using appropriate primers, the automated sequencing machine performs the sequence detection. Although not without its flaws, capillary sequencing is a robust method with a low error rate, and was the method chosen for the Human Genome Project (11).

Repeat detection, such as those in the *HTT* gene that causes Huntington's disease, employs the same principles, although sizing of the DNA fragment is ultimately performed by simultaneous comparison with a known standard run.

Sanger sequencing as a diagnostic technique is usually used in two scenarios: (i) when the genes causing the disease are known; (ii) when the disease genes are not yet described but several individuals, both affected and unaffected, from the same kindred are available for testing.

In the first scenario the genes are initially amplified by PCR followed by sequencing, determining their DNA sequence for the individual. Even in these cases, where genes have been described and the phenotype is suggestive of their involvement, one must bear in mind some of the limitations of this approach: large heterozygous deletions encompassing the region being sequenced are likely to go unnoticed, and the same holds true for duplications. Also, complete screening of genes with a large number of exons is typically too costly, and in these cases it is common for only a subset of exons to be tested. While this is common practice, it is worth noting that rare mutations may go unnoticed. *LRRK2,* one of the most common genetic causes of Parkinson's disease, contains 42 exons and screening is usually performed only for the two or three exons where mutations are most common; very few studies have screened the entire coding region of the gene, and it certainly is not practicable to do this on a routine basis.

In the second scenario a clear genetic component to the disease is present (e.g. family history), but the causative genes are either unknown or screening for the known gene(s) has been unsuccessful. In such cases it is possible to map the position of the gene by comparing fragments of DNA between affected and unaffected individuals in the family (a method known as family-based linkage). After this initial mapping has been performed, sequencing of the region is undertaken to identify the causal gene and mutation.

While Sanger sequencing is still widely used, there are limitations to the types of mutations it can detect that should be noted. In some recessive diseases it is possible that instead of one homozygous mutation underlying the disease, the subject presents with compound heterozygous mutations. Here, one allele presents one mutation while the other allele presents a different mutation. If these two mutations are positioned very close together, one can usually determine the phase. However, if they are located in different exons, and there are several thousand bases separating them, Sanger sequencing of the proband alone will not reveal the phase of these mutations. In these cases one typically needs to sequence additional family members, if they are available. This is often the case for *PRKN,* the most common recessive gene for Parkinson's disease. *PRKN* contains 12 exons and spans over 1.3 million bases, and mutations have been described in the majority of these exons, implying that two mutations may be separated by as many as a million base pairs.

Additionally, capillary sequencing is unable to detect some copy number variations. For example, a heterozygous deletion of an entire exon and flanking regions would be missed using common sequencing primers, since it would appear as if the individual simply had no heterozygous variants in that particular exon. If a disease can be caused by a combination of point mutations and copy number changes, this severely limits the accuracy of Sanger sequencing as a diagnostic tool for that particular disease.

A third limitation relates to sequencing more complex genomic regions. Two examples are the *GBA* and *CR1* genes. The former is known to harbour mutations which, when homozygous, cause Gaucher's disease and, when heterozygous, confer risk for Parkinson's disease (12), while the latter was one of the hits from a genome-wide association study in Alzheimer's disease (13). *GBA,* which is located on chromosome 1, is very close to a pseudo-gene, with which it shares approximately 96% homology (14, 15). Furthermore, a large number of known pathogenic mutations in *GBA* are present in the normal sequence of the pseudo-gene (16). In such a gene, exon sequencing is very complicated because of the similarity between sequences. Unless the primers are able to distinguish completely between the two regions, it is difficult to be absolutely certain which fragment is being sequenced. The second gene, *CR1,* is even more complex; it contains repetitions of entire exons that can harbour different mutations in the same individual.

Thus it is clear that while Sanger sequencing is a robust and widely used technology for genetic diagnosis, some limitations have become apparent as we have improved our understanding of the genetic basis of neurological diseases and should be taken into account when interpreting these results.

Whole-genome genotyping

Assaying about two million single nucleotide polymorphisms (SNPs) present in the human genome is currently a trivial and fairly inexpensive approach for many laboratories. The growth of this field in the past four years has been remarkable and we have now moved from assaying tens of markers to assaying millions which cover all the known common variability in the genome.

There are currently several platforms that allow high-throughput genotyping, but the Illumina Infinium Beadchips (Illumina Inc.) are arguably the ones with the largest user base. Very briefly, the Infinium protocol is based on genotyping chips (glass slides) containing probes that are complementary to the sequence adjacent to the SNP of interest. When hybridized to the test DNA, the probes are polymerase-extended to the SNP base using labelled nucleotides, which provide a way of detecting the nucleotide incorporated at that position. When coupled with image analysis hardware, it is possible to assay several million of these probes in a very short time span.

Genotyping chips were initially based on the HapMap project findings which depicted over 3.1 million SNP locations on the genome, compiled using 269 samples from four human populations (17). Probes were then selected that 'tagged' (i.e. were in close linkage disequilibrium) with the majority of these markers, allowing a genome-wide analysis while assaying only a subset of well-defined surrogate markers. This powerful technology not only allows genotyping of SNPs, but also facilitates the determination of copy number variation in an extraordinarily easy manner (Fig. 7.1).

The initial application of this technology was for genome-wide association studies (GWAS). Until that point, research into the genetic associations of disease was typically limited to the study of a handful of markers in a gene of interest. This obviously meant that without a correct assumption of a candidate gene, the study could prove to be meaningless. GWAS has enabled the evaluation

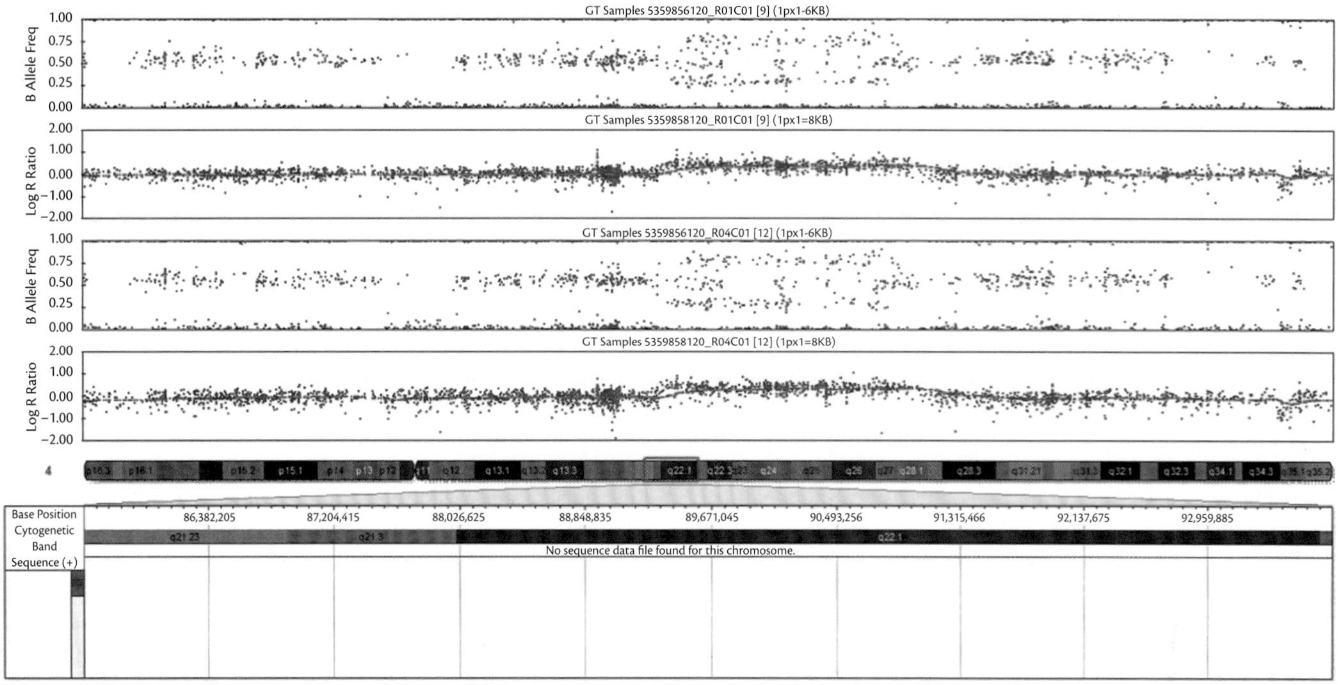

Fig. 7.1 GenomeStudio plot showing the two common metrics analysed (LogR ratio and B allele frequency). The first metric indicates the normalized intensity for each probe/SNP depicted by a single blue dot. In case of an increase in copy number (duplication, triplication, etc.) LogR ratio for that SNP becomes higher than the average value and this can easily be seen in these plots. The second metric depicts heterozygosity by outputting the B allele frequency. This allows rapid examination of regions of homozygosity. (GenomeStudio is a registered trademark of Illumina Inc.)

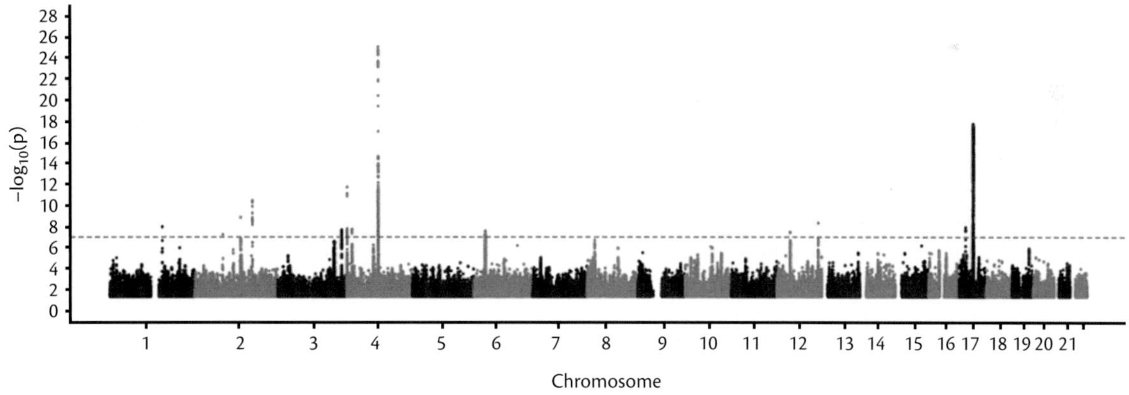

Fig. 7.2 Manhattan plot showing genome-wide association values. These plots have quickly become the standard for illustrating GWAS results. They allow genomic regions that appear to be associated with a particular phenotype to be detected in a quick and easy manner. Here, individual SNPs are plotted by position and association *p*-value. The higher the peak for a locus, the stronger is the association with disease.

of associations in a global manner without the need for a prior hypothesis, relying simply on the tenet that common sequence variants are responsible for common diseases (CV–CD). This approach has proved to be extremely successful, with new loci and genes now being identified for a variety of diseases on an almost monthly basis (Fig. 7.2).

Although this approach was purely directed at research goals, the implications for genetic diagnosis are also very significant. With the improvement in array design and decrease in costs, it is now possible to create custom assays that target relevant variation in a very cost-effective manner, such that one can create an array that targets all the known sequence variation in all the genes involved in a particular disease and assay all those variants in a single three-day run.

Furthermore, since the cost of such experiments is rapidly falling below the \$100 barrier, one can envisage this technology being used as an initial screen for all samples coming to a diagnostic laboratory. For example, a neurogenetics laboratory would assay all the genes known to be involved in neurological diseases for all samples received, providing information for all the known causes of neurological diseases in a single experiment that would cost ~\$100. This approach will very likely revolutionize diagnostic laboratories and greatly improve the speed and accuracy with which results are reported back to the clinician.

In addition to assaying sequence variants of interest, the array simultaneously assays for copy number changes. This has been shown to be a significant determinant of common neurological disorders; for example, the alpha-synuclein gene (*SNCA*) is not only known to contain pathogenic point mutations, but also duplication and triplication of the entire gene have been described (18, 19). In the same manner, the amyloid precursor protein gene (*APP*) associated with Alzheimer's disease has been shown to contain not only sequence variants, but also an increased number of copies (20). The ability to assay both types of variation in a single experiment will contribute greatly to improvement in genetic diagnostics.

Nonetheless, every technology has its limitations and genotyping arrays are not immune to this. While the fact that markers can be chosen to be included in the array offers great flexibility, it also means that any unknown variant will be missed by this method. This is particularly relevant for complex diseases where it is still believed that a significant proportion of genes causing the disease are yet to be found. Likewise, although the genes may be identified and a number of mutations discovered, novel mutations in the same gene would still be missed using this approach.

Another limitation of genotyping arrays relates to the probe set that is used. For each marker, the array contains a 50 bp probe complementary to the genomic sequence. If an unknown SNP is present within the length of this probe, the genotype result may not be accurate since the hybridization will not be completely efficient. This is a difficult issue to address since different samples will carry different benign rare variants which have no impact on pathobiology of disease. Before an array is designed, all markers go through a very thorough process of screening to ensure that they will be successful. However, if SNPs have not been described previously, there is no screening procedure that would detect this issue.

Similarly to Sanger sequencing, genomic regions that have homologous loci are also difficult to assay. Even though this is usually screened for before designing the array, if the variant to be assessed is within one of these high-homology regions, a probe with sufficient specificity will be difficult to design.

It is also worth noting that since this technology assays individual SNPs, chromosomal translocations are virtually impossible to detect, given that the only output obtained is signal intensity per individual marker, regardless of its position on the genome.

Although high-throughput genome-wide genotyping studies have yielded very exciting results, and the technology is now stable, robust, and very reproducible, the use of this approach has always been perceived as transitory and not as the ultimate analytical methodology. As we advance rapidly towards ever more cost-effective sequencing technology, it is expected that high-throughput genotyping will be replaced by whole-genome sequencing.

Massively parallel sequencing

In the past five years new chemistries and instruments have been developed to perform sequencing (so-called 'next-generation' or 'massively parallel' instruments), and such technology has already transformed the field. Their impact on genomics has been so dramatic that the very nature of genetic experimentation has shifted towards more comprehensive and complete analysis. The requirements for handling these data are also fundamentally different from those associated with Sanger sequencing, particularly the computational algorithms used, and their continuous improvement has enabled us to answer questions that range from interrogating a single base to large copy number variation on a genome-wide scale. This will ultimately change our understanding of the human genome in a radical manner.

The field of 'next-generation' sequencing started with three major players: Illumina (Genome Analyzer), Life Technologies (SOLiD), and Roche (454). All first-generation instruments have since seen major improvements and, in the case of Illumina, the majority of sequencing centres quickly updated to a successor of the Genome Analyzer, the HiSeq2000.

All three instruments are based on different chemistries, but they all share fundamental similarities that set them apart from capillary sequencing. Instead of processing up to 96 DNA fragments at a time (the maximum for Sanger sequencing machines), these instruments are able to process several millions of sequence reads in parallel. This throughput usually means that a single machine can successfully finish a mid-size project in just a few runs. Additionally, the DNA preparation for sequencing is straightforward and does not require complex cloning or amplification stages as used in capillary sequencing. Thus it is possible to avoid some of the bias issues that have plagued genome representation in several sequencing projects. Nevertheless, each of these technologies has its own set of biases. The typical workflow for sample preparation for any of these three technologies starts with breaking up genomic DNA into small fragments, to which specific adaptor 'oligos' are ligated at both ends; at this point, the sample is ready to be sequenced. A relatively small amount of starting DNA (typically up to a couple of micrograms) is needed to perform a complete experiment that can potentially sequence the entire genome of that sample. All three platforms also allow for sequencing both ends of each DNA fragment (paired ends), which is helpful for read mapping and *de novo* genome sequencing. Additionally, the data produced by these platforms is typically comprised of shorter reads (36–500 bp) compared with capillary sequencing (650–900 bp), which has an impact on several applications.

The Roche (454) GS FLX sequencer was first introduced commercially in 2004. This sequencer works on the principle of 'pyrosequencing', which uses the pyrophosphate molecule released on nucleotide incorporation by DNA polymerase to fuel a downstream set of reactions that ultimately produce light from the cleavage of oxyluciferin by luciferase (21). The current 454 instrument produces an average read length of approximately 400 bp per sample, with a throughput of about a billion bases per day.

Applied Biosystem's SOLiD sequencer was initially released in 2007 and relies on an innovative ligation-based chemistry (21). One of the main advantages of this approach is that it has one of the lowest error rates of all three technologies. The current SOLiD instrument, the 5500xl, has a throughput of 30 billion bases per day with read lengths of up to 75 bp.

In 2006 Illumina introduced their first instrument, the Genome Analyzer, which has since seen several improvements, increasing throughput and reducing the times per run (22). In 2010 a new instrument was released commercially which, although utilizing the same chemistry, improved throughput dramatically and quickly became the sequencer of choice for the vast majority of genome centres. Illumina's approach is based on the concept of 'sequencing by synthesis' (SBS) to produce sequence reads of 35–150 bp from tens of millions of surface-amplified DNA fragments simultaneously. The major features of this technology are the low turnaround time and the amount of data produced. At the time of writing, Illumina's HiSeq is capable of producing over 600 billion bases per eight-day run, with read lengths of up to 150 bp.

While the improvements in sequencing have been astonishing, clearly defying Moore's Law (23), the cost is still high enough to preclude whole-genome sequencing *en masse* at the present time. To this end, strategies need to be developed to leverage this technology and simultaneously provide cost-effectiveness. The first approach was derived from common sense: given that the portion of the genome that we can most easily understand is the coding region, sequencing should start by targeting this small portion—the so-called exome (24). Much like genotyping arrays, exome sequencing is a transitory approach that reflects the most cost-effective approach to 'next-generation' sequencing that is currently available.

Exome sequencing follows the same principle as described for the technologies above, but includes an additional step where the genomic DNA library is hybridized with a pool of short biotin-labelled oligonucleotides that were designed to be complementary to the entire collection of exons in the genome. These are then magnetically captured and the non-coding DNA is washed away. This creates a library that contains only DNA fragments representative of the coding region.

This approach has already permitted the identification of the genetic causes underlying a significant number of Mendelian diseases (24–29). While this is a powerful approach, there are some caveats. The first of these is that by sequencing the exome, a significant proportion of variation in regulatory regions that may play a role in the disease is missed. Additionally, no method has yet allowed for the sequencing of the entire collection of known exons. Typically, 15–20% of known coding exons are not captured as they are located in complex genomic regions, for which capture probes are difficult to design. Added to this percentage are all the exons that are not properly described or annotated in the current genome reference build. Moreover, since these technologies all use short-reads, determining phase is still a poorly addressed issue, unless relevant family members are available for testing, which increases costs linearly. The combination of short-reads with the fact that only small dispersed fragments of the genome are being sequenced also means that mid-size insertions or deletions are difficult to assess, particularly if they are heterozygous. The identification of ~1–5 bp deletions is quite accurate, but a heterozygous deletion of ~60–100 bp is less so.

In some cases, however, whole-genome sequencing has been performed instead. This has usually occurred when a small number of individuals, with a very defined and often rare phenotype, is being studied. The major differences in this approach relate to the cost of the analysis, handling much larger amounts of data, and ultimately interpreting these data. It is worth noting that, so far, all genome sequencing projects that have revealed new mutations could theoretically have arrived at the same result by performing exome sequencing, since the mutations were all coding and in known genes. This is not advocating exome sequencing in place of whole-genome sequencing; it simply shows that our understanding of the effects of genetic variability is still very much confined to the coding portion of the genome. As we continue to gather evidence for, and increase our knowledge of, functional effects of non-coding variability, a whole new range of novel, pathogenic, non-coding mutations is likely to be discovered.

In parallel with whole-exome and whole-genome sequencing, it is now also possible to sequence the entire transcriptome (the collection of RNA molecules, including mRNA, rRNA, tRNA, and non-coding RNA, usually called RNA-seq) of an individual (30). This is potentially a very powerful approach that is still in its early days, partly because the data analysis is more complex than that required for DNA sequencing. For example, a single gene will have several transcripts, created by alternative splicing, which may or may not have been previously described. This has implications for primary data analysis, particularly the mapping of reads to the genome, which means that if a read is uniquely aligned to the wrong gene, such as a paralog, this may result in false-positive variants being called. One of the added benefits of RNA-seq is that it detects both sequence variability and expression levels simultaneously. This means that tissue-specific genes will only be detected (for both expression and sequence variability) when using RNA extracted from that same tissue.

These high-throughput approaches may play a very significant role in the diagnostics laboratory in the next three to five years. One can certainly envisage a screening approach that relies on the genotyping of disease-specific markers using microarrays, while simultaneously whole-genome and transcriptome are being sequenced to detect novel variability. This approach is likely to be very successful in determining the genetic causes of a high proportion of diseases at a fraction of the total cost that novel/complex diseases face in their diagnostic work-up.

Single-molecule sequencing

The next major advance in genomics technology will be single-molecule sequencing. The premise behind this technique is that it will be capable of sequencing one DNA molecule at a time, whether that molecule is a constituent of an amplified sample or unamplified DNA. There are two primary advantages of single-molecule sequencing. First, individual fragments of DNA do not need to be amplified or, when they are, far fewer cycles of amplification are required. Secondly, sequencing can occur in real time, meaning that a complete human genome could be sequenced within minutes. Several approaches to single-molecule sequencing are currently being tested; these range from scanning probe techniques, to fluorescence techniques, to nanopore approaches (31–34). The last of these possibly has the greatest promise. The most advanced nanopore approach is that being developed by Oxford Nanopore, where a molecule of DNA is passed through an alpha-haemolysine pore with an exonuclease attached that cleaves the DNA molecule one base at a time. The bases are dropped through the nanopore, which is embedded in a membrane. As the DNA passes through the nanopore, the conductance across the membrane changes: different base pairs change the conductance in different ways, allowing each base to be accurately identified.

The implications of this technique are enormous. The ability to sequence one DNA molecule in its entirety (presumably parallelizing reactions will allow for increased coverage), with costs that are negligible compared with current methods, which allows an entire genome to be sequenced in a matter of hours, or even minutes, instead of weeks, and which allows one to clearly determine phase (since only one molecule is being sequenced at a time) is likely to revolutionize the field of genetics.

Future challenges: defining variability in human genomes

Our knowledge of the human genome has seen great improvements over the last few years with the arrival of these high-throughput technologies, but also as a result of the Human Genome and HapMap projects. This has allowed us to perform many genome-wide association and exome-sequencing studies that have elucidated, to some extent, the genetic basis of several complex neurological diseases. Although we understand genetic diversity among humans fairly well at the level of common variants, we still know very little about the amount and type of variation below that level of frequency. Since common variants have not fully explained all the heritability in these diseases, it is expected that less common and rarer alleles will also contribute. This is the case with some of the known genes for Parkinson's disease: common variability in *SNCA* confers risk for PD, and rare mutations are the cause of the disease in a few families. It will soon be possible to re-sequence large numbers of healthy controls to determine a baseline for 'normal' variation, which will be fundamental for future studies of complex diseases. This is one of the goals of the 1000 Genomes Project, although a much larger number of individuals, from a variety of genetic backgrounds, need to be sequenced to better capture the spectrum of variability in the human genome (35).

With the increase in knowledge, and especially in understanding, of human genome variability, we will also see great improvements in our ability to correctly annotate variability leading to functional changes. These annotations will add a whole new layer of data to genome variation, making these results much more readily interpretable in terms of their potential impact(s) on function and, ultimately, biology. This integrated knowledge will significantly enhance our ability to interpret the genome in the context of observed human phenotypes, eventually leading to the era of personalized genomics.

Towards the '$1000' genome and personalized medicine

These high-throughput technologies, by enabling vast data generation, together with our ever-increasing understanding of human genome variability and its impact on biology, will provide the groundwork for true genetic disease risk prediction and therapeutic approaches. Targeted treatments, which selectively block the impact of certain variants, might also be suggested.

Direct-to-consumer genetic test companies are the first approach to this paradigm. Here, any individual is able to send a sample of their DNA, from which the companies will generate whole-genome genotyping data. Although this is not a diagnostic test per se, the implications for diagnosis are obvious. Furthermore, the fact that such companies are providing this service and that customers are interested in it, shows that this approach appeals to the general population. This system has one severe limitation: only a very limited and selected subset of markers is medically actionable, since only known variants that it is possible to design assays for can be tested. This clearly suggests that, although genotyping methods may become one aspect of personalized medicine in the future, they will not be the cornerstone of personal genomics.

A mere three years ago, a whole genome sequence would cost ~$700 000; today that cost has dropped to ~$7 000 and it is expected that it will soon reach the $1000 mark, thus becoming a viable approach to clinical assays and a point of entry for health insurance or medical care. The question is whether we are able to keep pace with technology and be in a position to make sense of the raw data these technologies will generate.

Conclusions and future prospects

Despite the remarkable advances in genome analysis methods, the current methodologies have some limitations that should be highlighted. Even in monogenic diseases, where it would be expected that identifying a pathogenic mutation would be easiest, there are two major problems. The first relates to technology—for example, inhomogeneous coverage of the target region. This problem leads to a widely varying number of reads covering different regions of the exome which cause, in conjunction with unequal sequencing quality, the detection of false-positive and false-negative variants. Sanger re-sequencing can eliminate false-positive variants, but false-negative variants are potentially a major problem because if the filtering strategy relies on the detection of mutations in the same gene in different affected individuals, these might be missed. These problems are likely to be overcome with further technological progress. The main genetic problem is locus heterogeneity, which is the presence of multiple distinct disease genes/disease loci for one clinical phenotype. Some neurological disorders, such as Charcot–Marie–Tooth disease (with over 40 loci), hereditary ataxia, and hereditary spastic paraplegia, show a high degree of locus heterogeneity. The main biological problem is proving the causality of a mutation. Ultimately, causality has to be shown using cell and animal model systems, although currently segregation is usually the minimum requirement.

In cases where the causative genes are known and screening of these needs to be performed, using approaches like genome or exome sequencing will discover not only the causative mutation for the investigated disease, but also mutations causing other monogenic disorders and genetic risk factors for complex disorders. This creates an obvious ethical problem.

One of the most significant issues that still needs to be addressed is that of phase. None of the current technologies allows us to determine genome-wide maps of phased haplotypes, which means that we are still neglecting one of the most fundamental aspects of the human genome—its diploid nature.

The coming years will see a great increase in the description of variants found in exomes and genomes; some of these will simply be rare non-functional variants while others will have important functional implications for the biology of the human genome. The diagnostic power of whole-genome sequencing in the context of genetically heterogeneous Mendelian disease has already been shown (36) and it is likely that the identification of rare heterogeneous alleles, by means of whole-genome sequencing, will be the only way to definitively determine genetic contribution to the associated clinical phenotypes.

References

1. Ross CA, Tabrizi SJ. Huntington's disease: from molecular pathogenesis to clinical treatment. *Lancet Neurol* 2011; 10: 83–98.
2. Zimprich A, Biskup S, Leitner P, et al. Mutations in *LRRK2* cause autosomal-dominant parkinsonism with pleomorphic pathology. *Neuron* 2004; 44: 601–7.

3. Valente EM, Abou-Sleiman PM, Caputo V, et al. Hereditary early-onset Parkinson's disease caused by mutations in PINK1. *Science* 2004; 304: 1158–60.
4. Paisán-Ruíz C, Jain S, Evans EW, et al. Cloning of the gene containing mutations that cause *PARK8*-linked Parkinson's disease. *Neuron* 2004; 44: 595–600.
5. Bonifati V, Rizzu P, van Baren MJ, et al. Mutations in the DJ-1 gene associated with autosomal recessive early-onset parkinsonism. *Science* 2003; 299: 256–9.
6. Kitada T, Asakawa S, Hattori N, et al. Mutations in the *parkin* gene cause autosomal recessive juvenile parkinsonism. *Nature* 1998; 392: 605–8.
7. Polymeropoulos MH, Lavedan C, Leroy E, et al. Mutation in the alpha-synuclein gene identified in families with Parkinson's disease. *Science* 1997; 276: 2045–7.
8. West A, Periquet M, Lincoln S, et al. Complex relationship between Parkin mutations and Parkinson disease. *Am J Med Genet* 2002; 114: 584–91.
9. Sanger F, Nicklen S, Coulson AR. DNA sequencing with chain-terminating inhibitors. *Proc Natl Acad Sci USA* 1977; 74, 5463–7.
10. Sanger F, Air GM, Barrell BG, et al. Nucleotide sequence of bacteriophage phi X174 DNA. *Nature* 1977; 265: 687–95.
11. Lander ES, Linton LM, Birren B, et al. Initial sequencing and analysis of the human genome. *Nature* 2001; 409: 860–921.
12. Sidransky E, Nalls MA, Aasly JO, et al. Multicenter analysis of glucocerebrosidase mutations in Parkinson's disease. *N Engl J Med* 2009; 361, 1651–61.
13. Lambert JC, Heath S, Even G, et al. Genome-wide association study identifies variants at CLU and CR1 associated with Alzheimer's disease. *Nat Genet* 2009; 41: 1094–9.
14. Martínez-Arias R, Calafell F, Mateu E, Comas D, Andrés A, Bertranpetit J. Sequence variability of a human pseudogene. *Genome Res* 2001; 11: 1071–85.
15. Martinez-Arias R, Comas D, Mateu E, Bertranpetit J. Glucocerebrosidase pseudogene variation and Gaucher disease: recognizing pseudogene tracts in GBA alleles. *Hum Mutat* 2001; 17:191–8.
16. Hruska KS, LaMarca ME, Scott CR, Sidransky E. Gaucher disease: mutation and polymorphism spectrum in the glucocerebrosidase gene (GBA). *Hum Mutat* 2008; 29: 567–83.
17. The International HapMap Project. *Nature* 2003; 426: 789–96.
18. Singleton AB, Farrer M, Johnson J, et al. Alpha-synuclein locus triplication causes Parkinson's disease. *Science* 2003; 302: 841.
19. Chartier-Harlin MC, Kachergus J, Roumier C, et al. Alpha-synuclein locus duplication as a cause of familial Parkinson's disease. *Lancet* 2004; 364: 1167–9.
20. Rovelet-Lecrux A, Hannequin D, Raux G, et al. APP locus duplication causes autosomal dominant early-onset Alzheimer disease with cerebral amyloid angiopathy. *Nat Genet* 2006; 38: 24–6.
21. Margulies M, Egholm M, Altman WE, et al. Genome sequencing in microfabricated high-density picolitre reactors. *Nature* 2005; 437: 376–80.
22. Bentley DR, Balasubramanian S, Swerdlow HP, et al. Accurate whole human genome sequencing using reversible terminator chemistry. *Nature* 2008; 456: 53–9.
23. Moore GE. Cramming more components onto integrated circuits. *Proc IEEE* 1998; 86: 82–5.
24. Ng SB, Buckingham KJ, Lee C, et al. Exome sequencing identifies the cause of a Mendelian disorder. *Nat Genet* 2010; 42: 30–5.
25. Bilgüvar K, Oztürk AK, Louvi A, et al. Whole-exome sequencing identifies recessive WDR62 mutations in severe brain malformations. *Nature* 2010; 467: 207–10.
26. Varela I, Tarpey P, Raine K, et al. Exome sequencing identifies frequent mutation of the SWI/SNF complex gene *PBRM1* in renal carcinoma. *Nature* 2011; 469: 539–42.
27. Çalışkan M, Chong JX, Uricchio L, et al. Exome sequencing reveals a novel mutation for autosomal recessive non-syndromic mental retardation in the TECR gene on chromosome 19p13. *Hum Mol Genet* 2011; 20: 1285–9.
28. Johnson JO, Mandrioli J, Benatar M, et al. Exome sequencing reveals VCP mutations as a cause of familial ALS. *Neuron* 2010; 68: 857–64.
29. Wang JL, Yang X, Xia K, et al. TGM6 identified as a novel causative gene of spinocerebellar ataxias using exome sequencing. *Brain* 2010; 133: 3510–18.
30. Mortazavi A, Williams BA, McCue K, Schaeffer L, Wold B. Mapping and quantifying mammalian transcriptomes by RNA-Seq. *Nat Methods* 2008; 5: 621–8.
31. Lund J, Parviz BA. Scanning probe and nanopore DNA sequencing: core techniques and possibilities. *Methods Mol Biol* 2009; 578: 113–22.
32. Wallace EV, Stoddart D, Heron AJ, et al. Identification of epigenetic DNA modifications with a protein nanopore. *Chem Commun* 2010; 46: 8195–7.
33. Stoddart D, Heron AJ, Klingelhoefer J, Mikhailova E, Maglia G, Bayley H. Nucleobase recognition in ssDNA at the central constriction of the alpha-hemolysin pore. *Nano Lett* 2010; 10: 3633–7.
34. Maglia G, Heron AJ, Stoddart D, Japrung D, Bayley H. Analysis of single nucleic acid molecules with protein nanopores. *Methods Enzymol* 2010; 475: 591–623.
35. 1000 Genomes Project Consortium, Abecasis GR, Altshuler D, Auton A, et al. A map of human genome variation from population-scale sequencing. *Nature* 2010; 467: 1061–73.
36. Lupski JR, Reid JG, Gonzaga-Jauregui C, et al. Whole-genome sequencing in a patient with Charcot–Marie–Tooth neuropathy. *N Engl J Med* 2010; 362: 1181–91.

CHAPTER 8

Overview of Parkinsonism and Approach to Differential Diagnosis

Sabine Spielberger and Werner Poewe

Summary

Parkinsonism is one of the most common movement disorders and may be the clinical manifestation of a variety of neurodegenerative, structural, toxic, metabolic, infectious, and vascular disorders. Since therapy and prognosis differ considerably between different forms of parkinsonism, an early correct diagnosis is of great clinical significance but may be challenging on clinical grounds alone.

Ancillary tests for enhancement of diagnostic accuracy include drug-challenge testing to assess dopaminergic responsiveness, neuroimaging to evaluate nigrostriatal presynaptic dopaminergic function or evidence for structural abnormalities, and genetic testing to identify common genetic subtypes of Parkinson's disease. Therapeutic management of parkinsonism mainly depends on the underlying pathology. Levodopa is the single most effective way to treat the motor symptoms of Parkinson's disease, but it may also be at least partially effective in other types of parkinsonism, so that a trial with levodopa will be part of the treatment approach in most patients presenting with parkinsonism.

Essential background

Classification of parkinsonism

A parkinsonian syndrome is a presenting or important clinical feature in a variety of distinct conditions including neurodegenerative, metabolic, toxic, inflammatory, and autoimmune disorders, as well as vascular or neoplastic disorders. In addition, there are rare cases without an identifiable organic cause which satisfy criteria for psychogenic parkinsonism. For pragmatic clinical purposes, parkinsonian disorders are best grouped into two principal categories: degenerative parkinsonism, where a variety of sporadic and genetic degenerative diseases cause nigrostriatal neurodegeneration, and symptomatic or secondary parkinsonism, caused by non-degenerative lesions of the same system or other sites of the striatopallidothalamic-cortical motor circuitry (see Table 8.1). Several of these disorders are discussed in detail in other chapters in this book. In the absence of reliable and valid biomarkers, the differential diagnosis within this heterogenic group of parkinsonian syndromes is a matter of clinical acumen and judicious use of the ancillary investigations discussed below.

Epidemiology of parkinsonism

Parkinsonism is one of the most common movement disorders among the elderly. Published reports on the prevalence of parkinsonism estimate a range of 2–15% in the population aged over 65 (1–5), with incidence increasing with age. A community-based survey documented a prevalence rate of 52.4% for parkinsonism in the population over the age of 85 (2), and therefore, although it occurs worldwide, parkinsonism is more frequent in regions with longer life expectancy. By far the most common cause of parkinsonism is Parkinson's disease (PD), followed by drug-induced parkinsonism and vascular parkinsonism (1, 4). Atypical parkinsonian disorders, such as multiple system atrophy (MSA), progressive supranuclear palsy (PSP), and corticobasal syndrome (CBS), are rare causes of parkinsonism, with estimated prevalences ranging from 1 to 6 per 100 000 (6, 7).

Aetiopathogenesis

The aetiology of symptomatic forms of parkinsonism is diverse (see Table 8.1), but is usually definable in terms of functional or structural disorders affecting nigrostriatal dopamine transmission or downstream signalling pathways, although this is only partially understood in degenerative parkinsonism. Up to 5% of clinical cases of PD may be caused by Mendelian mutations, and recent genome-wide association studies (GWAS) have identified eleven risk loci associating with PD, some of which overlap with the known causative mutations such as alpha-synuclein (8). Taken together, however, such loci only about double a person's risk of developing PD, suggesting that there are multiple additional aetiological factors, both genetic and environmental. Nevertheless, genetic findings in PD suggest that dysfunction at the level of the mitochondria, synuclein processing, and endolysosomal trafficking are all likely to be important in PD pathogenesis. Aetiopathogenesis of other types of degenerative parkinsonism, such as MSA, PSP, or CBS, is even

Table 8.1 Overview of principal causes of parkinsonism

Neurodegenerative parkinsonism	
Sporadic	Sporadic Parkinson's disease (PD) Multiple system atrophy (MSA) Progressive supranuclear palsy (PSP) Corticobasal syndrome (CBS) Dementia with Lewy bodies (DLB)
Genetic	Genetic Parkinson's disease (PARK 1–18) Huntington's disease (Westphal variant) SCA mutations (SCA2, SCA3) Frontotemporal dementia with parkinsonism linked to chromosome 17 (FTDP-17) Wilson disease Neuronal brain iron accumulation syndrome (NBIA) Parkinsonism–amyotrophic lateral sclerosis–dementia complex of Guam PSP-like parkinsonism in Guadeloupe X-linked dystonia parkinsonism (DYT 3, XDP, Lubag) Dopa-responsive dystonia (DYT 5, Segawa syndrome) Rapid-onset dystonia parkinsonism (DYT 12) Dentatorubral-pallidoluysian atrophy Fragile X-associated tremor–ataxia syndrome Neuroacanthocytosis
Symptomatic parkinsonism	
Infectious	Post-encephalitic (encephalitis lethargica, Japanese B, post-streptococcal, other viral infections (HIV, PML)) Prion disease Toxoplasmosis
Toxic	Carbon monoxide Cyanide MPTP Manganese Methanol Rotenone
Drug-induced	Dopamine-receptor blockers Dopamine-depleting drugs Other drugs (e.g. valproic acid, calcium-channel blockers)
Brain tumours	Supratentorial tumours (e.g. frontal meningioma) Brainstem tumours (rare)
Metabolic	Hypoparathyroidism Extrapontine myelinolysis Chronic liver failure Fahr's disease
Miscellaneous	Normal pressure hydrocephalus Hemiatrophy-hemiparkinson syndrome Psychogenic

HIV, human immunodeficiency virus; MPTP, 1-methyl-4-phenyl-1,2,3-tetrahydropyridine ; PML, progressive multifocal leucoencephalopathy

less clear, but involves oligodendroglial alpha-synuclein pathology in MSA and neuronal tau pathology in PSP and CBS.

More detailed discussions are given in the corresponding chapters of this volume.

Pathophysiology

Regardless of aetiology, the principal pathophysiological abnormality underlying the cardinal motor features of parkinsonism—in particular bradykinesia—is related to dysfunctional motor loops connecting the prefrontal cortex, basal ganglia, and motor thalamus. According to a model of basal ganglia motor processing originally proposed and developed by Alexander and colleagues (9), the striatum plays a central role in processing sensorimotor information and relaying this to the internal segment of the globus pallidus (GPi), which in turn projects via inhibitory GABAergic projections to the motor segments of the ventral anterior thalamus from where glutamatergic facilitatory input reaches the motor planning and iniating structures of the prefrontal cortex (see Fig. 8.1a). This signalling circuit is controlled and modulated by the nigrostriatal dopamine projection, such that dopamine deficiency or pathologies affecting striatal dopamine receptors will lead to changes in the two principal striatopallidal output pathways targeting the GPi in a monosynaptic fashion (direct pathway) or via relays in the external pallidum (indirect pathway). The net effect of dysfunctional dopaminergic input onto these two striatal neuronal populations of projection neurons is increased firing of the GPi, resulting in

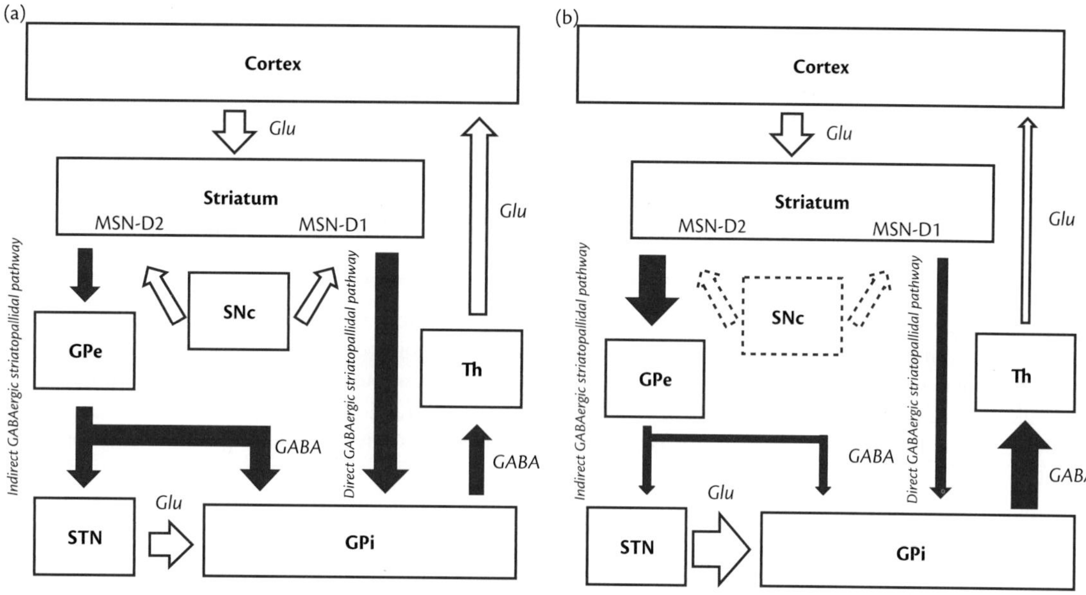

Fig. 8.1 (a) Basal ganglia motor loops with direct and indirect pathways. Black arrows indicate inhibition; white arrows indicate activation. SNc, substantia nigra pars compacta; GPe, globus pallidus externus; STN, subthalamic nucleus; GPi, globus pallidus internus; SNr, substantia nigra pars reticulata; Th, thalamus; Glu, glutamate; Enk, encephalin; SP, substance P; MSN, medium spiny neurons. (b) Impaired basal ganglia motor loops in patients with Parkinson's disease. Owing to neurodegeneration in the SNc, dopaminergic input into the striatum is reduced, resulting in a loss of excitatory dopaminergic drive on D1 receptors and inhibitory dopaminergic input on D2 receptors. The net result is increased GPi activity via direct and indirect pathways, leading to inhibition of Th and cortex.

increased inhibitory input into the motor thalamus, thus reducing thalamocortical motor drive with underactivity of the motor parts of the prefrontal cortex leading to impaired movement initiation, speed, and amplitude (see Fig. 8.1b). Similar effects may also be due to downstream events at the level of the pallidum, motor thalamus, or thalamocortical projections, as is the case in different types of secondary parkinsonism.

Clinical presentation

Cardinal features of parkinsonian syndromes

A parkinsonian syndrome is defined by the presence of *bradykinesia* in combination with at least one of the following signs: resting tremor, rigidity, and impaired postural reflexes, with the last of these not being the result of sensory, proprioceptive, or cerebellar dysfunction (10). According to the UK Parkinson's Disease Society Brain Bank criteria (QSBB criteria) bradykinesia is the anchor feature for parkinsonism and is used as an umbrella term including reduced movement speed (bradykinesia in the strict sense) and amplitude (hypokinesia), as well as slowness of movement initiation, and decrementing speed and amplitude with or without interruptions (akinesia) of sequential repetitive movements. Bradykinesia is the single most disabling motor feature of PD, impacting on virtually every aspect of activities of daily living, including handwriting, getting dressed, handling feeding utensils, hygiene, speech, and communication, as well as general mobility. Hypomimia with decreased blink rate, micrographia with decrementing script size within a sentence or even a word (see Fig. 8.2), or hypophonia with reduced volume of speech are clinical terms frequently used to describe isolated features of parkinsonian bradykinesia. Common early complaints of patients related to bradykinesia include handwriting difficulties, buttoning up a shirt, turning keys, or brushing their teeth, while relatives, colleagues, or friends may note changes in facial expression, a softer voice, or reduced arm swing or dragging of one leg while the patient is walking. With more advanced disease, getting up from an armchair or out of a car seat or turning around in bed, as well as problems with walking become more prominent among the symptoms reported in the patient interview. A peculiar and severely disabling feature of parkinsonian motor impairment, which is more aptly covered under the term of akinesia rather than bradykinesia, comprises difficulties of movement initiation, and maintenance of a flow of sequential or repetitive movements. This commonly manifests as hesitation when a patient is about to start walking or as sudden stops in a sequence of finger

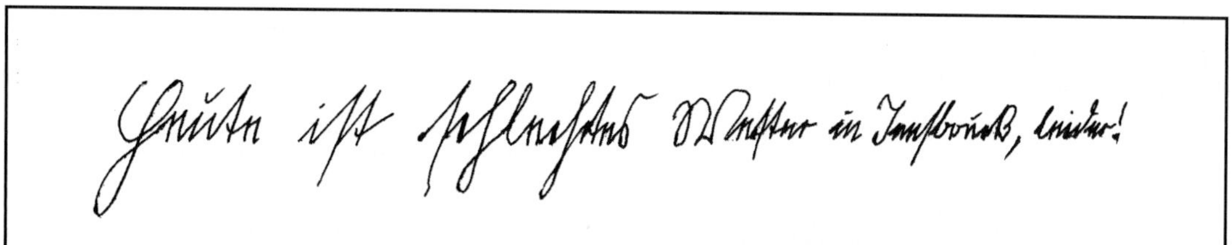

Fig. 8.2 Micrographia with decrementing script size in a patient with idiopathic PD.

tapping as well as during walking. The prototypical example of such motor blocks is freezing of gait (FoG), where the patient's feet appear to be glued to the ground while the trunk is moving forward. FoG is a major cause of falls in people with parkinsonian disorders and is commonly induced by changes in gait rhythmicity, such as turning, as well as by environmental stimuli such as narrow passages or people approaching in the opposite direction. An extreme form of start hesitation with freezing, where patients are unable to initiate walking but once under way may almost walk normally, has been described as 'gait ignition failure' (11).

Most patients presenting with bradykinetic parkinsonism also exhibit *muscular rigidity*, characterized by a steady resistance to passive movement which is independent of velocity and may include cogwheel-like rhythmic oscillations. Rigidity in parkinsonism is often described as lead-pipe rigidity since it is present to the same extent over the whole range of movement. It tends to aggravate when patients are asked to perform active movements of the opposite limb during rigidity testing. Parkinsonian rigidity can affect both limb and axial muscles, with somewhat different distributions in the different forms of parkinsonism.

Tremor (involuntary rhythmical sinusoidal oscillation of a body part) is the third cardinal motor feature of parkinsonism. The prototypical parkinsonian tremor is a 4–6 Hz resting tremor, which decreases or diminishes upon voluntary movements to revert after a new position is obtained (re-emergent tremor). It may be aggravated by fatigue, stress, or emotions. Unilateral onset and persistent asymmetry define the classical rest tremor of PD, with a subgroup of patients also showing additional postural tremor of higher frequency (12). In PD, rest tremor usually involves the limbs in isolation; head, chin, and voice tremor are uncommon. Similarly, classical 5 Hz rest tremor is uncommon in atypical degenerative parkinsonian disorders such as MSA or PSP, where irregular and jerky types of postural or kinetic tremor prevail.

The fourth cardinal feature of parkinsonism is *postural instability* and loss of postural reflexes, resulting in frequent falls. While postural instability and falls are frequent problems in advanced stages of PD, their early appearance is a hallmark in atypical parkinsonian disorders such as PSP, MSA, or CBS.

Additional clinical features

Apart from the defining cardinal motor features, patients with parkinsonian syndromes commonly show additional motor and non-motor signs that may often be helpful clinical clues to differential diagnosis depending on their type, severity, and time of presentation in the course of disease.

Dysarthria is common in all types of parkinsonism, but clinical presentation and severity differ. While some loss of volume and prosody is almost universal in PD speech, this does not significantly impair intelligibility until late in the disease course. Severe dysarthria with marked loss of volume and occasionally a high-pitched quavering voice with early loss of intelligibility are typical of MSA. Likewise, marked dysarthria is also an early feature of PSP. Depending on the cause, dysarthria may also be associated with early loss of intelligibility in some forms of symptomatic parkinsonism such as those seen in chronic manganese poisoning.

Dysphagia is also a late feature of PD, but is present earlier and to a more severe degree in PSP and MSA, where nasogastric or percutaneous gastrostomy tube feeding regularly becomes necessary (also to avoid aspiration pneumonia) within the first six to eight years of disease.

Postural deformities are also common to many types of parkinsonism. A stooped posture with flexion of the trunk is a hallmark of PD, while in MSA parkinsonism antecollis or mixed anterolaterocollis deviations are often seen in the absence of significant trunk flexion (13). However, patients with PSP typically show some degree of hyperextension of the neck and trunk, while severe degrees of trunk flexion, termed camptocormia, occur in PD and occasionally in MSA (14). The stooped posture of PD as well as hyperextension of the neck in PSP have been related to muscular rigidity, but there is ongoing controversy as to what extent antecollis posturing in MSA or camptocormia in PD might also be the result of dystonic muscle contractions or myopathy of extensor muscles (15, 16).

Dystonia is a rare presenting feature of idiopathic PD (17), but is not uncommon in autosomal recessive froms with young-onset disease like Parkin, Pink-1, and DJ-1 where focal limb dystonia has been reported in up to 40% of cases (18). Focal limb dystonia with strictly asymmetrical parkinsonism should raise suspicions of CBS; further examples of dystonia–parkinsonism syndromes include rare genetic disorders such as X-linked rapid-onset dystonia–parkinsonism (Lubag), PARK 9 (Kufor–Rakeb disease), PARK 16 or neurodegeneration with brain iron accumulation (NBIA), Wilson disease or secondary parkinsonian syndromes in manganese, carbon monoxide, or cyanide poisoning, basal ganglia infarcts, or drug-induced parkinsonism (see Table 8.2).

Myoclonus may rarely be observed as part of the spectrum of levodopa-induced involuntary movements in PD, but is otherwise incompatible with a diagnosis of idiopathic PD. Focal myoclonus of a dystonic limb is classically seen in CBS, and myoclonic jerking also causes the 'irregular' tremor commonly seen in patients with MSA.

Oculomotor disorders are usually inconspicuous in PD, where they may include slightly broken pursuit and some saccadic hypometria, but are defining features of some of the atypical parkinsonian disorders, including vertical gaze palsy in classical PSP or oculomotor dysmetria and gaze-evoked nystagmus in MSA.

Ataxia is a disease-defining accompaniment of parkinsonism in MSA, and some of the hereditary ataxias (spinocerebellar ataxias (SCAs)) may also cause a parkinsonian phenotype, in particular SCA3.

Apraxia is one of the focal cortical signs constituting a clinical hallmark of CBS, but an exclusion criterion for PD.

Dementia is a common late feature of idiopathic PD, affecting 70–80% of patients after prolonged disease of more than 10 years (19), while onset of dementia within 12 months of the first appearance of parkinsonism defines DLB. Parkinsonism–dementia combinations are also characteristic of several tauopathies, including frontotemporal dementia with parkinsonism linked to chromosome 17 (FTDP-17), CBS, and PSP, and may also occur in Alzheimer's disease.

Hallucinosis is a characteristic feature in both PD and DLB, where it includes minor forms with sensations of presence or passage in addition to well-formed visual hallucinations and, less commonly, auditory or tactile sensations. A recent study found that the occurrence of visual hallucinations had high specificity for the distinction between PD and DLB and other parkinsonian disorders like PSP, MSA, or vascular parkinsonism (20).

Autonomic failure, including orthostatic hypotension, male erectile dysfunction, and neurogenic bladder dysfunction, is a defining

Table 8.2 Conditions causing dystonia–parkinsonism

Sporadic
Parkinson's disease
Progressive supranuclear palsy
Multiple system atrophy
Corticobasal syndrome
Hemiatrophy–hemiparkinson syndrome
Toxic Carbon monoxide/cyanide Neuroleptics Manganese MPTP
Basal ganglia infarction
Inherited
X-linked dystonia–parkinsonism (Lubag, DYT3)
Dopa-responsive dystonia (DYT 5)
Rapid-onset dystonia–parkinsonism (DYT 12)
PARK 2
PARK 6
PARK 7
PARK 9 (Kufor–Rakeb disease)
PARK 16
NBIA 1 (Hallervorden–Spatz syndrome)
NBIA 2/PARK 14 (PLA2G6-related neurodegeneration)
Wilson disease
Huntington's disease
Neuroacanthocytosis
Spinocerebellar ataxia (SCA3)
GM 1 gangliosidosis
Rett syndrome

feature of MSA (21), but is also common in PD, where it occurs later in the disease course and is usually of lesser severity than in MSA.

Approach to differential diagnosis

Parkinsonism may be the clinical manifestation of a plethora of neurodegenerative, structural, toxic, metabolic, infectious, and vascular disorders (see Table 8.1). As prognosis and therapy differ considerably among parkinsonian syndromes, an early correct diagnosis is of great clinical significance. In patients presenting with the classical motor signs, including asymmetric rest tremor responding to levodopa and without atypical features, the diagnosis of PD is usually straightforward without the need for further tests. However, in the early stages of the disease, clinical overlap between PD and other neurodegenerative diseases, such as MSA, CBS, or PSP, can cause diagnostic difficulties. In a recent clinicopathological study of more than 100 cases of parkinsonism diagnosed and followed by experienced neurologists or geriatricians, specificity and positive predictive value for a post-mortem diagnosis of PD was above 90% after long-term clinical follow-up in a specialist setting. However, even in a movement disorder specialist setting, diagnostic reclassification during follow-up of patients with post-mortem confirmed PD occurred in about a third of cases, while this percentage was even higher in those with post-mortem confirmed diagnoses of one of the atypical disorders (22). Clinical misclassification rates are likely to be higher in a non-specialist setting, as exemplified by a large series of post-mortem confirmed PSP cases, of which a quarter had initially been referred as PD and only about 60% had received the correct diagnosis (23). While there are clinical pointers to aid differential diagnosis between PD and other neurodegenerative types of parkinsonism (see Table 8.3), ancillary tests are often needed to enhance diagnostic accuracy. These include drug challenge tests to assess dopaminergic responsiveness, neuroimaging to evaluate nigrostriatal presynaptic dopaminergic function or evidence for structural abnormalities as seen in many of the atypical or secondary parkinsonian disorders, or, still somewhat limited regarding use in clinical routine, genetic testing to identify the more common genetic subtypes of PD such as Parkin or LRRK2 parkinsonism.

Drug challenge testing

The responsiveness of motor symptoms to levodopa is a key feature of PD, and the sustained efficacy of levodopa even after years of treatment remains one of the major differences between PD and other forms of parkinsonism. Acute single-dose dopaminergic drug challenges using levodopa or the equipotent dopamine agonist apomorphine have been suggested as a useful tool in the differential diagnosis of PD (24). A positive response is usually defined as an improvement of more than 30% in the UPDRS motor section following acute challenges with 100–200 mg of levodopa or 2–3 mg of subcutaneous apomorphine (pre-treatment with oral domperidone 24 hours prior to testing is recommended to block the emetic effects of apomorphine). Unfortunately, the sensitivity and specificity of these acute drug-challenge tests in differentiating levodopa-responsive PD from poorly responsive atypical or secondary forms of parkinsonism are limited. The positive predictive values for the long-term response to levodopa were only 67% for apomorphine and 80% for levodopa, meaning that at least 20% of patients with levodopa-responsive parkinsonism during long-term treatment respond poorly to acute drug challenges (25). Also, patients with atypical parkinsonian disorders, such as MSA, PSP, or vascular parkinsonism, may show initial levodopa responsiveness in up to 50% of cases (26–28). In clinical practice, a negative outcome of acute dopaminergic testing should never discourage a trial of sustained treatment with levodopa at a sufficient dose (300–600 mg/day for at least 2 months, and even higher doses can be tried for clinically typical PD). In view of this, acute drug challenge testing is of limited use in clinical practice. In addition, it should be noted that, although similar diagnostic accuracies have been reported for single-dose drug challenges and chronic dopaminergic therapy (29), some guidelines discourage its use in the differential diagnosis of parkinsonian disorders (www.nice.org.uk).

Genetic testing

An increasing number of genetic loci, currently listed as PARK1–18, have been linked to PD, and mutations within six of these loci cause familial parkinsonism in a Mendelian fashion (SNCA, LRRK2, PARKIN, DJ1, PINK1, and ATP13A2), all but ATP13A2 clinically closely resembling idiopathic PD (30). Furthermore, polymorphic variations within two of these loci (SNCA, LRRK2) have been

Table 8.3 Differential diagnosis of parkinsonian syndromes

	PD	MSA	PSP	CBS	Vascular parkinsonism	Drug-induced parkinsonism
Family history	Occasionally positive	Rarely positive	Rarely positive	Rarely positive	Negative	Negative
Symmetry	Asymmetric	Asymmetric	Symmetric	Asymmetric	Asymmetric or symmetric	Asymmetric or symmetric
Akinesia	+	+	+	+	+	+
Classical resting tremor	+	–	+/–	–	+	+
Rigidity	+	+	Axial > limb	Axial < limb	+	+
Early postural instability	–	+	+	+	+/–	+/–
Early falls	–	+	+	+	–	–
Supranuclear gaze palsy	–	–	+	+	–	–
Early autonomic failure	–	+	+/–	+/–	–	–
Apraxia	–	–	+	+	–	–
Levodopa response	Excellent and sustained response	Transient and poor response	Transient and poor response	Poor response	Inconsistent response	Inconsistent response

validated as genetic risk factors for PD (31–33). In the absence of implications of a positive or negative test on patient management against a background of cost and unresolved ethical issues, genetic testing is currently not part of clinical routine in the diagnostic work-up of PD. This may well change for the more common mutations once selective and disease-modifying therapies begin to emerge. The chance of detecting a Parkin gene mutation in a subject with young-onset parkinsonism is less than 5% in sporadic cases, and the chance of identifying a mutation of LRRK2 in European patients with typical late-onset PD and a positive family history is about 7% (18, 34).

On the other hand, molecular genetic testing is an essential part of the diagnostic process in a variety of conditions presenting as 'parkinsonism-plus' disorders featuring various combinations of parkinsonism with dystonia, ataxia, pyramidal signs, and cognitive dysfunction including Wilson disease, SCA2 or SCA3, dopa-responsive dystonia (DYT3 and DYT5) or DYT12, NBIAs, or fragile X-associated tremor–ataxia syndrome (FXTAS) (see Table 8.4).

Olfactory testing

Hyposmia, referred to as difficulties in the detection, discrimination, and identification of odours, is a prominent and early symptom in PD and is found in up to 90% of patients (35). Notably, olfactory dysfunction seems to be unrelated to disease duration or the manifestation of motor symptoms of PD, and is not influenced by antiparkinsonian drugs. In contrast, olfactory function is normal in PSP, CBS, vascular parkinsonism, and essential tremor, and the deficit seems to be mild in MSA (36). A recent study has also shown that hyposmia discriminates between patients with parkinsonism who have abnormal nigrostriatal function as assessed by dopamine transporter (DAT) imaging and those who do not (scans without evidence of dopaminergic deficit (SWEDDs)) (37). Therefore olfactory testing may be useful in the differential diagnosis of parkinsonian syndromes. The most widely used test worldwide to date is the University of Pennsylvania Smell Identification Test (UPSIT) which contains some odours culture-specific for the North American population, while the test battery called Sniffin Sticks has been validated for the European population. It comprises subtests for olfactory discrimination, identification, and odour threshold, and has been successfully applied to PD patient cohorts (38).

Cardiovascular reflex testing

Since the presence of autonomic failure is a key feature of MSA, cardiovascular reflex testing, especially the verification of orthostatic hypotension in head-up tilt-table testing, has been put forward for the differentiation between PD and MSA. Indeed, orthostatic hypotension with a drop of blood pressure of more than 30 mmHg systolic or more than 15 mmHg diastolic in head-up tilt has been found in about 50% of patients with MSA but in only about 20% of PD patients (39). In addition, orthostatic drops in blood pressure are significantly higher in patients with MSA. Nevertheless, because of the overlap between the two entities, cardiovascular reflex testing is not conclusive in individual cases even at the earliest stages of disease.

Urodynamic assessment

Analogous to orthostatic hypotension, other features of autonomic failure, such as urodynamic and erectile dysfunctions, are much more common in MSA than in PD and PSP. Therefore characteristic patterns of abnormality, such as detrusor hyperreflexia and abnormal urethral sphincter function, have been assessed for differential diagnosis. Similarly, the use of sphincter electromyography, exhibiting denervation in MSA due to degeneration of Onuf's nucleus in the spinal cord (40), has been tested regarding its role in differential diagnosis. None of these parameters was able to reliably discriminate between MSA and PD in clinical trials (41).

Brain imaging

Neuroimaging techniques are the single most informative group of ancillary investigations in the diagnostic work-up of parkinsonism in clinical practice. While their use may seem unnecessary in patients with the classical clinical presentation of levodopa-responsive PD, they may yield important clues in many instances of clinical uncertainty; functional radiotracer imaging may distinguish between parkinsonian and non-parkinsoniam tremor syndromes, and structural imaging may reveal causes of secondary parkinsonism or give indications for MSA, PSP, or CBS.

Table 8.4 Rare hereditary neurodegenerative disorders causing symptomatic parkinsonism

Disorder	Genes (loci)	Clinical features
Frontotemporal dementia with parkinsonism linked to chromosome 17 (FDTP-17)	Microtubule-associated protein tau-gene (17q21.1)	Parkinsonism, vertical gaze palsy, dystonia, executive dysfunction, behavioural changes, language impairment, progressive dementia
Huntington's disease	Huntingtin gene (4p16.3)	Akinetic–rigid syndrome, often associated with early disease onset (Westphal variant)
SCA mutations		
SCA2	Ataxin-2 (12q24)	Ataxia, dystonia, pyramidal signs, neuropathy, myoclonus, tremor, parkinsonism (rarely responsive to levodopa)
SCA3 (Machado–Joseph disease)	Ataxin-3 (14q24.3-q31)	Ataxia, dystonia, chorea, spasticity, parkinsonism (rarely responsive to levodopa)
Wilson disease	ATP7B gene (13q14.3-q21.1)	Neurological presentation with tremor, dystonia, parkinsonism, cerebellar signs, gait disturbance and psychiatric disturbance, Kayser–Fleischer rings, hepatic manifestation, osteoporosis, haemolytic anaemia, skin hyperpigmentation
Fragile X-associated tremor–ataxia syndrome	FMR1 gene (Xq27.3)	Tremor, parkinsonism, ataxia
Dystonia-plus syndromes		
DYT3 (X-linked dystonia parkinsonism, Lubag)	TAF1-gene (Xq13)	Progressive generalized dystonia and parkinsonism, occasionally responsive to levodopa
DYT5 (Segawa syndrome, dopa-responsive dystonia)	GTP cyclohydrolase 1-gene (14q22.1-q22.2)	Young-onset dystonia parkinsonism, responsive to levodopa
DYT12 (rapid-onset dystonia parkinsonism)	ATP1A3 (19q12-q13.2)	Rapid onset of dystonia and parkinsonism in young adults
Neuronal brain iron accumulation syndromes		
NBIA type 1 (Hallervorden–Spatz disease, pantothenate kinase-associated neurodegeneration)	PANK 2 (20p13-p12.3)	Onset in the first decade, progressive generalized dystonia, dysarthria, spasticity, mental retardation; rarely presenting as rapidly progressive parkinsonism
NBIA type 2/PARK 14	PLA2G6 (22q13.1)	Infantile neuroaxonal dystrophy; may present as dopa-responsive parkinsonism with dystonia
Neuroferritinopathy	FTL 1 (19q13.3-q13.4)	Dystonia, chorea, occasionally parkinsonism
Parkinsonism–amyotrophic lateral sclerosis dementia complex of Guam	TRPM7 gene (15q21)	Parkinsonism, ALS, dementia
Fahr's syndrome (familial basal ganglia calcification)	IBGC1 (14q)	Progressive parkinsonism, dystonia, tremor, dementia
Neuroacanthocytosis	VPS13A gene (9q21)	Orofacial chorea, dystonia, tics, parkinsonism, axonal neuropathy, cognitive decline, cardiac manifestations (arrhythmias and cardiomyopathies)

ALS, amyotrophic lateral sclerosis.

Role of structural brain imaging

Although usually normal in classical PD, cranial computed tomography (cCT) should probably be performed as part of the routine diagnostic work-up in every patient presenting with parkinsonism to rule out secondary forms such as vascular parkinsonism, normal pressure hydrocephalus, structural basal ganglia pathology, or (rarely) frontal meningioma. Even in otherwise typical PD, vascular or other concomitant brain pathology revealed by structural imaging is of potential clinical relevance regarding drug treatment and prognosis.

Wherever possible, however, magnetic resonance imaging (MRI) should be the preferred imaging modality because of its superior solution and higher diagnostic sensitivity. In particular, MRI has far greater sensitivity for detecting basal ganglia pathology in conditions such as Wilson disease, NBIA, or manganism. In addition, only MRI has sufficient sensitivity to detect structural abnormalities suggesting atypical parkinsonism, such as midbrain atrophy and the 'penguin' or 'colibri' sign in PSP, putaminal and/or cerebellar and pontine atrophy in MSA, or asymmetrical parietal cortical atrophy in CBS (see Table 8.5 and Fig. 8.3).

Furthermore, advanced MRI techniques, such as diffusion-weighted imaging (DWI) and diffusion tensor imaging (DTI), are sensitive to changes in the integrity of neuronal tissue that are not associated with signal changes or atrophy on conventional MRI. Diffusivity changes have been described in the putamen in MSA and PSP patients, and increased diffusivity in the middle cerebellar peduncle has been proposed as a differential diagnostic MRI sign separating MSA from PSP (42).

Single photon emission computed tomography (SPECT)

Radiotracer imaging is able to provide information on functional changes of the nigrostriatal dopaminergic projection, as first shown with positron emission tomography (PET) using ^{18}F-fluorodopa as a tracer molecule in patients with PD (43). In contrast with PET, which has developed into a powerful research tool in parkinsonian disorders, SPECT is widely clinically available and, although it has lower spatial resolution and poorer signal-to-noise-ratio, it can also detect pre- and post-synaptic functional changes in the nigrostriatal dopaminergic system and elsewhere, depending on the tracers used. Currently, only

Table 8.5 Role of cCT and MRI in the differential diagnosis of parkinsonism

Imaging technique	Findings	Diagnostic relevance	Sensitivity	Specificity
cCT	Structural lesions	Discrimination of secondary causes of parkinsonism	Moderate–high	Moderate–high
	Cerebral micro/macroangiopathy	Discrimination of VP	Moderate–high	Low
	Dilated ventricles	Discrimination of NPH	High	High
	Cortical atrophy	Discrimination of DLB, CBS, FTDP-17	Moderate	Moderate
	Subcortical/infratentorial atrophy	Discrimination of MSA, PSP	Low	Moderate
Structural MRI	Structural lesions	Discrimination of secondary causes of parkinsonism	High	Moderate–high
	Cerebral micro/macroangiopathy	Discrimination of VP	High	Moderate–high
	Dilated ventricles	Discrimination of NPH	High	High
	Cortical atrophy	Discrimination of DLB, CBS, FTDP-17	Moderate–high	High
	Subcortical/infratentorial atrophy	Discrimination of MSA, PSP	Moderate–high	Moderate–high
	Subcortical signal alterations	Discrimination of MSA, PSP		
	Putaminal hypointensity in combination with a hyperintense putaminal rim	Discrimination of MSA		
	Hot cross bun sign	Discrimination of MSA		
	'Penguin' sign	Discrimination of PSP		
DWI/DTI	ADC putamen	Discrimination of MSA, PSP	High	High
	FA putamen	Discrimination of MSA	High	High
	ADC pons	Discrimination of MSA	Moderate	Moderate
	ADC superior cerebellar peduncle	Discrimination of PSP	High	High
	ADC middle cerebellar peduncle	Discrimination of MSA	Moderate–high	High
Planimetry	Reduced AP midbrain diameter	Discrimination of PSP	Moderate	Moderate–high
	Reduction of midbrain-to-pontine area ratio	Discrimination of MSA	High	High
Volumetry	Volume loss putamen	Discrimination of MSA	Moderate	Moderate–high
	Volume loss midbrain	Discrimination of PSP	Moderate–high	moderate–high

VP, vascular parkinsonism; NPH, normal pressure hydrocephalus; DLB, dementia with Lewy bodies; CBS, corticobasal syndrome; FTDP-17, frontotemporal dementia with parkinsonism linked to chromosome 17; MSA, multiple system atrophy; PSP, progressive supranuclear palsy; ADC, apparent diffusion coefficient; FA, fractional anisotropy; DWI, diffusion-weighted imaging; DTI, diffusion tensor imaging.

dopamine transporter SPECT imaging using the commercially available tracer FP-CIT is licensed as a routine procedure for differential diagnosis in parkinsonian disorders.

FP-CIT SPECT The SPECT technique most widely used in the differential diagnosis of parkinsonism is dopamine transporter (DAT) imaging. The commercially available tracer ^{123}I-FP-CIT (^{123}I-2-carbomethoxy-3-(4-iodophenyl)-*N*-(3-fluoropropyl)-nortropane) (DAT-Scan) binds specifically to presynaptic dopamine transporters of nigrostriatal nerve endings, and semiquantitative region of interest (ROI) based analysis of DAT-SPECT is able to identify reduced striatal tracer binding in PD and other parkinsonian syndromes associated with degeneration of the nigrostriatal projections (44). In PD, these changes are typically asymmetrical and correlate with disease duration and severity of motor symptoms (45, 46). DAT-SPECT is useful to distinguish PD from other tremor disorders without nigrostriatal neurodegeneration, such as essential or dystonic tremor, as well as from drug-induced parkinsonism, psychogenic parkinsonism, and levodopa-responsive dystonia presenting with parkinsonism (47). This imaging modality is also helpful in rejecting or confirming a possible diagnosis of neurodegenerative parkinsonism in subjects with equivocal or vague symptoms or atypical tremor presentations like unilateral postural tremor. SWEDDs can be taken as a firm exclusion of PD according to long-term follow-up data of a series of cases with this constellation. In contrast, DAT-SPECT is not able to distinguish reliably between patients with different types of degenerative parkinsonism, such as PD, MSA, PSP, or CBS, although novel image analysis techniques may improve this in future (48). Distinction between PD and vascular parkinsonism when using DAT-SPECT also seems imperfect (49).

IBZM-SPECT IBZM (^{123}I-3-iodo-6-methoxy benzamine) is a ligand which specifically binds to D2-receptors, enabling visualization of postsynaptic dopamine receptors within the striatum. Based on the sparing of striatal neurons in the pathology of PD and their involvement in other types of degenerative parkinsonism, such as MSA and PSP, postsynaptic dopamine receptor imaging has been proposed as a differential diagnostic tool (50). In early untreated PD patients, IBZM-SPECT studies revealed a relative increase in D2-binding, especially in the putamen contralateral to the more affected body side (51). In contrast, tracer uptake seems to be reduced even in the earliest stages of atypical parkinsonian conditions such as MSA and PSP (52). However, there is considerable overlap, particularly in early disease stages, where clinical differentiation is the most difficult, such that postsynaptic dopamine

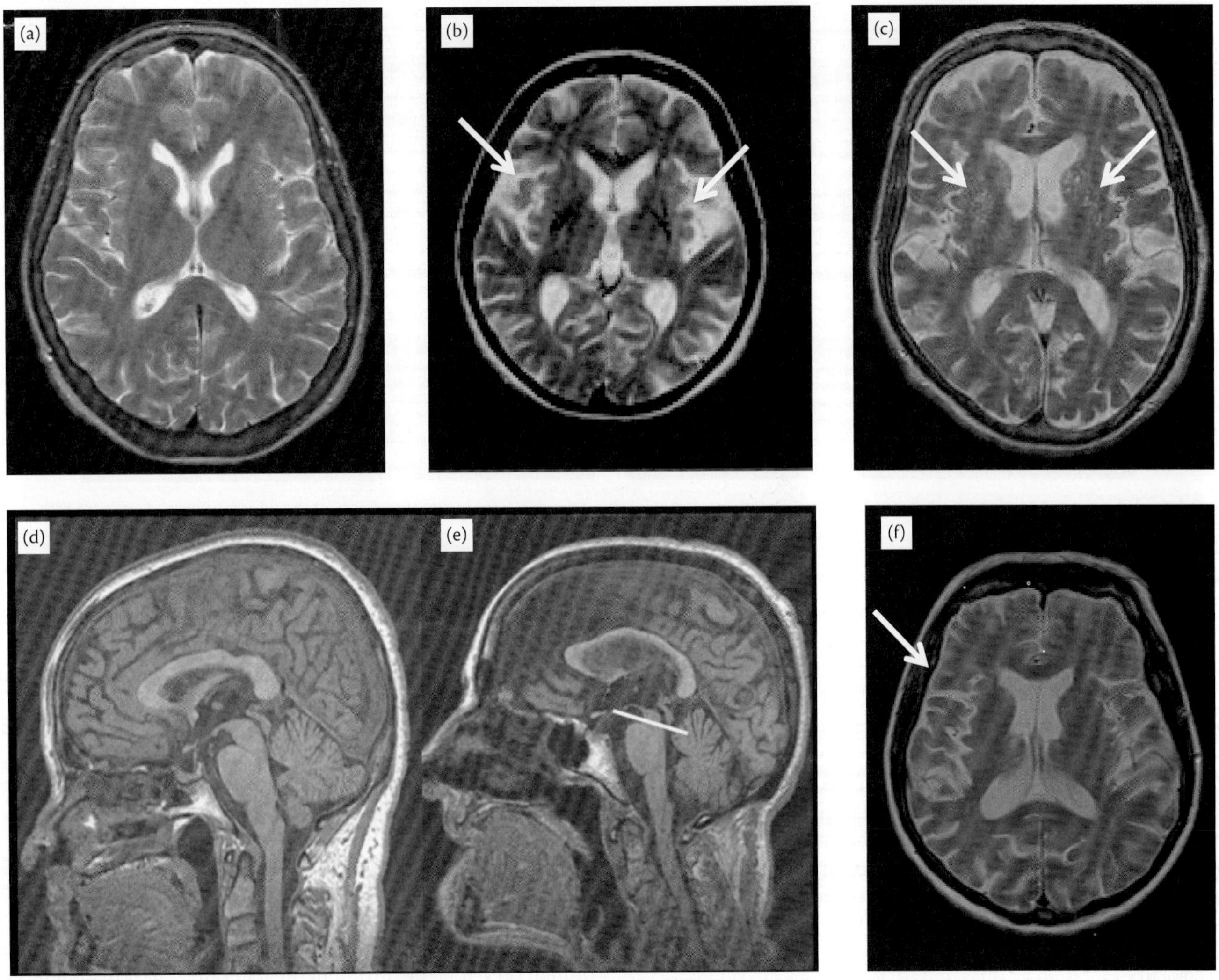

Fig. 8.3 (a) Normal MRI in a patient with idiopathic PD; (b) putaminal atrophy and putaminal hypointensity in a patient with MSA; (c) vascular lesions in a patient with vascular parkinsonism; (d) mid-sagittal T_1-weighted MRI in a patient with idiopathic PD; (e) mid-sagittal T_1-weighted MRI in a PSP patient, exhibiting marked midbrain atrophy without significant pontine atrophy (divided by white line) forming the silhouette of a penguin or colibri; (f) asymmetric parietal atrophy in a patient with CBS.

D2 receptor SPECT imaging has limited value in clinical practice, although high predictive values have been reported for the combined application of IBZM-SPECT and FP-CIT SPECT in the evaluation of PD and MSA (53).

MIBG-SPECT ^{123}I-MIBG (meta-iodobenzyl guanidine), an analogue of norepinephrine, is a tracer used to assess sympathetic cardiac innervation, which is significantly reduced even in early PD, while postganglionic sympathetic efferents are spared in MSA. Therefore MIBG-SPECT is potentially useful in the differential diagnosis of these types of degenerative parkinsonism, with reduced binding in PD versus normal cardiac uptake in MSA. However, there can be false-negative results in patients with PD without significant autonomic nervous system involvement (54).

Transcranial sonography

Transcranial sonography (TCS) can visualize the butterfly-shaped structure of the midbrain using an acoustic temporal bone window. About 90% of patients with idiopathic PD show increased areas of hyperechogenicity in the substantia nigra (SN) region of the midbrain with this technique (see Fig. 8.4), but this is not the case in patients with PSP and MSA who, unlike PD patients, have been reported to show increased areas of echogenicity in the lenticular nucleus (55). A recent study has proposed that hyperechogenicity of the SN in combination with normal echogenicities in the lenticular nucleus discriminates PD from PSP and MSA with a positive predictive value of over 90% (56). In addition, another recent study has demonstrated that midbrain hyperechogenicity is able to distinguish between PD patients and SWEDD patients (57). While these observations are certainly of great interest, the precise role of TCS in the diagnostic work-up of parkinsonism in clinical practice still needs to be defined.

Principles of management

The therapeutic management of parkinsonian disorders is complex and often involves multidisciplinary approaches combining medical therapies with non-pharmacological measures such as physiotherapy, speech therapy, or psychosocial counselling. In

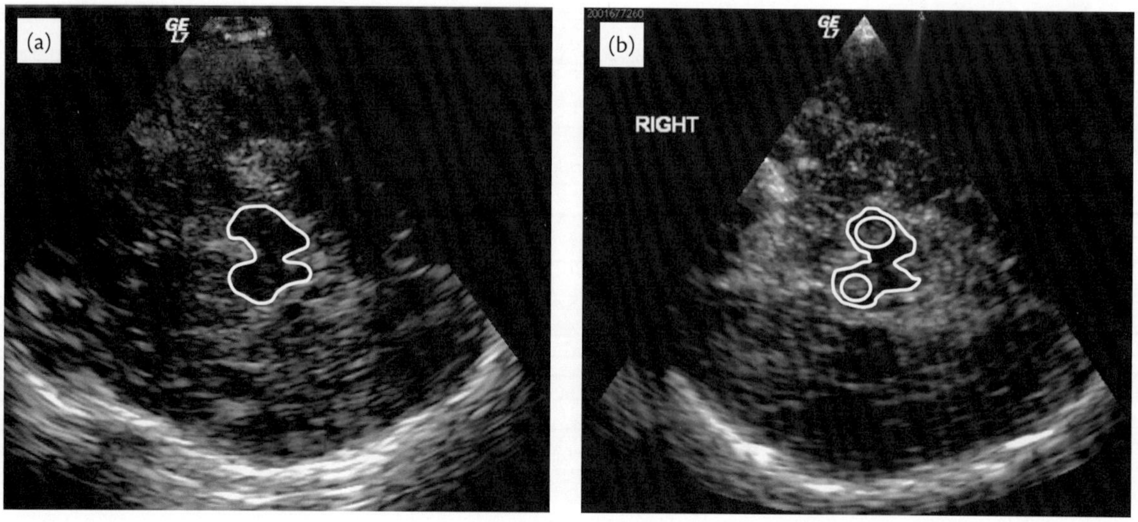

Fig. 8.4 (a) TCS visualization of the butterfly-shaped structure of the midbrain in a healthy subject; (b) hyperechogenicity of the substantia nigra in a patient with idiopathic PD.

addition, deep brain surgery has become an important modality for a subset of PD patients with drug-related complications. Details of these different approaches and their indications for the miscellaneous forms of degenerative and secondary parkinsonism can be found in the respective chapters of this volume. In principle, all available therapies for degenerative parkinsonian disorders are symptomatic, and so far no approach has been proved to slow or halt the underlying progression of disease. This can be different for some secondary types of parkinsonism where removal of a causative drug or tumour or eradication of an underlying infection (see Table 8.1) may even lead to complete remission. Despite all recent advances in the drug treatment of parkinsonism, levodopa substitution has remained the gold standard of symptomatic efficacy for PD, and is often at least partially effective in other types of degenerative or secondary parkinsonism. However, the magnitude of response is most pronounced in PD, such that levodopa responsiveness is part of the clinical diagnostic criteria of PD. Therefore, depending on the results of the diagnostic work-up, a trial of levodopa will be part of the treatment approach in most patients presenting with parkinsonism.

Key advances

The most important advances in the field of parkinsonism in recent years have been related to the genetics of PD and insights into pathophysiological pathways developing out of genetic discoveries (see Chapter 7). Clinicopathological studies have re-focused on clinical differential diagnosis between different types of degenerative parkinsonism, recognizing a parkinsonian variant of PSP (28) that can initially closely mimic PD, as well as the impossibility of reliably distinguishing between the tauopathies of PSP and CBS on clinical grounds alone (58). Important advances have also been made in the use of neuroimaging to aid differential diagnosis of parkinsonism, where dopamine transporter SPECT has become a routine clinical tool for distinguishing between PD and atypical tremor of other aetiology, and has introduced the new diagnostic concept of SWEDDs for patients presenting with signs of parkinsonism clinically but with 'scans without evidence of dopaminergic deficit' (59). Perhaps even more importantly, advanced MRI has shown promise of differentiating between the different types of degenerative parkinsonism early in the disease course, and transcranial ultrasound has entered the stage as a potential novel diagnostic imaging tool.

Future developments

A key priority of clinical research in parkinsonian disorders is again driven by the PD field and is likely to lead to new concepts for early diagnosis and at-risk definition, including 'pre-motor' signs of disease as well as molecular and imaging markers. Biomarkers for the different degenerative parkinsonian syndromes are also a major requirement for improved differential diagnosis, and studies of their progression include clinical trials of disease-modifying agents. Genetic and proteomic markers distinguishing between the different neurodegenerative disorders associated with parkinsonism are evolving, with some showing promising sensitivities and specificities (60, 61). High-field MR holds the promise of detecting early PD with high sensitivity and specificity (62), and transcranial ultrasound is being suggested as a future tool for screening for PD risk in the general population (63).

Conclusions

Diagnosing idiopathic PD can be a straightforward clinical exercise in cases presenting with a typical history and classical clinical features which subsequently show an excellent response to levodopa. In many cases, however, a patient with new-onset parkinsonism will require consideration of a broad spectrum of differential diagnoses, and diagnostic accuracy will often remain suboptimal. Judicious use of structural and functional neuroimaging techniques will often enhance accuracy of early diagnosis. Although in the case of PD this can be further refined by genetic testing in those with a family history and/or young onset of disease, there is no immediate management implication emanating from such testing and it is not currently part of routine diagnostic work-up. Simple as the elementary clinical definition of a parkinsonian syndrome may be, differential diagnosis of parkinsonism continues to require considerable clinical acumen in terms of careful assessment and weighing of the details in the history and the clinical findings as well as making optimal use of ancillary tests, avoiding unnecessary over-investigation. Even in the hands of movement disorder experts, clinical differential diagnosis between the early stages of PD and atypical degenerative parkinsonian disorders is often difficult, if not impossible, such that there is need for further refinement of diagnostic molecular or imaging markers for the different diseases.

Key points

- Parkinsonism is the presenting feature in a variety of diseases of different aetiologies including sporadic or genetic neurodegenerative disorders and structural basal ganglia lesions from infectious, inflammatory, vascular, neoplastic, and toxic causes.
- Clinical differential diagnosis is aided by patterns of topography and profile of cardinal motor features, specific combinations of neurological signs, and drug response characteristic of different forms of parkinsonism.
- Structural neuroimaging using MR, including advanced MR techniques as well as functional imaging using dopamine transporter (DAT) SPECT, is part of the clinical routine to aid early differential diagnosis. MR findings can provide clues for secondary parkinsonism and diffusion tensor MRI may enhance the distinction between PD and the atypical parkinsonism of MSA or PSP, while DAT imaging is useful to distinguish atypical tremors from PD or to confirm or reject degenerative parkinsonism in cases with clinically uncertain signs.
- Management of parkinsonism is multifaceted and multidisciplinary, depending on cause or subtype, but levodopa remains the single most effective agent to reduce the cardinal motor features.

References

1. Seijo-Martinez M, Castro del Rio M, Rodríguez Alvarez J, et al. Prevalence of parkinsonism and Parkinson's disease in the Arosa Island (Spain): a community-based door-to-door survey. *J Neurol Sci* 2011; 304: 49–54.
2. Bennett DA, Beckett LA, Murray AM, et al. Prevalence of parkinsonian signs and associated mortality in a community population of older people. *N Engl J Med* 1996; 334: 71–6.
3. Benito-León J, Bermejo-Pareja F, Rodríguez J, et al. Prevalence of PD and other types of parkinsonism in three elderly populations of central Spain. *Mov Disord* 2003; 18: 267–74.
4. Wenning GK, Kiechl S, Seppi K, et al. Prevalence of movement disorders in men and women aged 50–89 years (Bruneck Study cohort): a population-based study. *Lancet Neurol* 2005; 4: 815–20.
5. Bower JH, Maraganore DM, McDonnell SK, Rocca WA. Incidence and distribution of parkinsonism in Olmsted County, Minnesota, 1976–1990. *Neurology* 1999; 52: 214–20.
6. Schrag A, Ben-Shlomo Y, Quinn NP. Prevalence of progressive supranuclear palsy and multiple system atrophy: a cross-sectional study. *Lancet* 1999; 354: 1771–5.
7. Schrag A, Ben-Shlomo Y, Quinn NP. Cross sectional prevalence survey of idiopathic Parkinson's disease and Parkinsonism in London. *BMJ* 2000; 321: 21–2.
8. Nalls MA, Plagnol V, Hernandez DG, et al. Imputation of sequence variants for identification of genetic risks for Parkinson's disease: a meta-analysis of genome-wide association studies. *Lancet* 2011; 377: 641–9.
9. Alexander GE, DeLong MR, Strick PL. Parallel organization of functionally segregated circuits linking basal ganglia and cortex. *Annu Rev Neurosci* 1986; 9: 357–81.
10. Gibb WR, Lees AJ. The significance of the Lewy body in the diagnosis of idiopathic Parkinson's disease. *Neuropathol Appl Neurobiol* 1989; 15: 27–44.
11. Atchison PR, Thompson PD, Frackowiak RS, Marsden CD. The syndrome of gait ignition failure: a report of six cases. *Mov Disord* 1993; 8: 285–92.
12. Hallett M, Deuschl G. Are we making progress in the understanding of tremor in Parkinson's disease? *Ann Neurol* 2010; 68: 780–1.
13. Quinn N. Disproportionate antecollis in multiple system atrophy. *Lancet* 1989; i: 844.
14. Tolosa E, Compta Y. Dystonia in Parkinson's disease. *J Neurol* 2006; 253 (Suppl 7): VII7–13.
15. Wanschitz JV, Sawires M, Seppi K, et al. Axial myopathy in parkinsonism. *Mov Disord* 2011; 26: 1569–71.
16. Margraf NG, Wrede A, Rohr A, et al. Camptocormia in idiopathic Parkinson's disease: a focal myopathy of the paravertebral muscles. *Mov Disord* 2010; 25: 542–51.
17. Poewe WH, Lees AJ, Stern GM. Dystonia in Parkinson's disease: clinical and pharmacological features. *Ann Neurol* 1988; 23: 73–8.
18. Lücking CB, Dürr A, Bonifati V, et al. Association between early-onset Parkinson's disease and mutations in the parkin gene. *N Engl J Med* 2000; 342: 1560–7.
19. Hely MA, Reid WG, Adena MA, Halliday GM, Morris JG. The Sydney multicenter study of Parkinson's disease: the inevitability of dementia at 20 years. *Mov Disord* 2008; 23: 837–44.
20. Williams DR, Lees AJ. Visual hallucinations in the diagnosis of idiopathic Parkinson's disease: a retrospective autopsy study. *Lancet Neurol* 2005; 4: 605–10.
21. Gilman S, Wenning GK, Low PA, et al. Second consensus statement on the diagnosis of multiple system atrophy. *Neurology* 2008; 71: 670–6.
22. Hughes AJ, Daniel SE, Ben-Shlomo Y, Lees AJ. The accuracy of diagnosis of parkinsonian syndromes in a specialist movement disorder service. *Brain* 2002; 125: 861–70.
23. Nath U, Ben-Shlomo Y, Thomson RG, et al. The prevalence of progressive supranuclear palsy (Steele–Richardson–Olszewski syndrome) in the UK. *Brain* 2001; 124: 1438–49.
24. Merello M, Nouzeilles MI, Arce GP, Leiguarda R. Accuracy of acute levodopa challenge for clinical prediction of sustained long-term levodopa response as a major criterion for idiopathic Parkinson's disease diagnosis. *Mov Disord* 2002; 17: 795–8.
25. Hughes AJ, Lees AJ, Stern GM. Challenge tests to predict the dopaminergic response in untreated Parkinson's disease. *Neurology* 1991; 41: 1723–5.
26. Colosimo C, Pezzella FR. The symptomatic treatment of multiple system atrophy. *Eur J Neurol* 2002; 9: 195–9.
27. Zijlmans JC, Katzenschlager R, Daniel SE, Lees AJ. The L-dopa response in vascular parkinsonism. *J Neurol Neurosurg Psychiatry* 2004; 75: 545–7.
28. Williams DR, de Silva R, Paviour DC. Characteristics of two distinct clinical phenotypes in pathologically proven progressive supranuclear palsy: Richardson's syndrome and PSP-parkinsonism. *Brain* 2005; 128: 1247–58.
29. Clarke CE, Davies P. Systematic review of acute levodopa and apomorphine challenge tests in the diagnosis of idiopathic Parkinson's disease. *J Neurol Neurosurg Psychiatry* 2000; 69: 590–4.
30. Lesage S, Brice. Parkinson's disease: from monogenic forms to genetic susceptibility factors. *Hum Mol Genet* 2009; 18(R1): R48–59.

31. Mueller JC, Fuchs J, Hofer A, et al. Multiple regions of alpha-synuclein are associated with Parkinson's disease. *Ann Neurol* 2005; 57: 535–41.
32. Ross OA, Wu YR, Lee MC et al. Analysis of Lrrk2 R1628P as a risk factor for Parkinson's disease. *Ann Neurol* 2008; 64: 88–92.
33. Di Fonzo A, Wu-Chou YH, Lu CS, et al. A common missense variant in the LRRK2 gene, Gly2385Arg, associated with Parkinson's disease risk in Taiwan. *Neurogenetics* 2006; 7: 133–8.
34. Healy DG, Falchi M, O'Sullivan SS, et al. Phenotype, genotype, and worldwide genetic penetrance of LRRK2-associated Parkinson's disease: a case–control study. *Lancet Neurol* 2008; 7: 583–90.
35. Katzenschlager R, Lees AJ. Olfaction and Parkinson's syndromes: its role in differential diagnosis. *Curr Opin Neurol* 2004; 17: 417–23.
36. Wenning GK, Shephard B, Hawkes C, Petruckevitch A, Lees A, Quinn N. Olfactory function in atypical parkinsonian syndromes. *Acta Neurol Scand* 1995; 91: 247–50.
37. Silveira-Moriyama L, Schwingenschuh P, O'Donnell A, et al. Olfaction in patients with suspected parkinsonism and scans without evidence of dopaminergic deficit (SWEDDs). *J Neurol Neurosurg Psychiatry* 2009; 80: 744–8.
38. Boesveldt S, de Muinck Keizer RJ, Knol DL, Wolters ECh, Berendse HW. Extended testing across, not within, tasks raises diagnostic accuracy of smell testing in Parkinson's disease. *Mov Disord* 2009; 24: 85–90.
39. Wenning GK, Seppi K, Poewe W, et al. Differential association of orthostatic hypotension with the cerebellar versus parkinsonian presentation of multiple system atrophy. *Neurology* 2001; 56: A444.
40. Pramstaller PP, Wenning GK, Smith SJ, Beck RO, Quinn NP, Fowler CJ. Nerve conduction studies, skeletal muscle EMG, and sphincter EMG in multiple system atrophy. *J Neurol Neurosurg Psychiatry* 1995; 58: 618–21.
41. Riley DE, Chelimsky TC. Autonomic nervous system testing may not distinguish multiple system atrophy from Parkinson's disease. *J Neurol Neurosurg Psychiatry* 2003; 74: 56–60.
42. Mahlknecht P, Hotter A, Hussl A, Esterhammer R, Schocke M, Seppi K. Significance of MRI in diagnosis and differential diagnosis of Parkinson's disease. *Neurodegener Dis* 2010; 7: 300–18.
43. Calne DB, Langston JW, Martin WR, et al. Positron emission tomography after MPTP: observations relating to the cause of Parkinson's disease. *Nature* 1985; 317: 246–8.
44. Scherfler C, Nocker M. Dopamine transporter SPECT: how to remove subjectivity? *Mov Disord* 2009; 24 (Suppl 2): S721–4.
45. Benamer HT, Patterson J, Wyper DJ, Hadley DM, Macphee GJ, Grosset DG. Correlation of Parkinson's disease severity and duration with ^{123}I-FP-CIT SPECT striatal uptake. *Mov Disord* 2000; 15: 692–8.
46. Booij J, Tissingh G, Boer GJ, et al. (^{123}I)FP-CIT SPECT shows a pronounced decline of striatal dopamine transporter labelling in early and advanced Parkinson's disease. *J Neurol Neurosurg Psychiatry* 1997; 62: 133–40.
47. Scherfler C, Schwarz J, Antonini A, et al. Role of DAT-SPECT in the diagnostic work up of parkinsonism. *Mov Disord* 2007; 22: 1229–38.
48. Goebel G, Seppi K, Donnemiller E, et al. A novel computer-assisted image analysis of (^{123}I)beta-CIT SPECT images improves the diagnostic accuracy of parkinsonian disorders. *Eur J Nucl Med Mol Imaging* 2011; 38: 702–10.
49. Zijlmans J, Evans A, Fontes F, et al. (^{123}I) FP-CIT spect study in vascular parkinsonism and Parkinson's disease. *Mov Disord* 2007; 22: 1278–85.
50. Brücke T, Asenbaum S, Pirker W, et al. Measurement of the dopaminergic degeneration in Parkinson's disease with (^{123}I) beta-CIT and SPECT. Correlation with clinical findings and comparison with multiple system atrophy and progressive supranuclear palsy. *J Neural Transm Suppl* 1997; 50: 9–24.
51. Kaasinen V, Ruottinen HM, Någren K, Lehikoinen P, Oikonen V, Rinne JO. Upregulation of putaminal dopamine D2 receptors in early Parkinson's disease: a comparative PET study with (^{11}C) raclopride and (^{11}C)N-methylspiperone. *J Nucl Med* 2000; 41: 65–70.
52. van Royen E, Verhoeff NF, Speelman JD, Wolters EC, Kuiper MA, Janssen AG. Multiple system atrophy and progressive supranuclear palsy. Diminished striatal D2 dopamine receptor activity demonstrated by ^{123}I-IBZM single photon emission computed tomography. *Arch Neurol* 1993; 50: 513–16.
53. Plotkin M, Amthauer H, Klaffke S, et al. Combined ^{123}I-FP-CIT and 123I-IBZM SPECT for the diagnosis of parkinsonian syndromes: study on 72 patients. *J Neural Transm* 2005; 112: 677–92.
54. Courbon F, Brefel-Courbon C, Thalamas C, et al. Cardiac MIBG scintigraphy is a sensitive tool for detecting cardiac sympathetic denervation in Parkinson's disease. *Mov Disord* 2003; 18: 890–7.
55. Vlaar AM, Bouwmans A, Mess WH, Tromp SC, Weber WE. Transcranial duplex in the differential diagnosis of parkinsonian syndromes: a systematic review. *J Neurol* 2009; 256: 530–8.
56. Behnke S, Berg D, Naumann M, Becker G. Differentiation of Parkinson's disease and atypical parkinsonian syndromes by transcranial ultrasound. *J Neurol Neurosurg Psychiatry* 2005; 76: 423–5.
57. Stockner H, Schwingenschuh P, Djamshidian A, et al. Is transcranial sonography useful to distinguish scans without evidence of dopaminergic deficit patients from Parkinson's disease? *Mov Disord* 2012; 27: 1182–5.
58. Ling H, O'Sullivan SS, Holton JL, et al. Does corticobasal degeneration exist? A clinicopathological re-evaluation. *Brain* 2010; 133: 2045–57.
59. Marek K, Seibyl J. Beta-CIT scans without evidence of dopaminergic deficit (SWEDD) in the ELLDOPA-CIT and CALM-CIT study: long-term imaging assessment. *Neurology* 2003; 60 (Suppl 1): A293.
60. Mollenhauer B, Locascio JJ, Schulz-Schaeffer W, Sixel-Döring F, Trenkwalder C, Schlossmacher MG. Alpha-synuclein and tau concentrations in cerebrospinal fluid of patients presenting with parkinsonism: a cohort study. *Lancet Neurol* 2011; 10: 230–40.
61. Shi M, Bradner J, Hancock AM, et al. Cerebrospinal fluid biomarkers for Parkinson disease diagnosis and progression. *Ann Neurol* 2011; 69: 570–80.
62. Vaillancourt DE, Spraker MB, Prodoehl J, et al. High-resolution diffusion tensor imaging in the substantia nigra of *de novo* Parkinson disease. *Neurology* 2009; 72: 1378–84.
63. Berg D. Substantia nigra hyperechogenicity is a risk marker of Parkinson's disease: yes. *J Neural Transm* 2011; 118: 613–19.

CHAPTER 9

Parkinson's Disease: Premotor Features, Diagnosis, and Early Management

Anthony H.V. Schapira and David Gallagher

Introduction

Parkinson's disease (PD) is a neurodegenerative disease, the initial clinical features of which are the result of loss of dopaminergic neurons in the substantia nigra pars compacta (SNc) of the midbrain. As the disease progresses the involvement of additional brain areas in the degenerative process produces predominantly non-dopaminergic, non-motor features (e.g. cognitive decline and autonomic dysfunction). Although the classic clinical triad of bradykinesia, rigidity, and tremor still defines PD and enables a diagnosis, it is recognized that the disease process has evolved for many years if not decades, before these clinical features appear. Certain non-motor symptoms may appear before a diagnosis of PD can be made and these may represent risk factors for the disease or even prodromal PD. These features include hyposmia, rapid eye movement (REM) sleep behaviour disorder (RBD), depression, and constipation.

The discovery of dopamine deficiency in PD in the 1960s and the subsequent introduction of levodopa have provided patients with a significant improvement in both quality of life and life expectancy, but the treatment of non-motor features and slowing of disease progression remain important unmet needs. Thus the prodromal period of PD, in both its molecular and clinical perspectives, has become a major focus of attention of research (1).

Pathology of Parkinson's disease

Pathologically, PD is characterized by the loss of dopaminergic neurons in the SNc and the presence of alpha-synuclein-containing inclusions, Lewy bodies (LBs), and Lewy neurites, which can occur at a number of extra-nigral locations and involve non-dopaminergic neurotransmitter systems (2). The pathogenesis of PD is complex and involves mitochondrial dysfunction, oxidative stress, and free-radical-mediated neuronal damage, ubiquitin proteasome system (UPS) defects, excitotoxic cell damage, oligodendrocytic interaction, and nerve trophic factor depletion (3). The exact role of LBs in this process, whether toxic, neuroprotective, or an epiphenomenon, remains unclear. Nonetheless, autopsy studies of the topographic distribution of alpha-synuclein pathology provide important insights into neuroanatomical correlates of non-motor symptoms in PD and their temporal relationship to the onset of motor symptomatology. Braak and colleagues (2) have proposed a sequential staging of LB pathology in PD. Stage I involves the anterior olfactory structures and dorsal motor nucleus of the vagus (lower medulla). Involvement of the olfactory bulb and vagal nucleus have been proposed as neuropathological correlates for olfactory impairment and autonomic dysfunction (particularly gastrointestinal), respectively, which commonly occur in early PD and during the premotor phase of the disease. Stage II involves LB deposition in a number of brainstem nuclei, including the locus coeruleus, lower raphe nuclei, and reticular formation, but confined to the medulla and pontine tegmentum. These pathological changes have been implicated in the development of RBD and mood disorders in early PD. It is only during stages III–IV that, according to the Braak staging hypothesis, LBs appear in the substantia nigra pars compacta. In more advanced disease (stages V and VI) diffuse deposition of LBs in neocortical structures can occur.

However, it must be recognized that the caudal–rostral Braak concept refers to LB deposition and not neuronal degeneration, and the first sites to undergo actual neuronal loss are the SNc and premotor cortex. Furthermore, the pattern of LB spread described by Braak is thought to be seen in only half the autopsied cases of PD. Also, LB pathology is not unique to PD and related disorders (the alpha-synucleinopathies, dementia with Lewy bodies (DLB), and multiple system atrophy (MSA)), but can also occur in other degenerative neurological conditions, including neurodegeneration with brain iron accumulation (NBIA), subacute sclerosing panencephalitis, and Alzheimer's disease. Therefore LB formation may represent a non-specific downstream process encountered in different neurodegenerative disorders.

Prodromal or premotor clinical features of Parkinson's disease

Clinical features such as hyposmia, RBD, depression, and constipation can occur relatively commonly in the premotor, prediagnostic phase of PD (4). For example, in a large retrospective case-notes analysis of 433 pathologically proven PD patients, 21% had exclusively non-motor symptoms at presentation to their general practitioner, and of these 53% presented with pain, 16.5% with urinary problems, 12.1% with depression or anxiety, 5.5% with non-specific cognitive impairment without functional limitation or dementia, and 4.4% with fatigue (5). A number of patients in this study had inappropriate specialist referrals (orthopaedics, rheumatology, psychiatry, and urology), leading to unnecessary diagnostic and therapeutic interventions and delayed diagnosis of PD.

Risk association genes

The results of genome-wide association studies for PD confirm that alpha-synuclein, tau, and histocompatibility genes are risk factors for idiopathic/sporadic PD (6–8). Evidence is accumulating that glucocerebrosidase (GBA) mutations are numerically the most important risk factor for PD. Several studies have shown that GBA mutations are seen more commonly in PD patients than in age-matched controls (9). The Ashkenazi Jewish population has a particularly high frequency of PD related to GBA mutations (10). The link between GBA and PD has been reinforced by the increased frequency of mutations in post-mortem confirmed LB-positive PD (11). The published frequencies of GBA mutations in PD are likely to be an underestimate, as most studies have only tested for the two most frequent GBA mutations causing Gaucher's disease. Numerous mutations of the GBA gene impair enzyme activity and cause Gaucher's disease, and there may be GBA sequence changes that are exclusive to PD. As a conservative estimate, GBA mutations are associated with a five- to tenfold increase risk for PD.

Several genetic causes of familial PD have been identified (1, 12). However, even the autosomal dominant causes such as *LRRK2* mutations have variable penetrance, with a median age of onset in the early seventh decade. It is unclear at present whether single copies of the autosomal recessive genes predispose to PD. Current data suggest that these genetic causes account for only a small proportion (~5–10%) of PD patients although, taken together with the genetic risk factors, they indicate that a substantial proportion of the risk for PD can be explained on a genetic basis.

Despite the considerable and important advances in defining the genetic contribution to PD, we have not yet reached the stage where, other than in the autosomal dominant cases, genetic profile can be used to define risk for PD.

Olfaction

Several epidemiological studies have suggested that impaired olfaction is an early marker of idiopathic PD. In the Honolulu–Asia Aging Study, 2267 participants had olfactory testing at baseline and those in the lowest quartile of olfaction had a significantly increased age-adjusted risk of subsequently developing PD (odds ratio (OR) 5.2; 95% confidence interval (CI) 1.5–25.6) compared with the top two quartiles (13). In a two-year longitudinal study of first-degree relatives of patients with PD, olfactory testing was used to select normosmic and hyposmic individuals who then underwent dopamine transporter (DAT) single photon emission computed tomography (SPECT) (14). At two years, 10% of the hyposmic group who had shown markedly reduced DAT binding on SPECT imaging at baseline had developed clinical PD. In the remainder of the hyposmic group, despite no clinical evidence of parkinsonism, DAT binding had decreased more than in normosmic controls. In a further study of 30 subjects with idiopathic hyposmia, 11 demonstrated hyperechogenicity of the substantia nigra on transcranial sonography, but the majority had no motor features or signs suggestive of PD. Despite this, DAT SPECT was abnormal in five subjects and two had borderline binding ratios (15), suggestive of possible premotor PD.

The University of Pennsylvania Smell Identification Test (UPSIT), a 40-item odour identification test, has been extensively studied in PD. In a study of early PD (mean Hoehn and Yahr stage 1.4), a strong correlation between UPSIT scores and DAT SPECT imaging indices in the striatum as a whole (regression coefficient 0.66, $p = 0.001$), and particularly the putamen (0.74, $p < 0.001$), was demonstrated (16). Extrapolation of these findings into the premotor phase of PD is supported by epidemiological studies of smell loss antecedent to clinical PD and is consistent with the topographical distribution of LB in anterior olfactory structures in autopsy studies of early PD, suggesting a potential role for smell testing in the early diagnosis of PD.

UPSIT scores are significantly lower in PD than in both vascular parkinsonism and controls (17). In a study where olfaction in PD was compared with atypical parkinsonian syndromes (18), UPSIT scores were normal in progressive supranuclear palsy (PSP) and corticobasal degeneration (CBD) compared with controls, and there was only mild impairment in MSA. However, UPSIT scores were markedly reduced in the PD group and demonstrated good sensitivity (77%) and specificity (85%) in differentiating PD from atypical parkinsonism.

Sleep disorders and restless legs syndrome

RBD is a parasomnia characterized by dream enactment and loss of muscle atonia during REM sleep. Patients may be vocal and violent, posing a risk to their bed partner. Insights into the pathophysiology of RBD have been gained from brainstem structural lesions in humans, post-mortem autopsy studies, and animal models. RBD has been described in case reports in association with demyelination of the dorsal pontine tegmentum, an ischaemic pontine lesion, a pontomesencephalic cavernoma, and brainstem neurinoma (19). Incidental brainstem LB pathology has been demonstrated in an autopsied case of RBD (20). Proposed anatomical loci of RBD in humans, extrapolated from animal models, include the pre-coeruleus, sublaterodorsal nucleus, and lateral pontine tegmentum (19). These topographical locations correspond to brainstem regions that are involved before the development of striatal LB pathology (stages I and II) according to the Braak hypothesis. This may provide an explanation for the high prevalence of RBD in PD, with its occurrence often preceding motor impairment.

There have been a number of epidemiological studies showing an association between RBD and the development of PD or other neurodegenerative disorders. For example, in one study of 44 patients presenting to a sleep centre with idiopathic RBD (iRBD), confirmed by polysomnography, 20/44 (45%) subsequently developed a neurodegenerative disorder (in all cases alpha-synucleinopathy—PD in nine, DLB in six, and MSA in one) a mean 11.5 years after symptom onset and 5.1 years after formal diagnosis of RBD (21). In a second study, 57% of patients presenting to a sleep clinic with RBD had an underlying neurological disorder, and 52% of those with PD had symptoms of RBD preceding the development of motor symptoms (22).

Several imaging studies in iRBD have demonstrated early premotor basal ganglia changes. An imaging study assessing presynaptic DAT using ^{123}I-(*N*-3-iodopro-pene-2-yl-2β-carbomethoxy-3β-4-chlorophenyl tropane) (^{123}I-IPT) SPECT revealed significantly reduced striatal uptake in iRBD patients compared with controls, but less reduced than in symptomatic PD (23). ^{13}C-dihydrotetrabenazine positron emission tomography (PET) in patients with iRBD demonstrated reduced binding in all striatal nuclei, particularly the posterior putamen (24), and a cerebral perfusion study (^{99m}Tc-ethylene cysteinate dimer (ECD) SPECT) in iRBD showed increased perfusion bilaterally in the pons and putamen with reduced perfusion of the frontal and temporoparietal cortices, a metabolic picture consistent with that found in idiopathic PD (25).

These studies suggest that in patients with iRBD there is a predisposition to future development of alpha-synucleinopathies, including PD and MSA, and that early striatal and cortical metabolic changes may already be present, even years before the appearance of motor symptoms or clinical presentation of PD. Other disorders of sleep may also predict subsequent development of PD. A large population-based study (Honolulu–Asia Aging Study, N = 3078 (26)) revealed that daytime excessive somnolence was a risk factor (OR, 2.8; p = 0.014) for the development of PD.

Restless legs syndrome (RLS) is prevalent in PD, and in a proportion of patients precedes motor involvement (27). In a study of PD patients with RLS, PD/RLS occurred at an older age of onset, was less likely to be associated with a family history, and was associated with significantly lower ferritin levels than idiopathic RLS (iRLS) (27). When patients with iRLS were compared with patients in the early stages of PD using ^{123}I-IPT SPECT, no presynaptic dopaminergic neuronal loss was demonstrated in iRLS, and there was no difference from controls (28). The relationship between RLS and PD is most likely to represent a chance occurrence rather than a common pathogenesis.

Neuropsychiatric illness and cognitive impairment

LB deposition in brainstem loci, such as in the noradrenergic locus coeruleus and serotoninergic dorsal raphe nuclei, has been implicated in affective disorders, and this can precede basal midbrain involvement in PD. This may explain the high prevalence of depression in early PD that may precede development of motor symptoms (29). In a systematic review of psychiatric illness preceding motor symptoms in PD (30), two cohort studies, one nested case-control (NCC) study, and six case–control studies were identified for depression and PD. Five of the six case–control studies, both cohort studies, and the NCC showed a statistically significant association between a history of depression and subsequent development of PD. For example, a large retrospective cohort study (N = 105 406) (31) showed that, at diagnosis of PD, 9.2% of patients had a history of depression compared with 4.0% of controls (OR, 2.4; 95% CI, 2.1–2.7). In two other retrospective cohort studies, depressed subjects had a relative risk (RR) of 3.13 (95% CI, 1.95–5.01) of subsequently developing PD compared with controls in the first study (32), and a relative risk of developing PD of 2.20 (95% CI, 1.70–2.84) compared with a diabetes cohort and 2.24 (95% CI, 1.72–2.93) compared with an osteoarthritis cohort in the second study (33). A case–control study identified increased prevalence of premorbid anxiety disorder in PD compared with controls, and in a large prospective study (N = 35 815) using the Crown–Crisp phobic anxiety index there was an increased risk of developing PD (RR, 1.5; 95% CI, 1.0–2.1) in those with the highest level of anxiety at baseline (34).

Therefore depression and anxiety may be predictive of future development of PD. Several functional imaging studies in PD have demonstrated signal change in the brainstem which correlates with clinimetric indices of mood. For example, in a study using ^{123}I-βCIT SPECT, dorsal midbrain binding reflecting serotoninergic function was significantly correlated with Unified Parkinson's Disease Rating Scale (UPDRS) mood and mentation scores, but not with motor function (35). These imaging studies suggest that degeneration of serotoninergic and noradrenergic brainstem nuclei can occur in parallel or precede substantia nigra degeneration, leading to affective disorders in the early and premotor phase of PD.

Development of dementia is common in PD, particularly in the later stages. However, a number of studies using detailed neuropsychological assessments, including tests sensitive to frontal lobe function, have revealed that cognitive impairment, particularly dysexecutive, can occur early in PD (36). PD dementia (PDD) and DLB are distinguished by whether dementia occurs within a year of onset of motor symptoms, but this is an arbitrary distinction given the common neuropathology (alpha-synuclein containing LB deposition) and overlapping non-motor symptomatology of the two diseases. Imaging studies in PD have revealed that disruption of frontal–striatal dopaminergic connections can occur early in PD and are associated with abnormalities in frontal executive cognitive function (37–39).

Autonomic dysfunction

Autonomic features may occur early in PD and predate the onset of motor features. Epidemiological evidence suggests that constipation, in particular, may be an early premotor feature of PD. In the Honolulu Heart Program, 6790 subjects were questioned about their bowel habits, and in a 24-year follow-up period less than one bowel movement per day was associated with a greater risk of developing PD (RR, 4.1; 95% CI, 1.7–9.6; p = 0.001) compared with those whose bowels were opened twice per day (40). In a retrospective study, 44.6% of respondents described onset of constipation preceding motor symptoms with a mean latency of 18.7 years (41).

Sexual dysfunction is common in PD and includes difficulties with sexual arousal, reduced libido, erectile dysfunction, and anorgasmia (42). In a large retrospective epidemiological study (32 616 participants), men with erectile dysfunction had increased risk of subsequently developing PD (RR, 3.8; 95% CI, 2.4–6.0, p < 0.0001) (43). In another study, 23.3% of men and 21.9% of women reported that premorbid sexual dysfunction contributed to cessation of sexual activity following diagnosis of PD (42). In a large retrospective analysis of patients with pathologically proven PD (5), 3.5% of initial presentations were with urinary symptoms but without motor features of PD.

Orthostatic hypotension (OH) is common in PD, particularly in later disease, and can be a consequence of dopaminergic medication. However, in a study of patients with a clinical diagnosis of PD, in whom MSA had been excluded using imaging of myocardial sympathetic function (cardiac ^{18}F-fluorodopa SPECT), OH was of early onset (within a year of onset of motor symptoms) in 60%, and preceded motor involvement in 13% (44). Autopsy examinations have revealed early involvement (LB deposition) of central (medulla oblongata) and peripheral (sympathetic and parasympathetic) neurons that control autonomic function in PD, which may represent a pathological basis for early autonomic symptoms (45).

Neuroimaging in the premotor diagnosis of Parkinson's disease

All the symptoms described so far are relatively non-specific, occurring both in the general elderly population and in other neurodegenerative diseases including non-PD parkinsonism, and in the case of hyposmia in Alzheimer's disease (46–49). However, a composite of clinical premotor features may allow stratification for risk of future development of neurodegenerative disorders sufficient to direct appropriate use of imaging techniques to identify those with premotor dopamine deficits (50). SPECT imaging using ligands which bind to presynaptic DAT is widely used in practice to help diagnose PD, particularly in early disease or in patients presenting with subtle or atypical features. But DAT SPECT imaging could also have a role in presymptomatic diagnosis of at-risk individuals, for example those with susceptibility genes, hyposmia, or other premotor features. Other recent developments in imaging in PD include transcranial sonography. Hyperechogenicity of the substantia nigra on sonography has been demonstrated as an early marker of PD and is present in monogenetic forms of PD in the preclinical phase (51). However, substantia nigra hyperechogenicity has been shown in up to 10% of normal subjects, and the nigra cannot be visualized in a similar proportion, limiting the diagnostic utility of the test. Cardiac sympathetic denervation is a feature of Lewy body disorders, and extra-striatal imaging modalities, such as meta-iodobenzyl guanidine (MIBG) SPECT, have been demonstrated to be abnormal in early PD (52).

Biochemical markers for Parkinson's disease

Insights into the pathogenetic pathways involved in PD have enabled a number of candidate peripheral assays to be considered as potentially useful for calculating risk for PD. Blood markers for oxidative stress, including uric acid or urinary 8-dihydroxydeoxyguanosine, or platelet mitochondrial complex I activity may be abnormal in a proportion of cases. Whilst no single assay could distinguish PD from normal, a composite 'basket' of assays which might also include peripheral or cerebrospinal fluid (CSF) alpha-synuclein or DJ-1, together with the genetic markers and prodromal clinical features described above, might together help define and refine a population considered at high risk for PD.

The relevance of early diagnosis in Parkinson's disease

At present, the diagnosis of PD is predominantly based on clinical criteria which may, in appropriate circumstances, be supported by imaging of the dopamine nigrostriatal system. It is doubtful whether any of the clinical or biochemical features described in the previous section are capable of, or indeed even necessary for, discriminating PD from other parkinsonian syndromes. Genetic testing may confirm status in affected individuals in familial forms of PD, and may also identify family members at risk, although at the time of writing genetic testing for PD per se is not appropriate for PD.

The most important reason for establishing an individual's risk for PD is to enable early and effective intervention to prevent the onset or slow the development or progression of the disease. It is estimated from autopsy studies that at least 50% of dopaminergic neurons in the SNc will have been lost at diagnosis of PD, and that there is a negative exponential progression of the disease (53). The non-linear pattern of dopaminergic cell loss is consistent with clinical and imaging studies. In a longitudinal study using 18F-fluorodopa PET, change in fluorodopa signal was inversely related to PD duration at baseline (54). In a prospective study using UPDRS as a clinical marker of disease progression, rate of deterioration in motor scores decreased with advancing disease duration (55), although it is recognized that earlier-onset disease is associated with slower progression (56). Given that a rapid rate of SNc dopamine depletion occurs in the premotor phase, it could be inferred that, to derive most benefit, any potential disease-modifying therapy should be started before the onset of motor symptoms.

The diagnosis of Parkinson's disease

Motor features of PD

The classic early features of PD are bradykinesia, rigidity, and tremor. Postural instability and several additional motor and non-motor symptoms usually develop later in the disease.

Bradykinesia manifests in several ways, including difficulty or delay in initiating voluntary movement, multitasking, or undertaking rapid motor tasks in sequence. A poverty of movement becomes evident, especially to family and friends. This may be represented by a reduction in spontaneous gestures, decreased facial movement, and blinking. Involvement of the limbs may be seen, with impaired fine movements of a hand and in the dominant hand leads to progressive micrographia. There are problems with fastening buttons or brassieres, tying laces, and using a screwdriver.

The patient's gait becomes slow, small-stepped, and shuffling, with the patient sometimes 'chasing his own centre of gravity'. The arm on the affected side does not swing as much as the contralateral arm. The patient may complain of difficulty turning over in bed or rising from a chair. Freezing usually occurs later in the course of PD, but some patients experience 'gait ignition failure' especially when approaching a doorway.

Physical examination for bradykinesia will evaluate rapid alternating movements in the upper and lower limbs and, in idiopathic PD, show asymmetry of speed, amplitude, and rhythm in the early stages. Examples of helpful manoeuvres include finger- or heel-tapping, pronation–supination of the outstretched arms, and rapid flexion–extension of the extended fingers at the metacarpophalangeal joints.

Rigidity represents an increase in tone which is present throughout the range of movement and is independent of the speed at which the limb is moved. The tremor of PD may superimpose upon rigidity to produce cogwheeling, and this phenomenon may be absent if there is no tremor. Examination of the wrist with gentle flexion–extension movements is the best way to elicit cogwheeling, and this can be repeated at the elbow. Rigidity affects the patient's posture, producing a flexion at most joints including the spine which results in the simian posture typical of PD. An extreme form of this is known as camptocormia (57). Postural abnormalities also affect the distal limbs, with extension of the fingers and flexion of the metacarpophalangeal joints or dorsiflexion of the great toe (striatal hand or toe).

The development of an asymmetric intermittent resting tremor at 4–6 Hz is estimated to be a presenting feature in 70% of PD patients. In addition, there is often a small-amplitude postural tremor at a higher frequency (~12 Hz). The resting hand tremor is referred to as 'pill-rolling', in the style of the pharmacists of the nineteenth century who would prepare their tablets by hand. A tremor may affect other parts, including the foot or leg (in which it may first manifest), lips, jaw, and tongue (58). A head tremor, titubation, is more suggestive of essential tremor. The resting tremor is exacerbated by physical or emotional stress, and in the early stages can be voluntarily inhibited for short periods. The tremor usually becomes bilateral after about five or six years, although the tremor in the first affected side generally remains more severe (59).

Non-motor features of PD

The widespread and progressive neurodegeneration in the PD brain leads to the emergence of a variety of features that are collectively grouped under the title of non-motor symptoms. Some of these have already been discussed, as their emergence may precede motor symptoms and signs. The non-motor symptoms of PD range from cognitive problems, such as apathy, depression, anxiety disorders, and hallucinations, to fatigue, gait and balance disturbances, hypophonia, sleep disorders, sexual dysfunction, bowel problems, drenching sweats, sialorrhoea, and pain. These symptoms are often the most troubling for patients, and contribute significantly to morbidity and impaired quality of life (60, 61). Diplopia is a frequent symptom even in early PD, although the neurological basis is not known.

Abnormalities of sleep are common in PD and are the result of a combination of the natural consequences of ageing, the underlying disease pathology (62), motor and non-motor complications (63, 64), and drugs (65, 66). Disordered sleep often results in excessive daytime sleepiness (EDS), and this in turn may be compounded by the sedative effect of dopaminergic drugs (65, 66). EDS and involuntary dozing affect up to 50% of PD patients, and may be preclinical markers (67). In some patients, EDS has been linked with the development of sudden onset of sleep and a pattern reminiscent of narcolepsy with an abnormal sleep latency period (<5 min) in 30% of PD patients. Polysomnographic studies have showed transition from wakefulness to sleep stage 2 within seconds without the sudden onset of REM sleep (68, 69). Following reports of road traffic accidents caused by 'sudden irresistible attacks of sleep' in PD patients, a large body of research focused on the possible effects of dopaminergic drugs and disease progression and the occurrence of sudden onset of sleep (65, 69–71). The issue remains unclear, although EDS is now regarded as part of the non-motor complex of the disease progression in PD (72).

Sexual and bladder dysfunction are common and occur in both sexes. The dopaminergic treatment of PD may lead to increased sex drive, but the effects of the disease often result in impaired sexual performance (73). Bladder abnormalities in particular cause problems at night with nocturia, which when associated with bradykinesia during nocturnal OFF periods causes considerable discomfort.

Pain is a frequent symptom in PD, and some patients manifest especially with shoulder pain. Pain, anxiety, akathisia, respiratory distress, depressive mood swings, and slowed and impaired thought are symptoms which may be experienced during OFF periods and which will respond, at least in part, to dopaminergic therapy (74).

Treatment of early PD

Following a secure diagnosis of PD, it is important to educate the patient accordingly in the nature of their illness and the treatments available to them, as well as lifestyle changes that may be appropriate. Contact with an established national patient organization is often invaluable. Lines of communication to the patient's primary physician should be clearly established, and the patient should be provided with information on specialist nursing and physician care.

Non-pharmacological therapies for PD are important. Exercise therapy can improve and maintain function in PD patients, and should be encouraged. Laboratory studies suggest that exercise might also have protective effects on disease progression, but this remains to be established. It is also important for patients to maintain social and intellectual activities. The needs of the caregiver should also be considered. Their work load may be dramatically increased by caring for a person with PD, and there is an increased incidence of depression.

Pharmacological therapy in early PD is focused on oral drug treatment. There are several groups or classes of agent with proven efficacy in PD.

Levodopa

Levodopa is routinely administered in combination with a peripheral decarboxylase inhibitor to prevent its peripheral metabolism to dopamine and the development of nausea and vomiting due to activation of dopamine receptors in the area postrema which are not protected by the blood–brain barrier. Levodopa remains the most effective symptomatic oral treatment for PD, and the gold standard against which new therapies are compared. Almost all PD patients experience improvement, and failure to respond to an adequate trial should cause the diagnosis to be questioned. Levodopa benefits the classic motor features of PD, increases independence, prolongs employability, improves quality of life, and enhances lifespan (75).

However, there are important limitations on levodopa therapy. Acute side effects include nausea, vomiting, and orthostatic hypotension, but if they occur are usually transient and can usually be avoided by gradual titration. Motor complications (motor fluctuations and dyskinesia) develop in the majority of patients treated for more than five years, and can be disabling in some patients.

Levodopa-induced motor complications consist of fluctuations in motor response and involuntary movements known as dyskinesias. When patients initially take levodopa, the benefits are long-lasting (many hours) even though the drug has a short pharmacological half-life (60–90 min). However, with continued treatment the duration of benefit following an individual dose of levodopa becomes progressively shorter until it approaches the half-life of the drug. This is known as the wearing-off effect. At the same time, or subsequently, many patients develop dyskinesias. These tend to occur at the time of maximum levodopa benefit and plasma concentration (peak-dose dyskinesia). They are usually choreiform in nature, but can manifest as dystonia, myoclonus, or other movement disorders. They are usually mild, but can limit the ability to fully utilize levodopa to control PD features. In more advanced states the dyskinesias can be disabling, and patients may cycle between ON periods complicated by severe dyskinesias and OFF periods in which they suffer severe parkinsonism.

The precise cause of levodopa-induced motor complications is not known. However, the risk of dyskinesias is increased with the dose of levodopa; doses greater than 400 mg/day are associated with a significant risk for dyskinesia. Young patients are likewise at greater risk. The intermittent or pulsatile stimulation of dopamine receptors by levodopa causes molecular changes in striatal neurons, neurophysiological changes in pallidal neurons, and ultimately motor complications. It has been hypothesized that more continuous delivery of levodopa might prevent the development of motor complications.

Because of the risk of motor complications some physicians delay the introduction of levodopa and prefer to use alternative therapies in the early phases of the disease (see below). On the other hand, levodopa is the most effective therapy for PD and should not be withheld when satisfactory control cannot otherwise be achieved.

Behavioural alterations can be encountered in levodopa-treated patients. A dopamine dysregulation syndrome has been described where patients have a craving for levodopa and take frequent and unnecessary doses of the drug in an addictive manner. PD patients taking high doses of levodopa may also have purposeless and stereotyped behaviours such as the meaningless assembly and disassembly or collection and sorting of objects, known as punding. Hypersexuality and other impulse control disorders are occasionally encountered with levodopa, although these are more commonly seen in conjunction with dopamine agonists.

Dopamine agonists

Dopamine agonists are a diverse group of chemical agents which act directly on the dopamine receptor. Unlike levodopa, they do not require metabolism to an active product and do not undergo oxidative metabolism. Initial dopamine agonists were ergot derivatives (e.g. bromocriptine, pergolide, cabergoline), but these have been shown to be associated with ergot-related side effects, including cardiac valvular damage (76), and have largely been withdrawn from the market and replaced by second-generation non-ergot dopamine agonists (e.g. pramipexole, ropinirole, rotigotine). Dopamine agonists were initially introduced as adjuncts to levodopa to improve motor function and reduce OFF time in fluctuating patients. Subsequently, it was shown that initiation of PD therapy with a long-acting dopamine agonist was less likely than levodopa to induce dyskinesia. For this reason many physicians initiate PD therapy with a dopamine agonist, although supplemental levodopa is eventually required. Maintenance of the agonist therapy in combination with levodopa helps to keep the dose of the latter low and diminish the risk for subsequent dyskinesias.

Both ropinirole and pramipexole are available as once-daily oral formulations which combine effective treatment with ease of use and have confirmed patient preference (77). Rotigotine is a dopamine agonist that is administered as a transdermal patch and has the benefit of once-daily administration. Dopamine agonists can also be administered by continuous subcutaneous infusion and have been demonstrated to reduce both OFF time and dyskinesia in advanced patients.

Acute side effects of dopamine agonists include nausea, vomiting, and orthostatic hypotension. As with levodopa, these can usually be avoided by slow titration. Hallucinations and cognitive impairment are more common, particularly in the elderly with dopamine agonists more than levodopa. Sedation is a dose-related side effect of dopamine agonists, and sudden unintended episodes of falling asleep while driving have been reported. Patients should be informed about this potential problem and advised not to drive when tired. More recently, it has become evident that dopamine agonists are associated with a variety of impulse control disorders, including pathological gambling, hypersexuality, and compulsive eating, and shopping.

MAO-B inhibitors

Inhibitors of monoamine oxidase type B (MAO-B) block central dopamine metabolism and increase synaptic concentrations of the neurotransmitter. Selegiline and rasagiline are both relatively selective irreversible inhibitors of the MAO-B enzyme. Clinically, MAO-B inhibitors provide modest anti-parkinsonian benefits when used as monotherapy in early disease, and reduce OFF time when used as an adjunct to levodopa in patients with motor fluctuations. MAO-B inhibitors have the potential to block the oxidative metabolism of dopamine and thereby prevent oxidative stress. In addition, both selegiline and rasagiline incorporate a propargyl ring within their molecular structure which provides powerful anti-apoptotic effects in laboratory models. The DATATOP study showed that selegiline significantly delays the time until the emergence of disability necessitating the introduction of levodopa in early PD patients. However, it could not be determined whether this effect was due to a neuroprotective effect that slowed disease progression, or was merely a symptomatic effect that masked ongoing neurodegeneration. More recently, the ADAGIO study demonstrated that early treatment with rasagiline 1 mg/day provided benefits that could not be achieved with delayed treatment with the same drug. Positive results in this delayed-start study are consistent with the drug having a disease-modifying effect. However, the long-term clinical significance of this finding remains to be determined (78).

MAO-B inhibitors are generally safe and well-tolerated. They may increase dyskinesia in levodopa-treated patients, but this can usually be controlled by down-titrating levodopa. Selegiline is metabolized to form an amphetamine which can cause insomnia, but this can be avoided by administering the drug before noon. There are theoretical risks of a serotonin reaction in patients on selective serotonin-reuptake inhibitors (SSRIs), but again these are rarely encountered.

COMT inhibitors

When levodopa is administered in conjunction with a decarboxylase inhibitor, it is primarily metabolized by catechol-*O*-methyltransferase (COMT). Inhibitors of COMT increase the elimination half-life of levodopa and enhance its brain availability. Combining levodopa with a COMT inhibitor has been shown to reduce OFF time and to prolong ON time in fluctuating patients, while enhancing motor scores. Two COMT inhibitors (tolcapone and entacapone) have been approved, and a combination tablet of levodopa, carbidopa, and entacapone (Stalevo®) is available.

Side effects of COMT inhibitors are primarily dopaminergic (nausea, vomiting, increased dyskinesia) and can usually be controlled by down-titrating the dose of levodopa by 20–30%. Severe diarrhoea has been described with tolcapone, and to a lesser degree with entacapone, which necessitates stopping the medication in 5–10% of individuals. Cases of fatal hepatic toxicity have been reported with tolcapone, and accordingly periodic monitoring of liver function is required. This problem has not been encountered with entacapone. Discoloration of urine can be seen with both COMT inhibitors because of accumulation of a metabolite, but is of no clinical concern.

There has been interest in the possibility that initiating levodopa in combination with a COMT inhibitor will increase its half-life and provide more continuous delivery, thereby reducing the risk of motor complications. No benefit was detected in early PD patients in the recently completed STRIDE-PD study, and the main value of COMT inhibitors continues to be in patients who experience motor fluctuations.

Other medical therapies

Centrally acting anticholinergic drugs, such as trihexyphenidyl and benztropine, were used historically for the treatment for PD but lost favour with the introduction of dopaminergic agents. Their major clinical benefit is an effect on tremor, although it is not certain that this is superior to that which is obtained with other agents such as levodopa and dopamine agonists. Still, they can be helpful in individual patients. Their use is limited, particularly in the elderly, by their propensity to induce a variety of side effects including prostatism, glaucoma, and particularly cognitive impairment.

Amantadine has antiparkinsonian effects thought to be due to NMDA receptor antagonism. While some physicians use amantadine in patients with early disease for its mild symptomatic effects, it is most widely used as an anti-dyskinesia agent in patients with advanced PD. Indeed, it is the only oral agent that has been demonstrated in controlled studies to reduce dyskinesia while improving parkinsonian features, and this effect can be sustained in many patients. Side effects include livedo reticularis, weight gain, and, most importantly, dose-related impairment in cognitive function. Amantadine should always be discontinued gradually as patients can experience withdrawal symptoms.

Neuroprotection

Despite the many therapeutic agents available for the treatment of PD, patients still experience intolerable disability due to disease progression and the emergence of features such as falling and dementia that are not controlled with dopaminergic therapies. The development of a therapy that slows or stops disease progression is the most important need in PD therapeutics. Towards this end, there are many promising candidate agents based on targeting factors implicated in the pathogenesis of PD. However, no agent which unequivocally has a disease-modifying effect in PD has been determined. Obstacles to defining a disease-modifying drug include uncertainty as to the precise cause of the disease, and exactly what to target, and a relevant animal model that reflects the aetiopathogenesis of the disease in which to test promising compounds. With the identification of genes and proteins associated with familial PD, it is anticipated that there will be important progress in these areas in the near future. Equally challenging will be the development of an endpoint for clinical trials that provides a measure of the underlying disease state and is not confounded by symptomatic or pharmacological effects of the study intervention.

Some studies have had positive results consistent with the possibility that the drug has disease-modifying effects. As described above, selegiline delayed the development of disability necessitating levodopa in the DATATOP study, but this result could have been due to a previously unappreciated symptomatic effect of the drug that masked rather than protected against disease progression. Co-enzyme Q10 is thought to enhance mitochondrial function, and reduced the rate of decline of UPDRS scores in a pilot study. However, the study was underpowered and a symptomatic confound could not be excluded. The dopamine agonists ropinirole and pramipexole have anti-apoptotic effects in the laboratory, and slowed the rate of decline of a surrogate neuroimaging biomarker of dopamine function in comparison with levodopa. However, a pharmacological effect on the biomarker rather than true protection of dopamine neurons could not be excluded.

To avoid the problem of a confounding symptomatic effect, a delayed-start design has been proposed. This is a two-period study in which subjects are randomized to receive the active drug or placebo in the first period, while subjects in both groups receive the active drug in the second period. Benefits of the active drug at the end of period one could be due to symptomatic and/or disease-modifying effects. However, benefits of early treatment at the end of the second period, when both groups are receiving the same medication, is unlikely to be due to a symptomatic effect alone and is consistent with disease modification. This is substantiated by demonstrating that the rates of decline of motor scores in the early and delayed start groups are not converging, indicating that the benefit of early treatment is enduring. In the ADAGIO study, rasagiline 1 mg met all principal endpoints of the delayed-start study consistent with the possibility that the drug has a disease-modifying effect. However, the 2 mg dose failed in this same clinical trial, and the reason for these disparate effects remains to be clarified.

The importance of the delayed-start design is its potential to detect benefits of a putative neuroprotective agent that are not due to an early symptomatic effect and therefore must be due to disease modification. However, long-term studies are required to determine the clinical significance of the drug and assess its effect on cumulative disability.

Management of early PD

The management of PD should be tailored to the needs of the individual patient, and there is no single approach that is universally accepted (79, 80). Clearly, if an agent was demonstrated to have disease-modifying effects it would be initiated at the time of diagnosis. Several studies now suggest that it may be best to initiate symptomatic therapy early after diagnosis in order to maintain quality of life and to preserve compensatory mechanisms and provide benefits even in early disease. Levodopa remains the most effective symptomatic therapy for PD, and some recommend starting therapy early but with relatively low doses to minimize the risk of motor complications. Alternatively, many physicians select an alternative strategy in early patients, especially if they are younger, in order to reduce the risk of motor complications. A compromise is to begin with an MAO-B inhibitor or a dopamine agonist and reserve levodopa for when these drugs can no longer provide satisfactory control. In patients with more severe disability, in the elderly, where there is cognitive impairment, or where the diagnosis is uncertain, most physicians would elect to initiate therapy directly with levodopa. It is important not to deny patients levodopa in scenarios where they are not adequately controlled by alternative medications.

If motor complications develop, they can be treated by manipulating the frequency and dose of levodopa, or by combining lower doses of levodopa with a dopamine agonist, a COMT inhibitor, or an MAO-B inhibitor. Amantadine is the only drug that has been demonstrated to treat dyskinesia without worsening parkinsonism, but the benefits are not permanent. Efforts are being aimed at developing a long-acting continuous delivery oral or transdermal formulation of levodopa that mirrors the pharmacokinetic properties of a levodopa infusion. Such a formulation might provide all the benefits of levodopa without motor complications and avoid the need for polypharmacy and surgical interventions.

The non-dopaminergic features of PD remain an important target for future therapies. Agents that target non-dopaminergic systems, such as A2a antagonists, glutamate antagonists, cholinergic agents, and trophic factors, are all being actively investigated, but it is by no means clear that they will meaningfully influence non-dopaminergic symptoms. The best prospect is a neuroprotective therapy which might slow disease progression. While this has proved difficult to achieve with currently available drugs and clinical designs, there have been great advances that create opportunities for the future. Advances in genetics have defined new candidate targets. Transgenic animals which carry mutations associated with PD are likely to provide animal models for testing candidate neuroprotective agents that are more reliable than those which have been employed to date. Finally, it is hoped that new clinical trial designs will the delineation of disease-modifying effects and their clinical significance.

References

1. Schapira AH, Tolosa E. Molecular and clinical prodrome of Parkinson disease: implications for treatment. *Nat Rev Neurol* 2010; 6: 309–17.
2. Braak H, Bohl JR, Muller CM, Rub U, de Vos RA, Del TK. Stanley Fahn Lecture 2005. The staging procedure for the inclusion body pathology associated with sporadic Parkinson's disease reconsidered. *Mov Disord* 2006; 21: 2042–51.
3. Olanow CW. The pathogenesis of cell death in Parkinson's disease. *Mov Disord* 2007; 22 (Suppl 17): S335–42.
4. Gallagher DA, Schapira AH. Etiopathogenesis and treatment of Parkinson's disease. *Curr Top Med Chem* 2009; 9(10): 860–8.
5. O'Sullivan SS, Williams DR, Gallagher DA, Massey LA, Silveira-Moriyama L, Lees AJ. Nonmotor symptoms as presenting complaints in Parkinson's disease: a clinicopathological study. *Mov Disord* 2008; 23: 101–6.
6. Simon-Sanchez J, Schulte C, Bras JM, et al. Genome-wide association study reveals genetic risk underlying Parkinson's disease. *Nat Genet* 2009; 41: 1308–12.
7. Satake W, Nakabayashi Y, Mizuta I, et al. Genome-wide association study identifies common variants at four loci as genetic risk factors for Parkinson's disease. *Nat Genet* 2009; 41: 1303–7.
8. Hamza TH, Zabetian CP, Tenesa A, et al. Common genetic variation in the HLA region is associated with late-onset sporadic Parkinson's disease. *Nat Genet* 2010; 42: 781–5.
9. Velayati A, Yu WH, Sidransky E. The role of glucocerebrosidase mutations in Parkinson disease and Lewy body disorders. *Curr Neurol Neurosci Rep* 2010; 10: 190–8.
10. Aharon-Peretz J, Rosenbaum H, Gershoni-Baruch R. Mutations in the glucocerebrosidase gene and Parkinson's disease in Ashkenazi Jews. *N Engl J Med* 2004; 351: 1972–7.
11. Neumann J, Bras J, Deas E, et al. Glucocerebrosidase mutations in clinical and pathologically proven Parkinson's disease. *Brain* 2009; 132: 1783–94.
12. Schapira AH. Etiology of Parkinson's disease. *Neurology* 2006; 66 (Suppl 4): S10–23.
13. Ross GW, Petrovitch H, Abbott RD, et al. Association of olfactory dysfunction with risk for future Parkinson's disease. *Ann Neurol* 2008; 63: 167–73.
14. Ponsen MM, Stoffers D, Booij J, van Eck-Smit BL, Wolters EC, Berendse HW. Idiopathic hyposmia as a preclinical sign of Parkinson's disease. *Ann Neurol* 2004; 56: 173–81.
15. Sommer U, Hummel T, Cormann K, et al. Detection of presymptomatic Parkinson's disease: combining smell tests, transcranial sonography, and SPECT. *Mov Disord* 2004; 19: 1196–202.
16. Siderowf A, Newberg A, Chou KL, et al. (99mTc)TRODAT-1 SPECT imaging correlates with odor identification in early Parkinson disease. *Neurology* 2005; 64: 1716–20.
17. Katzenschlager R, Zijlmans J, Evans A, Watt H, Lees AJ. Olfactory function distinguishes vascular parkinsonism from Parkinson's disease. *J Neurol Neurosurg Psychiatry* 2004; 75: 1749–52.
18. Wenning GK, Shephard B, Hawkes C, Petruckevitch A, Lees A, Quinn N. Olfactory function in atypical parkinsonian syndromes. *Acta Neurol Scand* 1995; 91: 247–50.
19. Boeve BF, Silber MH, Saper CB, et al. Pathophysiology of REM sleep behaviour disorder and relevance to neurodegenerative disease. *Brain* 2007; 130: 2770–88.
20. Uchiyama M, Isse K, Tanaka K, et al. Incidental Lewy body disease in a patient with REM sleep behavior disorder. *Neurology* 1995; 45: 709–12.
21. Iranzo A, Molinuevo JL, Santamaria J, et al. Rapid-eye-movement sleep behaviour disorder as an early marker for a neurodegenerative disorder: a descriptive study. *Lancet Neurol* 2006; 5: 572–7.
22. Olson EJ, Boeve BF, Silber MH. Rapid eye movement sleep behaviour disorder: demographic, clinical and laboratory findings in 93 cases. *Brain* 2000; 123: 331–9.
23. Eisensehr I, Linke R, Noachtar S, Schwarz J, Gildehaus FJ, Tatsch K. Reduced striatal dopamine transporters in idiopathic rapid eye movement sleep behaviour disorder. Comparison with Parkinson's disease and controls. *Brain* 2000; 123: 1155–60.
24. Albin RL, Koeppe RA, Chervin RD, et al. Decreased striatal dopaminergic innervation in REM sleep behavior disorder. *Neurology* 2000; 55: 1410–12.
25. Mazza S, Soucy JP, Gravel P, et al. Assessing whole brain perfusion changes in patients with REM sleep behavior disorder. *Neurology* 2006; 67: 1618–22.
26. Abbott RD, Ross GW, White LR, et al. Excessive daytime sleepiness and subsequent development of Parkinson disease. *Neurology* 2005; 65: 1442–6.
27. Ondo WG, Vuong KD, Jankovic J. Exploring the relationship between Parkinson disease and restless legs syndrome. *Arch Neurol* 2002; 59: 421–4.
28. Linke R, Eisensehr I, Wetter TC, et al. Presynaptic dopaminergic function in patients with restless legs syndrome: are there common features with early Parkinson's disease? *Mov Disord* 2004; 19: 1158–62.
29. Shiba M, Bower JH, Maraganore DM, et al. Anxiety disorders and depressive disorders preceding Parkinson's disease: a case–control study. *Mov Disord* 2000; 15: 669–77.
30. Ishihara L, Brayne C. A systematic review of depression and mental illness preceding Parkinson's disease. *Acta Neurol Scand* 2006; 113: 211–20.
31. Leentjens AF, van den Akker M, Metsemakers JF, Lousberg R, Verhey FR. Higher incidence of depression preceding the onset of Parkinson's disease: a register study. *Mov Disord* 2003; 18: 414–18.
32. Schuurman AG, van den Akker M, Ensinck KT, et al. Increased risk of Parkinson's disease after depression: a retrospective cohort study. *Neurology* 2002; 58: 1501–4.

33. Nilsson FM, Kessing LV, Sorensen TM, Andersen PK, Bolwig TG. Major depressive disorder in Parkinson's disease: a register-based study. *Acta Psychiatr Scand* 2001; 106: 202–11.
34. Weisskopf MG, Chen H, Schwarzschild MA, Kawachi I, Ascherio A. Prospective study of phobic anxiety and risk of Parkinson's disease. *Mov Disord* 2003; 18: 646–51.
35. Murai T, Muller U, Werheid K, et al. *In vivo* evidence for differential association of striatal dopamine and midbrain serotonin systems with neuropsychiatric symptoms in Parkinson's disease. *J Neuropsychiatry Clin Neurosci* 2001; 13: 222–8.
36. Lees AJ, Smith E. Cognitive deficits in the early stages of Parkinson's disease. *Brain* 1983; 106: 257–70.
37. Bruck A, Aalto S, Nurmi E, Bergman J, Rinne JO. Cortical 6-(18F) fluoro-l-dopa uptake and frontal cognitive functions in early Parkinson's disease. *Neurobiol Aging* 2005; 26: 891–8.
38. Lewis SJ, Dove A, Robbins TW, Barker RA, Owen AM. Cognitive impairments in early Parkinson's disease are accompanied by reductions in activity in frontostriatal neural circuitry. *J Neurosci* 2003; 23: 6351–6.
39. Lange KW, Paul GM, Robbins TW, Marsden CD. l-dopa and frontal cognitive function in Parkinson's disease. *Adv Neurol* 1993; 60: 475–8.
40. Abbott RD, Petrovitch H, White LR, et al. Frequency of bowel movements and the future risk of Parkinson's disease. *Neurology* 2001; 57: 456–62.
41. Ueki A, Otsuka M. Life style risks of Parkinson's disease: association between decreased water intake and constipation. *J Neurol* 2004; 251 (Suppl 7): VII 18–23.
42. Bronner G, Royter V, Korczyn AD, Giladi N. Sexual dysfunction in Parkinson's disease. *J Sex Marital Ther* 2004; 30: 95–105.
43. Gao X, Chen H, Schwarzschild MA, et al. Erectile function and risk of Parkinson's disease. *Am J Epidemiol* 2007; 166: 1446–50.
44. Goldstein DS. Orthostatic hypotension as an early finding in Parkinson's disease. *Clin Auton Res* 2006; 16: 46–54.
45. Braak H, Sastre M, Bohl JR, de Vos RA, Del TK. Parkinson's disease: lesions in dorsal horn layer I, involvement of parasympathetic and sympathetic pre- and postganglionic neurons. *Acta Neuropathol* 2007; 113: 421–9.
46. Atli T, Keven K. Orthostatic hypotension in the healthy elderly. *Arch Gerontol Geriatr* 2006; 43: 313–17.
47. Deems DA, Doty RL, Settle RG, et al. Smell and taste disorders, a study of 750 patients from the University of Pennsylvania Smell and Taste Center. *Arch Otolaryngol Head Neck Surg* 1991; 117: 519–28.
48. McDougall FA, Kvaal K, Matthews FE, et al. Prevalence of depression in older people in England and Wales: the MRC CFA Study. *Psychol Med* 2007; 37: 1787–95.
49. Choung RS, Locke GR, III, Schleck CD, Zinsmeister AR, Talley NJ. Cumulative incidence of chronic constipation: a population-based study 1988–2003. *Aliment Pharmacol Ther* 2007; 26: 1521–8.
50. Jankovic J. Parkinson's disease: clinical features and diagnosis. *J Neurol Neurosurg Psychiatry* 2008; 79: 368–76.
51. Berg D. Transcranial sonography in the early and differential diagnosis of Parkinson's disease. *J Neural Transm Suppl* 2006; 70: 249–54.
52. Suzuki M, Kurita A, Hashimoto M, et al. Impaired myocardial 123I-metaiodobenzylguanidine uptake in Lewy body disease: comparison between dementia with Lewy bodies and Parkinson's disease. *J Neurol Sci* 2006; 240: 15–19.
53. Greffard S, Verny M, Bonnet AM, et al. Motor score of the Unified Parkinson Disease Rating Scale as a good predictor of Lewy body-associated neuronal loss in the substantia nigra. *Arch Neurol* 2006; 63: 584–8.
54. Hilker R, Schweitzer K, Coburger S, et al. Nonlinear progression of Parkinson disease as determined by serial positron emission tomographic imaging of striatal fluorodopa F18 activity. *Arch Neurol* 2005; 62: 378–82.
55. Schrag A, Dodel R, Spottke A, Bornschein B, Siebert U, Quinn NP. Rate of clinical progression in Parkinson's disease. A prospective study. *Mov Disord* 2007; 22: 938–45.
56. Schapira AH, Schrag A. Parkinson disease: Parkinson disease clinical subtypes and their implications. *Nat Rev Neurol* 2011; 7: 247–8.
57. Djaldetti R, Mosberg-Galili R, Sroka H, Merims D, Melamed E. Camptocormia (bent spine) in patients with Parkinson's disease—characterization and possible pathogenesis of an unusual phenomenon. *Mov Disord* 1999; 14: 443–7.
58. Hunker CJ, Abbs JH. Uniform frequency of parkinsonian resting tremor in the lips, jaw, tongue, and index finger. *Mov Disord* 1990; 5: 71–7.
59. Hoehn MM, Yahr MD. Parkinsonism: onset, progression and mortality. *Neurology* 1967; 17: 427–42.
60. Gallagher DA, Lees AJ, Schrag A. What are the most important nonmotor symptoms in patients with Parkinson's disease and are we missing them? *Mov Disord* 2010; 25: 2493–500.
61. Hely MA, Morris JG, Reid WG, Trafficante R. Sydney Multicenter Study of Parkinson's disease: non-l-dopa-responsive problems dominate at 15 years. *Mov Disord* 2005; 20: 190–9.
62. Jellinger KA. Pathology of Parkinson's disease. Changes other than the nigrostriatal pathway. *Mol Chem Neuropathol* 1991; 14: 153–97.
63. Lees AJ, Blackburn NA, Campbell VL. The nighttime problems of Parkinson's disease. *Clin Neuropharmacol* 1988; 11: 512–19.
64. van Hilten B, Hoff JI, Middelkoop HA, et al. Sleep disruption in Parkinson's disease. Assessment by continuous activity monitoring. *Arch Neurol* 1994; 51: 922–8.
65. Paus S, Brecht HM, Koster J, Seeger G, Klockgether T, Wullner U. Sleep attacks, daytime sleepiness, and dopamine agonists in Parkinson's disease. *Mov Disord* 2003; 18: 659–67.
66. Hobson DE, Lang AE, Martin WR, Razmy A, Rivest J, Fleming J. Excessive daytime sleepiness and sudden-onset sleep in Parkinson disease: a survey by the Canadian Movement Disorders Group. *JAMA* 2002; 287: 455–63.
67. Garcia-Borreguero D, Larrosa O, Bravo M. Parkinson's disease and sleep. *Sleep Med Rev* 2003; 7(2): 115–29.
68. Tracik F, Ebersbach G. Sudden daytime sleep onset in Parkinson's disease: polysomnographic recordings. *Mov Disord* 2001; 16: 500–6.
69. Ulivelli M, Rossi S, Lombardi C, et al. Polysomnographic characterization of pergolide-induced sleep attacks in idiopathic PD. *Neurology* 2002; 58: 462–5.
70. Frucht S, Rogers JD, Greene PE, Gordon MF, Fahn S. Falling asleep at the wheel: motor vehicle mishaps in persons taking pramipexole and ropinirole. *Neurology* 1999; 52: 1908–10.
71. Schapira AH. Sleep attacks (sleep episodes) with pergolide. *Lancet* 2000; 355: 1332–3.
72. Olanow CW, Schapira AH, Roth T. Waking up to sleep episodes in Parkinson's disease. *Mov Disord* 2000; 15: 212–15.
73. Basson R. Sex and idiopathic Parkinson's disease. *Adv Neurol* 2001; 86: 295–300.
74. Hillen ME, Sage JI. Nonmotor fluctuations in patients with Parkinson's disease. *Neurology* 1996; 47: 1180–3.
75. Schapira AH, Emre M, Jenner P, Poewe W. Levodopa in the treatment of Parkinson's disease. *Eur J Neurol* 2009; 16: 982–9.
76. Bhattacharyya S, Schapira AH, Mikhailidis DP, Davar J. Drug-induced fibrotic valvular heart disease. *Lancet* 2009; 374: 577–85.
77. Schapira AH, Barone P, Hauser RA, et al. Patient-reported convenience of once-daily versus three-times-daily dosing during long-term studies of pramipexole in early and advanced Parkinson's disease. *Eur J Neurol* 2013; 20: 50–6.
78. Schapira AH. Challenges to the development of disease-modifying therapies in Parkinson's disease. *Eur J Neurol* 2011; 18 (Suppl 1): 16–21.
79. Schapira AH. Treatment options in the modern management of Parkinson disease. *Arch Neurol* 2007; 64: 1083–8.
80. Schapira AH, Olanow CW. Drug selection and timing of initiation of treatment in early Parkinson's disease. *Ann Neurol* 2008; 64 (Suppl 2): S47–55.

CHAPTER 10

Parkinson's Disease: Advanced Disease, Motor Complications, and Management

Susan H. Fox, Binit Shah, Richard Walsh, and Anthony Lang

Introduction

The early stages of Parkinson's disease (PD) can be well managed with medical therapy. However, as the disease progresses, motor complications make it difficult to maintain adequate control of parkinsonian symptoms. Motor complications can broadly be divided into those which are amenable to dopaminergic therapies and those which tend to be refractory (see Table 10.1). The two main categories of levodopa-responsive motor complications are motor fluctuations and dyskinesia. Motor complications that are less responsive and often refractory to dopaminergic therapy include drug-resistant tremor, postural instability, freezing of gait, postural deformity, and speech problems. This chapter describes these motor complications and provides practical approaches to treatment and management.

The pathophysiology of motor complications

The development of drug-responsive motor complications occurs as a result of a combination of disease progression and chronic levodopa therapy. The plasma half-life of levodopa is short (~90 min); early in the disease this is buffered by the storage capabilities of remaining nigrostriatal neurons. Over time there is loss of presynaptic nigrostriatal dopaminergic input with more pulsatile stimulation of dopamine receptors. The consequent loss of the normal tonic stimulation of postsynaptic dopamine receptors results in pharmacodynamic changes in basal ganglia signalling pathways. In addition, there are peripheral and central pharmacokinetic factors that contribute further to the fluctuant response to levodopa (1). One means of defining the development of motor complications over time is the duration of antiparkinsonian response to levodopa. Thus, the antiparkinsonian response can be divided into what is termed the 'short-duration response' (SDR) and the 'long-duration response' (LDR) (2, 3). The SDR refers to levodopa benefit on PD symptoms which occurs in response to each individual dose of levodopa, whereas the LDR refers to maintained benefit of levodopa therapy beyond the normal half-life of an individual dose. The LDR is dominant in early PD, where patients with mild early disease are adequately controlled with only two to three daily doses of levodopa. Patients tend to note no temporal response to their medication doses and no 'wearing off', even if a dose is taken late or missed entirely. In advanced PD, the SDR is the more typical response to levodopa doses. In this case, PD patients are much more aware of the timing of individual levodopa doses. The maximum benefit of levodopa on PD symptoms may remain robust, but the duration of the effect shortens and the benefit is less consistent. Peripheral pharmacokinetics of levodopa in relation to absorption via the gastrointestinal (GI) tract can also play a significant role in the development of motor complications and will be discussed further below. The cause of drug-resistant motor complications in advanced PD is less clear, although progressive degenerative changes beyond the dopaminergic nigrostriatal system (e.g. within brainstem and cerebral cortex) are likely to be important. Full discussion of the pathophysiological changes that may occur in all forms of motor complications is beyond the scope of this chapter.

Drug-responsive motor complications

OFF state complications

Predictable wearing-off

The earliest encountered fluctuation in advancing PD is predictable wearing-off. As described above, the LDR effect begins to wane and the duration of benefit of each dose of levodopa becomes shorter. Akinesia on awakening in the morning may be the first sign of this that patients notice. Additionally, patients who forget doses or take them late will begin to recognize a re-emergence of problematic symptoms. Patients inevitably become more dependent on the need to rigidly adhere to their dose schedules. For some patients, factors such as exercise can further accelerate the wearing-off of

Table 10.1 Motor complications of advanced PD

OFF-state complications	On-state complications	Transitional state complications
Drug-responsive		
Predictable wearing-off	Peak-dose dyskinesia	Beginning-of-dose worsening and end-of-dose rebound
Sudden/unpredictable OFF	ON freezing	Diphasic dyskinesia
OFF freezing	Delayed ON	
OFF dystonia	Tachykinesia	
Dose failure/partial response		
Drug-resistant		
Gait and balance		
ON-period freezing		
Speech problems		
Refractory tremor		
Dysarthria and dysphagia		
Postural deformity		

the levodopa dose. A suggested algorithm for treating predictable wearing-off is shown in Fig. 10.1.

The treatment of predictable wearing-off involves maintaining a minimum effective level of levodopa throughout the day. Simply decreasing the dose interval to around 4 hours may be sufficient when wearing-off first begins. Alternatively, maintaining dose timings but increasing individual doses can also serve to increase the duration of action for levodopa, but with the risk of inducing dyskinesia. There may be an attraction to using a long-acting form of levodopa such as levodopa CR; however, double-blind randomized controlled trials (RCTs) comparing CR with standard levodopa have shown no benefit of such a strategy in reducing OFF

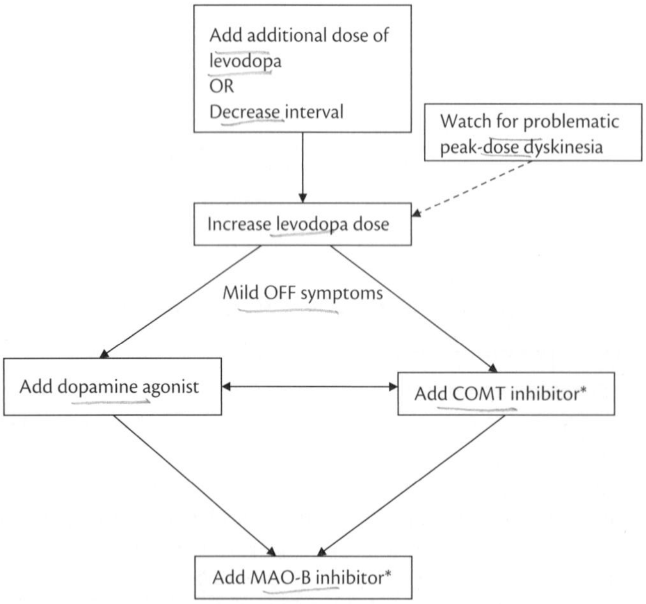

* The order of choosing these could be interchangeable

Fig. 10.1 Algorithm for managing predictable OFFs.

time (4, 5). The bioavailability of these longer acting preparations is 20–30% less than standard release preparations and patients require higher daily doses of levodopa, with a greater risk of dyskinesia (6). In addition, these preparations typically have a longer latency from drug intake to benefit, so patients may experience 'delayed-ON' problems.

Adding an inhibitor of catechol-*O*-methyltransferase (COMT), an enzyme involved in the breakdown of levodopa and dopamine, can help prolong the duration of action of levodopa and reduce OFF time. The peripheral COMT inhibitor entacapone has been demonstrated to reduce OFF time by an average of 1 hour per day (7). Retrospective analysis of four phase III RCTs (pooled $n = 977$) comparing RCTs of levodopa and entacapone with levodopa for 6 months followed by open-label addition of entacapone for up to 5 years showed maintained improvement in ON time (as measured by duration of action of first dose of the day) above baseline. However, 28% discontinued due to side effects including worsening of PD and dyskinesia (8). A combined formulation of levodopa–carbidopa and entacapone is also available and can help reduce the number of tablets patients take while achieving the same benefit as entacapone taken separately (9).

Tolcapone is another COMT inhibitor that has both central and peripheral actions and, because it has a longer half-life than entacapone, can be given three times daily regardless of levodopa timing (10). Tolcapone may be more efficacious than entacapone although no direct comparison has been performed. A meta-analysis of 14 studies with 2566 patients showed that tolcapone-treated patients had superior improvements in placebo-corrected ON time and OFF time compared with entacapone-treated patients (11). Tolcapone was withdrawn because of concerns related to liver toxicity in unmonitored patients. However, it has been reintroduced in several European countries and the US Food and Drug Administration (FDA) has modified monitoring requirements such that liver function testing is required every 2–4 weeks for 6 months and at the physician's discretion thereafter.

Monoamine oxidase B (MAO-B) is an enzyme which catalyses the oxidation and inactivation of monoamines, including dopamine. MAO-B inhibitors block this action and therefore prolong the effect of levodopa. The currently approved agents are selegiline and rasagiline. Selegiline is available in an oral ingestible tablet form and reduces OFF time by 1.6 hours per day (12). Concerns related to potential amphetamine metabolites led to development of a zydis form that disintegrates under the tongue and bypasses hepatic metabolism with reduced amphetamine metabolite production (13, 14). Evidence for benefit using this preparation is contradictory, with one study showing a significant effect on reducing total daily OFF time in patients with predictable wearing-off compared with placebo (15) and a second study showing no effect (16). Rasagiline is another MAO-B inhibitor that is not associated with the production of amphetamine metabolites (17). It can significantly reduce total daily OFF time by 1.18–1.8 hours (18, 19). No head-to-head comparison study between selegiline and rasagiline has been conducted.

Dopamine receptor agonists provide reliable long-acting dopamine receptor stimulation and are options for managing predictable wearing-off. The non-ergot agents ropinirole, ropinirole prolonged release (PR), pramipexole, and rotigotine, and the ergot-derived dopamine agonists pergolide, cabergoline, and bromocriptine, have all been shown to significantly reduce OFF time by an average of 1–1.5 hours per day and improve duration of ON time when combined with levodopa (20–27). To date, studies using once-daily pramipexole extended release (ER) in advanced PD for wearing-off have not been reported.

Dopamine agonists with a longer duration of action and/or once-daily dosing (e.g. cabergoline, ropinirole PR, pramipexole ER) or the transdermal rotigotine patch would appear to be more attractive options. However, to date, there appears to be no advantage to this strategy and improvement in OFF time appears comparable with other orally active dopamine agonists. A recent RCT comparing efficacy of the longer-acting version of ropinirole PR and regular ropinirole immediate release (IR) reported a significant benefit of ropinirole PR in the proportion of patients maintaining ≥20% reduction in OFF time (28), although the final dose of ropinirole was higher in the PR group than in the IR group, thus making comparisons difficult. The relative efficacy of all currently available add-on therapies to levodopa, including dopamine agonists, COMT inhibitors, or MAO-B inhibitors, is not clear because there is a lack of randomized comparator studies. One RCT has shown that rasagiline and entacapone are equally efficacious at reducing wearing-off (–1.18 hours/day for rasagiline and –1.2 hours/day for entacapone compared with –0.4 hours/day for placebo (19). A recent meta-analysis evaluating RCTs of add-on therapies using indirect comparisons showed that dopamine agonist therapy was more effective and reduced OFF time by 1.6 hours/day, compared with 0.8 hours/day with COMT inhibitors and 0.9 hours/day with MAO-B inhibitors (12). However, side effects were more frequent with dopamine agonists and COMT inhibitors than with MAO-B inhibitors (12).

Unpredictable OFFs, sudden OFFs, and ON–OFF fluctuations

Patients may experience unpredictable wearing-off that is unrelated to medication timing. When this wearing-off is rapid, occurring over seconds or minutes, it is termed 'sudden-OFF' (29). Triggers such as exercise or emotional stress may be present, but there is often no identifiable cause. Many advanced PD patients also encounter ON–OFF fluctuations, or 'yo-yoing' (29). These often rapid and unpredictable fluctuations between the ON and OFF states can be very debilitating.

Treatment of such fluctuations can be challenging. A practical approach to this problem is outlined in Fig. 10.2. For subjects on levodopa CR, one option is to convert to regular release levodopa; this ensures a more consistent onset and duration of effect, and allows for more precise dose titration. Increasing levodopa dose or frequency can then help to combat sudden OFFs and unpredictable OFFs, but one must be vigilant about worsening dyskinesia. Adding or increasing the dose of a dopamine agonist allows an increase in overall dopaminergic treatment with less risk of worsening dyskinesia. Indeed, adding a dopamine agonist may permit a reduction in levodopa dose and may even improve dyskinesia. Practically, however, side effects associated with dopamine agonists (see Table 10.3) often limit their use in this advanced PD population.

Rapid-onset oral forms of levodopa may be useful as 'rescue' for sudden-OFFs. These agents provide a more reliable rapid absorption and onset of effect (30). Preparations available include orally disintegrating levodopa–carbidopa and levodopa–benserazide, levodopa methylester, and levodopa ethylester (31). These levodopa preparations are not amenable to scheduled dosing because of the short duration of effect (1–1.5 hours) and are best used as intermittent rescue agents. An alternative when such soluble preparations are

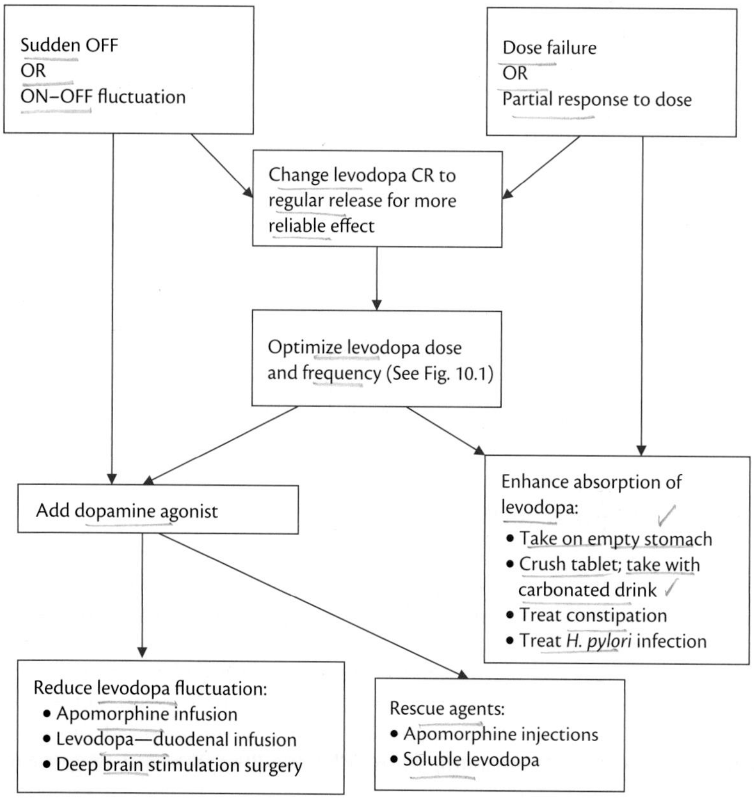

Fig. 10.2 Algorithm for managing unpredictable OFFs.

unavailable is to use a liquid levodopa preparation made by crushing levodopa–peripheral decarboxylase tablets, mixed together with water and ascorbic acid (vitamin C) as an antioxidant. This solution allows for minute dose adjustments and more rapid onset. The drawbacks to liquid levodopa include instability; the solution remains stable for less than 24 hours and must be refrigerated and kept away from light (32). Making up a new solution every day and storing and carrying it in portable containers can prove onerous. Patients and families often abandon this strategy soon after starting. Another rescue agent worthy of consideration is parenteral apomorphine. This is a dopamine agonist which has been used for many years in Europe for the treatment of ON–OFF fluctuations and sudden-OFF (33). A single subcutaneous injection can alleviate parkinsonian signs within 5–15 minutes and last for 1–1.5 hours (34). The dose needs to be determined for an individual patient and ranges from 3 to 10 mg. An open-label follow-up of 546 PD patients using subcutaneous apomorphine for OFF periods reported the most effective average dose to be 4 mg (35). Pre-treatment with oral antiemetics such as trimethobenzamide hydrochloride (300 mg tid) or domperidone (20 mg tid) is necessary given the pro-emetic effects of apomorphine. For subjects requiring several injections per day with persistent unpredictable ON–OFF fluctuations, apomorphine can also be given as a continuous subcutaneous infusion. Apomorphine infusions may be an alternative for individuals unsuitable for surgical treatments (see section below on treatments for unresponsive motor fluctuations).

Dose failure: no response to dose, delayed response, partial response

In early PD, patients may find that their response to levodopa is not greatly affected by diet or the relationship between meal and medication times. In advanced PD this typically changes, and maximizing levodopa absorption can be a key factor in reducing motor complications. The disease processes underlying PD, as well as intake of food per se, can lead to slowed gastric emptying with delay of levodopa transit and absorption in the small bowel. Constipation also results in slowed gastric emptying and worsens levodopa absorption. Other medications used in the treatment of PD, particularly anticholinergic agents, can further slow gastric emptying and bowel motility. Additionally, levodopa competes with dietary large amino acids for transport into the bloodstream and, in particular, across the blood–brain barrier.

A delayed ON is an increase in latency between taking a dose of levodopa and experiencing benefit from it (36). A partial response or entirely absent response to a dose of levodopa are called partial ON or dose failure (no-ON), respectively. These problems are often caused by deficient or delayed levodopa absorption in the GI tract. Delay in the action of one dose can sometimes result in simultaneous onset of effect with a subsequent dose, resulting in marked dyskinesias, further contributing to the wide variation in levodopa response. This effect can be further exacerbated by patients taking additional doses when they are concerned that a delay in onset means that a tablet has 'not worked'. A number of strategies can be tried in the hope of making the response to treatment more predictable:

- *Dietary protein intake.* Protein intake should be adjusted in such a way as to reduce interference with levodopa absorption. This can be accomplished by directing patients to avoid large protein loads at the morning meal and spread protein intake throughout the day.
- *Empty stomach.* Patients should also be instructed to take levodopa on an empty stomach (at least 30 minutes prior to food or 2 hours after) or with a light snack. If nausea is a problem, patients can be pretreated with an antiemetic agent with promotility properties, such as domperidone.
- *Constipation and anticholinergics.* Treating constipation and reducing or stopping anticholinergic treatment can provide improved GI motility and ease patient discomfort. In our experience, most standard stool softeners, osmotics, and stimulant laxatives are effective in managing constipation in PD.
- *Treatment of Helicobacter pylori.* infection is thought to cause a gastroduodenitis which interferes with levodopa absorption. There is recent evidence that eradication of *H. pylori* infection improves the efficacy of anti-PD therapy and hence reduces motor fluctuations (37, 38).
- *Soluble levodopa.* These preparations have a more rapid and reliable onset of action
- *Apomorphine.* Bypassing the GI system with parenteral apomorphine can avoid problems with levodopa gastrointestinal absorption entirely.

Acute deterioration of symptoms or persistence of unexplained dose failures in advanced PD without cause should raise suspicion of co-morbid pathologies (39). It is important to assess patients thoroughly for changes in compliance, intercurrent illness, or other factors which may affect PD control (Table 10.2).

Beginning-of-dose worsening and end-of-dose rebound

Patients can experience worsening of their symptoms soon after taking a levodopa dose, called 'beginning-of-dose worsening' (40). These symptoms, most commonly tremor, last for a short time (5–15 min) after which a more usual beneficial response ensues. Similarly, patients may also note an exacerbation or rebound of their symptoms as a dose of levodopa wears off, called 'end-of-dose rebound' (41). These rebounds can result in a phenomenon known as 'super-OFFs' where, as a dose of levodopa wears off, symptom severity is notably worse than in the early morning when the longest time has passed between levodopa doses. Fluctuating non-motor symptoms or non-motor fluctuations (e.g. pain, akathisia, behavioural changes) often complicate these super-OFFs, adding considerably to the patient's disability. Treating these symptoms is difficult. Adding a dose of levodopa while still in the ON state can help to avoid problematic wearing-off, but it often does so at the cost of increasing dyskinesia. Other approaches to treating motor fluctuations outlined above can all be tried with varying success. Referral for deep brain stimulation (DBS) should be considered when medication changes are unsuccessful for all the above motor complications.

OFF-period freezing

Freezing represents a transient inability to initiate or continue voluntary movement, usually lasting several seconds. Freezing is common in advanced PD but can occur at any stage. Early freezing should prompt consideration of an alternative diagnosis, such as progressive supranuclear palsy or vascular parkinsonism. Freezing can disrupt movement in any muscle group, but 'freezing of gait' (FoG) is the most common form observed and is an important contributor to the risk of falling. Freezing of gait can occur on initiation of gait (start hesitation), when turning, or

Table 10.2 Management of acute deterioration in advanced PD

1. Check for missed doses or inappropriate administration of dopamine receptor antagonists. This is most common in the perioperative setting.
2. A change of levodopa formulation between generic and proprietary brands can sometimes cause a change in clinical response, although this is uncommon and generally mild. A planned or inadvertent change from intermediate to controlled release formulation will reduce the bioavailability of administered levodopa by approximately 30%.
3. Constipation can affect absorption of levodopa and hence result in apparent worsening of underlying PD. A plain film of abdomen can help diagnose constipation, but this is usually clear from the history. Resolution can sometimes considerably improve individual dose responses.
4. If the pattern of lower limb weakness appears pyramidal or there is an unexplained deterioration of gait that is unresponsive to levodopa, always consider a cervical spine problem, particularly in the age group with advanced disease. Be particularly suspicious when dyskinesias below the neck resolve in the setting of new gait impairment.
5. Where there is also cognitive deterioration, eliminate other common causes of systemic upset in an elderly population, including electrolyte imbalance, dehydration, new drugs, and infections. Where there is a history of falls consider a CT brain scan to rule out a subdural haematoma. Long-standing drugs such as amantadine that were previously tolerated may subacutely become toxic due to changes in renal function or age-related changes in cerebral tolerance.

less commonly on reaching a destination such as approaching a chair to sit down. Another characteristic of freezing is responsiveness to triggers. Patients will often report increased incidence of freezing in situations where they must deal with restrictions in time (crossing the street with a changing light is often cited as an example) or space (a narrow doorway). A change in sensory inputs such as a transition from one colour of floor tile to another can also trigger freezing. The relationship of freezing to levodopa treatment is complex. It has been suggested that freezing is a side effect of levodopa treatment (42). Longer duration of levodopa treatment correlates with freezing, although this association may be more reflective of an association with greater disease severity rather than with levodopa per se (43). Freezing can be seen in both treated and untreated PD, supporting the notion that it is a disease-related phenomenon and not necessarily a motor complication of levodopa treatment, although in some patients high doses of levodopa or dopamine agonists clearly trigger or worsen freezing. Non-dopaminergic pathology may also be important as there appears to be a relationship with the emergence of balance and speech problems, which are typically unresponsive to levodopa treatment (see later section).

The underlying pathophysiology of freezing is unclear. Freezing episodes may be the tip of the iceberg, with evidence of subclinical stride-to-stride variation and progressive shortening of stride before freezing episodes in affected patients (44). This would suggest that freezing is not a paroxysmal gait disorder but part of a wider disorder of the timing and scaling of lower limb movements during walking. OFF-period freezing has been linked to abnormalities of temporal discrimination thresholds that normalize with levodopa (45). Cognitive load appears to be a factor in some cases, raising the possibility that an attentive deficit contributes to freezing when 'dual tasking' (46).

In the majority of patients freezing occurs in the OFF state, suggesting a relationship with low dopamine levels (47). This offers an important therapeutic avenue to begin with where this relationship can be gleaned from the history. Therefore management of OFF states can reduce OFF period freezing. There has been interest in the possibility that the MAO-B inhibitor selegiline may have an additional protective effect by reducing the risk of future freezing. A double-blind placebo-controlled follow-up of the DATATOP cohort found that fewer patients treated with selegiline went on to develop freezing (48). However, much of the therapeutic effect in patients with OFF period freezing is likely to be due to a symptomatic effect. Amantadine is another drug with a mild dopaminergic effect which may be helpful for freezing in some patients, although there is conflicting evidence (43, 49). ON period and unpredictable freezing and non-dopaminergic approaches to their management are dealt with later in this chapter.

OFF dystonia

Dystonia can occur during OFF periods or when dopaminergic therapy is wearing off. The prototypical time for this is upon awakening in the morning, known as 'early morning OFF dystonia' or 'early morning painful dystonia'. This tends to involve the extremities, particularly the feet, and toe curling or other fixed dystonic posture is commonly reported (50, 51). These problematic OFF times can be managed by having patients take levodopa prophylactically or as soon as symptoms begin. Soluble levodopa preparations, crushing levodopa tablets, or rescue injections of apomorphine can provide fast-acting options to reverse OFF symptoms. For early morning dystonia, patients can be instructed to set an alarm and take a dose of levodopa overnight. Levodopa CR at bedtime can provide benefit by providing some dopaminergic coverage by the time patients wake up. An algorithm for the management of dystonia in PD is reviewed later (see Fig. 10.4).

ON state complications

The long-term effectiveness of levodopa can become complicated by the development of involuntary movements—dyskinesia. Less frequently subjects can also experience some worsening of certain symptoms with levodopa, including freezing (ON-freezing) and increased speed of movements (tachykinesia).

Dyskinesia

It is important to determine the timing of dyskinesia in relation to the antiparkinsonian action of levodopa as treatment options will vary.

Peak-dose dyskinesia

Peak-dose dyskinesia is the most common form of dyskinesia and occurs at the time of the best ON response to levodopa, while less commonly 'square-wave' dyskinesia occurs throughout the entire duration of levodopa effect (52). Peak-dose dyskinetic movements are typically choreiform, often of the neck and limbs, but dystonic posturing is also common (53). Ballistic movements and myoclonus are rare. Dyskinesia often begins with limb and neck involvement on the side most affected by PD (54). As the disease progresses and dyskinesia becomes more prominent, facial dyskinesia and even diaphragmatic dyskinesia can be seen.

Treatment of peak-dose dyskinesia begins with first identifying the degree to which dyskinesias are problematic. Most patients on levodopa therapy will develop dyskinesias as some point (55); however, these dyskinesias are often not troublesome (56). Where dyskinesia is either physically limiting for patients, or presents unacceptable social embarrassment, treatment is required. A practical approach to managing dyskinesia is shown in Fig. 10.3. First, reducing the dose of levodopa should be attempted with close observation of the patient to assess for worsening parkinsonian disability. Along with decreasing individual doses of levodopa, increasing dose frequency may be required to avoid wearing-off. Using frequent small doses of levodopa runs the risk of causing a very unpredictable fluctuating motor state with multiple dose failures. Dopamine agonists may be used to enable a reduction in levodopa without worsening of dyskinesia. Another option is to reduce or discontinue the use of COMT inhibitors and MAO-B inhibitors. As PD advances and motor fluctuations are more problematic, these adjuvant agents provide less benefit than in earlier disease, they are more likely to induce dyskinesia, and stopping them may not adversely affect overall PD symptom control (12).

If the above steps fail to reduce problematic dyskinesia or lead to unacceptable worsening of PD symptoms, introducing a specific antidyskinesia agent should be considered. The most commonly used agent for this purpose is the non-selective *N*-methyl-D-aspartate (NMDA) receptor antagonist amantadine (100–400 mg/day), which has been shown to reduce dyskinesia without worsening parkinsonian symptoms (57, 58). Waning of benefit and tachyphylaxis can limit long-term use of amantadine. However, a recent study suggested ongoing benefit of amantadine for dyskinesia after a mean use of 4.8 years (59).

Clozapine is an atypical antipsychotic agent with a reduced propensity to worsen parkinsonian symptoms because it has less affinity for striatal dopamine D2 receptors than standard neuroleptics and non-dopaminergic properties (60). These properties have enabled clozapine to be safely used to treat PD psychosis. A single RCT demonstrated that clozapine reduced dyskinesia by 30%, although the effect was largely on resting and not activated dyskinesia (61). The possible adverse effect of agranulocytosis warrants frequent blood monitoring and thus can limit its convenience and use.

Botulinum toxin injections can be used for problematic or disabling focal dystonic dyskinesias. These are best used when there is a more fixed posture (especially accompanied by pain) where targeted injections can provide significant benefit without risk of bothersome weakness (62). The management of dystonia (both ON and OFF period) is summarized in Fig. 10.4.

Diphasic dyskinesia

Diphasic, or 'beginning-of-dose/end-of-dose', dyskinesia involves predominant lower extremity stereotypical alternating, jerking, dystonic, or ballistic kicking movements (53). These symptoms occur at low or intermediate levels of levodopa (i.e. when dopaminergic tone is increasing soon after a dose is given or decreasing as a dose is wearing off). Managing these symptoms can be challenging. Clinical experience suggests that the most effective option is to add a dopamine agonist to provide longer-acting dopamine receptor stimulation. To date, no RCTs have been performed to fully evaluate this approach. Agents used for predictable wearing-off typically do not work well for diphasic dyskinesia. Shortening the levodopa interval may work temporarily; however, the timing often quickly

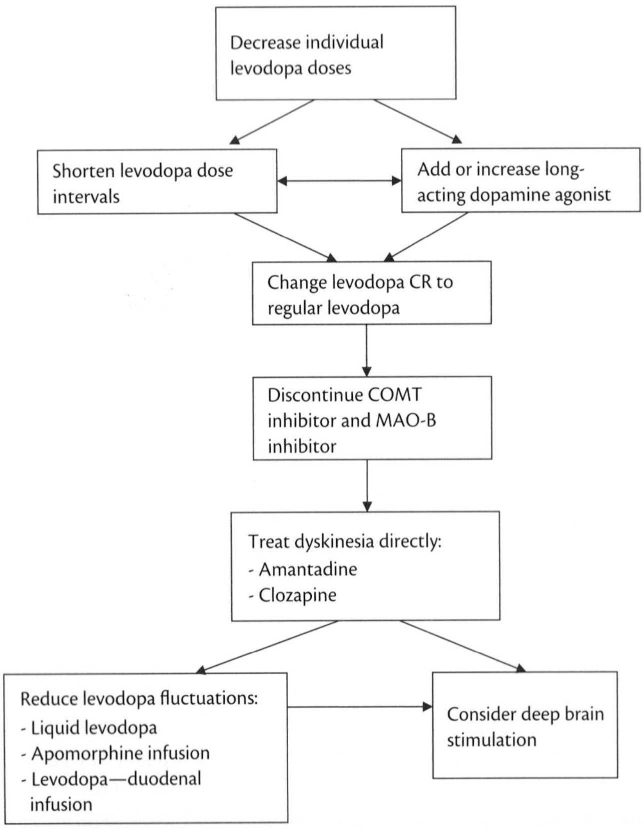

Fig. 10.3 Algorithm for managing peak-dose levodopa-induced dyskinesia.

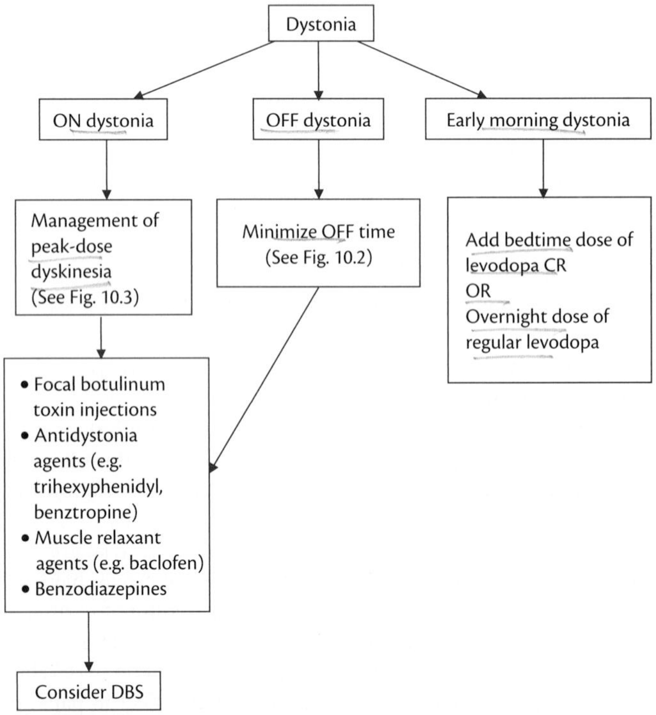

Fig. 10.4 Management of dystonia in PD.

resets with a relapse in symptoms after a short hiatus. A fast-acting rescue, in the form of a soluble or crushed levodopa or apomorphine injection, may shorten or help avoid this phenomenon entirely (63). Some patients will have a mixture of both diphasic and peak-dose dyskinesia, thus making management very difficult. If suitable, patients with diphasic dyskinesia may benefit from bilateral subthalamic nucleus (STN) DBS (64).

Tachykinesia

Some patients may experience an increase in speed in speaking (tachyphemia) and walking (tachyambulia). These are ON-period phenomena usually associated with higher doses of levodopa (65). If problematic, such symptoms should be managed in the same manner as peak-dose dyskinesia. Additionally, speech and physical therapy, paying particular attention to these issues, may provide some degree of benefit and should be explored.

Currently available agents for the management of drug-responsive motor complications, their adverse effects, and conclusions from current evidence based medicine (EBM) reviews from the American Academy of Neurology (AAN) Practice Parameters and Movement Disorder Society Evidence-Based Medicine Updates on Treatments of Motor Symptoms of PD are reviewed in Table 10.3. For recent reviews on new drugs in development for motor complications, see refs 66 and 67.

Table 10.3 Drug classes used for advanced PD motor symptoms, evidence for their use, and adverse effect profile

Motor complication	Class of drug	Drug(s)	AAN Practice Parameter recommendations (68)	Mov Disorder Society EBM recommendations 2002, 2005, 2011	Side effects
Predictable wearing-off	Dopamine receptor agonists	Ropinirole (up to 24mg/day), ropinirole PR Pramipexole (up to 4.5mg/day) Rotigotine patch (up to 6mg/24h) Bromocriptine (up to 100mg/day) Cabergoline (up to 3mg/day) Pergolide (voluntarily withdrawn)	Pergolide, pramipexole, and ropinirole should be considered for treatment of wearing-off (level B) Cabergoline may be considered (level C). Bromocriptine may be disregarded (level C) There is no evidence that one DA is superior to another	Ropinirole, ropinirole ER, pramipexole, pergolide, and rotigotine are efficacious Bromocriptine and cabergoline are probably efficacious	Common: nausea, postural hypotension, somnolence, hallucinations, lower extremity oedema, sleep fragmentation (68) Major: impulse control disorders (ICDs) including excessive or uncontrollable gambling, shopping, hypersexuality, and hyperphagia (69)
	COMT inhibitor	Entacapone (200mg/dose of levodopa up to 8 per day) Tolcapone (100mg tid)	Entacapone (level A) and tolcapone (level B) are effective at reducing wearing-off There is no evidence that one COMT inhibitor is superior to another	Entacapone and tolcapone are efficacious	Common: constipation, nausea/vomiting, dry mouth, somnolence Major: long-term follow-up of liver monitoring of tolcapone reported that mild increases in transaminases are common, but >3 times normal is rare (1–2%) with no mortality (70)
	Levodopa	Levodopa CR, DDCI controlled release	Levodopa–carbidopa CR is not helpful in treating motor fluctuations (level C)	Insufficient evidence	Similar to regular release levodopa–carbidopa
	MAO-B inhibitor	Selegiline (5–10mg) Rasagiline (1–2mg) Zydis selegiline (buccal absorption in order to minimize first-pass metabolism)	Rasagiline is effective at reducing wearing-off (level A) Selegiline (level C) No current evidence that one MAO inhibitor is superior to another	Insufficient evidence for selegiline and zydis selegiline in motor fluctuations Rasagiline is efficacious	Common: constipation, dizziness, hypotension, emesis Drug interaction: there is a theoretical risk of serotonin syndrome with MAO-B inhibitors and concurrent use of antidepressants (tricyclic and serotonin reuptake inhibitors). However, recent RCTs using rasagiline in PD patients also using antidepressants report no cases of serotonin syndrome (71) Tyramine effect: unlike MAO-A inhibitors, MAO-B inhibitors have not been shown to augment the hypertensive effects of tyramine ingestion (the 'cheese effect') (72). Theoretical risks should be explained to patients, but concerns should be allayed given the current evidence of safety

(Continued)

Table 10.3 (Continued)

Motor complication	Class of drug	Drug(s)	AAN Practice Parameter recommendations (68)	Mov Disorder Society EBM recommendations 2002, 2005, 2011	Side effects
Dose failure, no-ON response, sudden-OFFs; ON–OFF fluctuations	Levodopa	Dispersible: levodopa–benserazide Carbidopa: orally disintegrating tablets Levodopa methylester (melevodopa), levodopa ethylester (etilevodopa)		Insufficient evidence	Similar to regular release levodopa–carbidopa
		Stable suspension of levodopa and carbidopa in methyl cellulose by infusion via gastrojejunostomy		Probably efficacious	Acute complications include peritonitis, haemorrhage, local wound infection, and perioperative delirium in elderly patients Hardware issues are relatively common and include tube kinking, displacement, and occlusion Case reports of peripheral neuropathy/GBS with duodenal levodopa; possibly associated with vitamin B_6 deficiency—further studies are ongoing (73)
	Parenteral DA	Apomorphine—intermittent or (3–10mg) infusion (30–100mg/day) s.c.		Apomorphine is efficacious	Subcutaneous injections Nausea prevented/reduced using trimethobenzamide hydrochloride (300 mg tid) or domperidone (20mg tid) Hypotension, visual hallucinations and worsening psychosis, punding Infusional therapy: side effects as above plus subcutaneous nodules—treated with ultrasound and rotation of injection sites; olive-green discoloration of clothing
Dyskinesia	Non-subtype selective NMDA-receptor antagonist	Amantadine (100–400mg/d)	Amantadine may be effective (level C)	Efficacious	Psychosis, confusions, hallucinations, painful lower extremity oedema, and livedo reticularis Side effects: corneal lesions; myoclonus (dose/plasma-level dependent); care with renal disease
	Atypical antipsychotic	Clozapine (12.5–100mg/d)	Insufficient data to recommend clozapine	Efficacious	Agranulocytosis: required mandatory monitoring Sedation, postural hypotension

DA, dopamine agonist; DDCI, dopa decarboxylase inhibitor.

Treatment options for fluctuations refractory to oral therapies

Apomorphine infusion

Apomorphine is a potent dopamine agonist that can be administered by either intermittent subcutaneous (s.c.) injection for sudden-OFF periods (see above) or infused over 12–24 hours as a method of treating motor complications. The system requires a portable pump that is connected to a small needle usually inserted into the skin of the thigh or abdomen. The injection site is rotated to avoid the development of subcutaneous nodules. The main indication for apomorphine infusion would be for subjects with motor complications unsuitable for deep brain stimulation (DBS) of the subthalamic nucleus (discussed below). Apomorphine infusion is effective at reducing overall OFF time by 60–70% and can also improve dyskinesia (by up to 60%) by a mechanism other than simply permitting a reduction in levodopa dose (74). Despite this benefit, uptake in use of apomorphine is limited because of cost and practical issues related to skin viability (e.g. nodule formation), the availability of nursing support, and the need for an active caregiver.

It is important to emphasize to patients that apomorphine will not improve any symptoms that are not already responsive to levodopa. The total daily dose of levodopa required can be reduced by up to half in some patients, but monotherapy is usually not achievable for tolerability reasons. The side effects of apomorphine are similar to those of other dopamine agonists, with local effects specific to the parenteral infusion (Table 10.3).

Infusional levodopa–carbidopa intestinal gel

Infusional therapies using levodopa have been attempted over many years but have usually failed because of problems with the method of administration and the need for large volumes to dilute levodopa. A recent preparation using levodopa–carbidopa (20mg/5mg/ml) in a stable methylcellulose gel has overcome some of these issues. The levodopa gel is delivered through a gastrostomy tube with a jejunal extension by a pump carried by the patient. The gastrostomy is endoscopically placed, usually after a trial period of nasojejunal delivery, and can typically be initiated during a single hospital admission. A small study evaluated the efficacy of this preparation over 3 weeks when compared with conventional oral therapy, reporting a significant improvement in ON time without troublesome dyskinesia (75). A retrospective review of 64 patients with mean follow-up of 3.7 years (maximum 10.7 years) reported ongoing benefit (76). Although levodopa–carbidopa gel infusion is available in many countries, its efficacy has not been reported in an RCT; a large multi-centre double-blind double-placebo-controlled trial is ongoing in North America.

The large size of the pump required to infuse the viscous gel containing levodopa in suspension is a potential inconvenience and may deter some patients. Most patients start with the infusion running during waking hours only, but continuous infusion overnight can be used for troublesome nocturnal symptoms. Additional bolus doses can be given at any time of the day as required. The total daily dose of levodopa required can be reduced by 20–30% by the addition of a COMT inhibitor if not already being used. Ideally, patients are weaned off dopamine agonists as their long half-life is no longer of benefit in the setting of continuous levodopa delivery.

Complications associated with gastrostomy tube placement and its chronic use are not uncommon (Table 10.3). Acute medical problems associated with any surgery will be encountered in this patient group, many of whom will be elderly and considered unfit for DBS. With continuous use up to 63% of patients will experience technical hardware problems such as tube kinking, occlusion, or displacement (77). More recently, there have been reports of development of a subacute neuropathy in patients receiving jejunal levodopa infusion (73). This appears to be associated with biochemical disturbances in B vitamins and associated co-factors, although further clarification on the exact pathogenesis is required.

Technical consideration and cost may preclude widespread uptake in this treatment. However, infusional levodopa may be useful in advanced PD subjects intolerant of apomorphine because of confusion, hallucinations, intolerable infusion site complications, or hypotension, or for subjects who are considered poor surgical candidates because of age constraints or cognitive–behavioural concerns (78). Despite concerns in relation to potential tolerance and neuropsychiatric complications of continuous dopaminergic stimulation, infusional levodopa therapy appears to be well tolerated (79). In the recently reported experience of the French DUODOPA study group, over 50% of the study participants had cognitive impairment suggestive of PD dementia; however, the procedure was tolerated and no patient experiencing hallucinations prior to infusional therapy reported a worsening of this side effect (77). On the other hand, management of this form of therapy is very complex, and patients with moderate to severe dementia should probably not be considered as candidates.

Surgical options in advanced Parkinson's disease

Despite being developed as early as the 1940s, surgical therapy for PD faded from prominence after the advent of levodopa therapy. However, in the last two decades it has again emerged as a viable management option in PD. Better imaging techniques have allowed stereotactic targeting of deep brain structures and non-destructive stimulation has largely replaced irreversible lesioning. DBS has the added advantage of allowing postsurgical modification through adjustment of stimulation settings, and this is now accepted as being superior to the best medical therapy for the management of fluctuations and dyskinesias in advanced PD (80, 81). Stereotactic lesioning is still used in certain clinical scenarios, such as elderly patients in whom DBS is considered too high risk, and therefore will be addressed briefly below.

Patient selection is of paramount importance. Apart from tremor, DBS will provide no additional symptom relief over levodopa, but reducing the variability of this response (i.e. motor fluctuations) is the main target of this treatment. There is no absolute age cut-off for consideration of surgery, although many centres do not pursue surgical options in patients above the age of 70. Advancing age increases the probability of cognitive impairment, surgical comorbidities, and non-levodopa-responsive PD symptoms, such as postural impairment. Because of the risk of postoperative deterioration, cognitive impairment is the most common exclusion factor cited, although a recent report from a consortium of experts in the field failed to reach a consensus on the most appropriate measurement tools and exclusion criteria, and there is increasing interest in applying surgical treatment earlier in the course of the disease before patients are severely disabled by the symptoms known to be most responsive (82). As with much of the decision-making process, the timing of surgery needs to be individualized. Most patients undergoing DBS will have had over 10 years of disease by virtue of the natural history of evolving motor fluctuations. Early surgical intervention may provide better outcomes in terms of quality of life measures (83). A multidisciplinary approach to patient selection, including input from neurosurgery, neurology, neuropsychology, and psychiatry, is vital before a final decision on suitability is made.

Structures targeted in the management of PD and the rationale and evidence for targeting each will be discussed below along with guidelines for patient selection.

Subthalamotomy and subthalamic nucleus stimulation

The subthalamic nucleus (STN) is of interest as a target for surgical treatment given our knowledge of pathologically increased neuronal firing within it that may drive excessive inhibitory outputs via the indirect cortico-striato-pallido-thalamo-cortical pathway. However, although the STN was first chosen because it was believed that DBS has a lesion-like inhibitory effect on its target, the effects of DBS are clearly much more complicated than this and it must be acknowledged that there is still great uncertainty as to exactly how it works and whether its mechanism of action is the same in different anatomical targets. Subthalamotomy is rarely performed now because of the risk of producing contralateral hemiballism. This risk does not appear to be present with stimulation of the same target. There has previously been little evidence to guide the choice between the STN or the globus pallidus internus (GPi) as the prime surgical target in PD, although the STN is currently the more commonly chosen target. The recently reported Co-op Study of 299 patients randomized to either STN or GPi DBS found similar motor benefit in both groups at 24 months (84). Analysis of secondary endpoints suggested that patients with depression may benefit more from GPi DBS. Worsening verbal fluency and executive dysfunction have been reported following STN DBS, but these parameters were not evaluated in the Co-op Study (85). Therefore, it seems that, with all else being equal, individualization of the target for particular patients may depend on a number of non-motor features that should be evaluated prior to a final choice being made. Long-term follow-up will be critical in helping to resolve this debate as there is some evidence that patients with GPi stimulation may lose benefit after a period of two or more years, and such patients have responded to subsequent STN stimulation (86).

Pallidotomy and pallidal stimulation

This target is chosen because it receives glutaminergic neurons from the STN which is overactive in PD. Lesioning or stimulation of the GPi is sometimes chosen for its particular benefit in managing contralateral dyskinesia or dystonia. It can also be helpful for contralateral rigidity and tremor (87). As indicated above, it is unclear why lesioning and stimulation can produce similar results. Bilateral pallidotomy is associated with increased risk of cognitive dysfunction, dysarthria, and dysphagia (88, 89). As with thalamotomy, the propensity of bilateral lesioning to produce intolerable side effects has pushed bilateral GPi stimulation to the forefront. The GPi and STN are the two main targets for the management of motor fluctuations in advanced PD with no clear benefit of one over the other in terms of change in UPDRS motor scores (see below).

Thalamotomy and thalamic stimulation

Unilateral thalamotomy of the ventralis intermediate (VIM) nucleus has potent anti-tremor effects on the contralateral side and produces a reduction in contralateral rigidity. The latter effect is less impressive than the tremor response with reported improvements from 45.8 to 92% (90, 91) Bilateral thalamotomy is associated with an increased risk of irreversible dysarthria and dysphagia. Given this risk, bilateral thalamotomies are not commonly performed since DBS has become the standard of practice. DBS for PD tremor should not be restricted to patients with advanced disease, as younger patients with a shorter duration of disease but intractable drug-resistant tremor may also benefit greatly.

Other targets

Recently, novel target sites for DBS have been investigated. These include bilateral stimulation of the caudal zona incerta (cZI) and pedunculopontine nucleus (PPN). A study evaluating cZI in PD tremor, along with other tremor types, found marked reduction primarily in PD tremor, but also in bradykinesia and rigidity (92). However, it is unclear whether this effect was due to stimulation of the STN, given its proximity to the cZI. PPN stimulation is discussed later in this chapter. It may have a role in controlling axial symptoms and improving postural instability in PD (93).

Drug-resistant motor complications

The gratifying response of most symptoms to treatment in early PD is often in stark contrast to the predominance of symptoms that are not responsive to dopaminergic drugs in advanced disease. This is not restricted to the non-motor features that are addressed in Chapter 11. With advancing disease, axial motor features emerge that can be frustratingly refractory to treatment. Such symptoms include postural instability and dysphagia which carry a high morbidity and attributable mortality in advanced disease. In the Sydney Multicentre Study 81% of patients were experiencing falls at a disease duration of 15 years, 23% had sustained fractures, and 50% were experiencing choking episodes (94). These non-dopa-responsive features were deemed to be more disabling than the motor fluctuations that were also extremely common in this cohort. Measures to help management of these late motor features, typically resistant to levodopa, are discussed below.

Falls and postural instability

The impact of falling in PD can be huge, not only in terms of immediate risk of fractures and their associated complications but also on the psychological outlook of the patient. It is important to recognize that falls are commonly multifactorial in patients with long-standing disease, making both their management and the study of novel therapies difficult. Careful history taking with a reliable informant is, as always, important. Consideration should be given to the possibility that orthostatic hypotension may contribute to some falls and can be effectively managed by a reduction in hypotensive agents (including dopamine agonists) or the addition of drugs that increase vasomotor tone or circulating blood volume. Cognitive issues are also likely to play a significant role. Anecdotally, patients will often report a fall occurring when trying to perform two tasks at once (dual tasking) such as turning to pick up something from a worktop in the kitchen. Reduced attention to the act of maintaining an upright posture may be responsible when the automatic motor programmes that maintain postural control cannot be relied upon. There is limited evidence to support a trial of acetylcholinesterase inhibitors—drugs which may improve cognition or attention (95).

The majority of falls in advanced PD are due to postural instability, a primary disorder of balance that becomes increasingly common with advancing disease duration. Freezing of gait will often accompany postural instability but can occur independently. It is likely that involvement of non-dopaminergic neurons projecting to and from the basal ganglia contribute to the instability. The structural correlates of gait dysfunction in PD are poorly understood but there has been interest in pursuing alternative targets for DBS, in particular the PPN area. This is a poorly defined structure anatomically, made up predominantly of cholinergic neurons that are known to be destroyed in PD. The PPN has a number of efferent and afferent connections with the basal ganglia and surrounding brainstem nuclei. Blinded evaluations of stimulation, possibly influencing an excess of descending inhibitory control from the basal ganglia, have suggested limited benefit (93) and, clearly, further well-designed trials are needed before this target can be accepted for treatment-resistant axial features. The current mainstay of managing postural instability is physiotherapy and gait training. Often the very process of addressing postural instability in the clinic can lead to a reduction in falling frequency, as both patients and family become increasingly cautious. Input from physiotherapists with experience in managing PD can be particularly helpful as patients will learn adaptive mechanisms to prevent falls and can be trained to concentrate on maintaining stride length (96). Over time, however, the cognitive impairment that often accompanies the onset of axial motor symptoms can limit the benefit patients obtain from such training. Treatment to prevent osteoporosis is important to limit the consequences of falls in PD.

Unpredictable or ON-period freezing

ON-period freezing occurs when patients otherwise have little bradykinesia, rigidity, or tremor. Most patients with ON-period freezing also experience freezing during OFF periods, and this combination results in rather unpredictable freezing. These forms of freezing are particularly frustrating for both patient and physician to manage, typically being stubbornly unresponsive to drug treatment. Paradoxically, 'high-dose freezing' or 'hypotonic freezing' is a phenomenon that was described in some of the first patients treated with levodopa. A correlation between serum levodopa concentrations and akinesia was demonstrated (97). Some of these patients would have been treated with doses far higher than those in common usage today and the applicability to current practice is questionable. However, when faced with a patient receiving high individual doses of levodopa (or dopamine agonists), and where all other therapeutic avenues have been exhausted, a trial of lowering dopaminergic medication doses is not unreasonable. However, lowering levodopa may lead to worsening of other PD features. Thus a non-dopaminergic approach may be an option for ON-period freezing. Several of the non-dopaminergic treatments tried have targeted the attention deficits proposed to contribute to some forms of freezing. Others target monoaminergic neurotransmitters, including noradrenaline and serotonin which are also depleted in PD and may play a role in brainstem circuits serving gait stability. Non-dopaminergic approaches to freezing of gait include the following.

1. *Caffeine.* A non-selective adenosine receptor antagonist, caffeine has been studied as a non-dopaminergic treatment of freezing in PD. A dose of 100 mg daily improved the 'akinetic' subtype but tolerance developed (98). The mechanism of action is unclear, but it may be that improved attention is responsible, as opposed to a direct effect on basal ganglia as has been proposed for other adenosine antagonists in development for motor symptoms of PD (99).
2. *Methylphenidate.* This amphetamine derivative boosts brain noradrenaline and dopamine levels by blocking reuptake. In high doses, methylphenidate reduced freezing in patients with advanced disease who had previously undergone bilateral STN DBS (100). However, a recent study using 80 mg/day showed no effect on gait, suggesting that subjects with freezing are unlikely to benefit (101). In a similar manner to selegiline and caffeine, methylphenidate may be effective in part through a direct effect on attention (102).
3. *Antidepressant drugs.* Anxiety states can provoke freezing in PD. Treatment of anxiety intuitively may improve freezing unresponsive to dopaminergic drugs. A recent case report identified a patient with primary progressive freezing of gait who had a clear response to the serotonin–noradrenaline reuptake inhibitor (SNRI) antidepressant duloxetine but not to citalopram (103). Given the action of the former, this raises the question of a more specific role for noradrenaline in the mechanism of freezing in PD.
4. *Amantadine.* Anecdotally, success with amantadine has been reported where freezing of gait has been unresponsive to dopaminergic medications. However, there are no data from randomized placebo-controlled trials to support this assertion. A recent open-label non-randomized study using intravenous amantadine demonstrated a significant improvement in subjective freezing in five of six patients with PD that was unrelated to changes in UPDRS motor scores, suggesting a mechanism other than a dopaminergic effect (104). Replication in a blinded study is required.
5. *PPN DBS.* In a recent study of unilateral DBS of the PPN there was a suggestion that patients' subjective ratings of freezing and postural instability improved (93), but further studies are required to validate this.

Refractory tremor

The management of drug-resistant tremor is not exclusive to advanced PD but may become increasingly problematic and disabling as time progresses. Management can be difficult and often frustrating as the benefits of levodopa in treating bradykinesia and rigidity can be overshadowed by a recalcitrant tremor. Maximization of levodopa therapy is typically tried but is limited by dopaminergic side effects at higher doses, in particular dyskinesia that becomes ubiquitous in advanced disease. The potential benefit of an anticholinergic in patients with long-standing PD is often limited by the age profile of this population in whom tolerability is an issue. Importantly, unlike all other parkinsonian features, the absence of a levodopa response in the management of tremor does not predict a poor operative outcome should DBS be considered. However, a number of medical strategies can be tried.

1. *Dopamine agonists.* There is evidence to support the adjunctive use of a dopamine agonist to provide an additive benefit for PD tremor, even with concomitant reductions in levodopa dose (105). Anecdotally, some patients with little or no tremor response to levodopa can experience an improvement on an agonist.
2. *Amantadine.* Some patients will report improvement with use of this glutamate antagonist, although the mechanism of action is unclear. There is evidence from double-blinded studies that amantadine is a reasonable choice as a second-line agent in the treatment of parkinsonian tremor (106, 107). Antagonism of striatal glutaminergic projections or STN projections to the GPi, where pathological neuronal oscillations can be recorded, may be responsible.
3. *Clozapine.* Evidence exists for an anti-tremor effect of clozapine in PD tremor (108–110). In keeping with the use of clozapine in dyskinesia, the doses required are typically similar to that required for psychosis in PD, and therefore there can be additional improvement in sleep disturbance, anxiety, and hallucinations. A starting dose of 12.5 mg at night alone can be effective, and rarely is more than 50 mg daily required. However, mandatory blood monitoring precludes widespread use of clozapine.
4. *β-adrenergic antagonists.* Consideration of a β-adrenergic antagonist for tremor management in PD may be an option, especially if there is a postural component and when worsening with anxiety or stress is a major complaint. Despite widespread use, there is a paucity of evidence for this approach (111). Long-acting propranolol up to 160 mg daily is generally well tolerated, but care should be taken in advanced PD because of the risk of bradycardia and significant postural drop in blood pressure.
5. *Mirtazapine.* The antidepressant mirtazapine has anticholinergic and antiserotonergic properties that may help reduce tremor, but this has not been demonstrated in a randomized placebo-controlled trial (112, 113).

Dysarthria and dysphagia

Speech disturbance in PD is characterized by monotony of pitch and volume, loss of prosody, variability of rate, bursts of rapid unintelligible speech (tachyphemia), and imprecise consonants (114).

Hypophonia can also be an early symptom when improvement with levodopa treatment suggests a contribution from dopamine deficiency (115). Levodopa-induced oro-buccal-lingual dyskinesias in the ON state can also have a detrimental effect on speech output in PD.

Speech therapy is commonly used in the absence of a demonstrable levodopa response. Lee Silverman Voice Treatment (LSVT) is the only technique that has consistently shown benefit. This method involves an intensive programme of frequent training developed to promote an up-scaling of vocal amplitude by improving vocal cord adduction (116, 117). Sustained benefit on speech volume has been reported for up to two years after treatment; however, in clinical practice loss of benefit is often seen before this (118). Variable methodology, lack of adequate controls, and blinding makes application of trial data to the advanced PD population difficult. The response of dysarthria to functional neurosurgery is usually negative, although this complication is less common with DBS than with bilateral stereotactic lesions. Patients undergoing DBS should be warned about the possibility of increased speech and swallowing dysfunction postoperatively. In some patients this is temporary and can be addressed during postoperative programming.

Dysphagia in PD is increasingly common with longer disease duration. Up to 15% of patients can have silent aspiration in the absence of symptoms (119). Aspiration pneumonia is common in advanced disease, and contributes significantly to hospital admissions and the overall increased mortality (94). As with dysarthria, dopaminergic drugs and surgery do not provide consistent benefit, and the mainstay of management involves surveillance (including appropriate use of special swallowing studies by experienced speech pathologists), modification of diet, and provision of swallowing strategies. In some cases, the placement of percutaneous endoscopic gastrostomy may need to be considered.

Postural deformity

Camptocormia and head drop

Postural deformities, particularly those involving the axial skeleton, can complicate advanced PD and contribute significantly to disability. Camptocormia is characterized by extreme flexion of the thoracolumbar spine, sometimes up to 90°, that is most prominent when walking. It can be corrected by sitting, lying supine, or sometimes leaning against a wall (helping to differentiate it from fixed bony deformities). 'Head drop' is another descriptive term relating to pathological neck flexion. It is also seen in PD but, like camptocormia, is not specific to it, also being seen in multiple system atrophy, motor neuron disease, and myopathic disorders. The mechanism of head drop and camptocormia in PD is uncertain and there is no evidence to prove a shared pathogenesis. Some authors have proposed an extensor myopathy as the most likely mechanism, but others favour a form of dystonia or parkinsonian rigidity (120–123). Rarely, head drop has been associated with dopamine agonist toxicity (124).

Lateral flexion

This phenomenon was described as scoliosis of Parkinson's disease by Duvoisin and Marsden in 1975 and is sometimes referred to as the 'Pisa syndrome', although this term was originally coined to describe a similar postural abnormality which can complicate neuroleptic treatment (125). As with camptocormia and head drop, the pathophysiology of lateral flexion is poorly understood, with an absence of consistent abnormality on imaging or neurophysiology. Tonic activity in paravertebral muscles both ipsilateral and contralateral to the side of flexion has been described along with contralateral dystonic activation in six of ten patients in one case series (126). In keeping with this, contralateral hypertrophy has been identified on MRI of paravertebral muscles (127). It is unclear why contralateral muscle activity should predominate, although pathological dystonic co-contraction has been proposed.

Striatal limb deformity

Striatal hand and foot deformities tend to be seen more commonly in advanced disease, but can be an uncommon early or even presenting feature (128). The striatal hand deformity is characterized by flexion at the metacarpophalangeal joints, extension at the interphalangeal joints, and flexion at the distal phalangeal joints that can be associated with subluxation. Ulnar deviation can be a feature that may lead to misdiagnosis as rheumatoid arthritis, although pain and swelling are not seen. The striatal toe of a PD patient is hyperextended at the hallux and can be part of a 'striatal foot', with flexion of the other toes and an equinovarus deformity of the ankle. The striatal toe can sometimes be mistaken for a Babinski response, although the absence of toe fanning and parkinsonian rigidity in the same limb can help discriminate. The pathophysiology of these deformities is unknown, but they probably represent a form of dystonia. Rigidity may contribute, and over time contractures can develop.

Management

Camptocormia is generally unresponsive to levodopa, but improvement in up to 20% of cases has been reported (129). There are reported cases of improvement with botulinum toxin injection to the rectus abdomini muscles (130). Botulinum toxin is also useful for a striatal limb that is causing pain or where a striatal toe makes it difficult to wear a shoe. Camptocormia has been treated using a backpack as a form of sensory trick (131). Concurrent antipsychotic drugs should be withdrawn if possible because of their association with drug-induced axial dystonia. If axial posturing develops after the introduction of a dopamine agonist, discontinuation should also be considered (124). Surgical correction may provide some benefit for severe symptoms, although complications are common in this advanced PD population (132).

Conclusion

Motor complications are an inevitable feature of advanced PD. Management strategies should focus on the elimination of fluctuations in drug response where possible. As the disease progresses, and with advancing patient age, return from further manipulation of the drug regimen is diminished and marked by complications. In such individuals, bilateral STN DBS is the best therapeutic option, with infusion therapies as possible alternatives. A good knowledge of drug indications and side effects as well as recognizing complications which could be levodopa-responsive will allow the clinician to make timely and effective choices.

Top clinical tips

- It is important to distinguish motor complications which are levodopa-responsive from those that are not. Having patients or family members keep a detailed diary of symptoms in relation to their drug doses can provide quite helpful information about this. For those symptoms which are levodopa-responsive, the aim should be smoothing out the drug response to target the therapeutic window.
- Avoid overly aggressive treatment of peak-dose dyskinesia. Focus on disabling or painful dyskinesia, but remember that most patients prefer to have better control of PD symptoms and find dyskinesia less bothersome. Indeed, many advanced PD patients have no useful ON without some degree of dyskinesia.
- Do not chase non-disabling OFF symptoms. Treatment should be geared towards maximizing function. Pursuing mild OFF symptoms with escalating doses of levodopa may lead to more problematic dyskinesia and fluctuation without practical improvement.
- Less is sometimes more. It is important always to evaluate the efficacy of all anti-PD agents frequently. Adjuvant medications (e.g. dopamine agonists, amantadine, COMT inhibitors, and MAO-B inhibitors) may cause more adverse effects than benefits. Further simplifying drug regimens allows for fewer adverse effects and better patient understanding and compliance.
- Consideration of deep brain stimulation (DBS) should not be thought of as a last resort. Discussing this option earlier in the disease course will allow for greater patient understanding and less resistance when DBS is deemed appropriate. This can also expedite surgical management before possible cognitive problems can present a contraindication.
- Do not be afraid to utilize levodopa more, as reliable responses to medication are ideal. Agents such as levodopa controlled release (CR) do not have consistent pharmacokinetics and make managing fluctuations more difficult. Changing from CR to regular levodopa allows for more precise medication adjustments.

References

1. Obeso JA, Rodriguez-Oroz MC, Goetz CG, et al. Missing pieces in the Parkinson's disease puzzle. *Nature Med* 2010; 16: 653–61.
2. Nutt JG, Holford NHG. The response to levodopa in Parkinson's disease: imposing pharmacological law and order. *Ann Neurol* 1996; 39: 561–73.
3. Obeso JA, Rodriguez-Oroz MC, Chana P, Lera G, Rodriguez M, Olanow CW. The evolution and origin of motor complications in Parkinson's disease. *Neurology* 2000; 55: S13–20.
4. Macmahon DG, Sachdev D, Boddie HG, Ellis CJ, Kendal BR, Blackburn NA. A comparison of the effects of controlled-release levodopa (Madopar CR) with conventional levodopa in late Parkinson's disease. *J Neurol Neurosurg Psychiatry* 1990; 53: 220–3.
5. Jankovic J, Schwartz K, Vander LC. Comparison of Sinemet CR4 and standard Sinemet: double blind and long-term open trial in parkinsonian patients with fluctuations. *Mov Disord* 1989; 4: 303–9.
6. Lieberman A, Gopinathan G, Miller E, Neophytides A, Baumann G, Chin L. Randomized double-blind cross-over study of Sinemet-controlled release (CR4 50/200) versus Sinemet 25/100 in Parkinson's disease. *Eur Neurol* 1990; 30: 75–8.
7. Parkinson Study Group. Entacapone improves motor fluctuations in levodopa-treated Parkinson's disease patients. *Ann Neurol* 1997; 42: 747–55.
8. Brooks DJ, Leinonen M, Kuoppamaki M, Nissinen H. Five-year efficacy and safety of levodopa/DDCI and entacapone in patients with Parkinson's disease. *J Neural Transm* 2008; 115: 843–9.
9. Brooks DJ, Agid Y, Eggert K, et al. Treatment of end-of-dose wearing-off in Parkinson's disease: Stalevo(R) (levodopa/carbidopa/entacapone) and levodopa/DDCI given in combination with Comtess(R)/Comtan(R) (Entacapone) provide equivalent improvements in symptom control superior to that of traditional levodopa/DDCI treatment. *Eur Neurol* 2005; 53: 197–202.
10. Factor SA, Molho ES, Feustel PJ, Brown DL, Evans SM. Long-term comparative experience with tolcapone and entacapone in advanced Parkinson's disease. *Clin Neuropharmacol* 2001; 24: 295–9.
11. Lees AJ. Evidence-based efficacy comparison of tolcapone and entacapone as adjunctive therapy in Parkinson's disease. *CNS Neurosci Ther* 2008; 14: 83–93.
12. Stowe R, Ives N, Clarke CE, et al. Meta-analysis of the comparative efficacy and safety of adjuvant treatment to levodopa in later Parkinson's disease. *Mov Disord* 2011; 26: 587–98.
13. Clarke A, Brewer F, Johnson ES, et al. A new formulation of selegiline: improved bioavailability and selectivity for MAO-B inhibition. *J Neural Transm* 2003; 110: 1241–55.
14. Archibald NK, Clarke MP, Mosimann UP, Burn DJ. The retina in Parkinson's disease. *Brain* 2009; 132: 1128–45.
15. Waters CH, Sethi KD, Hauser RA, Molho E, Bertoni JA; Zydis Selegiline Study Group. Zydis selegiline reduces off time in Parkinson's disease patients with motor fluctuations: a 3-month, randomized, placebo-controlled study. *Mov Disord* 2004; 19: 426–32.
16. Ondo WG, Sethi KD, Kricorian G. Selegiline orally disintegrating tablets in patients with Parkinson disease and 'wearing off' symptoms. *Clin Neuropharmacol* 2007; 30: 295–300.
17. Finberg JP, Lamensdorf I, Weinstock M, Schwartz M, Youdim MB. Pharmacology of rasagiline (*N*-propargyl-1R-aminoindan). *Adv Neurol* 1999; 80: 495–9.
18. Schwid SR, Shoulson I, Stern M, et al. A randomized placebo-controlled trial of rasagiline in levodopa-treated patients with Parkinson disease and motor fluctuations: the PRESTO study. *Arch Neurol* 2005; 62: 241–8.
19. Rascol O, Brooks DJ, Melamed E, et al. Rasagiline as an adjunct to levodopa in patients with Parkinson's disease and motor fluctuations (LARGO, Lasting effect in Adjunct therapy with Rasagiline Given Once daily, study): a randomised, double-blind, parallel-group trial. *Lancet* 2005; 365: 947–54.
20. Hoehn MM, Elton RL. Low dosages of bromocriptine added to levodopa in Parkinson's disease. *Neurology* 1985; 35: 199–206.
21. Lieberman A, Imke S, Muenter M, et al. Multicenter study of cabergoline, a long-acting dopamine receptor agonist, in Parkinson's disease patients with fluctuating responses to levodopa/carbidopa. *Neurology* 1993; 43: 1981–4.
22. Rascol O, Lees AJ, Senard JM, et al. A placebo-controlled study of ropinirole, a new D_2 agonist, in the treatment of motor fluctuations of L-DOPA-treated Parkinsonian patients. *Adv Neurol* 1996; 69: 531–4.
23. Pinter MM, Pogarell O, Oertel WH. Efficacy, safety, and tolerance of the non-ergoline dopamine agonist pramipexole in the treatment of advanced Parkinson's disease: a double blind, placebo controlled, randomised, multicentre study. *J Neurol Neurosurg Psychiatry* 1999; 66: 436–41.
24. LeWitt PA, Boroojerdi B, MacMahon D, Patton J, Jankovic J. Overnight switch from oral dopaminergic agonists to transdermal rotigotine patch in subjects with Parkinson disease. *Clin Neuropharmacol* 2007; 30: 256–65.
25. LeWitt PA, Lyons KE, Pahwa R. Advanced Parkinson disease treated with rotigotine transdermal system—PREFER Study. *Neurology* 2007; 68: 1262–7.

26. Poewe WH, Rascol O, Quinn N, et al. Efficacy of pramipexole and transdermal rotigotine in advanced Parkinson's disease: a double-blind, double-dummy, randomised controlled trial. *Lancet Neurol* 2007; 6: 513–20.
27. Pahwa R, Stacy MA, Factor SA, et al. Ropinirole 24-hour prolonged release: randomized, controlled study in advanced Parkinson disease. *Neurology* 2007; 68: 1108–15.
28. Stocchi F. Continuous dopaminergic stimulation and novel formulations of dopamine agonists. *J Neurol* 2011; 258 (Suppl 2): S316–22.
29. Fahn S. 'On-off' phenomenon with levodopa therapy in parkinsonism: clinical and pharmacologic correlations and the effect of intramuscular pyridoxine. *Neurology* 1974; 431–41.
30. Stocchi F, Nordera G, Marsden CD. Strategies for treating patients with advanced Parkinson's disease with disastrous fluctuations and dyskinesias. *Clin Neuropharmacol* 1997; 20: 95–115.
31. Stocchi F, Marconi S. Factors associated with motor fluctuations and dyskinesia in Parkinson disease: potential role of a new melevodopa plus carbidopa formulation (Sirio). *Clin Neuropharmacol* 2010; 33: 198–203.
32. Kurth MC, Tetrud JW, Irwin I, Lyness WH, Langston JW. Oral levodopa/carbidopa solution versus tablets in Parkinson's patients with severe fluctuations: a pilot study. *Neurology* 1993; 43: 1036–9.
33. Stibe CMH, Lees AJ, Kempster PA, Stern GM. Subcutaneous apomorphine in Parkinsonian on–off oscillations. *Lancet* 1988; 403–6.
34. Pahwa R, Koller WC, Trosch RM, Sherry JH. Subcutaneous apomorphine in patients with advanced Parkinson's disease: a dose-escalation study with randomized, double-blind, placebo-controlled crossover evaluation of a single dose. *J Neurol Sci* 2007; 258: 137–43.
35. LeWitt PA, Ondo WG, VanLunen B, Bottini PB. Open-label study assessment of safety and adverse effects of subcutaneous apomorphine injections in treating 'off' episodes in advanced Parkinson disease. *Clin Neuropharmacol* 2009; 32: 89–93.
36. Melamed E, Bitton V, Zelig O. Delayed onset of responses to single doses of L-dopa in parkinsonian fluctuators on long-term L-dopa therapy. *Clin Neuropharmacol* 1986; 9: 182–8.
37. Dobbs SM, Dobbs RJ, Weller C, et al. Differential effect of *Helicobacter pylori* eradication on time-trends in brady/hypokinesia and rigidity in idiopathic parkinsonism. *Helicobacter* 2010; 15: 279–94.
38. Pierantozzi M, Pietroiusti A, Brusa L, et al. *Helicobacter pylori* eradication and L-dopa absorption in patients with PD and motor fluctuations. *Neurology* 2006; 66: 1824–9.
39. Robottom BJ, Weiner WJ, Factor SA. Movement disorders emergencies. Part 1: Hypokinetic disorders. *Arch Neurol* 2011; 68: 567–72.
40. Merello M, Lees AJ. Beginning-of-dose motor deterioration following the acute administration of levodopa and apomorphine in Parkinson's disease. *J Neurol Neurosurg Psychiatry* 1992; 55: 1024–6.
41. Nutt JG, Gancher ST, Woodward WR. Does an inhibitory action of levodopa contribute to motor fluctuations? *Neurology* 1988; 38: 1553–7.
42. Ambani LM, Van Woert MH. Start hesitation—a side effect of long-term levodopa therapy. *N Engl J Med* 1973; 288: 1113–15.
43. Giladi N, Treves TA, Simon ES, et al. Freezing of gait in patients with advanced Parkinson's disease. *J Neur Transm* 2001; 108: 53–61.
44. Hausdorff JM, Schaafsma JD, Balash Y, Bartels AL, Gurevich T, Giladi N. Impaired regulation of stride variability in Parkinson's disease subjects with freezing of gait. *Exp Brain Res* 2003; 149: 187–94.
45. Lee MS, Kim HS, Lyoo CH. 'Off' gait freezing and temporal discrimination threshold in patients with Parkinson disease. *Neurology* 2005; 64: 670–4.
46. Camicioli R, Oken BS, Sexton G, Kaye JA, Nutt JG. Verbal fluency task affects gait in Parkinson's disease with motor freezing. *J Geriatr Psychiatry Neurol* 1998; 11: 181–5.
47. Schaafsma JD, Balash Y, Gurevich T, Bartels AL, Hausdorff JM, Giladi N. Characterization of freezing of gait subtypes and the response of each to levodopa in Parkinson's disease. *Eur J Neurol* 2003; 10: 391–8.
48. Shoulson I, Oakes D, Fahn S, et al. Impact of sustained deprenyl (selegiline) in levodopa-treated Parkinson's disease: a randomized placebo-controlled extension of the deprenyl and tocopherol antioxidative therapy of parkinsonism trial. *Ann Neurol* 2002; 51: 604–12.
49. Macht M, Kaussner Y, Moller JC, et al. Predictors of freezing in Parkinson's disease: a survey of 6620 patients. *Mov Disord* 2007; 27: 953–6.
50. Poewe WH, Wenning GK. The natural history of Parkinson's disease. *Ann Neurol* 1998; 44: S1–9.
51. Melamed E. Early-morning dystonia. A late side effect of long-term levodopa therapy in Parkinson's disease. *Arch Neurol* 1979; 36: 308–10.
52. Nutt JG. Levodopa-induced dyskinesia: review, observations, and speculations. *Neurology* 1990; 40: 340–5.
53. Luquin MR, Scipioni O, Vaamonde J, Gershanik O, Obeso JA. Levodopa-induced dyskinesias in Parkinson's disease: clinical and pharmacological classification. *Mov Disord* 1992; 7: 117–24.
54. Marconi R, Lefebvre-Caparros D, Bonnet AM, Vidailhet M, Dubois B, Agid Y. Levodopa-induced dyskinesias in Parkinson's disease phenomenology and pathophysiology. *Mov Disord* 1994; 9: 2–12.
55. Van Gerpen JA, Kumar N, Bower JH, Weigand S, Ahlskog JE. Levodopa-associated dyskinesia risk among Parkinson disease patients in Olmsted County, Minnesota, 1976–1990. *Arch Neurol* 2006; 63: 205–9.
56. Hung SW, Adeli GM, Arenovich T, Fox SH, Lang AE. Patient perception of dyskinesia in Parkinson's disease. *J Neurol Neurosurg Psychiatry* 2010; 81: 1112–15.
57. Verhagen Metman VL, del Dotto P, van den Munckhof P, Fang J, Mouradian MM, Chase TN. Amantadine as treatment for dyskinesias and motor fluctuations in PD. *Neurology* 1998; 50: 1323–6.
58. Snow BJ, Macdonald L, Mcauley D, Wallis W. The effect of amantadine on levodopa-induced dyskinesias in Parkinson's disease: a double-blind, placebo-controlled study. *Clin Neuropharmacol* 2000; 23: 82–5.
59. Wolf E, Seppi K, Katzenschlager R, et al. Long-term antidyskinetic efficacy of amantadine in Parkinson's disease. *Mov Disord* 2010; 25: 1357–63.
60. Seeman P, Tallerico T. Antipsychotic drugs which elicit little or no parkinsonism bind more loosely than dopamine to brain D2 receptors, yet occupy high levels of these receptors. *Mol Psychiatry* 1998; 3: 123–34.
61. Durif F, Debilly B, Galitzky M, et al. Clozapine improves dyskinesias in Parkinson disease: a double-blind, placebo-controlled study. *Neurology* 2004; 62: 381–8.
62. Espay AJ, Vaughan JE, Shukla R, et al. Botulinum toxin type A for levodopa-induced cervical dyskinesias in Parkinson's disease: unfavorable risk–benefit ratio. *Mov Disord* 2011; 26: 913–14.
63. Espay AJ. Management of motor complications in Parkinson disease: current and emerging therapies. *Neurol Clin* 2010; 28: 913–25.
64. Kim HJ, Lee JY, Kim JY, Kim DG, Paek SH, Jeon BS. Effect of bilateral subthalamic deep brain stimulation on diphasic dyskinesia. *Clin Neurol Neurosurg* 2008; 110: 328–32.
65. Giladi N, Kao R, Fahn S. Freezing phenomenon in patients with parkinsonian syndromes. *Mov Disord* 1997; 12: 302–5.
66. Fox SH, Brotchie JM, Lang AE. Non-dopaminergic treatments in development for Parkinson's disease. *Lancet Neurol* 2008; 7: 927–38.
67. Meissner WG, Frasier M, Gasser T, et al. Priorities in Parkinson's disease research. *Nat Rev Drug Discov* 2011; 10: 377–93.
68. Pahwa R, Factor SA, Lyons KE, et al. Practice parameter: Treatment of Parkinson disease with motor fluctuations and dyskinesia (an evidence-based review). Report of the Quality Standards Subcommittee of the American Academy of Neurology. *Neurology* 2006; 66: 983–95.
69. Voon V, Hassan K, Zurowski M, et al. Prospective prevalence of pathologic gambling and medication association in Parkinson disease. *Neurology* 2006; 66: 1750–2.
70. Lees AJ, Ratziu V, Tolosa E, Oertel WH. Safety and tolerability of adjunctive tolcapone treatment in patients with early Parkinson's disease. *J Neurol Neurosurg Psychiatry* 2007; 78: 944–8.
71. Olanow CW, Hauser RA, Jankovic J, et al. A randomized, double-blind, placebo-controlled, delayed start study to assess rasagiline as a disease modifying therapy in Parkinson's disease (the ADAGIO Study): rationale, design, and baseline characteristics. *Mov Disord* 2008; 23: 2194–201.

72. DeMarcaida JA, Schwid SR, White WB, et al. Effects of tyramine administration in Parkinson's disease patients treated with selective MAO-B inhibitor rasagiline. *Mov Disord* 2006; 21:1716–21.
73. Urban PP, Wellach I, Faiss S, et al. Subacute axonal neuropathy in Parkinson's disease with cobalamin and vitamin B6 deficiency under duodopa therapy. *Mov Disord* 2010; 25: 1748–52.
74. Garcia Ruiz PJ, Sesar IA, Ares PB, et al. Efficacy of long-term continuous subcutaneous apomorphine infusion in advanced Parkinson's disease with motor fluctuations: a multicenter study. *Mov Disord* 2008; 23: 1130–6.
75. Nyholm D, Remahl AIMN, Dizdar N, et al. Duodenal levodopa infusion monotherapy vs oral polypharmacy in advanced Parkinson disease. *Neurology* 2005; 64: 216–23.
76. Nyholm D, Lewander T, Johansson A, LeWitt PA, Lundqvist C, Aquilonius SM. Enteral levodopa/carbidopa infusion in advanced Parkinson disease: long-term exposure. *Clin Neuropharmacol* 2008; 31: 63–73.
77. Devos D, French DUODOPA Study Group. Patient profile, indications, efficacy and safety of duodenal levodopa infusion in advanced Parkinson's disease. *Mov Disord* 2009; 24: 993–1000.
78. Merola A, Zibetti M, Angrisano S, Rizzi L, Lanotte M, Lopiano L. Comparison of subthalamic nucleus deep brain stimulation and Duodopa in the treatment of advanced Parkinson's disease. *Mov Disord* 2011; 26: 664–70.
79. Nyholm D, Jansson R, Willows T, Remahl IN. Long-term 24-hour duodenal infusion of levodopa: outcome and dose requirements. *Neurology* 2005; 65: 1506–7.
80. Deuschl G, Schade-Brittinger C, Krack P, et al. A randomized trial of deep-brain stimulation for Parkinson's disease. *N Engl J Med* 2006; 355: 896–908.
81. Weaver FM, Follett K, Stern M, et al. Bilateral deep brain stimulation vs best medical therapy for patients with advanced Parkinson disease: a randomized controlled trial. *JAMA* 2009; 301: 63–73.
82. Bronstein JM, Tagliati M, Alterman RL, et al. Deep brain stimulation for Parkinson disease: an expert consensus and review of key issues. *Arch Neurol* 2011; 68: 165.
83. Schupbach WM, Maltete D, Houeto JL, et al. Neurosurgery at an earlier stage of Parkinson disease: a randomized, controlled trial. *Neurology* 2007; 68: 267–71.
84. Follett KA, Weaver FM, Stern M, et al. Pallidal versus subthalamic deep-brain stimulation for Parkinson's disease. *N Engl J Med* 2010; 362: 2077–91.
85. Saint-Cyr JA, Trépanier LL, Kumar R, Lozano AM, Lang AE. Neuropsychological consequences of chronic bilateral stimulation of the subthalamic nucleus in Parkinson's disease. *Brain* 2000; 123: 2091–108.
86. Volkmann J, Allert N, Voges J, Sturm V, Schnitzler A, Freund HJ. Long-term results of bilateral pallidal stimulation in Parkinson's disease. *Ann Neurol* 2004; 55: 871–5.
87. Das K, Benzil DL, Rovit RL, Murali R, Couldwell WT. Irving S. Cooper (1922–1985): a pioneer in functional neurosurgery. *J Neurosurg* 1998; 89: 865–73.
88. Giller CA, Dewey RB, Ginsburg MI, Mendelsohn DB, Berk AM. Stereotactic pallidotomy and thalamotomy using individual variations of anatomic landmarks for localization. *Neurosurgery* 1998; 42: 56–62.
89. Scott R, Gregory R, Hines N, et al. Neuropsychological, neurological and functional outcome following pallidotomy for Parkinson's disease: a consecutive series of eight simultaneous bilateral and twelve unilateral procedures. *Brain* 1998; 121: 659–75.
90. Matsumoto K, Shichijo F, Fukami T. Long-term follow-up review of cases of Parkinson's disease after unilateral or bilateral thalamotomy. *J Neurosurg* 1984; 60: 1033–44.
91. Osenbach AK, Burchiel KJ. Thalamotomy: indications, techniques and results. In: Germano IM (ed.), *Neurosurgical treatment of movement disorders*, pp. 107–29. Park Ridge, IL: AANS, 1998.
92. Plaha P, Ben Shlomo Y, Patel NK, Gill SS. Stimulation of the caudal zona incerta is superior to stimulation of the subthalamic nucleus in improving contralateral parkinsonism. *Brain* 2006; 129: 1732–47.
93. Moro E, Hamani C, Poon YY, et al. Unilateral pedunculopontine stimulation improves falls in Parkinson's disease. *Brain* 2010; 133: 215–24.
94. Hely MA, Morris JGL, Reid WGJ, Trafficante R. Sydney multicenter study of Parkinson's disease: non-L-dopa-responsive problems dominate at 15 years. *Mov Disord* 2005; 20: 190–9.
95. Chung KA, Lobb BM, Nutt JG, Horak FB. Effects of a central cholinesterase inhibitor on reducing falls in Parkinson disease. *Neurology* 2010; 75: 1263–9.
96. Smania N, Corato E, Tinazzi M, et al. Effect of balance training on postural instability in patients with idiopathic Parkinson's disease. *Neurorehabil Neural Repair* 2010; 24: 826–34.
97. Barbeau A. Six years of high-level levodopa therapy in severely akinetic Parkinsonian patients. *Arch Neurol* 1976; 33: 333–8.
98. Kitagawa M, Houzen H, Tashiro K. Effects of caffeine on the freezing of gait in Parkinson's disease. *Mov Disord* 2007; 22: 710–12.
99. Hauser RA, Cantillon M, Pourcher E, et al. Preladenant in patients with Parkinson's disease and motor fluctuations: a phase 2, double-blind, randomised trial. *Lancet Neurol* 2011; 10: 221–9.
100. Devos D, Krystkowiak P, Clement F, et al. Improvement of gait by chronic, high doses of methylphenidate in patients with advanced Parkinson's disease. *J Neurol Neurosurg Psychiatry* 2007; 78: 470–5.
101. Espay AJ, Dwivedi AK, Payne M, et al. Methylphenidate for gait impairment in Parkinson disease: A randomized clinical trial. *Neurology* 2011; 76: 1256–62.
102. Auriel E, Hausdorff JA, Giladi N. Methylphenidate for the treatment of Parkinson disease and other neurological disorders. *Clin Neuropharmacol* 2009; 32: 75–81.
103. Morgante F, Fasano A. Improvement with duloxetine in primary progressive freezing gait. *Neurology* 2010; 75: 2130–2.
104. Kim YE, Yun JY, Jeon BS. Effect of intravenous amantadine on dopaminergic-drug-resistant freezing of gait. *Parkinsonism Relat Disord* 2011; 17: 491–2.
105. Elble RJ. Tremor and dopamine agonists. *Neurology* 2002; 58: S57–62.
106. Butzer JF, Silver DE, Sahs AL. Amantadine in Parkinson's disease. A double-blind, placebo-controlled, crossover study with long-term follow-up. *Neurology* 1975; 25: 603–6.
107. Koller WC. Pharmacologic treatment of parkinsonian tremor. *Arch Neurol* 1986; 43: 126–7.
108. Bonuccelli U, Ceravolo R, Salvetti S, et al. Clozapine in Parkinson's disease tremor: effects of acute and chronic administration. *Neurology* 1997; 49: 1587–90.
109. Friedman JH, Koller WC, Lannon MC, Busenbark K, Swanson-Hyland E, Smith D. Benztropine versus clozapine for the treatment of tremor in Parkinson's disease. *Neurology* 1997; 48: 1077–81.
110. Trosch RM, Friedman JH, Lannon MC, et al. Clozapine use in Parkinson's disease: a retrospective analysis of a large multicentered clinical experience. *Mov Disord* 1998; 13: 377–82.
111. Crosby NJ, Deane KH, Clarke CE. Beta-blocker therapy for tremor in Parkinson's disease. *Cochrane Database Syst Rev* 2003; (1): CD003361.
112. Gordon PH, Pullman SL, Louis ED, Frucht SJ, Fahn S. Mirtazapine in Parkinsonian tremor. *Parkinsonism Relat Disord* 2002; 9: 125–6.
113. Pact V, Giduz T. Mirtazapine treats resting tremor, essential tremor, and levodopa-induced dyskinesias. *Neurology* 1999; 53: 1154.
114. Pinto S, Ozsancak C, Tripoliti E, Thobois S, Limousin-Dowsey P, Auzou P. Treatments for dysarthria in Parkinson's disease. *Lancet Neurol* 2004; 3: 547–56.
115. Wolfe VI, Garvin JS, Bacon M, Waldrop W. Speech changes in Parkinson's disease during treatment with L-dopa. *J Commun Disord* 1975; 8: 271–9.

116. Deane KH, Whurr R, Playford ED, Ben Shlomo Y, Clarke CE. A comparison of speech and language therapy techniques for dysarthria in Parkinson's disease. *Cochrane Database Syst Rev* 2001; (2): CD002814.
117. Ramig LO, Countryman S, O'Brien C, Hoehn M, Thompson L. Intensive speech treatment for patients with Parkinson's disease: short- and long-term comparison of two techniques. *Neurology* 1996; 47: 1496–504.
118. Ramig LO, Sapir S, Countryman S, et al. Intensive voice treatment (LSVT(R)) for patients with Parkinson's disease: a 2 year follow up. *J Neurol Neurosurg Psychiatry* 2001; 71: 493–8.
119. Ali GN, Wallace KL, Schwartz R, DeCarle DJ, Zagami AS, Cook IJ. Mechanisms of oral–pharyngeal dysphagia in patients with Parkinson's disease. *Gastroenterology* 1996; 110: 383–92.
120. Jankovic J. Camptocormia, head drop and other bent spine syndromes: heterogeneous etiology and pathogenesis of parkinsonian deformities. *Mov Disord* 2010; 25: 527–8.
121. Margraf NG, Wrede A, Rohr A, et al. Camptocormia in idiopathic Parkinson's disease: a focal myopathy of the paravertebral muscles. *Mov Disord* 2010; 25: 542–51.
122. Spuler S, Krug H, Klein C, et al. Myopathy causing camptocormia in idiopathic Parkinson's disease: a multidisciplinary approach. *Mov Disord* 2010; 25: 552–9.
123. van de Warrenburg BPC, Cordivari C, Ryan AM, et al. The phenomenon of disproportionate antecollis in Parkinson's disease and multiple system atrophy. *Mov Disord* 2007; 22: 2325–31.
124. Uzawa A, Mori M, Kojima S, et al. Dopamine agonist-induced antecollis in Parkinson's disease. *Mov Disord* 2009; 24: 2408–11.
125. Suzuki E, Obata M, Yoshida Y, Miyaoka H. Tardive dyskinesia with risperidone and anticholinergics. *Am J Psychiatry* 2002; 159: 1948.
126. di Matteo A, Fasano A, Squintani G, et al. Lateral trunk flexion in Parkinson's disease: EMG features disclose two different underlying pathophysiological mechanisms. *J Neurol* 2011; 258: 740–5.
127. Yokochi F. Lateral flexion in Parkinson's disease and Pisa syndrome. *J Neurol* 2006; 253: 17–20.
128. Ashour R, Tintner R, Jankovic J. Striatal deformities of the hand and foot in Parkinson's disease. *Lancet Neurol* 2005; 4: 423–31.
129. Bloch F, Houeto JL, Tezenas du Montcel S, et al. Parkinson's disease with camptocormia. *J Neurol Neurosurg Psychiatry* 2006; 77: 1223–8.
130. Fietzek UM, Schroeteler FE, CeballosBaumann AO. Goal attainment after treatment of parkinsonian camptocormia with botulinum toxin. *Mov Disord* 2009; 24: 2027–8.
131. Gerton BK, Theeler B, Samii A. Backpack treatment for camptocormia. *Mov Disord* 2010; 25: 247–8.
132. Wadia PM, Tan G, Munhoz RP, Fox SH, Lewis SJ, Lang AE. Surgical correction of kyphosis in patients with camptocormia due to Parkinson's disease: a retrospective evaluation. *J Neurol Neurosurg Psychiatry* 2011; 82: 364–8.

CHAPTER 11

Non-motor Symptom Management in Parkinson's Disease

Eduardo Tolosa, Carles Gaig, and Lillian Acevedo

Introduction

Interest in non-motor symptoms (NMS) in Parkinson's disease (PD) has increased in recent years. Unlike the classic motor symptoms that can respond to dopaminergic treatment and functional neurosurgery, NMS generally fail to improve with currently available treatments. Consequently, they are a major source of disability and frequently impact negatively upon the patient's quality of life. Interest in NMS in PD has also increased after it became evident that some NMS antedate the classic motor signs of PD. Information on the nature of NMS in premotor PD may provide information about the causes of PD and in the study of drugs with neuroprotective potential.

Many NMS are caused by PD-related lesions in the brain involving non dopaminergic structures (Table 11.1). Examples of such non-dopaminergic NMS include dementia, fatigue, smell loss, constipation, and REM behaviour disorder (RBD). Even though most NMS are thought to be primarily non-dopaminergic, they may be influenced by dopaminergic drugs. Examples of NMS that may respond in part to dopaminergic drugs are insomnia and other nocturnal problems, urinary urgency, depression, and in general NMS occurring during the OFF state.

Several NMS in PD are related to treatment. A number of medications, as well as deep brain stimulation (DBS), can produce or potentiate NMS, and acknowledgement of this is important for adequate management. Examples of NMS induced or aggravated by medications in PD are orthostatic hypotension (OH), hallucinations and excessive daytime sleepiness (EDS) associated with dopaminergic treatment, and memory problems related to anticholinergics.

In this chapter emphasis will be placed upon those NMS considered to be an intrinsic part of the PD process, including smell disturbances, dysautonomia, pain and other sensory symptoms, sleep disturbances, apathy and depression, and fatigue. Some less common or less disabling NMS, such as seborrhoeic dermatitis or hyperhidrosis, and particularly those NMS mostly related to treatment, such as skin erosions or skin nodules associated with DBS or apomorphine are listed in Table 11.2. The occurrence of NMS in premotor PD is briefly discussed at the end of the chapter.

Sleep disturbances

Nocturnal sleep problems such as sleep fragmentation and early awakening, or parasomnias like RBD and EDS, are frequent in PD and may have a major impact on patients' quality of life (1–5). They occur more commonly in advanced than in early PD, mostly because of a combination of factors which include an increase in dopaminergic treatment, worsening of motor performance, and neurodegeneration of systems other than the nigrostriatal pathway that are important in regulating the sleep–wake cycle (6, 7). Disturbances such as RBD or EDS can antedate the development of the motor symptoms of PD by several years (5).

Insomnia

Insomnia is present in up to 55% of patients with PD (8–10). Sleep fragmentation and early awakening are the most frequent causes of insomnia in PD. Several factors can cause insomnia in PD, and defining the relevant ones in a given patient may be challenging (1, 11, 12). Fragmented sleep and early awakening can be related to nocturnal akinesia (difficulties in turning in bed), but also to bouts of nocturnal tremor and dyskinesias (OFF-period dystonia). Sensory disturbances such as pain due to immobility or pain related to OFF periods, as well as restless-leg-like symptoms, may also disturb the patient. Nocturia can lead to sleep fragmentation (1). Mental depression and anxiety are other frequent contributory factors (9, 10). In addition, selegiline and amantadine are known to cause insomnia, and dopaminergic drugs such as the dopamine agonists or levodopa may have an awakening effect when administered at night. Fragmented sleep can also be related to obstructive sleep apnoea (OSA) (13).

Specific measures to treat insomnia include modification of antiparkinsonian treatment, such as reduction of selegiline or

Table 11.1 Non-motor symptoms and presumed neuropathological substrate

Non-motor symptoms	Underlying brain structures
Smell loss	Olfactory bulb; anterior olfactory nucleus; amygdala; perirhinal cortex
Autonomic dysfunction	Amygdala; dorsal nucleus of the vagus; intermediolateral column of the spinal cord; sympathetic ganglia; enteric plexus neurons; autonomic neurons in the thoracic and sacral spinal cord, heart, and gastrointestinal and genitourinary tracts
Sleep disturbances	Nucleus subcoeruleus; pedunculopontine nucleus; thalamus; hypothalamus
Behavioural/emotional dysfunction	Locus coeruleus; raphe nuclei; amygdala; limbic cortex; mesolimbic and mesocortical cortex
Hallucinations, psychosis	Amygdala; limbic cortex
Dementia and cognitive dysfunction	Frontal and ventral temporal lobe/neocortex, hippocampus, amygdala, nucleus basalis of Meynert, locus coeruleus

Table 11.2 Pain, cutaneous disturbances, and other less well-known NMS

Pain and sensory symptoms
◆ Non-fluctuating: continuous, not related to timing of antiparkinson drugs
◆ Musculoskeletal or radicular–neuropathic types of neck, lower back, or limb pain
• Central primary pain in a limb
• Akathisic discomfort
◆ Associated with motor fluctuations
• OFF related:
central primary pain in limb, low back, unusual body sites; angina-like chest pain; burning mouth syndrome; genital pain; abdominal pain
OFF dystonia (usually in the foot)
akathisic discomfort
RLS-like symptoms
• ON related:
associated to ON-dyskinesias
akathisia
Cutaneous problems
◆ Facial seborrhoea (seborrhoeic dermatitis)
◆ Possible increased risk of skin cancer
◆ Malignant melanoma (unrelated to dopaminergic treatment)
◆ Keratosis and basal cell carcinoma
◆ Adverse event of antiparkinsonian therapy
◆ Amantadine-induced livedo reticularis
◆ Leg oedema (dopamine agonists)
◆ Erythromelalgia-like (dopamine agonists)
◆ Subcutaneous nodules related to s.c. apomorphine injections
◆ Skin erosion over implants in deep brain stimulation
Ocular and visual disturbances
◆ Dry eyes (xerostomia, related to autonomic dysfunction)
◆ Diplopia, blurred vision
Other
◆ Weight loss, weight gain (possibly drug-induced), rhinorrhoea, ageusia

amantadine, or optimization of antiparkinsonian treatment at night to minimize nocturnal motor or sensory symptoms. Agents with a long half-life or sustained effect, such as rotigotine or ropinirole 24-hour prolonged release, can be useful for attenuating OFF periods during the night (14, 15). Nocturia has to be improved, if possible, and depression and anxiety treated. Adding a hypnotic is another option (16).

REM sleep behaviour disorder

RBD is a parasomnia characterized by recurrent episodes of vigorous dream-enacting behaviours associated with nightmares and abnormally increased phasic and/or tonic electromyographic (EMG) activity during REM sleep. In these dreams, patients are usually threatened or attacked by people or animals, and they react verbally or physically to the offender (17). Frequency and intensity of abnormal behaviours and dreams may vary during the night (they are usually worst at the end of the night), between different nights, and from one patient to another. In some patients these abnormal dream-enacting behaviours can be severe and cause injury to the patient or their bed partner, resulting in fractures, lacerations, or contusions. In other cases, the RBD is less severe in its expression. In most instances patients are unaware of these behaviours, which are reported by the bed partner (18).

Polysomnography with audiovisual recording (VPSG), demonstrating either abnormal movements or excessive EMG activity during REM sleep, is needed to confirm the diagnosis of RBD. VPSG is also helpful in ruling out conditions such as OSA, somnambulism, nocturnal epilepsy, hallucinations, confusional awakenings, or prominent periodic leg movements, which can mimic RBD-like behaviours (5, 19).

When diagnosis is based solely on clinical history, RBD frequency in PD is 15–46% (4, 20, 21). If RBD diagnosis is performed using VPSG, the frequency is somewhat higher, ranging from 46 to 58% (22–25). RBD may occur more often in the rigid–akinetic than in the tremor-predominant subtype of PD (26, 27). Whether RBD is more common in patients with dementia is unclear, but some studies have suggested that the presence of RBD is associated with cognitive impairment and represents a risk factor for dementia (28). RBD also occurs in patients with PD associated with *parkin* gene mutations (29). RBD in PD is probably best explained by dysfunction of the neural systems that regulate REM sleep, particularly those located in the brainstem including the locus coeruleus and pedunculopontine tegmental nucleus (17, 30).

Most patients with RBD respond to clonazepam at doses of 0.5–2 mg taken at night in a single dose (17). There is no clear evidence that dopaminergic agents influence the development, evolution, or severity of RBD (26). However, initiation of levodopa has been reported to improve RBD in some patients. In others, reduction of total daily dose of levodopa or other dopaminergic agents, such as the MAO-B inhibitors, may improve or eliminate the symptoms.

Excessive daytime sleepiness

The presence of EDS in PD has been reported to vary from 12 to 84% of patients (2, 3, 6, 10). Patients may complain of a constant feeling of sleepiness, or describe episodes of sudden, irresistible, and overwhelming sleepiness without awareness of falling asleep, which have been labelled sleep 'attacks' or episodes of sudden onset of sleep (31). Sleep attacks have been reported in 0.5–20% of patients with PD on a background of EDS (2, 3, 6, 10). A subgroup of patients (15–39%) with somnolence-present sleep-onset REM periods (SOREMPs) on the Multiple Sleep Latency Test (MSLT) and are said to have a narcolepsy-like phenotype (32, 33).

However, in contrast with narcolepsy, hypocretin-1 levels in the cerebrospinal fluid (CSF) are normal in most PD patients (34–37).

EDS in PD has been attributed to neurodegenerative changes in brain areas that regulate the sleep–wake cycle, including the locus coeruleus, the dopaminergic midbrain ventral tegmental area, the pedunculopontine tegmental nuclei, and the hypocretin-producing neurons in the lateral hypothalamus (38–40). Supporting the notion of a 'central' hypersomnia in PD is the fact that EDS is more frequent in patients with advanced PD or in those patients in whom the neuropathological process is more extensive, for example PD patients with dementia (6, 7, 37, 41–42).

EDS is also a well-known side effect of dopamine agonists (43). It has been reported to occur with ergot and non-ergot dopamine agonists (44–46). Levodopa monotherapy can also induce somnolence, although less frequently than in combination with dopamine agonists (47, 48).

Treatment of EDS in PD will depend on the underlying causative factors (Table 11.3). However, an important step is to inform the patient about the potential dangers of driving and other activities until the EDS has resolved or improved. The next step is to assess whether or not EDS is pharmacologically mediated. If sleepiness seems to be related to dopaminergic drugs, one should try to reduce the dose, switch to another dopaminergic drug, or even stop the offending drug, although this may worsen motor function. Other measures that need to be taken are outlined in Table 11.3. EDS can be treated with awake-promoting agents such as modafinil 200–400 mg/daily (49). However, the efficacy of this drug in treating EDS in PD has only been assessed in three small double-blind placebo-controlled trials, which have shown conflicting results (50–52). A recent open-label study suggested that sodium oxybate, a drug that has been approved for treating narcolepsy, could improve EDS in PD (53).

Smell loss in Parkinson's disease

Smell loss is frequent in PD and involves several functions such as impairment of odour detection, identification, and discrimination. Smell loss causes little disability and is rarely mentioned spontaneously by the patient, but if it is specifically asked about or tested for, olfactory impairment is demonstrated in up to 90% of PD patients (54–57). The olfactory deficit in PD is independent of disease severity and duration, being present in recently diagnosed and untreated PD patients, and does not vary between the ON and OFF states (54–55, 58). Hyposmia has been considered an early marker for PD, since it can antedate the motor signs of the disease (59, 60). Hyposmia in PD is attributed to involvement of the olfactory system by Lewy-type pathology. The olfactory bulb is the most frequently affected area, followed by the anterior olfactory nucleus and the primary olfactory cortex (61).

Some studies have found significantly better olfactory function in tremor-dominant PD than in akinetic–rigid or postural instability gait difficulty predominant PD subtypes (62, 63). Recent studies suggest that the degree of olfactory dysfunction in PD can correlate with increased autonomic dysfunction, reduced cognitive functioning, and the presence of psychotic symptoms (64–67).

Hyposmia can be useful in differentiating PD from other parkinsonian or tremor syndromes since olfactory function is preserved or mildly impaired in atypical parkinsonian disorders, such as multiple system atrophy (MSA), progressive supranuclear palsy, or corticobasal degeneration (54, 56, 68), or in secondary parkinsonism,

Table 11.3 Excessive daytime sleepiness in Parkinson's disease: causes and management

Causes	Management and treatment
Dopaminergic drugs	
EDS occurs more frequently with DA than levodopa Frequency of EDS is similar with all (instead of oral) DA currently in use	Consider dose reduction or gradual suppression of DA or other dopaminergic drugs or switching to another DA Risk of worsening of motor symptoms
Sedative drugs	
Neuroleptics, benzodiazepines, antihistamines, etc.	Careful check of all current medication Consider dose reduction or suppression of offending drug
Motor disturbances at night	
Nocturnal akinesia, rigidity or tremor Dyskinesias	Optimize antiparkinsonian treatment (e.g. add a nocturnal dose of levodopa)
Nocturnal sensory symptoms	
Pain: secondary to immobility, rigidity, cramps OFF-period dystonia (early morning) Restless-legs-like symptoms	Optimize antiparkinsonian treatment (e.g. levodopa); extended released or transdermal DA at bedtime
OSA syndrome	
Unclear if this occurs more frequently in PD than in the general population	Inquire about intense snoring, gasping, and respiratory pauses during sleep If OSA is suspected, nocturnal PSG is indicated CPAP mask eliminates OSA
PD-related hypersomnia	
Sleepiness can be caused by PD itself Some PD patients with EDS may have a narcoleptic-like phenotype	PSG followed by a MSLT (presence of >2 SOREMPs) may be present (narcolepsy-like phenotype) Treatment with wake-promoting agents such as modafinil can be helpful

EDS, excessive daytime sleepiness; DA, dopamine agonist; OSA, obstructive sleep apnoea; PSG, polysomnography; CPAP, continuous positive airways pressure; MSLT, Multiple Sleep Latency Test; SOREMP, sleep-onset REM period.

such as vascular or drug-induced parkinsonism (69). Smell is also preserved in essential tremor (70). Interestingly, patients with *parkin*-associated PD, which usually demonstrates nigral degeneration without Lewy bodies (LB) on neuropathological examination, tend to have intact olfactory function (71). In *LRRK2*-related PD, another genetic form of parkinsonism that has heterogeneous neuropathology, smell loss also appears to occur less frequently than in idiopathic PD (72, 73). In contrast, and similarly to classic PD, subjects with dementia with Lewy bodies (DLB) usually present with severe loss of smell (74), supporting the concept that hyposmia could be a marker of an underlying LB disorder.

Dysautonomia in Parkinson's disease

Dysautonomia in PD is frequent and includes gastrointestinal (GI), urogenital, cardiovascular, and thermoregulatory dysfunction (Table 11.4) (75, 76). Estimated prevalence of autonomic dysfunction in PD ranges from 14 to 80% (75), and disabling dysautonomic symptoms are present in up to 50% of patients (76).

The presence of dysautonomia in PD has been correlated with age, disease severity, and use of dopaminergic drugs. Symptomatic dysautonomia is more severe as the disease advances; however, dysautonomia is also frequent in recently diagnosed and untreated PD (77, 78). In some early PD patients, dysautonomic symptoms can be prominent, mimicking pure autonomic failure or MSA (79, 80). In addition, some dysautonomic symptoms may even predate the development of the cardinal motor signs of the disease (81). Dysautonomia is also frequent in genetically determined PD variants, including *alpha-synuclein*, *PINK-1*, and *LRRK2* gene mutations (82–85), and even in cases of parkinsonism related to *parkin* gene mutations which usually lack LB pathology (86, 87).

Table 11.4 Dysautonomic symptoms in Parkinson's disease

Gastrointestinal dysfunction
Hypersalivation (also related to swallowing difficulties)
Dysphagia
Regurgitation, nausea
Epigastric discomfort or bloating, heavy digestion (gastroparesis)
Constipation
Incomplete emptying, painful defecation, anismus
Bowel pseudo-occlusion (Ogilvie's syndrome), sigmoid volvulus
Urinary dysfunction
Urinary frequency and urgency
Urge incontinence
Nocturia
Difficulty with initiation of urination
Urinary retention
Sexual dysfunction
Erectile dysfunction
Impaired ejaculation
Reduced vaginal sensitivity and decreased mucosal lubrication
Cardiovascular dysfunction
Orthostatic hypotension
Postprandial hypotension
Thermoregulatory dysfunction
Sweating abnormalities (can be localized and asymmetric)
Hyperhidrosis (may occur in association with OFF periods, ON dyskinesias, or unrelated to motor fluctuations)
Hypohidrosis
Heat/cold intolerance

Although dysautonomia in PD can sometimes occur as a side effect of treatment, in most cases it can be attributed to the disease process itself. The neuropathological lesions in PD can involve the central and peripheral postganglionic autonomic nervous system, leading to autonomic dysfunction. LB and neuronal loss have been found in the dorsal nucleus of the vagus, the intermediate ventrolateral columns of the spinal cord, and Onuf's nucleus, and within the cardiac sympathetic plexus and enteric autonomic nervous system (80, 88–94). Early involvement of these structures would explain why some of these dysautonomic symptoms could occur as a premotor feature of PD (95–97).

Gastrointestinal dysfunction

GI symptoms are more frequent in PD than in age-matched controls, and include excess salivation, dysphagia, constipation, and other symptoms related to reduced GI motility, such as regurgitation, nausea, and epigastric discomfort or bloating secondary to gastroparesis (98, 99). Nausea is often related to dopaminergic medication, but impaired gastric emptying may also play a role (100). Gastroparesis also has relevant pharmacokinetic implications in PD, since delayed gastric emptying may cause increased exposure of levodopa to dopa-decarboxylase in the gastric mucosa and reduce absorption of the drug, leading to an erratic pharmacological response (99). Reduced GI motility may worsen with disease progression, and eventually can be life-threatening in some patients in association with fatal gastroparesis, Ogilvie's megacolon, and sigmoid volvulus (101, 102).

Constipation is very common and is present in up to 60% of PD patients (76, 103). Slowed or delayed colonic transit seems to be the main pathophysiological mechanism underpinning decreased bowel movement frequency (99). PD patients may also have additional difficulties with the act of defecation, such as painful or incomplete emptying, because of hypertonus in the perianal musculature, poor ability to voluntarily contract the external anal sphincter, or poor ability to activate pelvic muscles during OFF periods (104–106). In addition, problems with defecation can be aggravated by associated puborectalis dystonia or anismus (107, 108).

Treatment of constipation should include general measures of bowel hygiene such as dietary modifications, with increase in dietary fibre and fluid intake, and reduction or discontinuation of anticholinergic drugs. Some laxatives (macrogol, dietary herbal extracts) and prokinetic drugs (tegaserod, mosapride) have been specifically tested in PD in double-blind controlled randomized trials or observational short series, with promising results (49, 106, 109–112). Domperidone, a peripheral dopamine antagonist, may improve gastric emptying and reduce dopaminergic-drug-related GI symptoms (113). Dopamine receptor blockers with central activity, such as metoclopramide and clebopride, should be avoided. Other pro-kinetic drugs, such as erythromycin or ondansetron, could be useful but have not been specifically tested in PD. Treatment with botulinum toxin in pelvic musculature may have some benefit in cases with anismus (114). If GI symptoms are refractory, one should consider referral for additional investigations to rule out other causes, including common and readily treatable conditions such as *Helicobacter pylori* infection or peptic ulceration.

Genitourinary dysfunction

Poor bladder control can be one of the most troublesome non-motor symptoms of PD. Increased frequency, urinary urgency, urge incontinence, nocturia, and voiding difficulties are common in PD (115–117). Urinary symptoms are particularly frequent in the advanced stages and appear with a mean latency in relation to the onset of motor symptoms of about 144 months, in contrast with 12 months in MSA (118). However, a recent study in early untreated PD found storage problems (urinary urgency, day- and night-time urinary frequency (nocturia), and urge/stress/mixed incontinence) in 64% of subjects (119). Urinary symptoms have also been reported to antedate the onset of motor signs (120).

Increased frequency, urinary urgency, and urge incontinence result from detrusor over activity. The cause of nocturia, which occurs in about 60% of patients, has not been well established (115, 121). Less frequently, detrusor hypoactivity may result in delayed bladder emptying and difficulty with initiation of urination. Urodynamic testing may be helpful in identifying the type of urinary dysfunction and guiding appropriate treatment (115, 121). Both urinary retention and incontinence may lead to recurrent urinary infections.

Sexual dysfunction in PD occurs frequently in both men and women. Erectile dysfunction and impairment of ejaculation can be present in up to 79% of PD males (76, 121–123). In a recent retrospective study in 32 000 subjects, erectile dysfunction was associated with a higher risk of developing PD (124). Less frequently, exaggerated penile erection can occur as a consequence of dopaminergic treatment (125, 126). Reduced vaginal sensitivity and decreased mucosal lubrication has also been described in women with PD. Diminished libido and hypersexuality are also frequent, but these types of sexual dysfunction in PD appear to be related to mood disorders or behavioural abnormalities in the setting of an impulse control disorder and dopaminergic drugs.

Standard agents to treat neurogenic bladder dysfunction, such as peripherally acting anticholinergic drugs (oxybutinin, tolterodine, darifenacin, solifenacin, and trospium) and alpha-1 agonists (prazosin), can be used for urinary urgency and incontinence in PD, although controlled clinical trials in this population are lacking (49). Care should be exercised to avoid exacerbating existing cognitive impairment by prescribing drugs which have minimal 'central' anticholinergic actions. Urological referral should be considered, particularly in refractory or severe cases, to detect primary urinary pathology such as prostatic hypertrophy. Coffee and other natural diuretics, as well as a large water intake before bedtime, should be avoided in order to minimize nocturia. Evidence in support of intranasal desmopressin spray for nocturia is lacking (127). Sildenafil has been found to be efficacious in the treatment of erectile dysfunction and can be considered in patients with PD (49, 128, 129).

Cardiovascular dysfunction

Orthostatic hypotension (OH) is the main cardiovascular symptom. It is defined as a drop in more than 20 mmHg systolic pressure or 10 mmHg diastolic pressure when changing position from lying to standing (130). OH occurs in 20–50% of patients with PD; postprandial hypotension can also occur, but is less common. Except for the different circumstances in which they occur, the symptoms are similar, with somnolence, light-headedness, coat-hanger neck pain, and syncope (131, 132).

OH can contribute to falls and other accidental trauma. Cardiovascular dysautonomia worsens with disease progression. In the Sydney Multicentre Study of PD, a cohort of newly diagnosed patients was followed over 20 years (133). At 15 years follow-up, symptomatic postural hypotension occurred in 35%, increasing to 48% at 20 years follow-up (134). Symptomatic OH can occur even early in the course of the disease (135). Bonuccelli found a decrease of more than 20 mmHg in systolic blood pressure on standing in 7/51 (14%) patients with PD. Prominent OH in a parkinsonian patient is considered a red flag for MSA, and differentiation of early PD with symptomatic OH and MSA can be challenging.

OH and postprandial hypotension can be attributed to sympathetic neurocirculatory failure from generalized sympathetic denervation secondary to PD pathology (136–137), although dopaminergic medications may cause, or even aggravate, OH and postprandial hypotension (138). Cardiovascular abnormalities can occur in the absence of OH in PD, as shown by asymptomatic cardiac and vasomotor sympathetic dysfunction demonstrated by studying heart rate variability and 24-hour blood pressure monitoring (137, 139, 140). Extensive cardiac sympathetic denervation has been shown in most PD patients, using meta-iodobenzyl guanidine (MIBG) SPECT, even in the early stages of the disease (141–145). The degree of tracer uptake seems to correlate with disease progression (146, 147) and the rigid–akinetic PD subtype (148), but not with dysautonomic symptoms (144, 149). Several MIBG and pathological studies indicate that impaired sympathetic postganglionic function constitutes a marker of LB disorders compared with other parkinsonian syndromes without underlying LB pathology (97, 150–152). MIBG SPECT can be useful in the differentiation of PD with prominent OH from MSA.

Treatment of OH includes pharmacological and non-pharmacological measures used in the management of other conditions, alhough there are insufficient data to support or refute these treatments in PD (49). General measures include frequent small meals, increased salt and fluid intake, head-up bed tilt (by 10–30°) at night, thigh- or waist-high elastic stockings, portable chairs, and avoiding triggers or aggravating factors, such as alcohol intake, a warm environment, and increments of antihypertensive drugs (153–155). If OH is related to, or aggravated by, dopaminergic medications dose reduction of these drugs can be useful, although it may lead to worsening of motor symptoms. Domperidone may be of help in dopamine-agonist-related OH (155, 156). Agents that increase blood pressure, such as salt-retaining mineralocorticoids (e.g. fludrocortisone) or the alpha-adrenergic agonist midrodrine, can be useful (156–159). It is important to monitor blood pressure when using these agents, as they may cause supine or nocturnal hypertension. The anticholinesterase agent pyridostigmine has been reported to improve neurogenic OH without worsening supine hypertension (160), but this drug has not been formally tested in PD. Octreotide, a somatostatin agonist, may be of help in treating postprandial hypotension, but also has not been specifically studied in PD (161).

Neuropsychiatric symptoms

Neuropsychiatric symptoms (NPS) occur in the majority of patients at some point during the disease course, sometimes even before the diagnosis of PD has been established (162). The most common and important NPS are depression, anxiety, apathy, and psychosis (163). They have important consequences for the patient's quality of life and daily functioning (164), and they also have a negative impact on the quality of life of caregivers. They are frequently under-recognized and, consequently, are undertreated. Biological and psychological factors have been implicated in the pathogenesis of NPS in PD; frequently they occur as a complication of dopaminergic therapy.

Disease-associated NPS

Depression

The diagnosis of depression in PD may be difficult because of overlapping symptoms in the two disorders. The clinical 'gold-standard' diagnosis is frequently based on the application of the criteria of the *Diagnostic and Statistical Manual Version IV* (DSM-IV). These criteria may underestimate the real prevalence of depression in PD. To improve diagnostic assessment, the National Institute of Neurological Disorders and Stroke (NINDS)–National Institute of Mental Health (NIMH) working group on depression and PD has given specific recommendations (Table 11.5) (165).

A recent systematic review (166) of 36 studies concluded that, in PD, major depressive disorder is present in 17%, depressive symptoms in 22%, and dysthymia in 13%. Depression increases disability and caregiver distress and is the strongest predictor of quality of life in PD patients (167). The identification of depressive symptoms in PD by the treating neurologist is less accurate than in other groups of patients. Furthermore, once diagnosed, only 20–26% of depressed PD subjects will receive appropriate pharmacological treatment (168). Ravina and colleagues have shown that depression may cause patients to appear worse than they are, may cause doctors to start antiparkinsonian treatment before it is needed, and can cause poor daily functioning (169).

Depression in PD is thought to reflect disturbances in the monoaminergic pathways between brainstem nuclei and prefrontal and orbitofrontal cortical areas (170). A combination of dopaminergic, norepinephrinergic, and serotonergic pathways in the limbic system has been also implicated (171).

Few controlled studies exist with regard to the efficiency of antidepressants in PD. Tricyclic antidepressants may be more effective than SSRIs in the treatment of depression in PD, but the benefits are limited by a higher rate of side effects (172). The dopamine agonist pramipexole has been shown to have antidepressant effects in both unipolar and bipolar depression (173). A recent double-blind placebo-controlled study showed that pramipexole had a mild but significant antidepressant effect in PD, 80% of which could be attributed to a direct effect on depression and 20% to an indirect effect via improvement in motor function (174). A good strategy in the management of depression in PD is to optimize dopaminergic treatment first before adding an antidepressant (175).

There are certain situations in PD in which depression is particularly prominent and should be carefully looked for. This includes reactive depression at the time of first diagnosis, OFF period depression in patients with motor fluctuations (176), depression occurring in the setting of dopamine agonist cessation (dopamine agonist withdrawal syndrome) (177), and DBS-related depression (178) which on rare occasions may lead to suicide.

Table 11.5 NINDS/NIMH Work Group recommendations for improving the diagnosis of depression in PD (165)

(a) Use the inclusive approach rather than an aetiological strategy
(b) Eliminate 'the effects of a medical general condition' as a criterion of exclusion
(c) Subsyndromal depression should be included as a diagnostic category in research studies
(d) Specify the timing of assessment (ON versus – OFF periods)
(e) Anhedonia should only be diagnosed based on loss of pleasure rather than loss of interest (as it overlaps with apathy) for diagnosis of minor depression/ subsyndromal depression
(f) Informants should be used if possible when assessing cognitively impaired patients

Anxiety and apathy

Anxiety disorders are common in PD (179, 180), with many studies showing a high co-morbidity with depression. The most frequent anxiety disorders observed are generalized anxiety disorder, panic attacks, and phobias (181). Increasing anxiety has been associated with non-motor fluctuations, occurring particularly during OFF periods (179, 180). Therefore PD medication adjustment to avoid OFFs can decrease the duration and severity of anxiety (182). Occasionally, anxiety syndromes and mania have been reported as a side effect of dopamine agonists and high-dose levodopa treatment.

Apathy is defined as a set of behavioural, emotional, and cognitive features that involve reduced interest and motivation in goal-directed behaviours, indifference, and flattened affect (183). It is a common non-motor disturbance in PD, reported to occur in up to 70% in some studies (184, 185). It can be present early in the disease course and is frequently, but not always, associated with depression and cognitive impairment (186). Apathy in PD is more likely to be a consequence of neurodegeneration than psychological reaction or adaption to disability, and was rated one of the most distressing behavioural features by caregivers of demented patients with PD (184, 185). Disruption of non-motor basal ganglia connections to the mesial frontal anterior cingulate cortex has been suggested to underpin apathy in PD (187). Management is often difficult because patients are indifferent to the need to attend to their own health (188). Improvement in apathy may be effected by managing other conditions such as depression and dementia (189). Apathy occurring in the setting of chronic stimulation of the subthalamic nucleus can improve with dopamine agonists (190).

Fatigue

Fatigue is defined by two components: a feeling of tiredness, weariness, or exhaustion, and a reduction in the capacity to perform a task as a result of continuous performance of the same task (191). It is considered pathological when it is chronic, brought on by no or minimal exertion, does not fully improve with rest, and causes disability (192). Fatigue as defined above can be one of the most disabling symptoms reported by PD patients. Despite its prevalence (reported to occur in up two-thirds of patients) (193, 194) and negative impact, it is under-recognized clinically (195). It may be present early in the course of PD and may even predate the onset of motor features (196, 197).

In PD, fatigue onset and duration is not related to type of motor symptoms or disease severity, and is often exacerbated by physical, psychological, or social stressors (194, 196). Fatigue cannot be explained by EDS or poor sleep. In a recent study, the strongest predictors of fatigue in PD were symptoms of anxiety, depression, and impaired motivation (198). The Parkinson's Fatigue Scale (PFS) was developed as a disease-specific scale and has been validated in several countries (199). Alterations of the hypothalamic–pituitary–adrenal axis and dysfunction of frontal striatothalamocortical loops have been proposed as mechanisms underlying fatigue in PD (200, 201). Fatigue lacks specific treatment. An important step is to clarify to the patient and their caregivers that the symptom is a genuine and frequent manifestation of PD (202).

Psychosis

Psychotic symptoms are very common in PD, with increased risk in those with higher age at onset and need for high doses of dopaminergic drugs. Psychotic symptoms in PD include hallucinations, illusions, and paranoid delusions (203, 204). Reported prevalence rates of hallucinations vary, probably because of differences in patient selection and study design, ranging from 16 to 75% in prospective cross-sectional studies. Delusions affect 1–35% of subjects with PD (205).Visual hallucinations (VHs) are the most common psychotic symptoms observed in PD, but hallucinations can occur in all sensory domains (206). They tend to be persistent and progressive (207). Their prevalence increases with duration of disease, particularly if dementia develops. The presence of VHs in PD patients is a strong predictor of functional impairment, greater caregiver stress, and higher admission rates to nursing homes (208).

VHs are initially often minor, but may become formed; they are usually non-threatening, and insight is often retained with a clear sensorium. However, they may become severe and frightening, and insight can be lost. Typical VHs consist of human forms and animals, often mobile, which appear and vanish suddenly. The figures do not usually disturb the patients, who rarely involve themselves in the activities of the hallucinations (209). The awareness of the presence of another person (*Anwesenheit*) and the sensation of movement in the peripheral visual field (passage hallucinations) are sometimes considered pre-hallucinatory symptoms (203).

Delusions, which occur in approximately 5% of non-demented and 15% of demented patients with PD (163), are most commonly paranoid with contents of persecution, jealousy, spousal infidelity, and fears of impoverishment. Usually these beliefs are held with strong conviction, and such delusions can be extremely disruptive for the relationship between caregiver and patient. They almost always require treatment.

The pathophysiology of psychosis in PD is complex. Multiple external and internal factors may interact to produce the psychotic symptoms, such as visual impairment (210), sleep dysregulation with intrusion of REM fragments into wakefulness (211), overactivation of mesolimbic systems, and monoaminergic–cholinergic imbalance (212, 213). VHs occur mostly on medication. However, the dose and duration of treatment do not greatly influence the development of hallucinations, suggesting that other factors are more important. The most consistent risk factor has been cognitive impairment (214). Age, duration of disease, disease severity, depression, REM sleep disorder or daytime somnolence, and poor visual acuity have been associated with hallucinations only in some studies (215).

Non-pharmacological strategies are of the utmost importance in the management of psychotic symptoms in PD. These include:

a) identification and management of co-morbid medical conditions such as pain, dehydration, or infection (216);
b) psycho-educative approaches such as distraction or redirecting attention;
c) environmental interventions such as improving ambient light conditions and providing visual aids (217).

Reduction of polypharmacy should be considered, since this is an independent risk factor for the development of psychotic symptoms in PD. Narcotics, hypnotics, antidepressants, and anxiolytics, as well as dopaminergic medications, may contribute to the expression of psychosis. A gradual removal of anti-PD drugs is recommended: initially anticholinergics, MAO-B inhibitors, amantadine, and dopamine agonists, then catechol-*O*-methyltransferase (COMT) inhibitors, and finally levodopa.

Two atypical neuroleptics, quetiapine and clozapine, are frequently used in the management of psychosis in PD. Quetiapine is an atypical antipsychotic with a similar structure to clozapine, but it has the advantage of not requiring blood monitoring. It combines a strong antagonism for 5-HT2 receptors with a weak antagonism for D2 receptors. Four of five placebo-controlled studies found that quetiapine was not effective in PD psychosis (218–222). The only positive study excluded patients with delusions. Despite this, many physicians believe that quetiapine is effective and the American Academy of Neurology's task force on PD treatment recommends quetiapine as a treatment option after clozapine has been considered (223). Clozapine improves psychotic symptoms without worsening motor symptoms (224, 225). Nevertheless, its use is limited because of the risk of agranulocytosis and the requirement for regular blood monitoring. The recommended initial daily dose is 6.25–12.5 mg, with an increase of 12.5 mg every 4–7 days. Risperidone and olanzapine are effective in psychosis, but are not recommended because of significant motor worsening (226, 227). Some positive outcomes with cholinesterase inhibitors have been reported in a small series of PD patients with psychosis, with or without significant cognitive impairment. Further studies to assess the efficacy of these agents are required (228, 229).

Treatment-related NPS

Antiparkinsonian medication can produce or worsen psychosis (see previous section), but may also cause delirium (e.g. amantadine and anticholinergics), mood disturbances (e.g. hypomania secondary to levodopa), impulse control disorders (ICDs), and a variety of related behavioural disorders such as the dopamine dysregulation syndrome (DDS) and punding.

ICDs are defined by DSM IV criteria as the failure to resist an impulse, drive, or temptation and to perform an act that is harmful to the person or to others (230). Several such behaviours have been described in PD, including pathological gambling, compulsive shopping, hypersexuality, and compulsive eating. They often occur without causing distress and are frequently hidden by patients.

The most extensive evaluation of ICDs in PD is the multicentre North American DOMINION cross-sectional study (n = 3090 patients), which reported a six-month ICD prevalence of 13.6%. This study demonstrated a strong class association between ICDs and dopamine agonist use, and a weaker association with higher L-dopa dose, but not with agonist dose (231).

ICDs are frequently under-recognized in clinical practice (232). One study found that only 25% of PD patients with an active ICD were identified clinically (232). Risk factors for development of ICDs besides treatment with DA agonists, are early age of PD onset, personal or familial history of alcoholism or gambling, an impulsive or novelty-seeking premorbid personality, and male sex (233). Several mechanisms are implicated in the pathophysiology of ICDs, including interference with the normal pattern of dopamine release, stimulation of dopamine receptors (specifically, limbic D3 receptors), and chronic dopaminergic stimulation, resulting in neuronal sensitization.

DDS refers to the compulsive use of dopaminergic medication beyond the dose required for optimal control of motor disability and in the face of a mounting number of harmful physical, psychiatric, and social sequelae (234). The prevalence of DDS has been reported to be 4% (234). Novelty-seeking personality, high depression score, alcohol intake, and age of PD onset are independent predictors of DDS (235). The role of dopamine in the reward system and addiction has been proposed to underpin DDS (236). Patients commonly identify aversive dysphoric OFF mood states as a primary motivation to use their drugs compulsively (237). Supportive of addiction theories, one study utilizing positron emission tomography (PET) showed that PD patients with DDS had enhanced levodopa-induced ventral striatal dopamine release, perhaps due to sensitization (238). Not all patients with DDS have an ICD, although the majority of those with DDS also exhibit punding (239). Unfortunately, patients with DDS do not recognize the self-induced harm and demand increasing quantities of medication despite the development of complications (i.e. dyskinesias and OFF state dysphoria) (240).

Punding is defined as the display of aimless stereotyped behaviours performed for long periods of time at the expense of other activities (241). It was first described among amphetamine and cocaine abusers (242, 243). Nowadays, the most frequent cause of punding is dopaminergic drug treatment. In PD, punding prevalence studies show results ranging from 2 to 14% (239, 244), though it is considered an under-reported complication (245). It has also been described in 7% of patients with restless legs syndrome taking dopamine agonists (246). Punding is associated with high doses of dopaminergic drugs, but not with any specific subtype (233, 247). It has been described more frequently in males (13–40% higher proportion) and younger patients (239, 248).

Management of treatment-related complex behavioural disturbances

It is important for physicians to be aware of the neuropsychiatric side effects of dopaminergic therapy and to actively screen for them. Before initiation of therapy with dopamine agonists patients should be warned of the potential risk of these behaviours, and those considered to be 'at risk' should be closely monitored (233). ICD behaviours often resolve after discontinuing agonist treatment (249), but in many patients the parkinsonism worsens and some may develop a dopamine agonist withdrawal syndrome (177). If parkinsonism worsens, it may be prudent to increase levodopa concomitantly. The role of amantadine in managing ICDs is not yet resolved because of contradictory data (250).

In DDS, the strategy is reversed and levodopa should be reduced initially with a subsequent increase in dopamine agonist treatment if motor symptoms worsen. Patients with DDS are often poorly compliant, and therefore external control of dosing by pharmacies and families/caregivers is important. Regarding additional pharmacological options, antidepressants for obsessive thoughts, and antipsychotic treatment for manic or aberrant behaviour, may be considered (234). DBS of the subthalamic nucleus may allow dopaminergic drug reduction and therefore lead to improvement in these symptoms (251, 252); rarely, DDS and ICDs may worsen or develop for the first time after DBS surgery (253).

The pathophysiological mechanisms underlying punding are not well understood, and as a consequence the optimal therapeutic strategy is unclear. A reduction in the dose of levodopa or dopamine agonist is the first step. Atypical antipsychotics or selective serotonin-reuptake inhibitors (SSRIs) have been suggested (248, 254).

NPS and deep brain stimulation. NPS are well known side effects of DBS (240). In the immediate postoperative period they can be related to individual preoperative vulnerability, dopaminergic medication withdrawal, electrical stimulation effects, medication interacting with stimulation, and psychological changes. At later stages after DBS, most NPS are related to disease progression (255).

Apathy is a relatively common postoperative symptom, with ten studies having found increased apathy after surgery (256–259). A clear relation between apathy and DBS target—subthalamic nucleus (STN) or globus pallidus internus (GPi)—has not been established. Transient apathy early in the postoperative period is commonly part of the dopaminergic or psychostimulant withdrawal syndrome, and usually responds to increasing levodopa (260, 261). Postoperative hypomania–mania has been reported in 4–15% of patients following STN DBS, generally occurring within the first three postoperative months (262–264). This commonly improves with a decrease in either stimulation voltage or dopaminergic medication (264, 265). Premorbid depression, emotional lability, or a family history of bipolar disorders have been implicated as predisposing factors (266, 267).

The risk of suicidal behaviour has been reported to increase significantly in the first four years after STN DBS. Thus, it is one of the most important potentially preventable risks for mortality following DBS for PD (268). Postoperative depression, being single, and a previous history of ICD or DDS are associated with an increased risk of attempted suicide (268). In the recently reported Veterans Affairs Cooperative Studies Program 468 study, depression worsened with STN DBS but improved with GPi DBS (269). Clinically, pre- and post-DBS psychiatric monitoring is important, especially the appearance of depressive symptoms (268). There is still no consensus on individual psychiatric symptoms as exclusion criteria for DBS surgery (270).

Cognitive changes and dementia in Parkinson's disease

Cognitive impairment and dementia are among the most common non-motor disturbances occurring in PD. Mild cognitive changes occur in up to 20% of early untreated patients (271). These changes may underpin complaints such as memory problems or attention and planning disturbances. Currently, it is fashionable to categorize these mild changes as mild cognitive impairment (MCI). Depending on the type of cognitive changes present, MCI in PD has been classified as amnestic or non-amnestic (single or multiple domain) (272). Of great interest are results of studies suggesting that mild cognitive changes may predict the development of dementia (273).

Dementia is a serious, typically late, complication of PD and has been termed PD dementia (PDD). Point prevalence of dementia in PD has been estimated at around 30%, and approximately 10% of patients develop dementia annually (274). Two recent longitudinal studies with 12 and 20 years of follow-up, respectively, have shown that over 80% of patients eventually develop dementia (134, 275). The mean duration of PD before dementia develops is approximately 10 years, although it can vary considerably. Risk factors for dementia include older age, more severe parkinsonism, predominance of gait disturbances and postural instability, presence of hallucinations, and MCI documented at first evaluation (276, 277). The role of genetic factors in the development of dementia in PD is less clear. Variants of the *APOE* and *MAPT* genes have been linked with an increased risk of dementia in PD, but these results are controversial (278).

Clinical features

The clinical features of PDD comprise an insidious onset and slowly progressive course of cognitive impairment occurring on a background of loss of response to dopaminergic drugs, including levodopa. Behavioural and neuropsychiatric symptoms, including depression, also occur frequently in patients with PDD.

Cognitive changes

PDD is best summarized as a 'dysexecutive' syndrome (deficits in abstract thinking, planning, mental flexibility, judgement, and initiative) with impairment of visuospatial abilities and memory.

Deficits in attention are also consistently present in PDD, and attention may fluctuate with waxing and waning of vigilance similar to that described in DLB (279, 280). Memory impairment is a common feature, and memory complaints are the presenting cognitive problem in 67% of patients with PDD. Memory deficits affect verbal, non-verbal, and visual domains (279, 281). Impairment of learning of new information is less severe than that reported for Alzheimer's disease (AD).

PDD patients consistently show impairment in visuospatial functions (282, 283) with poor drawing ability that correlates with the Mini Mental State Examination (MMSE) score. Language and praxis, so-called instrumental functions, are affected to a lesser degree than in AD. Significant dysphasia or dyspraxia is very unusual in PDD and should call the diagnosis of PDD into question.

Behavioural and neuropsychiatric disturbances

Hallucinations and delusions commonly occur in PDD patients, as do depression and apathy. In a community-based study major depression occurred in 13% of PDD subjects (284). Major depression with suicidal ideation is rare. Sad affect, apathy, and loss of interest are widely encountered. Anxiety also occurs frequently and may overlap with depression in the same subject. Hypomanic mood disorders are uncommon, as are problems with anger or aggression.

Psychotic symptoms are common in PDD. Visual hallucinations occur in up to 55% of PDD patients (284) and are infrequently reported spontaneously in the clinic. In PD patients without dementia, hallucinations are a major predictor of subsequent dementia (275) and nursing home placement (208). They may be relatively 'benign' and non-threatening, but delusional misinterpretation of the hallucinatory phenomena frequently occurs when dementia develops. Delusions occur in approximately 30% of PDD patients and are mainly paranoid in type, dealing with persecution and spousal infidelity (284). Apathy is associated with PDD in approximately 25% of subjects (285, 286).

Diagnostic investigations

Group differences between PDD and PD patients without dementia have been documented in structural and functional imaging (287), as well as in electrophysiological studies. However, none of these techniques can be recommended for routine diagnostic purposes because of inadequate specificity.

Tau-protein levels have been found to be higher and Abeta42 lower in patients with PDD compared with PD patients and normal controls (288). Further studies with larger samples and more detailed assessments are needed to clarify the role of CSF markers in the diagnosis of cognitive impairment and dementia in PD.

Neuropathology

Recent studies have reported the presence of abundant LBs in the cerebral cortex PDD (289, 290). However, although the presence of cortical and subcortical Lewy pathology is likely to be causative, this link is controversial. Braak et al. (291) showed that even in stage 3 (i.e. in the virtual absence of cortical LB involvement), a third of patients already had impaired cognition, mostly of moderate severity. Colosimo et al. (292) described a series of PD patients with considerable limbic and/or neocortical LB involvement but without major cognitive impairment. In autopsy studies, PDD has been associated with neuronal loss in the locus coeruleus, medial SNc, ventral tegmental area, and nucleus basalis of Meynert. Although some authors have emphasized impaired mesolimbic and mesocortical dopaminergic function in PDD, a severe cortical cholinergic deficit, independent of co-existing Alzheimer disease changes, is the most consistent neurochemical finding associated with PDD (293). Additional Alzheimer pathological burden in PDD is generally low but probably exacerbates the overall disease process, as does ageing (294).

Diagnosis and assessment

In clinical practice, PDD often goes unrecognized and, as a result, is not appropriately treated. Cognitive changes occur gradually and it is frequently difficult to separate early dementia from the cognitive changes occurring in elderly subjects. Difficulties also arise since the clinical presentation is heterogeneous. Delusion and hallucinations may be prominent in some patients, while apathy and somnolence accompany early dementia in others. The presence of motor deficits (e.g. dysarthria, bradykinesia) interferes with the assessment of cognition and also makes it difficult to assess the functional consequences of the cognitive changes. In any event, it is not uncommon to overestimate the cognitive status of the patient on a routine clinical visit. Conversational speech and content of conversation may seem normal, and only a more detailed cognitive assessment, which may require considerable time, highlights the presence of cognitive changes.

Dementia diagnosis in PD has been commonly based on the DSM-IV criteria for dementia, and a standard bedside test is the

MMSE. However, DSM-IV criteria fail to capture several of the core features of PDD. Functional decline related to cognitive dysfunction, as required by DSM criteria, may be difficult to discern because of motor difficulties. The MMSE does not detect dysexecutive disturbances well. The Mattis Dementia Rating Scale and the Montreal Cognitive Assessment (MoCA) are probably more appropriate than the MMSE for this group of subjects. The Neuropsychiatric Inventory is a scripted interview of caregivers, providing ratings of ten behaviours common in dementia syndromes (295), and is frequently used in the evaluation of PDD patients.

The Movement Disorder Society has recently published guidelines that provide practical help to diagnose PDD (296). These guidelines emphasize the use of bedside tools that do not require neuropsychological expertise to administer or interpret. The information needed to arrive at the diagnosis requires the clear demonstration that cognitive impairment negatively impacts daily living. Acute confusion, major depression, or features compatible with vascular dementia preclude the diagnosis of PDD.

Management

Attention to motor, cognitive, neuropsychiatric, and sleep domains needs special attention in patients with PDD (Box 11.1). In many subjects the response to levodopa is reduced, and trying to maintain control of motor symptoms may be less effective than in the earlier stages of PD, while the risk of precipitating or aggravating cognitive and psychiatric symptoms is increased.

Box 11.1 Management of dementia in PD

General measures

- Maintain the patients in a familiar structured setting.
- Judicious use of day care centres and caregivers at home.
- Minimize pharmacological treatment.
- Manage behavioural distrubances.

Pharmacological treatment of associated behavioural disturbances

- Reduce doses of antiparkinsonian drugs as much as possible. The majority of these drugs can induce or worsen psychosis in demented patients. Monotherapy with levodopa is recommended.
- Atypical antipsychotics quetiapine (12.5–125mg/day) or clozapine (50–100mg/day) for management of hallucinations, confusion, and other psychotic symptoms.
- Acetylcholinesterase inhibitors can lessen hallucinations, attention disturbances, and sleep disturbances.
- Antidepressants: SSRIs and SSNIs can improve depression and anxiety. Tricyclic antidepressants should be avoided because of their central anticholinergic properties.
- Sleep disturbances:
  - RBD generally responds to clonazepam (0.25–1.0mg). This drug can worsen obstructive sleep apnoea. Consider melatonin as a second-line drug.
  - Insomnia may improve with quetiapine (25–100mg at bedtime).
  - Excessive daytime sleepiness may improve with modafinil or methylphenidate but worsening of psychosis may occur.

Non-pharmacological measures are important, as well as providing adequate information to the patient and family. These measures include appropriate physical and mental activation, and avoidance of aggravating factors (e.g. inappropriate environment). Conditions which can trigger or aggravate mental dysfunction should be excluded (e.g. depression, adverse effects of drugs given for PD, or co-morbid conditions) (297).

The management of sleep disturbances and dysautonomia, as well as specific treatments for psychiatric and behavioural symptoms, is outlined in earlier sections of this chapter.

Cholinesterase inhibitors are the main class of drugs available for the specific treatment of cognitive impairment. They inhibit the enzyme acetylcholinesterase which results in an increase of acetylcholine half-life and enhances cholinergic transmission. Two small double-blind placebo-controlled trials appeared to demonstrate modest cognitive benefits for donepezil (298, 299). However, only one large (n = 541) double-blind placebo-controlled cholinesterase inhibitor trial has been published to date (300). Statistically significant effects of rivastigmine capsules versus placebo on a range of primary and secondary outcome measures were observed, including cognitive performance, attention, executive function, activities of daily living (ADLs), and behavioural symptoms.

Donepezil, rivastigmine, and galantamine are widely approved for the treatment of AD, but rivastigmine is the only pharmacological agent currently approved for the treatment of mild to moderate PDD in Europe, the USA, and Canada. In the USA, a patch containing rivastigmine was the first transdermal treatment approved for both AD and PDD (301). The cholinesterase inhibitors are generally well tolerated. In addition, to the GI side effects, hypersalivation, rhinorrhoea, and lacrimation occur in 15% of PDD patients, and postural hypotension, falls, and syncope in up to 10%. Worsening of parkinsonism (tremor) can occur, but is rarely clinically significant (302).

The *N*-methyl-D-aspartate (NMDA) antagonist memantine is approved for the treatment of moderate to severe AD. Two relatively small randomized trials in patients with either PDD or DLB demonstrated benefit for memantine, although the effects were very modest (303, 304). A larger randomized double-blind placebo-controlled study in subjects with mild to moderate PDD or DLB failed to show significant differences between the two treatments in patients with PDD. The drug was well tolerated in both studies (305).

A joint task force of the European Federation of Neurological Societies and the European Section of the Movement Disorder Society provided their recommendations for the therapeutic management of PDD in 2011. Most of the recommendations are off-label, and include (a) discontinuation of potential aggravators (e.g. anticholinergics, amantadine, benzodiazepines), (b) adding a cholinesterase inhibitor (rivastigmine, donepezil, galantamine), and (c) adding or substituting memantine if cholinesterase inhibitors are not tolerated or lack efficacy (306).

References

1. Lees AJ, Blackburn NA, Campbell VL. The nighttime problems of Parkinson's disease. *Clin Neuropharmacol* 1988; 11: 512–19.
2. Factor SA, McAlarney T, Sanchez-Ramos JR, Weiner WJ. Sleep disorders and sleep effect in Parkinson's disease. *Mov Disord* 1990; 5: 280–5.

3. van Hilten JJ, Weggeman M, van der Velde EA, Kerkhof GA, van Dijk JG, Roos RA. Sleep, excessive daytime sleepiness and fatigue in Parkinson's disease. *J Neural Transm Park Dis Dement Sect* 1993; 5: 235–44.
4. Comella CL, Nardine TM, Diederich NJ, Stebbins GT. Sleep-related violence, injury, and REM sleep behavior disorder in Parkinson's disease. *Neurology* 1998 Aug; 51(2): 526–9.
5. Iranzo A, Santamaria J, Rye DB, Valldeoriola F, Marti MJ, Munoz E, et al. Characteristics of idiopathic REM sleep behavior disorder and that associated with MSA and PD. *Neurology* 2005; 65: 247–52.
6. Tandberg E, Larsen JP, Karlsen K. Excessive daytime sleepiness and sleep benefit in Parkinson's disease: a community-based study. *Mov Disord* 1999; 14: 922–7.
7. Gjerstad MD, Alves G, Wentzel-Larsen T, Aarsland D, Larsen JP. Excessive daytime sleepiness in Parkinson disease: is it the drugs or the disease? *Neurology* 2006; 67: 853–8.
8. Tandberg E, Larsen JP, Karlsen K. A community-based study of sleep disorders in patients with Parkinson's disease. *Mov Disord* 1998; 13: 895–9.
9. Gjerstad MD, Wentzel-Larsen T, Aarsland D, Larsen JP. Insomnia in Parkinson's disease: frequency and progression over time. *J Neurol Neurosurg Psychiatry* 2007; 78: 476–9.
10. Verbaan D, van Rooden SM, Visser M, Marinus J, van Hilten JJ. Nighttime sleep problems and daytime sleepiness in Parkinson's disease. *Mov Disord* 2008; 23: 35–41.
11. van Hilten B, Hoff JI, Middelkoop HA, et al. Sleep disruption in Parkinson's disease. Assessment by continuous activity monitoring. *Arch Neurol* 1994; 51: 922–8.
12. Kumar S, Bhatia M, Behari M. Sleep disorders in Parkinson's disease. *Mov Disord* 2002; 17: 775–81.
13. Maria B, Sophia S, Michalis M, et al. Sleep breathing disorders in patients with idiopathic Parkinson's disease. *Respir Med* 2003; 97: 1151–7.
14. Trenkwalder C, Kies B, Rudzinska M, et al. Rotigotine effects on early morning motor function and sleep in Parkinson's disease: a double-blind, randomized, placebo-controlled study (RECOVER). *Mov Disord* 2011; 26: 90–9.
15. Pahwa R, Stacy MA, Factor SA, et al. Ropinirole 24-hour prolonged release: randomized, controlled study in advanced Parkinson disease. *Neurology* 2007; 68: 1108–15.
16. Menza M, Dobkin RD, Marin H, et al. Treatment of insomnia in Parkinson's disease: a controlled trial of eszopiclone and placebo. *Mov Disord* 2010; 25(11): 1708–14.
17. Iranzo A, Santamaria J, Tolosa E. The clinical and pathophysiological relevance of REM sleep behavior disorder in neurodegenerative diseases. *Sleep Med Rev* 2009; 13: 385–401.
18. Schenck CH, Mahowald MW. REM sleep behavior disorder: clinical, developmental, and neuroscience perspectives 16 years after its formal identification in SLEEP. *Sleep* 2002; 25: 120–38.
19. Poryazova R, Waldvogel D, Bassetti CL. Sleepwalking in patients with Parkinson disease. *Arch Neurol* 2007; 64: 1524–7.
20. Scaglione C, Vignatelli L, Plazzi G, et al. REM sleep behaviour disorder in Parkinson's disease: a questionnaire-based study. *Neurol Sci* 2005; 25: 316–21.
21. Meral H, Aydemir T, Ozer F, et al. Relationship between visual hallucinations and REM sleep behavior disorder in patients with Parkinson's disease. *Clin Neurol Neurosurg* 2007; 109: 862–7.
22. Wetter TC, Trenkwalder C, Gershanik O, Hogl B. Polysomnographic measures in Parkinson's disease: a comparison between patients with and without REM sleep disturbances. *Wien Klin Wochenschr* 2001; 113: 249–53.
23. Gagnon JF, Bedard MA, Fantini ML, et al. REM sleep behavior disorder and REM sleep without atonia in Parkinson's disease. *Neurology* 2002; 59: 585–9.
24. Diederich NJ, Vaillant M, Mancuso G, Lyen P, Tiete J. Progressive sleep 'destructuring' in Parkinson's disease. A polysomnographic study in 46 patients. *Sleep Med* 2005; 6: 313–18.
25. De Cock VC, Vidailhet M, Leu S, et al. Restoration of normal motor control in Parkinson's disease during REM sleep. *Brain* 2007; 130: 450–6.
26. Kumru H, Iranzo A, Carrasco E, et al. Lack of effects of pramipexole on REM sleep behavior disorder in Parkinson disease. *Sleep* 2008; 31: 1418–21.
27. Postuma RB, Gagnon JF, Vendette M, Charland K, Montplaisir J. REM sleep behaviour disorder in Parkinson's disease is associated with specific motor features. *J Neurol Neurosurg Psychiatry* 2008; 79: 1117–21.
28. Vendette M, Gagnon JF, Decary A, et al. REM sleep behavior disorder predicts cognitive impairment in Parkinson disease without dementia. *Neurology* 2007; 69: 1843–9.
29. Kumru H, Santamaria J, Tolosa E, et al. Rapid eye movement sleep behavior disorder in parkinsonism with parkin mutations. *Ann Neurol* 2004; 56: 599–603.
30. Boeve BF, Dickson DW, Olson EJ, et al. Insights into REM sleep behavior disorder pathophysiology in brainstem-predominant Lewy body disease. *Sleep Med* 2007; 8: 60–4.
31. Frucht SJ, Greene PE, Fahn S. Sleep episodes in Parkinson's disease: a wake-up call. *Mov Disord* 2000; 15: 601–3.
32. Rye DB, Bliwise DL, Dihenia B, Gurecki P. FAST TRACK: daytime sleepiness in Parkinson's disease. *J Sleep Res* 2000; 9: 63–9.
33. Arnulf I, Konofal E, Merino-Andreu M, et al. Parkinson's disease and sleepiness: an integral part of PD. *Neurology* 2002; 58: 1019–24.
34. Ripley B, Overeem S, Fujiki N, et al. CSF hypocretin/orexin levels in narcolepsy and other neurological conditions. *Neurology* 2001; 57: 2253–8.
35. Overeem S, van Hilten JJ, Ripley B, Mignot E, Nishino S, Lammers GJ. Normal hypocretin-1 levels in Parkinson's disease patients with excessive daytime sleepiness. *Neurology* 2002; 58: 498–9.
36. Baumann C, Ferini-Strambi L, Waldvogel D, Werth E, Bassetti CL. Parkinsonism with excessive daytime sleepiness—a narcolepsy-like disorder? *J Neurol* 2005; 252: 139–45.
37. Compta Y, Santamaria J, Ratti L, et al. Cerebrospinal hypocretin, daytime sleepiness and sleep architecture in Parkinson's disease dementia. *Brain* 2009; 132: 3308–17.
38. Rye DB. The two faces of Eve: dopamine's modulation of wakefulness and sleep. *Neurology* 2004; 63 (Suppl 3): S2–7.
39. Fronczek R, Overeem S, Lee SY, et al. Hypocretin (orexin) loss in Parkinson's disease. *Brain* 2007; 130: 1577–85.
40. Thannickal TC, Lai YY, Siegel JM. Hypocretin (orexin) cell loss in Parkinson's disease. *Brain* 2007; 130: 1586–95.
41. Fabbrini G, Barbanti P, Aurilia C, Vanacore N, Pauletti C, Meco G. Excessive daytime sleepiness in de novo and treated Parkinson's disease. *Mov Disord* 2002; 17: 1026–30.
42. Gjerstad MD, Aarsland D, Larsen JP. Development of daytime somnolence over time in Parkinson's disease. *Neurology* 2002; 58: 1544–6.
43. Frucht S, Rogers JD, Greene PE, Gordon MF, Fahn S. Falling asleep at the wheel: motor vehicle mishaps in persons taking pramipexole and ropinirole. *Neurology* 1999; 52: 1908–10.
44. Ferreira JJ, Galitzky M, Montastruc JL, Rascol O. Sleep attacks and Parkinson's disease treatment. *Lancet* 2000; 355: 1333–4.
45. Schapira AH. Sleep attacks (sleep episodes) with pergolide. *Lancet* 2000; 355: 1332–3.
46. Hobson DE, Lang AE, Martin WR, Razmy A, Rivest J, Fleming J. Excessive daytime sleepiness and sudden-onset sleep in Parkinson disease: a survey by the Canadian Movement Disorders Group. *JAMA* 2002; 287: 455–63.
47. Ferreira JJ, Thalamas C, Montastruc JL, Castro-Caldas A, Rascol O. Levodopa monotherapy can induce 'sleep attacks' in Parkinson's disease patients. *J Neurol* 2001; 248: 426–7.
48. Holloway RG, Shoulson I, Fahn S, et al. Pramipexole vs levodopa as initial treatment for Parkinson disease: a 4-year randomized controlled trial. *Arch Neurol* 2004; 61: 1044–53.

49. Zesiewicz TA, Sullivan KL, Arnulf I, et al. Practice Parameter. Treatment of nonmotor symptoms of Parkinson disease: report of the Quality Standards Subcommittee of the American Academy of Neurology. *Neurology* 2010; 74: 924–31.
50. Hogl B, Saletu M, Brandauer E, et al. Modafinil for the treatment of daytime sleepiness in Parkinson's disease: a double-blind, randomized, crossover, placebo-controlled polygraphic trial. *Sleep* 2002; 25: 905–9.
51. Adler CH, Caviness JN, Hentz JG, Lind M, Tiede J. Randomized trial of modafinil for treating subjective daytime sleepiness in patients with Parkinson's disease. *Mov Disord* 2003; 18: 287–93.
52. Ondo WG, Fayle R, Atassi F, Jankovic J. Modafinil for daytime somnolence in Parkinson's disease: double blind, placebo controlled parallel trial. *J Neurol Neurosurg Psychiatry* 2005; 76: 1636–9.
53. Ondo WG, Perkins T, Swick T, et al. Sodium oxybate for excessive daytime sleepiness in Parkinson disease: an open-label polysomnographic study. *Arch Neurol* 2008; 65: 1337–40.
54. Doty RL, Stern MB, Pfeiffer C, Gollomp SM, Hurtig HI. Bilateral olfactory dysfunction in early stage treated and untreated idiopathic Parkinson's disease. *J Neurol Neurosurg Psychiatry* 1992; 55: 138–42.
55. Katzenschlager R, Lees AJ. Olfaction and Parkinson's syndromes: its role in differential diagnosis. *Curr Opin Neurol* 2004; 17: 417–23.
56. Muller A, Mungersdorf M, Reichmann H, Strehle G, Hummel T. Olfactory function in Parkinsonian syndromes. *J Clin Neurosci* 2002; 9: 521–4.
57. Henderson JM, Lu Y, Wang S, Cartwright H, Halliday GM. Olfactory deficits and sleep disturbances in Parkinson's disease: a case–control survey. *J Neurol Neurosurg Psychiatry* 2003; 74: 956–8.
58. Saifee T, Lees AJ, Silveira-Moriyama L. Olfactory function in Parkinson's disease in ON versus OFF states. *J Neurol Neurosurg Psychiatry* 2010; 81: 1293–5.
59. Ponsen MM, Stoffers D, Booij J, van Eck-Smit BL, Wolters E, Berendse HW. Idiopathic hyposmia as a preclinical sign of Parkinson's disease. *Ann Neurol* 2004; 56: 173–81.
60. Ross GW, Petrovitch H, Abbott RD, et al. Association of olfactory dysfunction with risk for future Parkinson's disease. *Ann Neurol* 2008; 63: 167–73.
61. Benarroch EE. Olfactory system: functional organization and involvement in neurodegenerative disease. *Neurology* 2010; 75: 1104–9.
62. Stern MB, Doty RL, Dotti M, et al. Olfactory function in Parkinson's disease subtypes. *Neurology* 1994; 44: 266–8.
63. Iijima M, Kobayakawa T, Saito S, et al. Differences in odor identification among clinical subtypes of Parkinson's disease. *Eur J Neurol* 2011; 18: 425–9.
64. Goldstein DS, Sewell L, Holmes C. Association of anosmia with autonomic failure in Parkinson disease. *Neurology* 2010; 74: 245–51.
65. Bohnen NI, Muller ML, Kotagal V, et al. Olfactory dysfunction, central cholinergic integrity and cognitive impairment in Parkinson's disease. *Brain* 2010; 133: 1747–54.
66. Damholdt MF, Borghammer P, Larsen L, Ostergaard K. Odor identification deficits identify Parkinson's disease patients with poor cognitive performance. *Mov Disord* 2011; 26: 2045–50.
67. Morley JF, Weintraub D, Mamikonyan E, Moberg PJ, Siderowf AD, Duda JE. Olfactory dysfunction is associated with neuropsychiatric manifestations in Parkinson's disease. *Mov Disord* 2011; 26: 2051–7.
68. Wenning GK, Shephard B, Hawkes C, Petruckevitch A, Lees A, Quinn N. Olfactory function in atypical parkinsonian syndromes. *Acta Neurol Scand* 1995; 91: 247–50.
69. Katzenschlager R, Zijlmans J, Evans A, Watt H, Lees AJ. Olfactory function distinguishes vascular parkinsonism from Parkinson's disease. *J Neurol Neurosurg Psychiatry* 2004; 75: 1749–52.
70. Louis ED, Bromley SM, Jurewicz EC, Watner D. Olfactory dysfunction in essential tremor: a deficit unrelated to disease duration or severity. *Neurology* 2002; 59: 1631–3.
71. Khan NL, Katzenschlager R, Watt H, et al. Olfaction differentiates parkin disease from early-onset parkinsonism and Parkinson disease. *Neurology* 2004; 62: 1224–6.
72. Healy DG, Falchi M, O'Sullivan SS, et al. Phenotype, genotype, and worldwide genetic penetrance of LRRK2-associated Parkinson's disease: a case–control study. *Lancet Neurol* 2008; 7: 583–90.
73. Silveira-Moriyama L, Munhoz RP, de J Carvalho M, et al. Olfactory heterogeneity in LRRK2 related Parkinsonism. *Mov Disord* 2010; 25: 2879–83.
74. McShane RH, Nagy Z, Esiri MM, et al. Anosmia in dementia is associated with Lewy bodies rather than Alzheimer's pathology. *J Neurol Neurosurg Psychiatry* 2001; 70: 739–43.
75. Jost WH. Autonomic dysfunctions in idiopathic Parkinson's disease. *J Neurol* 2003; 250 (Suppl 1): I28–30.
76. Magerkurth C, Schnitzer R, Braune S. Symptoms of autonomic failure in Parkinson's disease: prevalence and impact on daily life. *Clin Auton Res* 2005; 15: 76–82.
77. Bonuccelli U, Lucetti C, Del Dotto P, et al. Orthostatic hypotension in de novo Parkinson disease. *Arch Neurol* 2003; 60: 1400–4.
78. Muller B, Larsen JP, Wentzel-Larsen T, Skeie GO, Tysnes OB. Autonomic and sensory symptoms and signs in incident, untreated Parkinson's disease: frequent but mild. *Mov Disord* 2011; 26: 65–72.
79. Kaufmann H, Nahm K, Purohit D, Wolfe D. Autonomic failure as the initial presentation of Parkinson disease and dementia with Lewy bodies. *Neurology* 2004; 63: 1093–5.
80. O'Sullivan SS, Holton JL, Massey LA, Williams DR, Revesz T, Lees AJ. Parkinson's disease with Onuf's nucleus involvement mimicking multiple system atrophy. *J Neurol Neurosurg Psychiatry* 2008; 79: 232–4.
81. Abbott RD, Ross GW, Petrovitch H, et al. Bowel movement frequency in late-life and incidental Lewy bodies. *Mov Disord* 2007; 22: 1581–6.
82. Papapetropoulos S, Paschalis C, Athanassiadou A, et al. Clinical phenotype in patients with alpha-synuclein Parkinson's disease living in Greece in comparison with patients with sporadic Parkinson's disease. *J Neurol Neurosurg Psychiatry* 2001; 70: 662–5.
83. Singleton A, Gwinn-Hardy K, Sharabi Y, et al. Association between cardiac denervation and parkinsonism caused by alpha-synuclein gene triplication. *Brain* 2004; 127: 768–72.
84. Albanese A, Valente EM, Romito LM, Bellacchio E, Elia AE, Dallapiccola B. The PINK1 phenotype can be indistinguishable from idiopathic Parkinson disease. *Neurology* 2005; 64: 1958–60.
85. Goldstein DS, Imrich R, Peckham E, et al. Neurocirculatory and nigrostriatal abnormalities in Parkinson disease from LRRK2 mutation. *Neurology* 2007; 69: 1580–4.
86. Khan NL, Graham E, Critchley P, et al. Parkin disease: a phenotypic study of a large case series. *Brain* 2003; 126: 1279–92.
87. Kagi G, Klein C, Wood NW, et al. Nonmotor symptoms in Parkin gene-related parkinsonism. *Mov Disord* 2010; 25: 1279–84.
88. Qualman SJ, Haupt HM, Yang P, Hamilton SR. Esophageal Lewy bodies associated with ganglion cell loss in achalasia: similarity to Parkinson's disease. *Gastroenterology* 1984; 87: 848–56.
89. Kupsky WJ, Grimes MM, Sweeting J, Bertsch R, Cote LJ. Parkinson's disease and megacolon: concentric hyaline inclusions (Lewy bodies) in enteric ganglion cells. *Neurology* 1987; 37: 1253–5.
90. Jackson M, Lennox G, Balsitis M, Lowe J. Lewy body dysphagia. *J Neurol Neurosurg Psychiatry* 1995; 58: 756–8.
91. Singaram C, Ashraf W, Gaumnitz EA, et al. Dopaminergic defect of enteric nervous system in Parkinson's disease patients with chronic constipation. *Lancet* 1995; 346: 861–4.
92. Wakabayashi K, Takahashi H. The intermediolateral nucleus and Clarke's column in Parkinson's disease. *Acta Neuropathol* 1997; 94: 287–9.
93. Iwanaga K, Wakabayashi K, Yoshimoto M, et al. Lewy body-type degeneration in cardiac plexus in Parkinson's and incidental Lewy body diseases. *Neurology* 1999 12;52: 1269–71.

94. Benarroch EE, Schmeichel AM, Parisi JE. Involvement of the ventrolateral medulla in parkinsonism with autonomic failure. *Neurology* 2000; 54: 963–8.
95. Braak H, de Vos RA, Bohl J, Del Tredici K. Gastric alpha-synuclein immunoreactive inclusions in Meissner's and Auerbach's plexuses in cases staged for Parkinson's disease-related brain pathology. *Neurosci Lett* 2006; 396: 67–72.
96. Minguez-Castellanos A, Chamorro CE, Escamilla-Sevilla F, et al. Do alpha-synuclein aggregates in autonomic plexuses predate Lewy body disorders? A cohort study. *Neurology* 2007; 68: 2012–18.
97. Orimo S, Uchihara T, Nakamura A, et al. Axonal alpha-synuclein aggregates herald centripetal degeneration of cardiac sympathetic nerve in Parkinson's disease. *Brain* 2008; 131: 642–50.
98. Edwards LL, Pfeiffer RF, Quigley EM, Hofman R, Balluff M. Gastrointestinal symptoms in Parkinson's disease. *Mov Disord* 1991; 6: 151–6.
99. Pfeiffer RF. Gastrointestinal dysfunction in Parkinson's disease. *Lancet Neurol* 2003; 2: 107–16.
100. Hardoff R, Sula M, Tamir A, et al. Gastric emptying time and gastric motility in patients with Parkinson's disease. *Mov Disord* 2001; 16: 1041–7.
101. Sonnenberg A, Tsou VT, Muller AD. The 'institutional colon': a frequent colonic dysmotility in psychiatric and neurologic disease. *Am J Gastroenterol* 1994; 89: 62–6.
102. Hermanowicz N. Fatal gastroparesis in a patient with Parkinson's disease. *Mov Disord* 2008; 23: 152–3.
103. Kaye J, Gage H, Kimber A, Storey L, Trend P. Excess burden of constipation in Parkinson's disease: a pilot study. *Mov Disord* 2006; 21: 1270–3.
104. Ashraf W, Wszolek ZK, Pfeiffer RF, et al. Anorectal function in fluctuating (on-off) Parkinson's disease: evaluation by combined anorectal manometry and electromyography. *Mov Disord* 1995; 10: 650–7.
105. Bassotti G, Maggio D, Battaglia E, et al. Manometric investigation of anorectal function in early and late stage Parkinson's disease. *J Neurol Neurosurg Psychiatry* 2000; 68: 768–70.
106. Sakakibara R, Odaka T, Lui Z, et al. Dietary herb extract dai-kenchu-to ameliorates constipation in parkinsonian patients (Parkinson's disease and multiple system atrophy). *Mov Disord* 2005; 20: 261–2.
107. Mathers SE, Kempster PA, Swash M, Lees AJ. Constipation and paradoxical puborectalis contraction in anismus and Parkinson's disease: a dystonic phenomenon? *J Neurol Neurosurg Psychiatry* 1988; 51: 1503–7.
108. Ashraf W, Pfeiffer RF, Quigley EM. Anorectal manometry in the assessment of anorectal function in Parkinson's disease: a comparison with chronic idiopathic constipation. *Mov Disord* 1994; 9: 655–63.
109. Eichhorn TE, Oertel WH. Macrogol 3350/electrolyte improves constipation in Parkinson's disease and multiple system atrophy. *Mov Disord* 2001; 16: 1176–7.
110. Liu Z, Sakakibara R, Odaka T, et al. Mosapride citrate, a novel 5-HT4 agonist and partial 5-HT3 antagonist, ameliorates constipation in parkinsonian patients. *Mov Disord* 2005; 20: 680–6.
111. Sullivan KL, Staffetti JF, Hauser RA, Dunne PB, Zesiewicz TA. Tegaserod (Zelnorm) for the treatment of constipation in Parkinson's disease. *Mov Disord* 2006 Jan; 21: 115–16.
112. Zangaglia R, Martignoni E, Glorioso M, et al. Macrogol for the treatment of constipation in Parkinson's disease: a randomized placebo-controlled study. *Mov Disord* 2007; 22: 1239–44.
113. Soykan I, Sarosiek I, Shifflett J, Wooten GF, McCallum RW. Effect of chronic oral domperidone therapy on gastrointestinal symptoms and gastric emptying in patients with Parkinson's disease. *Mov Disord* 1997; 12: 952–7.
114. Albanese A, Brisinda G, Bentivoglio AR, Maria G. Treatment of outlet obstruction constipation in Parkinson's disease with botulinum neurotoxin A. *Am J Gastroenterol* 2003; 98: 1439–40.
115. Araki I, Kuno S. Assessment of voiding dysfunction in Parkinson's disease by the international prostate symptom score. *J Neurol Neurosurg Psychiatry* 2000; 68: 429–33.
116. Sakakibara R, Shinotoh H, Uchiyama T, et al. Questionnaire-based assessment of pelvic organ dysfunction in Parkinson's disease. *Auton Neurosci* 2001; 92: 76–85.
117. Campos-Sousa RN, Quagliato E, da Silva BB, de Carvalho RM, Jr, Ribeiro SC, de Carvalho DF. Urinary symptoms in Parkinson's disease: prevalence and associated factors. *Arq Neuropsiquiatr* 2003; 61: 359–63.
118. Wenning GK, Scherfler C, Granata R, et al. Time course of symptomatic orthostatic hypotension and urinary incontinence in patients with postmortem confirmed parkinsonian syndromes: a clinicopathological study. *J Neurol Neurosurg Psychiatry* 1999; 67: 620–3.
119. Uchiyama T, Sakakibara R, Yamamoto T, et al. Urinary dysfunction in early and untreated Parkinson's disease. *J Neurol Neurosurg Psychiatry* 2011; 82: 1382–6.
120. O'Sullivan SS, Williams DR, Gallagher DA, Massey LA, Silveira-Moriyama L, Lees AJ. Nonmotor symptoms as presenting complaints in Parkinson's disease: A clinicopathological study. *Mov Disord* 2008; 23: 101–6.
121. Ransmayr GN, Holliger S, Schletterer K, et al. Lower urinary tract symptoms in dementia with Lewy bodies, Parkinson disease, and Alzheimer disease. *Neurology* 2008; 70: 299–303.
122. Welsh M, Hung L, Waters CH. Sexuality in women with Parkinson's disease. *Mov Disord* 1997; 12: 923–7.
123. Bronner G, Royter V, Korczyn AD, Giladi N. Sexual dysfunction in Parkinson's disease. *J Sex Marital Ther* 2004; 30: 95–105.
124. Gao X, Chen H, Schwarzschild MA, et al. Erectile function and risk of Parkinson's disease. *Am J Epidemiol* 2007; 166: 1446–50.
125. Jimenez-Jimenez FJ, Tallon-Barranco A, Cabrera-Valdivia F, Gasalla T, Orti-Pareja M, Zurdo M. Fluctuating penile erection related with levodopa therapy. *Neurology* 1999; 52: 210.
126. Kanovsky P, Bares M, Pohanka M, Rektor I. Penile erections and hypersexuality induced by pergolide treatment in advanced, fluctuating Parkinson's disease. *J Neurol* 2002; 249: 112–14.
127. Suchowersky O, Furtado S, Rohs G. Beneficial effect of intranasal desmopressin for nocturnal polyuria in Parkinson's disease. *Mov Disord* 1995; 10: 337–40.
128. Zesiewicz TA, Helal M, Hauser RA. Sildenafil citrate (Viagra) for the treatment of erectile dysfunction in men with Parkinson's disease. *Mov Disord* 2000; 15: 305–8.
129. Hussain IF, Brady CM, Swinn MJ, Mathias CJ, Fowler CJ. Treatment of erectile dysfunction with sildenafil citrate (Viagra) in parkinsonism due to Parkinson's disease or multiple system atrophy with observations on orthostatic hypotension. *J Neurol Neurosurg Psychiatry* 2001; 71: 371–4.
130. O'Mara G, Lyons D. Postprandial hypotension. *Clin Geriatr Med* 2002; 18: 307–21.
131. Bleasdale-Barr KM, Mathias CJ. Neck and other muscle pains in autonomic failure: their association with orthostatic hypotension. *J R Soc Med* 1998; 91: 355–9.
132. Oka H, Yoshioka M, Onouchi K, et al. Characteristics of orthostatic hypotension in Parkinson's disease. *Brain* 2007; 130: 2425–32.
133. Hely MA, Reid WG, Adena MA, Halliday GM, Morris JG. The Sydney multicenter study of Parkinson's disease: the inevitability of dementia at 20 years. *Mov Disord* 2008; 23: 837–44.
134. Hely MA, Morris JG, Reid WG, Trafficante R. Sydney Multicenter Study of Parkinson's disease: non-l-dopa-responsive problems dominate at 15 years. *Mov Disord* 2005; 20: 190–9.
135. Goldstein DS. Orthostatic hypotension as an early finding in Parkinson's disease. *Clin Auton Res* 2006; 16: 46–54.
136. Goldstein DS, Holmes CS, Dendi R, Bruce SR, Li ST. Orthostatic hypotension from sympathetic denervation in Parkinson's disease. *Neurology* 2002; 58: 1247–55.
137. Oka H, Toyoda C, Yogo M, Mochio S. Cardiovascular dysautonomia in de novo Parkinson's disease without orthostatic hypotension. *Eur J Neurol* 2011; 18: 286–92.

138. Kujawa K, Leurgans S, Raman R, Blasucci L, Goetz CG. Acute orthostatic hypotension when starting dopamine agonists in Parkinson's disease. *Arch Neurol* 2000; 57: 1461–3.
139. Holmberg B, Kallio M, Johnels B, Elam M. Cardiovascular reflex testing contributes to clinical evaluation and differential diagnosis of Parkinsonian syndromes. *Mov Disord* 2001; 16: 217–25.
140. Ejaz AA, Sekhon IS, Munjal S. Characteristic findings on 24-h ambulatory blood pressure monitoring in a series of patients with Parkinson's disease. *Eur J Intern Med* 2006; 17: 417–20.
141. Yoshita M, Hayashi M, Hirai S. Decreased myocardial accumulation of ^{123}I-meta-iodobenzyl guanidine in Parkinson's disease. *Nucl Med Commun* 1998; 19: 137–42.
142. Orimo S, Ozawa E, Nakade S, Sugimoto T, Mizusawa H. ^{123}I-metaiodobenzylguanidine myocardial scintigraphy in Parkinson's disease. *J Neurol Neurosurg Psychiatry* 1999; 67: 189–94.
143. Braune S, Reinhardt M, Schnitzer R, Riedel A, Lucking CH. Cardiac uptake of [^{123}I]MIBG separates Parkinson's disease from multiple system atrophy. *Neurology* 1999; 53: 1020–5.
144. Takatsu H, Nishida H, Matsuo H, et al. Cardiac sympathetic denervation from the early stage of Parkinson's disease: clinical and experimental studies with radiolabeled MIBG. *J Nucl Med* 2000; 41: 71–7.
145. Courbon F, Brefel-Courbon C, Thalamas C, et al. Cardiac MIBG scintigraphy is a sensitive tool for detecting cardiac sympathetic denervation in Parkinson's disease. *Mov Disord* 2003; 18: 890–7.
146. Li ST, Dendi R, Holmes C, Goldstein DS. Progressive loss of cardiac sympathetic innervation in Parkinson's disease. *Ann Neurol* 2002; 52: 220–3.
147. Hamada K, Hirayama M, Watanabe H, et al. Onset age and severity of motor impairment are associated with reduction of myocardial ^{123}I-MIBG uptake in Parkinson's disease. *J Neurol Neurosurg Psychiatry* 2003; 74: 423–6.
148. Spiegel J, Hellwig D, Farmakis G, et al. Myocardial sympathetic degeneration correlates with clinical phenotype of Parkinson's disease. *Mov Disord* 2007; 22: 1004–8.
149. Matsui H, Nishinaka K, Oda M, Komatsu K, Kubori T, Udaka F. Does cardiac metaiodobenzylguanidine (MIBG) uptake in Parkinson's disease correlate with major autonomic symptoms? *Parkinsonism Relat Disord* 2006; 12: 284–8.
150. Orimo S, Ozawa E, Oka T, et al. Different histopathology accounting for a decrease in myocardial MIBG uptake in PD and MSA. *Neurology* 2001; 57: 1140–1.
151. Orimo S, Oka T, Miura H, et al. Sympathetic cardiac denervation in Parkinson's disease and pure autonomic failure but not in multiple system atrophy. *J Neurol Neurosurg Psychiatry* 2002; 73: 776–7.
152. Kashihara K, Ohno M, Kawada S, Okumura Y. Reduced cardiac uptake and enhanced washout of ^{123}I-MIBG in pure autonomic failure occurs conjointly with Parkinson's disease and dementia with Lewy bodies. *J Nucl Med* 2006; 47: 1099–101.
153. Smit AA, Wieling W, Opfer-Gehrking TL, van Emmerik-Levelt HM, Low PA. Patients' choice of portable folding chairs to reduce symptoms of orthostatic hypotension. *Clin Auton Res* 1999; 9: 341–4.
154. Hasegawa Y, Hakusui S, Hirayama M, et al. Clinical effects of elastic bandage on neurogenic orthostatic hypotension. *J Gravit Physiol* 2000; 7: 159–60.
155. Lang AE. Acute orthostatic hypotension when starting dopamine agonist therapy in parkinson disease: the role of domperidone therapy. *Arch Neurol* 2001; 58: 835.
156. Schoffer KL, Henderson RD, O'Maley K, O'Sullivan JD. Nonpharmacological treatment, fludrocortisone, and domperidone for orthostatic hypotension in Parkinson's disease. *Mov Disord* 2007; 22: 1543–9.
157. Jankovic J, Gilden JL, Hiner BC, et al. Neurogenic orthostatic hypotension: a double-blind, placebo-controlled study with midodrine. *Am J Med* 1993; 95: 38–48.
158. Low PA, Gilden JL, Freeman R, Sheng KN, McElligott MA. Efficacy of midodrine for neurogenic orthostatic hypotension. Reply. *JAMA* 1997; 278: 388.
159. Hakamaki T, Rajala T, Lehtonen A. Ambulatory 24-hour blood pressure recordings in patients with Parkinson's disease with or without fludrocortisone. *Int J Clin Pharmacol Ther* 1998; 36: 367–9.
160. Singer W, Sandroni P, Opfer-Gehrking TL, et al. Pyridostigmine treatment trial in neurogenic orthostatic hypotension. *Arch Neurol* 2006; 63: 513–18.
161. Senard JM, Brefel-Courbon C, Rascol O, Montastruc JL. Orthostatic hypotension in patients with Parkinson's disease: pathophysiology and management. *Drugs Aging* 2001; 18: 495–505.
162. Shiba M, Bower JH, Maraganore DM, et al. Anxiety disorders and depressive disorders preceding Parkinson's disease: a case-control study. *Mov Disord* 2000; 15: 669–77.
163. Aarsland D, Larsen JP, Lim NG, et al. Range of neuropsychiatric disturbances in patients with Parkinson's disease. *J Neurol Neurosurg Psychiatry* 1999; 67: 492–6.
164. McKinlay A, Grace RC, Dalrymple-Alford JC, Anderson T, Fink J, Roger D. A profile of neuropsychiatric problems and their relationship to quality of life for Parkinson's disease patients without dementia. *Parkinsonism Relat Disord* 2008; 14: 37–42.
165. Marsh L, McDonald WM, Cummings J, Ravina B. Provisional diagnostic criteria for depression in Parkinson's disease: report of an NINDS/NIMH Work Group. *Mov Disord* 2006; 21: 148–58.
166. Reijnders JS, Ehrt U, Weber WE, Aarsland D, Leentjens AF. A systematic review of prevalence studies of depression in Parkinson's disease. *Mov Disord* 2008; 23: 183–9, quiz 313.
167. Schrag A, Jahanshahi M, Quinn N. What contributes to quality of life in patients with Parkinson's disease? *J Neurol Neurosurg Psychiatry* 2000; 69: 308–12.
168. Weintraub D, Moberg PJ, Duda JE, Katz IR, Stern MB. Recognition and treatment of depression in Parkinson's disease. *J Geriatr Psychiatry Neurol* 2003; 16: 178–83.
169. Ravina B, Camicioli R, Como PG, et al. The impact of depressive symptoms in early Parkinson disease. *Neurology* 2007; 69: 342–7.
170. Braak H, Braak E. Pathoanatomy of Parkinson's disease. *J Neurol* 2000; 247 (Suppl 2): II3–10.
171. Remy P, Doder M, Lees A, Turjanski N, Brooks D. Depression in Parkinson's disease: loss of dopamine and noradrenaline innervation in the limbic system. *Brain* 2005; 128: 1314–22.
172. Serrano-Duenas M. [A comparison between low doses of amitriptyline and low doses of fluoxetin used in the control of depression in patients suffering from Parkinson's disease]. *Rev Neurol* 2002; 35: 1010–14.
173. Aiken CB. Pramipexole in psychiatry: a systematic review of the literature. *J Clin Psychiatry* 2007; 68: 1230–6.
174. Barone P, Poewe W, Albrecht S, et al. Pramipexole for the treatment of depressive symptoms in patients with Parkinson's disease: a randomised, double-blind, placebo-controlled trial. *Lancet Neurol* 2010; 9: 573–80.
175. Barone P. Treatment of depressive symptoms in Parkinson's disease. *Eur J Neurol* 2011; 18 (Suppl 1): 11–15.
176. Witjas T, Kaphan E, Azulay JP, et al. Nonmotor fluctuations in Parkinson's disease: frequent and disabling. *Neurology* 2002; 59: 408–13.
177. Rabinak CA, Nirenberg MJ. Dopamine agonist withdrawal syndrome in Parkinson disease. *Arch Neurol* 2010; 67: 58–63.
178. Bejjani BP, Damier P, Arnulf I, et al. Transient acute depression induced by high-frequency deep-brain stimulation. *N Engl J Med* 1999; 340: 1476–80.
179. Pontone GM, Williams JR, Anderson KE, et al. Prevalence of anxiety disorders and anxiety subtypes in patients with Parkinson's disease. *Mov Disord* 2009; 24: 1333–8.
180. Dissanayaka NN, Sellbach A, Matheson S, et al. Anxiety disorders in Parkinson's disease: prevalence and risk factors. *Mov Disord* 2010; 25: 838–45.
181. Mondolo F, Jahanshahi M, Grana A, Biasutti E, Cacciatori E, Di Benedetto P. Evaluation of anxiety in Parkinson's disease with some commonly used rating scales. *Neurol Sci* 2007; 28: 270–5.

182. Weintraub D, Burn DJ. Parkinson's disease: the quintessential neuropsychiatric disorder. *Mov Disord* 2011; 26: 1022–31.
183. Marin RS. Apathy: concept, syndrome, neural mechanisms, and treatment. *Semin Clin Neuropsychiatry* 1996; 1: 304–14.
184. Starkstein SE, Mayberg HS, Preziosi TJ, Andrezejewski P, Leiguarda R, Robinson RG. Reliability, validity, and clinical correlates of apathy in Parkinson's disease. *J Neuropsychiatry Clin Neurosci* 1992; 4: 134–9.
185. Starkstein SE, Merello M, Jorge R, Brockman S, Bruce D, Power B. The syndromal validity and nosological position of apathy in Parkinson's disease. *Mov Disord* 2009; 24: 1211–16.
186. Kirsch-Darrow L, Fernandez HH, Marsiske M, Okun MS, Bowers D. Dissociating apathy and depression in Parkinson disease. *Neurology* 2006; 67: 33–8.
187. Brown RG, Pluck G. Negative symptoms: the 'pathology' of motivation and goal-directed behaviour. *Trends Neurosci* 2000; 23: 412–17.
188. Campbell J. Treatment strategies in amotivated patients. *Psychiatr Ann* 1997; 27: 44–9.
189. Aarsland D, Marsh L, Schrag A. Neuropsychiatric symptoms in Parkinson's disease. *Mov Disord* 2009; 24: 2175–86.
190. Czernecki V, Schupbach M, Yaici S, et al. Apathy following subthalamic stimulation in Parkinson disease: a dopamine responsive symptom. *Mov Disord* 2008; 23: 964–9.
191. Ryan T. *Work and effort: the psychology of production*. New York: Ronald Press, 1947.
192. Fukuda K, Straus SE, Hickie I, Sharpe MC, Dobbins JG, Komaroff A. The chronic fatigue syndrome: a comprehensive approach to its definition and study. International Chronic Fatigue Syndrome Study Group. *Ann Intern Med* 1994; 121: 953–9.
193. Friedman J, Friedman H. Fatigue in Parkinson's disease. *Neurology* 1993; 43: 2016–18.
194. Friedman JH, Brown RG, Comella C, et al. Fatigue in Parkinson's disease: a review. *Mov Disord* 2007; 22: 297–308.
195. Shulman LM, Taback RL, Rabinstein AA, Weiner WJ. Non-recognition of depression and other non-motor symptoms in Parkinson's disease. *Parkinsonism Relat Disord* 2002; 8: 193–7.
196. Lou JS, Kearns G, Oken B, Sexton G, Nutt J. Exacerbated physical fatigue and mental fatigue in Parkinson's disease. *Mov Disord* 2001; 16: 190–6.
197. Schifitto G, Friedman JH, Oakes D. Fatigue in ELLDOPA. Paper presented at the World Congress on Parkinson's Disease, Washington, DC, 22–26 February 2006.
198. Hagell P, Brundin L. Towards an understanding of fatigue in Parkinson disease. *J Neurol Neurosurg Psychiatry* 2009; 80: 489–92.
199. Brown RG, Dittner A, Findley L, Wessely SC. The Parkinson fatigue scale. *Parkinsonism Relat Disord* 2005; 11: 49–55.
200. Chaudhuri A, Behan PO. Fatigue and basal ganglia. *J Neurol Sci* 2000; 179: 34–42.
201. Chaudhuri A, Behan PO. Fatigue in neurological disorders. *Lancet* 2004; 363: 978–88.
202. Kluger BMF. Fatigue in Parkinson's disease. In: Chaudhuri KR, Tolosa E, Schapira A, Poewe W. (eds) *Non-motor symptoms of Parkinson's disease*. New York: Oxford University Press, 2009.
203. Fenelon G, Mahieux F, Huon R, Ziegler M. Hallucinations in Parkinson's disease: prevalence, phenomenology and risk factors. *Brain* 2000; 123: 733–45.
204. Sanchez-Ramos JR, Ortoll R, Paulson GW. Visual hallucinations associated with Parkinson disease. *Arch Neurol* 1996; 53: 1265–8.
205. Fenelon G. Psychosis in Parkinson's disease: phenomenology, frequency, risk factors, and current understanding of pathophysiologic mechanisms. *CNS Spectr* 2008;13: 18–25.
206. Graham JM, Grunewald RA, Sagar HJ. Hallucinosis in idiopathic Parkinson's disease. *J Neurol Neurosurg Psychiatry* 1997; 63: 434–40.
207. Factor SA, Feustel PJ, Friedman JH, et al. Longitudinal outcome of Parkinson's disease patients with psychosis. *Neurology* 2003; 60: 1756–61.
208. Aarsland D, Larsen JP, Tandberg E, Laake K. Predictors of nursing home placement in Parkinson's disease: a population-based, prospective study. *J Am Geriatr Soc* 2000; 48: 938–42.
209. Diederich NJ, Goetz CG, Stebbins GT. Repeated visual hallucinations in Parkinson's disease as disturbed external/internal perceptions: focused review and a new integrative model. *Mov Disord* 2005; 20: 130–40.
210. Matsui H, Udaka F, Tamura A, et al. Impaired visual acuity as a risk factor for visual hallucinations in Parkinson's disease. *J Geriatr Psychiatry Neurol* 2006; 19: 36–40.
211. Comella CL, Tanner CM, Ristanovic RK. Polysomnographic sleep measures in Parkinson's disease patients with treatment-induced hallucinations. *Ann Neurol* 1993; 34: 710–14.
212. Goetz CG, Tanner CM, Klawans HL. Pharmacology of hallucinations induced by long-term drug therapy. *Am J Psychiatry* 1982; 139: 494–7.
213. Onofrj M, Thomas A, Bonanni L. New approaches to understanding hallucinations in Parkinson's disease: phenomenology and possible origins. *Expert Rev Neurother* 2007; 7: 1731–50.
214. Aarsland D, Larsen JP, Cummins JL, Laake K. Prevalence and clinical correlates of psychotic symptoms in Parkinson disease: a community-based study. *Arch Neurol* 1999; 56: 595–601.
215. Schrag A. Psychiatric aspects of Parkinson's disease—an update. *J Neurol* 2004; 251: 795–804.
216. Wint DP, Okun MS, Fernandez HH. Psychosis in Parkinson's disease. *J Geriatr Psychiatry Neurol* 2004; 17: 127–36.
217. Diederich NJ, Pieri V, Goetz CG. Coping strategies for visual hallucinations in Parkinson's disease. *Mov Disord* 2003; 18: 831–2.
218. Ondo WG, Tintner R, Voung KD, Lai D, Ringholz G. Double-blind, placebo-controlled, unforced titration parallel trial of quetiapine for dopaminergic-induced hallucinations in Parkinson's disease. *Mov Disord* 2005; 20: 958–63.
219. Rabey JM, Prokhorov T, Miniovitz A, Dobronevsky E, Klein C. Effect of quetiapine in psychotic Parkinson's disease patients: a double-blind labeled study of 3 months' duration. *Mov Disord* 2007; 22: 313–18.
220. Shotbolt P, Samuel M, Fox C, David AS. A randomized controlled trial of quetiapine for psychosis in Parkinson's disease. *Neuropsychiatr Dis Treat* 2009; 5: 327–32.
221. Fernandez HH, Okun MS, Rodriguez RL, et al. Quetiapine improves visual hallucinations in Parkinson disease but not through normalization of sleep architecture: results from a double-blind clinical-polysomnography study. *Int J Neurosci* 2009; 119: 2196–205.
222. Kurlan R, Cummings J, Raman R, Thal L. Quetiapine for agitation or psychosis in patients with dementia and parkinsonism. *Neurology* 2007; 68: 1356–63.
223. Miyasaki JM, Shannon K, Voon V, et al. Practice Parameter: evaluation and treatment of depression, psychosis, and dementia in Parkinson disease (an evidence-based review): report of the Quality Standards Subcommittee of the American Academy of Neurology. *Neurology* 2006; 66: 996–1002.
224. Low-dose clozapine for the treatment of drug-induced psychosis in Parkinson's disease. The Parkinson Study Group. *N Engl J Med* 1999; 340: 757–63.
225. Clozapine in drug-induced psychosis in Parkinson's disease. The French Clozapine Parkinson Study Group. *Lancet* 1999; 353: 2041–2.
226. Factor SA, Molho ES, Friedman JH. Risperidone and Parkinson's disease. *Mov Disord* 2002; 17: 221–2.
227. Ondo WG, Levy JK, Vuong KD, Hunter C, Jankovic J. Olanzapine treatment for dopaminergic-induced hallucinations. *Mov Disord* 2002; 17: 1031–5.
228. Kurita A, Ochiai Y, Kono Y, Suzuki M, Inoue K. The beneficial effect of donepezil on visual hallucinations in three patients with Parkinson's disease. *J Geriatr Psychiatry Neurol* 2003; 16: 184–8.
229. Sobow T. Parkinson's disease-related visual hallucinations unresponsive to atypical antipsychotics treated with cholinesterase inhibitors: a case series. *Neurol Neurochir Pol* 2007; 41: 276–9.

230. American Psychiatric Association. *Diagnostic and statistical manual of mental disorders IV.* Washington, DC: American Psychiatric Association, 1994.
231. Weintraub D, Koester J, Potenza MN, et al. Impulse control disorders in Parkinson disease: a cross-sectional study of 3090 patients. *Arch Neurol* 2010; 67: 589–95.
232. Weintraub D, Siderowf AD, Potenza MN, et al. Association of dopamine agonist use with impulse control disorders in Parkinson disease. *Arch Neurol* 2006; 63: 969–73.
233. Voon V, Fox SH. Medication-related impulse control and repetitive behaviors in Parkinson disease. *Arch Neurol* 2007; 64: 1089–96.
234. Giovannoni G, O'Sullivan JD, Turner K, Manson AJ, Lees AJ. Hedonistic homeostatic dysregulation in patients with Parkinson's disease on dopamine replacement therapies. *J Neurol Neurosurg Psychiatry* 2000; 68: 423–8.
235. Evans AH, Lawrence AD, Potts J, Appel S, Lees AJ. Factors influencing susceptibility to compulsive dopaminergic drug use in Parkinson disease. *Neurology* 2005; 65: 1570–4.
236. Evans AH, Lees AJ. Dopamine dysregulation syndrome in Parkinson's disease. *Curr Opin Neurol* 2004; 17: 393–8.
237. Evans AH, Lawrence AD, Cresswell SA, Katzenschlager R, Lees AJ. Compulsive use of dopaminergic drug therapy in Parkinson's disease: reward and anti-reward. *Mov Disord* 2010; 25: 867–76.
238. Evans AH, Pavese N, Lawrence AD, et al. Compulsive drug use linked to sensitized ventral striatal dopamine transmission. *Ann Neurol* 2006; 59: 852–8.
239. Evans AH, Katzenschlager R, Paviour D, et al. Punding in Parkinson's disease: its relation to the dopamine dysregulation syndrome. *Mov Disord* 2004; 19: 397–405.
240. Park A, Stacy M. Dopamine-induced nonmotor symptoms of Parkinson's disease. *Parkinsons Dis* 2011; 2011: 485063.
241. Ferrara JM, Stacy M. Impulse-control disorders in Parkinson's disease. *CNS Spectr* 2008; 13: 690–8.
242. Rylander G. Psychoses and the punding and choreiform syndromes in addiction to central stimulant drugs. *Psychiatr Neurol Neurochir* 1972; 75: 203–12.
243. Fasano A, Barra A, Nicosia P, et al. Cocaine addiction: from habits to stereotypical-repetitive behaviors and punding. *Drug Alcohol Depend* 2008; 96: 178–82.
244. Miyasaki JM, Al Hassan K, Lang AE, Voon V. Punding prevalence in Parkinson's disease. *Mov Disord* 2007; 22: 1179–81.
245. Spencer AH, Rickards H, Fasano A, Cavanna AE. The prevalence and clinical characteristics of punding in Parkinson's disease. *Mov Disord* 2011; 26: 578–86.
246. Cornelius JR, Tippmann-Peikert M, Slocumb NL, Frerichs CF, Silber MH. Impulse control disorders with the use of dopaminergic agents in restless legs syndrome: a case–control study. *Sleep* 2010; 33: 81–7.
247. Black KJ, Friedman JH. Repetitive and impulsive behaviors in treated Parkinson disease. *Neurology* 2006; 67: 1118–19.
248. Miwa H. Stereotyped behaviours or punding in Parkinson's disease. *J Neurol* 2007; 254: 61–7.
249. Mamikonyan E, Siderowf AD, Duda JE, et al. Long-term follow-up of impulse control disorders in Parkinson's disease. *Mov Disord* 2008; 23: 75–80.
250. Weintraub D, Sohr M, Potenza MN, et al. Amantadine use associated with impulse control disorders in Parkinson disease in cross-sectional study. *Ann Neurol* 2010; 68: 963–8.
251. Ardouin C, Voon V, Worbe Y, et al. Pathological gambling in Parkinson's disease improves on chronic subthalamic nucleus stimulation. *Mov Disord* 2006; 21: 1941–6.
252. Bandini F, Primavera A, Pizzorno M, Cocito L. Using STN DBS and medication reduction as a strategy to treat pathological gambling in Parkinson's disease. *Parkinsonism Relat Disord* 2007; 13: 369–71.
253. Lim SY, O'Sullivan SS, Kotschet K, et al. Dopamine dysregulation syndrome, impulse control disorders and punding after deep brain stimulation surgery for Parkinson's disease. *J Clin Neurosci* 2009; 16: 1148–52.
254. Bonvin C, Horvath J, Christe B, Landis T, Burkhard PR. Compulsive singing: another aspect of punding in Parkinson's disease. *Ann Neurol* 2007; 62: 525–8.
255. Voon V, Kubu C, Krack P, Houeto JL, Troster AI. Deep brain stimulation: neuropsychological and neuropsychiatric issues. *Mov Disord* 2006; 21 (Suppl 14): S305–27.
256. Le Jeune F, Drapier D, Bourguignon A, et al. Subthalamic nucleus stimulation in Parkinson disease induces apathy: a PET study. *Neurology* 2009; 73: 1746–51.
257. Drapier D, Drapier S, Sauleau P, et al. Does subthalamic nucleus stimulation induce apathy in Parkinson's disease? *J Neurol* 2006; 253: 1083–91.
258. Porat O, Cohen OS, Schwartz R, Hassin-Baer S. Association of preoperative symptom profile with psychiatric symptoms following subthalamic nucleus stimulation in patients with Parkinson's disease. *J Neuropsychiatry Clin Neurosci* 2009; 21: 398–405.
259. Denheyer M, Kiss ZH, Haffenden AM. Behavioral effects of subthalamic deep brain stimulation in Parkinson's disease. *Neuropsychologia* 2009; 47: 3203–9.
260. Kalechstein AD, Newton TF, Leavengood AH. Apathy syndrome in cocaine dependence. *Psychiatry Res* 2002; 109: 97–100.
261. Funkiewiez A, Ardouin C, Krack P, et al. Acute psychotropic effects of bilateral subthalamic nucleus stimulation and levodopa in Parkinson's disease. *Mov Disord* 2003; 18: 524–30.
262. Krack P, Batir A, Van Blercom N, et al. Five-year follow-up of bilateral stimulation of the subthalamic nucleus in advanced Parkinson's disease. *N Engl J Med* 2003; 349: 1925–34.
263. Herzog J, Volkmann J, Krack P, et al. Two-year follow-up of subthalamic deep brain stimulation in Parkinson's disease. *Mov Disord* 2003; 18: 1332–7.
264. Romito LM, Raja M, Daniele A, et al. Transient mania with hypersexuality after surgery for high frequency stimulation of the subthalamic nucleus in Parkinson's disease. *Mov Disord* 2002; 17: 1371–4.
265. Krack P, Fraix V, Mendes A, Benabid AL, Pollak P. Postoperative management of subthalamic nucleus stimulation for Parkinson's disease. *Mov Disord* 2002; 17 (Suppl 3): S188–97.
266. Krack P, Kumar R, Ardouin C, et al. Mirthful laughter induced by subthalamic nucleus stimulation. *Mov Disord* 2001; 16: 867–75.
267. Herzog J, Reiff J, Krack P, et al. Manic episode with psychotic symptoms induced by subthalamic nucleus stimulation in a patient with Parkinson's disease. *Mov Disord* 2003; 18: 1382–4.
268. Voon V, Krack P, Lang AE, et al. A multicentre study on suicide outcomes following subthalamic stimulation for Parkinson's disease. *Brain* 2008; 131: 2720–8.
269. Follett KA, Weaver FM, Stern M, et al. Pallidal versus subthalamic deep-brain stimulation for Parkinson's disease. *N Engl J Med* 2010; 362: 2077–91.
270. Lang AE, Houeto JL, Krack P, Kubu C, Lyons KE, Moro E, et al. Deep brain stimulation: preoperative issues. *Mov Disord* 2006; 21 (Suppl 14): S171–96.
271. Foltynie T, Brayne CE, Robbins TW, Barker RA. The cognitive ability of an incident cohort of Parkinson's patients in the UK. The CamPaIGN study. *Brain* 2004; 127: 550–60.
272. Aarsland D, Bronnick K, Larsen JP, Tysnes OB, Alves G. Cognitive impairment in incident, untreated Parkinson disease: the Norwegian ParkWest study. *Neurology* 2009; 72: 1121–6.
273. Janvin CC, Aarsland D, Larsen JP. Cognitive predictors of dementia in Parkinson's disease: a community-based, 4-year longitudinal study. *J Geriatr Psychiatry Neurol* 2005; 18: 149–54.
274. Aarsland D, Perry R, Brown A, Larsen JP, Ballard C. Neuropathology of dementia in Parkinson's disease: a prospective, community-based study. *Ann Neurol* 2005; 58: 773–6.

275. Aarsland D, Andersen K, Larsen JP, Lolk A, Kragh-Sorensen P. Prevalence and characteristics of dementia in Parkinson disease: an 8-year prospective study. *Arch Neurol* 2003; 60: 387–92.
276. Levy G, Schupf N, Tang MX, et al. Combined effect of age and severity on the risk of dementia in Parkinson's disease. *Ann Neurol* 2002; 51: 722–9.
277. Aarsland D, Kvaloy JT, Andersen K, et al. The effect of age of onset of PD on risk of dementia. *J Neurol* 2007; 254: 38–45.
278. Camicioli R, Rajput A, Rajput M, Reece C, Payami H, Hao C. Apolipoprotein E epsilon4 and catechol-O-methyltransferase alleles in autopsy-proven Parkinson's disease: relationship to dementia and hallucinations. *Mov Disord* 2005; 20: 989–94.
279. Noe E, Marder K, Bell KL, Jacobs DM, Manly JJ, Stern Y. Comparison of dementia with Lewy bodies to Alzheimer's disease and Parkinson's disease with dementia. *Mov Disord* 2004; 19: 60–7.
280. Ballard CG, Aarsland D, McKeith I, et al. Fluctuations in attention: PD dementia vs DLB with parkinsonism. *Neurology* 2002; 59: 1714–20.
281. Higginson CI, Wheelock VL, Carroll KE, Sigvardt KA. Recognition memory in Parkinson's disease with and without dementia: evidence inconsistent with the retrieval deficit hypothesis. *J Clin Exp Neuropsychol* 2005; 27: 516–28.
282. Starkstein SE, Sabe L, Petracca G, et al. Neuropsychological and psychiatric differences between Alzheimer's disease and Parkinson's disease with dementia. *J Neurol Neurosurg Psychiatry* 1996; 61: 381–7.
283. Mosimann UP, Mather G, Wesnes KA, O'Brien JT, Burn DJ, McKeith IG. Visual perception in Parkinson disease dementia and dementia with Lewy bodies. *Neurology* 2004; 63: 2091–6.
284. Aarsland D, Ballard C, Larsen JP, McKeith I. A comparative study of psychiatric symptoms in dementia with Lewy bodies and Parkinson's disease with and without dementia. *Int J Geriatr Psychiatry* 2001; 16: 528–36.
285. Pluck GC, Brown RG. Apathy in Parkinson's disease. *J Neurol Neurosurg Psychiatry* 2002; 73: 636–42.
286. Aarsland D, Bronnick K, Alves G, et al. The spectrum of neuropsychiatric symptoms in patients with early untreated Parkinson's disease. *J Neurol Neurosurg Psychiatry* 2009; 80: 928–30.
287. Junque C, Ramirez-Ruiz B, Tolosa E, et al. Amygdalar and hippocampal MRI volumetric reductions in Parkinson's disease with dementia. *Mov Disord* 2005; 20: 540–4.
288. Mollenhauer B, Trenkwalder C, von Ahsen N, et al. Beta-amyloid 1–42 and tau-protein in cerebrospinal fluid of patients with Parkinson's disease dementia. *Dement Geriatr Cogn Disord* 2006; 22: 200–8.
289. Apaydin H, Ahlskog JE, Parisi JE, Boeve BF, Dickson DW. Parkinson disease neuropathology: later-developing dementia and loss of the levodopa response. *Arch Neurol* 2002; 59: 102–12.
290. Aarsland D, Perry R, Brown A, Larsen JP, Ballard C. Neuropathology of dementia in Parkinson's disease: a prospective, community-based study. Annals of neurology. *Ann Neurol* 2005; 58(5):773–6.
291. Braak H, Rub U, Jansen Steur EN, Del Tredici K, de Vos RA. Cognitive status correlates with neuropathologic stage in Parkinson disease. *Neurology* 2005; 64: 1404–10.
292. Colosimo C, Hughes AJ, Kilford L, Lees AJ. Lewy body cortical involvement may not always predict dementia in Parkinson's disease. *J Neurol Neurosurg Psychiatry* 2003; 74: 852–6.
293. Bohnen NI, Kaufer DI, Ivanco LS, et al. Cortical cholinergic function is more severely affected in parkinsonian dementia than in Alzheimer disease: an in vivo positron emission tomographic study. *Arch Neurol* 2003; 60: 1745–8.
294. Levy G. The relationship of Parkinson disease with aging. *Arch Neurol* 2007; 64: 1242–6.
295. Cummings JL, Mega M, Gray K, Rosenberg-Thompson S, Carusi DA, Gornbein J. The Neuropsychiatric Inventory: comprehensive assessment of psychopathology in dementia. *Neurology* 1994; 44: 2308–14.
296. Emre M, Aarsland D, Brown R, et al. Clinical diagnostic criteria for dementia associated with Parkinson's disease. *Mov Disord* 2007; 22: 1689–1707, quiz 837.
297. McKeith I, Emre M. Management of Parkinson's disease dementia and dementia with Lewy bodies. In: Emre M (ed.) *Cognitive impairment and dementia in Parkinson's disease*, pp. 245–56. New York: Oxford University Press, 2010.
298. Aarsland D, Laake K, Larsen JP, Janvin C. Donepezil for cognitive impairment in Parkinson's disease: a randomised controlled study. *J Neurol Neurosurg Psychiatry* 2002; 72: 708–12.
299. Leroi I, Brandt J, Reich SG, et al. Randomized placebo-controlled trial of donepezil in cognitive impairment in Parkinson's disease. *Int J Geriatr Psychiatry* 2004; 19: 1–8.
300. Emre M, Aarsland D, Albanese A, et al. Rivastigmine for dementia associated with Parkinson's disease. *N Engl J Med* 2004; 351: 2509–18.
301. Poewe W, Gauthier S, Aarsland D, et al. Diagnosis and management of Parkinson's disease dementia. *Int J Clin Pract* 2008; 62: 1581–7.
302. Thomas AJ, Burn DJ, Rowan EN, et al. A comparison of the efficacy of donepezil in Parkinson's disease with dementia and dementia with Lewy bodies. *Int J Geriatr Psychiatry* 2005; 20: 938–44.
303. Leroi I, Overshott R, Byrne EJ, Daniel E, Burns A. Randomized controlled trial of memantine in dementia associated with Parkinson's disease. *Mov Disord* 2009; 24: 1217–21.
304. Aarsland D, Ballard C, Walker Z, et al. Memantine in patients with Parkinson's disease dementia or dementia with Lewy bodies: a double-blind, placebo-controlled, multicentre trial. *Lancet Neurol* 2009; 8: 613–18.
305. Emre M, Tsolaki M, Bonuccelli U, et al. Memantine for patients with Parkinson's disease dementia or dementia with Lewy bodies: a randomised, double-blind, placebo-controlled trial. *Lancet Neurol* 2010; 9: 969–77.
306. Oertel W, Berardelli A, Bloem B. Late (complicated) Parkinson's disease. In: Gilhus M, Barnes MP, Brainin M (eds) *European Handbook of Neurological Management* (2nd edn), pp. 237–67. Chichester: Wiley-Blackwell, 2011.

CHAPTER 12

The Many Faces of Parkinsonism: A Review of the Parkinson Look-alike Syndromes

Susanne A. Schneider and Christine Klein

Introduction

Parkinson's disease (PD) has many faces. Indeed, the phenotypic variability is even greater for syndromes of parkinsonism presenting with atypical or other neurological features. Because of the long list of differential diagnoses, physicians may face a challenge when confronted with a parkinsonian patient. In addition to idiopathic PD and secondary forms, numerous genetic causes of parkinsonism, sometimes mimicking idiopathic PD, have been identified in recent years. These include mutations in genes which have been grouped together under the umbrella of 'PARK disorders' such as *alpha-Synuclein* (PARK1/PARK4), *Parkin* (PARK2), *PINK1* (PARK6), *DJ-1* (PARK7), *LRRK2* (PARK8), *ATP13A2* (PARK9), and *PLA2G6* (PARK14) as well as numerous other non-PARK genes. While the well-established monogenic forms with PARK acronyms have been reviewed extensively (1–4), these other inherited conditions of parkinsonism have received less attention. We wish to draw attention to these latter conditions in this chapter.

We chose to group the various causes of heritable parkinsonian syndromes according to presence of classic or atypical parkinsonism. We use the term 'classic parkinsonism' for cases with the typical clinical characteristics of rest tremor, bradykinesia, and rigidity (not all features are mandatory), an excellent and sustained therapeutic levodopa response, and the frequent development of motor complications after several years of levodopa therapy (5). 'Parkinsonism' refers to patients who display some parkinsonian signs but also exhibit atypical or other neurological features. Based on these findings, conditions have been classified into three subgroups in order to account for the high degree of clinical and genetic heterogeneity (Table 12.1).

Financial disclosure: CK is supported by a Lichtenberg grant from the Volkswagen Foundation and a Career Development Award from the Hermann and Lilly Schilling Foundation.

A. Disorders which have been assigned a PARK locus that present with either classic parkinsonism or parkinsonism with additional atypical features.

B. Classic parkinsonism due to mutations in a non-PARK or 'other-than-PARK' gene (e.g. a *DYT* or *SCA* gene) where parkinsonism is a well-recognized concomitant or even an isolated feature.

C. Atypical parkinsonism in genetic disorders which are usually characterized by features other than parkinsonism.

We will summarize the clinical characteristics and main genetic findings. Pathological data or results of investigations (such as imaging or electrophysiology) will be mentioned if they are useful for differentiation from other diseases (see also Table 12.2).

PARK-associated disorders with signs of parkinsonism with or without atypical features

Mutations in PARK genes have unequivocally been linked with parkinsonism. *LRRK2*-associated parkinsonism (PARK8) clinically resembles idiopathic PD most closely (6). *LRRK2* mutations are inherited in an autosomal dominant fashion. The majority of patients carry the same specific genetic alteration (the G2019S mutation). Notably, patients with homozygous mutations do not show overt clinical differences compared to those with homozygous mutations. Thus, there do not seem to be major gene dosage effects (7). In addition to familial cases, *LRRK2* has recently been confirmed as a risk locus for PD in a genome-wide association study in a mixed patient cohort from the USA and Europe (8). Thus, *LRRK2* mutations should be considered in patients with a positive family history suggestive of dominant

Table 12.1 Overview of inherited forms of parkinsonism, grouped into three categories to account for the high degree of clinical and genetic heterogeneity

Subgroup	Gene/protein/locus	Comment, clinical correlate
'PARK syndromes' with atypical features	*Parkin*/PARK2	Early-onset parkinsonism with slower disease course
	PINK1/PARK6	
	DJ-1/PARK7	
	SNCA/PARK1+4	Early-onset parkinsonism with rapid progression and dementia
	ATP13A2/PARK9	Juvenile parkinsonism with rapid progression, pyramidal signs, supranuclear gaze palsy, and dementia; iron accumulation in some
	PLA2G6/PARK14/NBIA type 2	Early-onset pyramidal extrapyramidal syndrome Early-onset form: infantile neuroaxonal dystrophy (INAD) MRI with or without iron deposition
(Classic) parkinsonism due to mutations in non-PARK or 'other than-PARK' genes (e.g. *DYT* or *SCA* gene) where parkinsonism is a well-recognized concomitant or even an isolated feature	*TAF1*/DYT3	X-linked dystonia parkinsonism; Lubag
	GTP cyclohydrolase I and *tyrosine-hydroxylase*/DYT5	Dopa-responsive dystonia, Segawa's disease
	ATP1A3/DYT12	Rapid-onset dystonia-parkinsonism
	PRKRA/DYT16	Dystonia (parkinsonism)
	SCA types 2, 3, 6, 8, 17	Ataxia, parkinsonism may be present
	Glucocerebrosidase	Gaucher disease
	Mitochondrial gene mutations	Often complex syndromes
Atypical parkinsonism in genetic disorders which are usually characterized by features other than parkinsonism	*FMR1*	Fragile X-associated tremor–ataxia syndrome
	MAPT	Frontotemporal dementia parkinsonism linked to chromosome 17
	Progranulin	
	Prion protein	Creutzfeldt–Jakob disease
	ATP7B	Wilson disease
	PANK2/NBIA type 1	Panthothenate-kinase-2-associated neurodegeneration
	FBXO7	Extrapyramidal–pyramidal syndrome
	CHAC	Chorea–acanthocytosis
	FTL1	Neuroferritinopathy
	Huntingtin	Huntington's disease, Westphal variant
	JPH3	Huntington's disease-like 2, Westphal variant
	HFE	Haemochromatosis

CHAC, chorea–acanthocytosis; FBXO7, F-box protein 7; FTL1, ferritin light chain; *FMR1*, fragile-X mental retardation 1; *JPH3*, junctophilin-3; *MAPT*, microtubule-associated protein tau; *PANK2*, pantothenate kinase 2; *PINK1*, PTEN induced putative kinase 1; *PRKRA*, protein kinase interferon-inducible double-stranded RNA-dependent activator; SCA, spinocerebellar ataxia; SNCA, α-synuclein; *TAF1*, TATA-box binding protein–associated factor 1

or recessive inheritance as well as in sporadic cases (for further review of PARK8, see ref. 9) and in particular in North Africans and Ashkenazi Jews.

In young-onset cases mutations in the genes encoding *Parkin*/PARK2, *PINK1*/PARK6 and *DJ-1*/PARK7 should be considered as they can also resemble classic PD. They are characterized by a good response to levodopa and have a rather benign disease course (10, 11). Dystonia, mild hyperreflexia, and psychiatric features may be present in some patients and can be a diagnostic clue (12–14). Most data are available for the *Parkin* variant which is by far the most common cause of early-onset parkinsonism, accounting for nearly 80% of patients with onset before age 30 (10). Less is known about the *PINK1* or *DJ-1* type. These recessive parkinsonian disorders are being studied with great interest as a number of patients carrying only one mutated allele (rather than the expected two) have been identified who may provide important insights into the pathophysiology of idiopathic PD (15). However, owing to space limitations, these disorders and their role will not be discussed further in this chapter.

The recessive forms of PARK9- and PARK14-associated parkinsonism are examples of more complex phenotypes. Homozygous mutations in the *ATP13A2*/PARK9 gene were found to cause Kufor–Rakeb disease (16), a syndrome of juvenile atypical parkinsonism with rapid progression which is responsive to levodopa treatment in initial stages, but with early development of dyskinesias and additional neurological features including pyramidal signs and dementia (17). The most striking clinical features on examination are a bradykinetic–rigid syndrome, axial rigidity, spasticity, pyramidal weakness and Babinski signs, a supranuclear vertical gaze palsy, slow vertical and horizontal saccades, and facial, faucial, and finger mini-myoclonus (17–19).

Numerous cytoplasmic inclusion bodies within the Schwann, perineurial, and epineurials, but not in axons, were present in a sural nerve biopsy (20). On electron microscopy assessment, the

Table 12.2 Additional investigations which may be useful in the process of the diagnostic work-up

Test	Result	Disorder
Laboratory tests		
Peripheral blood smear	Acanthocytes	ChAc, MLS, also reported rarely in HDL2 and PKAN
Serum biochemistry	Elevated CK	MLS, ChAc
	Elevated LFTs	ChAc, MLS, Wilson disease
Erythrocyte antigen markers	Absent Kx, reduced Kell antigen expression	MLS
CSF	N14-3-3, tau, NSE, S100b, PrP^{Sc}	CJD (PRNP)
Urinary tests	Elevated urinary copper	Wilson disease
Neurophysiology		
Neuromuscular testing	Sensory and motor neuropathy	ChAc, MLS
NCS	Peripheral neuropathy	ChAc, MLS; PLA2G6-associated neurodegeneration, Niemann–Pick
EEG and polysomnography	Temporal abnormalities and seizure onset	ChAc
	Sleep fragmentation and poor sleep efficiency	ChAc, MLS
	Periodic bi- and triphasic sharp wave complexes	CJD (PRNP)
Ophthalmological assessment	Pigmentary retinal degeneration	PKAN
	Optic nerve atrophy	INAD (PLA2G6)
Neuroimaging		
MRI	Marked atrophy of the caudate nucleus and putamen, to a lesser extent of the cortex	HD, HDL2, ChAc, MLS
	Calcification	Fahr's disease
	Iron deposition in the globus pallidus	PKAN ('eye of the tiger' sign), PLA2G6 (PARK14), Kufor–Rakeb disease (PAR9), aceruloplasminaemia, neuroferritinopathy
	Generalized atrophy	PLA2G6-associated neurodegeneration, Kufor–Rakeb disease
	Symmetric hyperintensities in putamen and caudate	CJD (PRNP)
	T_2-signal intensity of the middle cerebellar peduncles	FXTAS
PET	Markedly reduced metabolic activity in the striatum on fluorodeoxyglucose PET	HD, ChAc, MLS
Pathology, histology		
Neuropathology	Atrophy of the caudate, putamen, to a lesser extent globus pallidus, neuronal cell loss and astrocytic gliosis in the striatum	HD, HDL2, ChAc, MLS
	Ubiquitin-immunoreactive neuronal intranuclear inclusions	HDL2
	Mosaic astrocytosis in the striatum	DYT3 (Lubag)
	Eosinophilic intranuclear, neuronal, and astrocytic inclusions; Purkinje cell loss	FXTAS
	Tau-positive inclusions	MAPT
	TDP43-positive inclusions	PGRN, DCTN1
Muscle/nerve biopsy	Spheroid bodies	*PLA2G6*-associated neurodegeneration
	Irregular primary lysosomes	Kufor–Rakeb disease
	Granular inclusion bodies	Neuroferritinopathy

ChAc, chorea–acanthocytosis; CK, creatine kinase; CJD, Creutzfeldt–Jakob disease; CSF, cerebrospinal fluid; DCTN1, dynactin1; EEG, electroencephalography; FXTAS, fragile X-associated tremor–ataxia syndrome; HD, Huntington's disease; HDL2, Huntington's disease looks like disease type 2; INAD, infantile neuroaxonal dystrophy; MAPT, microtubule-associated protein tau, MLS, McLeod neuroacanthocytosis syndrome; MRI, magnetic resonance imaging; NSE, neuron-specific enolase; PET, positron emission tomography; PKAN, pantothenate-kinase-associated neurodegeneration; PRNP, prion protein; PrPSc, scrapie prion protein; TDP43, TAR DNA-binding protein 43.

Based on data from Klein et al. (169).

inclusions were found to be membrane-bound, irregular, and occasionally folded. Overall, there was resemblance to irregular primary lysosomes, in line with the function of the encoded protein. ATP13A2 encodes a predominantly neuronal lysosomal type 5 P-type ATPase. Some patients may have cerebral iron accumulation as demonstrated by T_2*-weighted MRI (21, 22). Thus the condition falls into the group of syndromes with neurodegeneration with brain iron accumulation (see below). Heterozygous mutations in the *ATP13A2* gene have been associated with a more benign phenotype, resembling young-onset PD, akin to the Parkin type

(23, 24). Interestingly, mutations in the *ATP13A2* gene were recently also identified in animal models of neuronal ceroid lipofuscinosis (NCL), but screening humans with the compatible phenotype of Kuf's disease did not reveal mutations (25).

Similarly, homozygous mutations in *PLA2G6*/PARK14 are a cause of complex parkinsonism, dystonia with additional pyramidal involvement, and other complicating features, with both adolescent and adult onset (26). In children, *PLA2G6* mutations cause infantile neuroaxonal dystrophy (INAD) and are another important cause of brain iron accumulation (27). In the adult-onset cases described recently, parkinsonism was characterized by the presence of tremor, including a pill-rolling rest component, rigidity, and severe bradykinesia, with a good response to levodopa. However, there was early development of dyskinesias. Cerebellar signs and sensory abnormalities, which are often prominent in the early childhood variant of INAD, were absent. DAT SPECT imaging was abnormal and both Lewy body and tau pathology were observed in molecularly confirmed cases (20).

Other forms of PARK-associated parkinsonism include the autosomal dominantly inherited *alpha-synuclein*-associated variant (*SNCA/PARK1*). In addition to mutations, duplications and triplications have been identified. It has been suggested that duplications lead to late-onset autonomic dysfunction and parkinsonism, whereas triplications and point mutations are associated with early-onset PD and dementia (28). The latter form tends to produce more severe parkinsonism with a rapid course and a reduced life span (29). The *alpha-synuclein* gene codes for a protein that is abundantly expressed in neurons, where it is believed to participate in the maturation of presynaptic vesicles and to function as a negative co-regulator of neurotransmitter release (30).

Classic parkinsonism due to mutations in 'other-than-PARK' genes or other genes

Numerous 'other-than-PARK' disorders may also present with classic parkinsonism as a concomitant or even isolated feature, clinically mimicking idiopathic PD. Of these, some associated genes are not assigned to any list while others may have been added to 'other-than-PARK' lists, for example the DYT or SCA compilations (reflecting that their usual presentation is not with parkinsonism).

Dystonia syndromes: dystonia–parkinsonism, and parkinsonism in dystonia-plus syndromes

Dystonias are hyperkinetic movement disorders characterized by involuntary twisting and repetitive movements and abnormal postures (31). Monogenic dystonias have been grouped together in the DYT classification which currently holds 21 forms assigned to 21 DYT loci. Three of these present with combined features of dystonia and parkinsonism ('dystonia–parkinsonism'), i.e. DYT3 (X-linked dystonia–parkinsonism, Lubag), DYT5 (dopa-responsive dystonia, Segawa's disease), and DYT12 (rapid-onset dystonia–parkinsonism). Although in DYT16 parkinsonism has been reported in carriers of *PRKRA* mutations (32), this appeared to be isolated bradykinesia which was not levodopa-responsive and occurred in the context of severe dystonia. Therefore it remains to be seen whether true parkinsonism is indeed a clinical feature of DYT16.

X-linked recessive dystonia–parkinsonism (DYT3, XDP, Lubag) in the Philippines

DYT3 dystonia is an X-linked recessive form of dystonia found in the Philippines. There is complete penetrance by the end of the fifth decade. While XDP typically affects males, rarely women may also be affected, possibly due to severe X-inactivation or based on homozygosity for the mutation. While DYT3 has been associated with specific sequence changes in the *TAF1* gene (33), analysis of peripheral blood lymphocytes may fail to reveal mutations or alterations in gene expression, and therefore these may not be suitable surrogate disease markers for DYT3. It has been proposed that ancestral DYT3 haplotype and disease-specific SVA (short interspersed nuclear elements, variable number of tandem repeats, and Alu composite) retrotransposon insertion may be useful for genetic counselling (34).

The average age of onset in women (52 years) is higher than in men and may be as late as 75 years (35). Dystonic symptoms in DYT3 usually start focally in adulthood (36), and subsequently progress and generalize. Parkinsonism is a frequent concurrent feature (37). In a study of 42 DYT3 patients, 36% of the cases showed at least one of the cardinal signs of PD (36). Parkinsonism may even precede the onset of dystonia, be the predominant phenotype (38), and remain an isolated feature (39). It has been suggested that predominant or isolated parkinsonism may constitute a more benign phenotype of XDP (38, 39). Parkinsonism may improve with levodopa in the early stages, but becomes less responsive or unresponsive over time. Compared with males, parkinsonism is relatively common among women with XDP.

Investigations in XPD patients show hyperechogenicity of the substantia nigra on transcranial ultrasound, moderately decreased putaminal dopamine transporter activity on FP-CIT SPECT, and decreased dopamine D2 receptor expression, as demonstrated by IBZM SPECT (40). Positron emission tomography reveals selectively reduced striatal glucose metabolism. Fluorodopa uptake is normal, suggesting that the origin of the extrapyramidal symptoms is localized postsynaptically to the nigrostriatal pathway (41). The imaging findings are in line with the post-mortem findings of a striatal degeneration in a mosaic pattern with evidence for selective loss of striosomal neurons with multifocal mosaic astrocytosis in the caudate nucleus and lateral putamen (42).

Dopa-responsive dystonia (DYT5, Segawa's disease)

The syndrome of dopa-responsive dystonia (DRD) encompasses both autosomal dominant and autosomal recessive forms. Of these, the dominantly inherited DRD variants are more frequent and are often caused by mutations in the *GTP cyclohydrolase I* (*GCHI*) gene (*DYT5a*). Recessive variants are rarer (*DYT5b*) and associated with mutations in the *tyrosine hydroxylase* (*TH*) gene and other genes.

GCHI encodes the enzyme GTPCH that catalyses the first step in the biosynthesis of tetrahydrobiopterin (43). In patients, there is a decrease in GTPCH activity, leading to dopamine depletion and explaining the remarkable therapeutic effect of levodopa substitution. TH and other DRD-associated enzymes are functionally involved in the same metabolic pathways, in line with the overlapping clinical phenotypes.

DRD is usually characterized by childhood onset of dystonia, diurnal fluctuation of symptoms, and a dramatic response to levodopa therapy. Later in the course of the disease, parkinsonian features frequently occur (44). Rarely, both *TH* (45, 46) and *GCHI* mutations (47) may present as a levodopa-responsive, infantile hypokinetic rigid syndrome. However, *TH* mutations tend to present with a more severe phenotype with mild mental retardation and pronounced signs of dopamine deficiency including tremor, hypersensitivity to levodopa, oculogyric crises, akinesia, rigidity, and dystonia (48). In contrast, carriers of *GCHI* mutations may also show more typical late-onset isolated classic parkinsonism (49), but patients usually report a positive family history for DRD (50, 51). Similar to the dystonic symptoms, classical parkinsonism in DRD responds well to levodopa therapy but, unlike in idiopathic PD, patients do not usually develop severe long-term motor fluctuations and dyskinesias (52, 53). While the response to levodopa treatment seems to set in more slowly and persists longer in subjects with DRD than in patients with PD, re-emergence of parkinsonian signs upon withdrawal of levodopa occurs at similar rates in the two conditions (54).

If parkinsonism is prominent, an important differential diagnosis of DRD is early-onset parkinsonism due to mutations in one of the recessive 'PARK' genes, and in both conditions leg dystonia responsive to levodopa may be a presenting sign. For example, *Parkin* mutations may account for some cases of '*GCHI* mutation-negative DRD' (55). As molecular testing for both *GCHI* and *Parkin* mutations is time-consuming and expensive, transcranial sonography is being explored regarding its potential to distinguish *Parkin* and *GCHI* mutation carriers based on the presence (*Parkin*) or absence (*GCHI*) of hyperechogenicity of the substantia nigra (56). Biochemical studies with CSF analysis (57) and functional imaging may also help to differentiate the two syndromes. Early-onset DRD patients show normal fluorodopa uptake on PET studies (58) and normal dopamine transporter imaging on SPECT, but these are expected be abnormal in the PARK-associated disorders (59). Pathological data in DRD are limited. It appears that there is a reduction of melanin pigment in the substantia nigra, which is more pronounced in the lateral than the medial aspect, in a pattern similar to neuronal loss in PD. However, there are no Lewy bodies, and dopaminergic neurons and noradrenergic neurons in the substantia nigra and the locus coeruleus, respectively, are normal in number but severely hypomelanized (60, 61).

Rapid-onset dystonia–parkinsonism (DYT12)

Mutations in the *Na⁺/K⁺-ATPase alpha 3* gene (*ATP1A3*) cause rapid-onset dystonia–parkinsonism (RDP) (62, 63). Mean age of onset is in adolescence or young adulthood, and the mode of inheritance is autosomal dominant with reduced penetrance (64, 65). Symptoms usually manifest over hours to weeks, and may be followed by moderate or no progression. Some patients report mild (focal) dystonia preceding the onset (66, 67). RDP is clinically characterized by orofacial dystonia, dysarthria, dysphagia, and involuntary dystonic spasms, predominantly of the upper limbs with superimposed parkinsonian features, primarily bradykinesia and postural instability (66) with or without rigidity (68). Other features of classic parkinsonism, such as rest tremor and response to dopaminergic medication, are not a typical feature (66, 69). A presentation which could be more easily confused with PD has recently been described in a genetically proven patient with gradual onset of unilateral bradykinesia and rigidity at age 38 years, which did not improve on levodopa therapy. This was followed by overnight onset of oromandibular dystonia, 3.5 years after his first clinical presentation with parkinsonism (70). In a recent study, using a mouse model of RDP, the cerebellum was observed to be the primary instigator of dystonia; aberrant cerebellar activity altered basal ganglia function, which in turn caused dystonia (71). Most recently, mutations in *ATP1A3* were also identified as a major cause of alternating hemiplegia of childhood.

Spinocerebellar ataxias

Inherited autosomal dominantly inherited ataxias represent a clinically and genetically heterogeneous group of neurodegenerative disorders in which progressive degeneration of the cerebellum and spinocerebellar tracts of the spinal cord are associated with a variable combination of signs of central and peripheral nervous system involvement (72). To date, SCAs have been associated with at least 37 gene loci (73) (see also http://www.ncbi.nlm.nih.gov/omim). Extrapyramidal features, including parkinsonism, have been described in several of them. For example, it may occur as a prominent sign in SCA2, SCA3, SCA8, and SCA17, or as a mild additional feature in SCA6, which is usually considered a 'pure ataxia' (74), and other SCAs.

SCA2 may present with levodopa-responsive parkinsonism in patients from different genetic backgrounds (75), and seems to be particularly frequent among patients of Asian origin in whom it accounts for about 10% of familial parkinsonism (76). The parkinsonian phenotype consists of rest tremor, rigidity, and bradykinesia in conjunction with mild dysarthria, ataxic gait, and instability, particularly in later stages of the condition (76). Although most SCA2 patients have a positive family history of ataxia or ataxia plus parkinsonism (77), rarely SCA2 families with phenotypic familial homogeneity of classic parkinsonism (77, 78) have also been described. SCA2 is a polyglutamine disease associated with an increased number of CAG/CAA repeats. The configuration of the repeat expansion has recently been shown to play an important role in phenotypic variability. While uninterrupted SCA2 repeat expansions cause an ataxic presentation, parkinsonism is associated with CAA interruptions and shorter repeats (79, 80).

Overall, repeat expansions in SCA genes are a rare cause of parkinsonism (81). One family with SCA3 showed at least two of the cardinal features of parkinsonism without any atypical signs and a good response to levodopa (82). However, although ataxia may be negligible in SCA3 (83), parkinsonism is usually accompanied by peripheral neuropathy (84, 85), dystonia, and spasticity (83). Neuropathology studies of SCA3 showed nigral involvement, which probably accounts for the parkinsonism and the good levodopa response (86). A small number of patients with isolated levodopa-responsive parkinsonism have been described as carrying trinucleotide repeat expansions in the *Ataxin8* and *TBP* genes, adding SCA8 and SCA17 to the (rare) differential diagnosis of parkinsonism (87, 88). To our knowledge there are no data on pathological findings of patients with SCA mutations who have presented with a parkinsonian phenotype.

Mitochondrial gene mutations

Mitochondrial syndromes may be phenotypically complex, including disorders from a variety of medical subspecialties such as diabetes mellitus, deafness, and visual disturbance, in addition to neurological features. Genetically, mitochondrial diseases may be due to mutations in either mtDNA (associated with strictly maternal inheritance) or nDNA (nuclear encoded, Mendelian inheritance).

With respect to parkinsonism, the aforementioned proteins PINK1, DJ-1, and Omi/HtrA2 are nuclear encoded and form a link to mitochondria (89, 90). Furthermore, movement disorders are associated with mutations in the nuclear genes *DNA polymerase gamma* (*POLG*) and the *PEO1* (encoding Twinkle) genes. POLG disorders have a broad phenotypic range, including mitochondrial recessive ataxia syndrome without ophthalmoplegia (MIRAS), and sensory ataxic neuropathy, dysarthria, and ophthalmoparesis (SANDO) (91). Myoclonus is the main movement disorder presentation in POLG disorders, but parkinsonism with features similar to PD, including asymmetrical onset, resting tremor, and response to levodopa, may occur (91–93). Parkinsonism is typically preceded several years earlier by the development of ophthalmoplegia, but may also be the presenting feature (94). Fluorodopa PET imaging shows reduced tracer uptake in the caudate and putamen. Marked neuronal loss in the substantia nigra has been demonstrated on pathological examination, although Lewy bodies are absent.

Similarly, there is phenotypic heterogeneity for *PEO1* mutations (91), and infantile-onset SCA, SANDO syndrome, and a form of hepatocerebral mtDNA depletion syndrome have all been described. Parkinsonism with a history of reduced smell function was observed in an autosomal dominant pedigree with progressive external ophthalmoplegia. There was reduced uptake in the striatum bilaterally on ^{123}I-FP-CIT SPECT imaging.

Furthermore, maternally inherited 'mitochondrial parkinsonism', associated with mutations in the *Cytochrome b* gene, the *12sRNA* gene, and *tRNA* genes, has been identified in single families (95, 96). However, patients from such families usually present with additional signs, such as deafness and neuropathy. Overall, mitochondrial disease appears to be an exceedingly rare cause of classic parkinsonism.

The role of *Glucocerebrosidase*

Finally, mutations in the *Glucocerebrosidase* (*GBA*) gene are an increasingly recognized cause of parkinsonism. Historically, it was the presence of parkinsonian features in some cases with Gaucher disease and the identification of *GBA* mutations in individuals with PD that revealed the link between Gaucher disease and parkinsonism. Therefore this gene shares features with two of our categories and will be discussed here as causing parkinsonism alone (category B) in otherwise healthy individuals, and will also initiate a discussion of category C with mutations causing atypical parkinsonism in patients with classic Gaucher disease (97, 98).

Mutations in the *Glucocerebrosidase* gene: association with classic parkinsonism

Gaucher disease is the most common of the lipidoses and is one of the most frequently inherited disorders among Ashkenazi Jews. It is due to recessively inherited deficiency of the lysosomal enzyme glucocerebrosidase (GBA).

Family studies revealed that obligate or confirmed carriers of *GBA* mutations from 10 families developed parkinsonism (99). In addition, *GBA* mutations increase the risk of developing idiopathic PD, and mutations were found in 8–14% of autopsy-proven PD cases (100, 101). In fact, GBA variants are currently the most common genetic risk factor associated with parkinsonism, and both homozygous and heterozygous *GBA* mutations appear to predispose to parkinsonism (102). The phenotypic spectrum of parkinsonism associated with *GBA* mutations ranges from early-onset treatment-refractory parkinsonism, through classic parkinsonism, to features consistent with Lewy body dementia (103, 104).

The role of *GBA* mutations appears to be highly ethnically dependent (105). They have been found, mostly in the heterozygous state, in 29–31% of patients with classic parkinsonism from Israel (106), in 12% of a Venezuelan cohort with very early onset (107), in 6% of a sample of Canadian patients with a Caucasian background (108), in 4.3% of ethnic Chinese (109), and in only 2.3% of a Norwegian PD population (110). The last of these studies found similar rates of functional mutations in the GBA protein in controls (1.7%) (111). The age of onset was found to be either similar (105) between patients with parkinsonism with or without heterozygous *GBA* mutations (112) or slightly reduced (106). It was concluded that both severe and mild *GBA* mutations markedly increased the risk of developing PD (106). With respect to response to treatment, even carriers of two mutations, who otherwise benefit from enzyme replacement therapy, may require dopaminergic therapy to treat their parkinsonism adequately (113).

Atypical parkinsonism in genetic disorders that are usually mainly characterized by features other than parkinsonism

Parkinsonian features in patients with classical Gaucher disease

Typical features of Gaucher disease are painless hepatomegaly and splenomegaly. Other neurological symptoms and signs may include myoclonus, oculomotor apraxia, dementia, and convulsions. Parkinsonism may also develop in patients with otherwise typical Gaucher disease and two mutated *GBA* alleles (97, 98).

Fragile X-associated tremor–ataxia syndrome (FXTAS)

FXTAS is a neurodegenerative disorder occurring largely, but not exclusively, in men. It is caused by moderate expansions (55–200 repeats, so-called pre-mutation range) of a CGG trinucleotide in the *FMRI* gene (114, 115). Longer repeat lengths cause fragile X syndrome.

The core clinical features of FXTAS are action tremor and cerebellar gait ataxia, with an average age of onset of 60 years. Parkinsonism, primarily rigidity, is one of the frequent associated findings and is a minor clinical component of the proposed diagnostic criteria for FXTAS. In fact, parkinsonism has been among the most frequent false diagnoses given to patients with FXTAS (116). However, the phenotype usually differs from that of classic parkinsonism (117, 118) in that other features, including dementia, neuropathy, and dysautonomia, may also be present.

Increased T_2 signal intensity in the middle cerebellar peduncles on MRI imaging (MCP sign) is present in a majority of patients. Similar signal alterations are found in deep and subependymal cerebral white matter, along with general cortical and subcortical atrophy. Autopsy studies have revealed eosinophilic intranuclear, neuronal, and astrocytic inclusions in the brain and brainstem as the major neuropathological feature, together with loss of Purkinje cells and regional vacuolation of the cerebral white matter (119).

Familial dementias

Cognitive decline is common in idiopathic PD (120), and is particularly marked in some of the genetic parkinsonian disorders (e.g. Kufor–Rakeb disease). However, not only is there considerable clinical and pathological overlap between 'PD with dementia' and 'dementia with Lewy bodies' (DLB), and between DLB and Alzheimer's disease (AD), but parkinsonism may also be a feature in primary dementia syndromes including AD and the frontotemporal dementias (FTDs) (121).

Dominantly inherited *Presenilin 1* mutations are a cause of dementia, and early-onset levodopa-responsive parkinsonism, in combination with progressive cognitive decline, has been an early sign in single cases (122, 123). In FTDs, particularly 'frontotemporal dementia and parkinsonism linked to chromosome 17' (FTDP-17) associated with mutations in the *Tau* (*MAPT*) gene or the *Progranulin* (*PGRN*) gene, the three major clinical features of FTDP-17 include behavioural disturbances, cognitive impairment, and parkinsonism (124, 125). Prominent young-onset parkinsonism may be the earliest feature in some patients (126, 127). Age of onset is usually in the third to fifth decade. Overall, there is marked interfamilial, and even intrafamilial, phenotypic variability.

Mutations in autosomal dominantly inherited *Dynactin* cause motor neuron disease and frontotemporal dementia. Recently, mutations in this gene have been associated with Perry syndrome (128) which is clinically characterized by rapidly progressive parkinsonism, hypoventilation, depression, and severe weight loss. Parkinsonism is poorly or only transiently levodopa-responsive. The mean age of onset is 47 years and mean age at death is 52 years (129). Brain pathology reveals severe neuronal loss in the substantia nigra without Lewy bodies, in addition to TDP-43-positive neuronal inclusions, dystrophic neurites, and axonal spheroids in a predominantly pallidonigral distribution (129).

Prion disease

Human prion diseases are mostly sporadic. Inherited forms due to point mutations and insertions within the *prion protein* (*PRNP*) gene represent about 10% of cases (130). Early symptoms of genetic Creutzfeldt–Jakob disease (CJD) are somewhat non-specific (personality changes, disturbance of sleep and appetite). Eventually the triad of dementia, myoclonus, and ataxia emerges. Additional pyramidal and extrapyramidal signs may be part of the phenotype. Rarely, parkinsonism, sometimes levodopa-responsive, may predominate (131), but it has not been described as an isolated or initial symptom in CJD.

Wilson disease

Wilson disease (WD), which is due to mutations in the *ATP7B* gene (132), is an autosomal recessive disorder of impaired formation of ceruloplasmin, leading to copper accumulation in the liver, brain, kidney, and cornea. WD usually manifests in the first decade of life, although late onset may occur. A large series investigating 136 patients with neurological signs identified that parkinsonism was the most common manifestation in both juveniles and adults. However, most cases had additional signs that were not compatible with classical parkinsonism (133).

It has been hypothesized that a single mutated *ATP7B* allele may act as a risk factor for (late-onset) parkinsonism (134, 135). Diagnostic work-up should include serum and 24-hour urine copper, serum ceruloplasmin, free copper estimation, slit-lamp examination, and, if necessary, a liver biopsy. Genetic testing is not used for screening purposes because it is labour intensive, but it can confirm the exact mutation. Importantly, parkinsonism as well as the other features of WD respond well to specific treatment for WD. Wilson disease is described in further detail in Chapter 23.

Brain iron accumulation conditions

Iron overload increases oxidative stress and may lead to neurodegeneration presenting with parkinsonism.

Panthothenate kinase-associated neurodegeneration

Panthothenate kinase-associated neurodegeneration (PKAN) is a core disorder of syndromes with neurodegeneration with brain iron accumulation (NBIA) type 1. This rare autosomal recessively inherited disease is due to *PANK2* gene mutations (136) encoding pantothenate kinase, the key regulatory enzyme in co-enzyme A synthesis. Classic PKAN manifests in the first decade with severe extrapyramidal signs and progresses rapidly to loss of ambulation within 15 years. The most common clinical features are dysarthria, dystonia, corticospinal signs causing gait disturbance, behavioural and cognitive problems. Parkinsonian features include rigidity in the majority of patients, and sometimes tremor and freezing of gait (137). In contrast, atypical PKAN usually begins in the second or third decade, and is associated with fewer extrapyramidal signs and slower progression, and patients usually retain ambulatory function. Very rarely, atypical PKAN may present as early-onset parkinsonism (136). However, screening of 67 PD patients with affected siblings or an early age of onset has not revealed any *PANK2* mutation carriers (138).

Brain MRI may be an important clue to the diagnosis, as it shows pallidal hypointensity with a central area of hyperintensity ('eye of the tiger' sign) on T_2-weighted images.

PLA2G6-assocatiated neurodegeneration

This cause of neurodegeneration of brain iron accumulation (NBIA type 2) has been dealt with under *PARK14*.

Neuroferritinopathy

The phenotype of neuroferritinopathy due to mutations in the *ferritin light chain* (*FTL1*) gene is usually dominated by dystonia or chorea. Parkinsonism may also develop (139, 140).

Aceruloplasminaemia

This autosomal recessive disorder affecting iron metabolism due to mutations of the *ceruloplasmin* gene shows marked accumulation of iron in the liver, pancreas, retina, and basal ganglia. Clinically, it is characterized by the combination of movement disorders, dementia, and diabetes mellitus (141).

Further NBIA disorders

There have been additional single-case reports of NBIA with late-onset levodopa-responsive parkinsonism with an as yet undetermined genetic basis (142, 143). Rest tremor was asymmetric with a re-emergent component. There was development of levodopa-induced dyskinesias and good benefit from deep brain stimulation (143). MRI showed an 'eye of the tiger' sign, but genetic testing was negative for known genes.

FBXO7-associated neurodegeneration

This rare syndrome, which has recently been described, is characterized by childhood-onset dystonia with, in some cases, additional parkinsonism with bradykinesia and rigidity but no tremor. Parkinsonism was responsive to dopaminergic treatment with the development of dyskinesia (144, 145). In the third decade all family members developed lower limb spasticity. Dopamine transporter SPECT (FP-CIT) scan revealed severely reduced presynaptic nigrostriatal deficits (145), and assessment using transcranial magnetic stimulation showed abnormal cortical motor conduction time. Other investigations, including routine blood tests, ocular examination, brain and spinal MRI, IBZM-SPECT scanning (a measure of postsynaptic striatal dopamine binding), EEG, EMG, and a muscle biopsy, were normal (144, 145). Overall, little is yet known about this syndrome.

Fahr's disease

Bilateral striopallidodentate calcification, also referred to as Fahr's disease, is characterized by basal ganglia and extra-basal ganglia brain calcifications, parkinsonism, and neuropsychiatric symptoms. Causes are multiple and include inherited variants (146). An idiopathic case with progressive cognitive impairment, frontal lobe dysfunction, mild leg spasticity, levodopa-responsive parkinsonism, and marked basal ganglia hyperechogenicity on transcranial sonography has been reported (147).

Huntington's disease

The autosomal dominant trinucleotide disorder Huntington's disease (HD), due to CAG repeat expansions in the *huntingtin* gene (148, 149) is the most important cause of inherited chorea characterized by cognitive decline and psychiatric, oculomotor, and motor abnormalities, in addition to prominent chorea. Onset is typically in adulthood. However, the Westphal variant of HD is a distinct presentation characterized by a rigid–hypokinetic syndrome and is usually associated with young onset age. Juvenile HD (i.e. onset age 20 years or younger) accounts for 5–10% of all HD cases (150–152). While fine postural trunk and limb tremor may be seen (153), rest tremor has not been described. Some children show cerebellar signs or dystonia; eye movement disturbances are prominent, and behavioural problems and cognitive decline are common, sometimes as presenting features. Seizures have been reported in about 30% of juvenile cases, whereas they are rare in adult-onset patients. Very rarely, adult-onset patients may also present with classical parkinsonism without chorea in the initial stages of their illness (154). In rare instances, late-onset HD may mimic levodopa-responsive parkinsonism (155) or mild cardiovascular dysautonomia, which may mimic multiple system atrophy (156). In recent years, phenocopies of HD have been recognized (157) and, similar to HD, progression to a hypokinetic parkinsonian phenotype (157) and 'Westphal variants' have been described. Huntington's disease is discussed in more detail in Chapter 20.

Neuroacanthocytosis

Neuroacanthocytosis refers to a group of neurological syndromes characterized by abnormally spiculated red blood cells (see also Chapter 21). The core syndrome, chorea–acanthocytosis, is an autosomal recessive disorder associated with the *CHAC* gene that encodes chorein (158). The main motor signs are facial hyperkinesias, dysarthria, and dysphagia with frequent involuntary vocalizations, chorea, and, less often, dystonia. The hyperkinetic state can gradually progress to parkinsonism (159, 160) and is observed in about a third of patients (161). Very rarely parkinsonism is the presenting feature (162). Cognitive changes, seizures, and peripheral neuropathy may be present (161). McLeod syndrome, an X-linked form of neuroacanthocytosis associated with abnormalities in the Kell antigens on red blood cells, may also have a parkinsonian phenotype (163).

Miscellaneous conditions

In addition to the conditions described above, there are other diseases which may present with parkinsonism and should be considered in the differential diagnosis. Some of these cannot be discussed in detail because of space restrictions. They include hereditary haemochromatosis due to mutations in the *HFE* gene (164), neurometabolic disorders, such as Niemann–Pick type C, due to mutations in the *NPC1* gene (for a review, see ref. 52), and individual cases of hereditary spastic paraplegia (165) which may sometimes present with parkinsonism. Atypical parkinsonism has been reported in Rett syndrome (166), and dystonia–parkinsonism has been reported in the course of the immunodeficiency disorder X-linked agammaglobulinaemia (167). There are also reports of individual families with parkinsonism due to as yet unknown gene defects (168).

Acknowledgements

CK is supported by a Lichtenberg grant from the Volkswagen Foundation and a Career Development Award from the Hermann and Lilly Schilling Foundation. SAS is supported by the German Research Foundation.

References

1. Klein C, Lohmann-Hedrich K. Impact of recent genetic findings in Parkinson's disease. *Curr Opin Neurol* 2007; 20: 453–64.
2. Tan EK, Skipper LM. Pathogenic mutations in Parkinson disease. *Hum Mutat* 2007; 28: 641–53.
3. Hardy J, Cai H, Cookson MR, Gwinn-Hardy K, Singleton A. Genetics of Parkinson's disease and parkinsonism. *Ann Neurol* 2006; 60: 389–98.
4. Dodson MW, Guo M. Pink1, Parkin, DJ-1 and mitochondrial dysfunction in Parkinson's disease. *Curr Opin Neurobiol* 2007; 17: 331–7.
5. Galpern WR, Lang AE. Interface between tauopathies and synucleinopathies: a tale of two proteins. *Ann Neurol* 2006; 59: 449–58.
6. Haugrauvoll K, Rademakers R, Kachergus J, et al. Familial parkinsonism due to the R1441C mutation in LRRK2 is clinically similar to sporadic Parkinson's disease. *Neurology* 2008; 70: 1456–60.
7. Ishihara L, Warren L, Gibson R, et al. Clinical features of Parkinson disease patients with homozygous leucine-rich repeat kinase 2 G2019S mutations. *Arch Neurol* 2006; 63: 1250–4.
8. Nalls MA, Plagnol V, Hernandez DG, et al. Imputation of sequence variants for identification of genetic risks for Parkinson's disease: a meta-analysis of genome-wide association studies. *Lancet* 2011; 377: 641–9.
9. Healy DG, Falchi M, O'Sullivan SS, et al. Phenotype, genotype, and worldwide genetic penetrance of LRRK2-associated Parkinson's disease: a case-control study. *Lancet Neurol* 2008; 7: 583–90.
10. Lucking CB, Durr A, Bonifati V, et al. Association between early-onset Parkinson's disease and mutations in the parkin gene. French Parkinson's Disease Genetics Study Group. *N Engl J Med* 2000; 342: 1560–7.

11. Lohmann E, Periquet M, Bonifati V, et al. How much phenotypic variation can be attributed to parkin genotype? *Ann Neurol* 2003; 54: 176–85.
12. Abou-Sleiman PM, Muqit MM, McDonald NQ, et al. A heterozygous effect for PINK1 mutations in Parkinson's disease? *Ann Neurol* 2006; 60: 414–19.
13. Steinlechner S, Stahlberg J, Volkel B, et al. Co-occurrence of affective and schizophrenia spectrum disorders with PINK1 mutations. *J Neurol Neurosurg Psychiatry* 2007; 78: 532–5.
14. Criscuolo C, Volpe G, De Rosa A, et al. PINK1 homozygous W437X mutation in a patient with apparent dominant transmission of parkinsonism. *Mov Disord* 2006; 21: 1265–7.
15. Klein C, Schlossmacher MG. Parkinson disease, 10 years after its genetic revolution. Multiple clues to a complex disorder. *Neurology* 2007; 69: 2093–104.
16. Ramirez A, Heimbach A, Grundemann J, et al. Hereditary parkinsonism with dementia is caused by mutations in ATP13A2, encoding a lysosomal type 5 P-type ATPase. *Nat Genet* 2006; 38: 1184–91.
17. Williams DR, Hadeed A, al-Din AS, Wreikat AL, Lees AJ. Kufor–Rakeb disease: autosomal recessive, levodopa-responsive parkinsonism with pyramidal degeneration, supranuclear gaze palsy, and dementia. *Mov Disord* 2005; 20: 1264–71.
18. Lees AJ, Singleton AB. Clinical heterogeneity of ATP13A2 linked disease (Kufor–Rakeb) justifies a PARK designation. *Neurology* 2007; 68: 1553–4.
19. Machner B, Sprenger A, Behrens MI, et al. Eye movement disorders in ATP13A2 mutation carriers (PARK9). *Mov Disord* 2010; 25: 2687–9.
20. Paisan-Ruiz C, Li A, Schneider SA, et al. Widespread Lewy body and tau accumulation in childhood and adult onset dystonia–parkinsonism cases with PLA2G6 mutations. *Neurobiol Aging* 2010; 33: 814–23.
21. Schneider SA, Paisan-Ruiz C, Quinn NP, et al. ATP13A2 mutations (PARK9) cause neurodegeneration with brain iron accumulation. *Mov Disord* 2010; 25: 979–84.
22. Bruggemann N, Hagenah J, Reetz K, et al. Recessively inherited parkinsonism: effect of ATP13A2 mutations on the clinical and neuroimaging phenotype. *Arch Neurol* 2010; 67: 1357–63.
23. Di Fonzo A, Chien HF, Socal M, et al. ATP13A2 missense mutations in juvenile parkinsonism and young onset Parkinson disease. *Neurology* 2007; 68: 1557–62.
24. Fong CY, Rolfs A, Schwarzbraun T, Klein C, O'Callaghan FJ. Juvenile parkinsonism associated with heterozygous frameshift ATP13A2 gene mutation. *Eur J Paediatr Neurol* 2011; 15: 271–5.
25. Farias F, Zeng R, Johnson G, et al. A truncating mutation in ARP12A2 is responsible for adult-onset neuronal ceroid lipofuscinosis in Tibetan terriers. *Neurobiol Dis* 2011 .
26. Paisan-Ruiz C, Bhatia KP, Li A, Hernandez D, Davis M, Wood NW, et al. Characterization of PLA2G6 as a locus for dystonia–parkinsonism. *Ann Neurol* 2008; 48: 468–74.
27. Khateeb S, Flusser H, Ofir R, et al. PLA2G6 mutation underlies infantile neuroaxonal dystrophy. *Am J Hum Genet* 2006; 79: 942–8.
28. Fuchs J, Nilsson C, Kachergus J, et al. Phenotypic variation in a large Swedish pedigree due to SNCA duplication and triplication. *Neurology* 2007; 68: 916–22.
29. Golbe LI, Di Iorio G, Sanges G, et al. Clinical genetic analysis of Parkinson's disease in the Contursi kindred. *Ann Neurol* 1996; 40: 767–75.
30. Vekrellis K, Rideout HJ, Stefanis L. Neurobiology of alpha-Synuclein. *Mol Neurobiol* 2004; 30: 1–22.
31. Fahn S, Bressman SB, Marsden CD. Classification of dystonia. *Adv Neurol* 1998; 78: 1–10.
32. Camargos S, Scholz S, Simon-Sanchez J, et al. DYT16, a novel young-onset dystonia–parkinsonism disorder: identification of a segregating mutation in the stress-response protein PRKRA. *Lancet Neurol* 2008; 7: 207–15.
33. Makino S, Kaji R, Ando S, et al. Reduced neuron-specific expression of the TAF1 gene is associated with X-linked dystonia–parkinsonism. *Am J Hum Genet* 2007; 80: 393–406.
34. Deng H, Le W, Shahed J, Xie W, Jankovic J. Mutation analysis of the parkin and PINK1 genes in American Caucasian early-onset Parkinson disease families. *Neurosci Lett* 2008; 430: 18–22.
35. Evidente VG, Nolte D, Niemann S, Advincula J, Mayo MC, Natividad FF, et al. Phenotypic and molecular analyses of X-linked dystonia–parkinsonism ('lubag') in women. *Arch Neurol* 2004; 61: 1956–9.
36. Lee LV, Kupke KG, Caballar-Gonzaga F, Hebron-Ortiz M, Muller U. The phenotype of the X-linked dystonia–parkinsonism syndrome. An assessment of 42 cases in the Philippines. *Medicine (Baltimore)* 1991; 70: 179–87.
37. Müller U, Steinberger D, Nemeth A. Clinical and molecular genetics of primary dystonias. *Neurogenetics* 1998; 1: 165–77.
38. Evidente VG, Advincula J, Esteban R, et al. Phenomenology of 'lubag' or X-linked dystonia–parkinsonism. *Mov Disord* 2002; 17: 1271–7.
39. Gwinn-Hardy K. Genetics of parkinsonism. *Mov Disord* 2002; 17: 645–56.
40. Tackenberg B, Metz A, Unger M, et al. Nigrostriatal dysfunction in X-linked dystonia–parkinsonism (DYT3). *Mov Disord* 2007; 22: 900–2.
41. Eidelberg D, Takikawa S, Wilhelmsen K, et al. Positron emission tomographic findings in Filipino X-linked dystonia–parkinsonism. *Ann Neurol* 1993; 34: 185–91.
42. Waters CH, Faust PL, Powers J, et al. Neuropathology of lubag (X-linked dystonia–parkinsonism). *Mov Disord* 1993; 8: 387–90.
43. Nar H, Huber R, Auerbach G, et al. Active site topology and reaction mechanism of GTP cyclohydrolase I. *Proc Natl Acad Sci USA* 1995; 92: 12120–5.
44. Segawa M, Hosaka A, Miyagawa F, Nomura Y, Imai H. Hereditary progressive dystonia with marked diurnal fluctuation. *Adv Neurol* 1976; 14: 215–33.
45. Brautigam C, Steenbergen-Spanjers GC, Hoffmann GF, et al. Biochemical and molecular genetic characteristics of the severe form of tyrosine hydroxylase deficiency. *Clin Chem* 1999; 45: 2073–8.
46. de Rijk-van Andel J, Gabreels F, Geurtz G, et al. L-dopa-responsive infantile hypokinetic rigid parkinsonism due to tyrosine hydroxylase deficiency. *Neurology* 2000; 55: 1926–8.
47. Lopez-Laso E, Camino R, Mateos ME, et al. Dopa-responsive infantile hypokinetic rigid syndrome due to dominant guanosine triphosphate cyclohydrolase 1 deficiency. *J Neurol Sci* 2007; 256: 90–3.
48. Grattan-Smith PJ, Wevers RA, Steenbergen-Spanjers GC, Fung VS, Earl J, Wilcken B. Tyrosine hydroxylase deficiency: clinical manifestations of catecholamine insufficiency in infancy. *Mov Disord* 2002; 17: 354–9.
49. Nygaard TG, Trugman JM, de Yebenes JG, Fahn S. Dopa-responsive dystonia: the spectrum of clinical manifestations in a large North American family. *Neurology* 1990; 40: 66–9.
50. Bandmann O, Daniel S, Marsden CD, Wood NW, Harding AE. The GTP-cyclohydrolase I gene in atypical parkinsonian patients: a clinico-genetic study. *J Neurol Sci* 1996; 141: 27–32.
51. Hertz JM, Ostergaard K, Juncker I, et al. Low frequency of Parkin, Tyrosine Hydroxylase, and GTP Cyclohydrolase I gene mutations in a Danish population of early-onset Parkinson's disease. *Eur J Neurol* 2006; 13: 385–90.
52. Paviour DC, Surtees RA, Lees AJ. Diagnostic considerations in juvenile parkinsonism. *Mov Disord* 2004; 19: 123–35.
53. Trender-Gerhard I, Sweeney MG, Schwingenschuh P, et al. Autosomal-dominant GTPCH1-deficient DRD: clinical characteristics and long-term outcome of 34 patients. *J Neurol Neurosurg Psychiatry* 2009; 80: 839–45.
54. Nutt JG, Nygaard TG. Response to levodopa treatment in dopa-responsive dystonia. *Arch Neurol* 2001; 58: 905–10.
55. Tassin J, Durr A, Bonnet AM, et al. Levodopa-responsive dystonia. GTP cyclohydrolase I or parkin mutations? *Brain* 2000; 123: 1112–21.
56. Hagenah JM, Hedrich K, Becker B, Pramstaller PP, Seidel G, Klein C. Distinguishing early-onset PD from dopa-responsive dystonia with transcranial sonography. *Neurology* 2006; 66: 1951–2.

57. Nagatsu T, Ichinose H. GTP cyclohydrolase I gene, tetrahydrobiopterin, and tyrosine hydroxylase gene: their relations to dystonia and parkinsonism. *Neurochem Res* 1996; 21: 245–50.
58. Turjanski N, Bhatia K, Burn DJ, Sawle GV, Marsden CD, Brooks DJ. Comparison of striatal ^{18}F-dopa uptake in adult-onset dystonia–parkinsonism, Parkinson's disease, and dopa-responsive dystonia. *Neurology* 1993; 43: 1563–8.
59. Marshall V, Grosset D. Role of dopamine transporter imaging in routine clinical practice. *Mov Disord* 2003; 18: 1415–23.
60. Grotzsch H, Pizzolato GP, Ghika J, et al. Neuropathology of a case of dopa-responsive dystonia associated with a new genetic locus, DYT14. *Neurology* 2002; 58: 1839–42.
61. Nygaard TG, Wooten GF. Dopa-responsive dystonia: some pieces of the puzzle are still missing. *Neurology* 1998; 50: 853–5.
62. de Carvalho Aguiar P, Sweadner KJ, Penniston JT, et al. Mutations in the Na^+/K^+-ATPase alpha3 gene ATP1A3 are associated with rapid-onset dystonia–parkinsonism. *Neuron* 2004; 43: 169–75.
63. Rodacker V, Toustrup-Jensen M, Vilsen B. Mutations Phe785Leu and Thr618Met in Na^+,K^+-ATPase, associated with familial rapid-onset dystonia–parkinsonism, interfere with Na^+ interaction by distinct mechanisms. *J Biol Chem* 2006; 281: 18539–48.
64. Brashear A, DeLeon D, Bressman SB, Thyagarajan D, Farlow MR, Dobyns WB. Rapid-onset dystonia–parkinsonism in a second family. *Neurology* 1997; 48: 1066–9.
65. Dobyns WB, Ozelius LJ, Kramer PL, et al. Rapid-onset dystonia–parkinsonism. *Neurology* 1993; 43: 2596–602.
66. Brashear A, Dobyns WB, de Carvalho Aguiar P, et al. The phenotypic spectrum of rapid-onset dystonia–parkinsonism (RDP) and mutations in the ATP1A3 gene. *Brain* 2007; 130: 828–35.
67. Zaremba J, Mierzewska H, Lysiak Z, Kramer P, Ozelius LJ, Brashear A. Rapid-onset dystonia–parkinsonism: a fourth family consistent with linkage to chromosome 19q13. *Mov Disord* 2004; 19: 1506–10.
68. Lee JY, Gollamudi S, Ozelius LJ, Kim JY, Jeon BS. ATP1A3 mutation in the first Asian case of rapid-onset dystonia–parkinsonism. *Mov Disord* 2007; 22: 1808–9.
69. McKeon A, Ozelius LJ, Hardiman O, Greenway MJ, Pittock SJ. Heterogeneity of presentation and outcome in the Irish rapid-onset dystonia-Parkinsonism kindred. *Mov Disord* 2007; 22: 1325–7.
70. Kamphuis DJ, Koelman H, Lees AJ, Tijssen MA. Sporadic rapid-onset dystonia–parkinsonism presenting as Parkinson's disease. *Mov Disord* 2006; 21: 118–19.
71. Calderon DP, Fremont R, Kraenzlin F, Khodakhah K. The neural substrates of rapid-onset dystonia–parkinsonism. *Nat Neurosci* 2011; 14: 357–65.
72. Taroni F, DiDonato S. Pathways to motor incoordination: the inherited ataxias. *Nat Rev Neurosci* 2004; 5: 641–55.
73. Orr H, Zoghbi H. Trinucleotide repeat disorders. *Annu Rev Neurosci* 2007; 30: 575–621.
74. Schols L, Kruger R, Amoiridis G, Przuntek H, Epplen JT, Riess O. Spinocerebellar ataxia type 6: genotype and phenotype in German kindreds. *J Neurol Neurosurg Psychiatry* 1998; 64: 67–73.
75. Gwinn-Hardy K, Chen JY, Liu HC, et al. Spinocerebellar ataxia type 2 with parkinsonism in ethnic Chinese. *Neurology* 2000; 55: 800–5.
76. Lu CS, Chang HC, Kuo PC, et al. The parkinsonian phenotype of spinocerebellar ataxia type 3 in a Taiwanese family. *Parkinsonism Relat Disord* 2004; 10: 369–73.
77. Furtado S, Farrer M, Tsuboi Y, et al. SCA-2 presenting as parkinsonism in an Alberta family: clinical, genetic, and PET findings. *Neurology* 2002; 59: 1625–7.
78. Shan DE, Liu RS, Sun CM, Lee SJ, Liao KK, Soong BW. Presence of spinocerebellar ataxia type 2 gene mutation in a patient with apparently sporadic Parkinson's disease: clinical implications. *Mov Disord* 2004; 19: 1357–60.
79. Charles P, Camuzat A, Benammar N, et al. Are interrupted SCA2 CAG repeat expansions responsible for parkinsonism? *Neurology* 2007; 69: 1970–5.
80. Kim JM, Hong S, Kim GP, et al. Importance of low-range CAG expansion and CAA interruption in SCA2 Parkinsonism. *Arch Neurol* 2007; 64: 1510–18.
81. Lim SW, Zhao Y, Chua E, et al. Genetic analysis of SCA2, 3 and 17 in idiopathic Parkinson's disease. *Neurosci Lett* 2006; 403: 11–14.
82. Gwinn-Hardy K, Singleton A, O'Suilleabhain P, et al. Spinocerebellar ataxia type 3 phenotypically resembling parkinson disease in a black family. *Arch Neurol* 2001; 58: 296–9.
83. Giunti P, Sweeney MG, Harding AE. Detection of the Machado–Joseph disease/spinocerebellar ataxia three trinucleotide repeat expansion in families with autosomal dominant motor disorders, including the Drew family of Walworth. *Brain* 1995; 118: 1077–85.
84. Tuite PJ, Rogaeva EA, St George-Hyslop PH, Lang AE. Dopa-responsive parkinsonism phenotype of Machado–Joseph disease: confirmation of 14q CAG expansion. *Ann Neurol* 1995; 38: 684–7.
85. Yoritaka A, Nakagawa-Hattori Y, Hattori N, Kitahara A, Mizuno Y. A large Japanese family with Machado–Joseph disease: clinical and genetic analysis. *Acta Neurol ScandActa Neurol Scand* 1999; 99: 241–4.
86. Yamada M, Sato T, Tsuji S, Takahashi H. CAG repeat disorder models and human neuropathology: similarities and differences. *Acta Neuropathol* 2008; 115: 71–86.
87. Wu YR, Lin HY, Chen CM, et al. Genetic testing in spinocerebellar ataxia in Taiwan: expansions of trinucleotide repeats in SCA8 and SCA17 are associated with typical Parkinson's disease. *Clin Genet* 2004; 65: 209–14.
88. Wu YR, Fung HC, Lee-Chen GJ, et al. Analysis of polyglutamine-coding repeats in the TATA-binding protein in different neurodegenerative diseases. *J Neural Transm* 2005; 112: 539–46.
89. Schapira AH. Mitochondrial disease. *Lancet* 2006; 368: 70–82.
90. Muqit MM, Gandhi S, Wood NW. Mitochondria in Parkinson disease: back in fashion with a little help from genetics. *Arch Neurol* 2006; 63: 649–54.
91. Moustris A, Edwards MJ, Bhatia KP. Movement disorders and mitochondrial disease. *Handb Clin Neurol* 2011; 100: 173–92.
92. Mancuso M, Filosto M, Bellan M, et al. POLG mutations causing ophthalmoplegia, sensorimotor polyneuropathy, ataxia, and deafness. *Neurology* 2004; 62: 316–18.
93. Luoma P, Melberg A, Rinne JO, et al. Parkinsonism, premature menopause, and mitochondrial DNA polymerase gamma mutations: clinical and molecular genetic study. *Lancet* 2004; 364: 875–82.
94. Davidzon G, Greene P, Mancuso M, et al. Early-onset familial parkinsonism due to POLG mutations. *Ann Neurol* 2006; 59: 859–62.
95. Thyagarajan D, Bressman S, Bruno C, et al. A novel mitochondrial 12SrRNA point mutation in parkinsonism, deafness, and neuropathy. *Ann Neurol* 2000; 48: 730–6.
96. Grasbon-Frodl EM, Kosel S, Sprinzl M, von Eitzen U, Mehraein P, Graeber MB. Two novel point mutations of mitochondrial tRNA genes in histologically confirmed Parkinson disease. *Neurogenetics* 1999; 2: 121–7.
97. Aharon-Peretz J, Rosenbaum H, Gershoni-Baruch R. Mutations in the glucocerebrosidase gene and Parkinson's disease in Ashkenazi Jews. *N Engl J Med* 2004; 351: 1972–7.
98. Goker-Alpan O, Giasson BI, Eblan MJ, et al. Glucocerebrosidase mutations are an important risk factor for Lewy body disorders. *Neurology* 2006; 67: 908–10.
99. Goker-Alpan O, Schiffmann R, LaMarca ME, Nussbaum RL, McInerney-Leo A, Sidransky E. Parkinsonism among Gaucher disease carriers. *J Med Genet* 2004; 41: 937–40.
100. Lwin A, Orvisky E, Goker-Alpan O, LaMarca ME, Sidransky E. Glucocerebrosidase mutations in subjects with parkinsonism. *Mol Genet Metab* 2004; 81: 70–3.
101. Eblan MJ, Walker JM, Sidransky E. The glucocerebrosidase gene and Parkinson's disease in Ashkenazi Jews. *N Engl J Med* 2005; 352: 728–31.
102. Sidransky E. Heterozygosity for a Mendelian disorder as a risk factor for complex disease. *Clin Genet* 2006; 70: 275–82.

103. Bembi B, Zambito Marsala S, Sidransky E, et al. Gaucher's disease with Parkinson's disease: clinical and pathological aspects. *Neurology* 2003; 61: 99–101.
104. Goker-Alpan O, Lopez G, Vithayathil J, Davis J, Hallett M, Sidransky E. The spectrum of parkinsonian manifestations associated with glucocerebrosidase mutations. *Arch Neurol* 2008; 65: 1353–7.
105. Clark LN, Ross BM, Wang Y, et al. Mutations in the glucocerebrosidase gene are associated with early-onset Parkinson disease. *Neurology* 2007; 69: 1270–7.
106. Gan-Or Z, Giladi N, Rozovski U, et al. Genotype-phenotype correlations between GBA mutations and Parkinson disease risk and onset. *Neurology* 2008; 70: 2277–83.
107. Eblan MJ, Nguyen J, Ziegler SG, et al. Glucocerebrosidase mutations are also found in subjects with early-onset parkinsonism from Venezuela. *Mov Disord* 2006; 21: 282–3.
108. Sato C, Morgan A, Lang AE, et al. Analysis of the glucocerebrosidase gene in Parkinson's disease. *Mov Disord* 2005; 20: 367–70.
109. Ziegler SG, Eblan MJ, Gutti U, et al. Glucocerebrosidase mutations in Chinese subjects from Taiwan with sporadic Parkinson disease. *Mol Genet Metab* 2007; 91: 195–200.
110. Nichols WC, Pankratz N, Marek DK, et al. Mutations in GBA are associated with familial Parkinson disease susceptibility and age at onset. *Neurology* 2009; 72: 310–16.
111. Toft M, Pielsticker L, Ross OA, Aasly JO, Farrer MJ. Glucocerebrosidase gene mutations and Parkinson disease in the Norwegian population. *Neurology* 2006; 66: 415–17.
112. Aharon-Peretz J, Badarny S, Rosenbaum H, Gershoni-Baruch R. Mutations in the glucocerebrosidase gene and Parkinson disease: phenotype-genotype correlation. *Neurology* 2005; 65: 1460–1.
113. Tayebi N, Callahan M, Madike V, et al. Gaucher disease and parkinsonism: a phenotypic and genotypic characterization. *Mol Genet Metab* 2001; 73: 313–21.
114. Hagerman RJ, Leehey M, Heinrichs W, et al. Intention tremor, parkinsonism, and generalized brain atrophy in male carriers of fragile X. *Neurology* 2001; 57: 127–30.
115. Jacquemont S, Hagerman RJ, Hagerman PJ, Leehey MA. Fragile-X syndrome and fragile X-associated tremor/ataxia syndrome: two faces of FMR1. *Lancet Neurol* 2007; 6: 45–55.
116. Hall DA, Berry-Kravis E, Jacquemont S, et al. Initial diagnoses given to persons with the fragile X associated tremor/ataxia syndrome (FXTAS). *Neurology* 2005; 65: 299–301.
117. Berry-Kravis E, Lewin F, Wuu J, et al. Tremor and ataxia in fragile X premutation carriers: blinded videotape study. *Ann Neurol* 2003; 53: 616–23.
118. Berry-Kravis E, Abrams L, Coffey SM, et al. Fragile X-associated tremor/ataxia syndrome: clinical features, genetics, and testing guidelines. *Mov Disord* 2007; 22: 2018–30.
119. Greco CM, Berman RF, Martin RM, et al. Neuropathology of fragile X-associated tremor/ataxia syndrome (FXTAS). *Brain* 2006; 129: 243–55.
120. Hely MA, Reid WG, Adena MA, Halliday GM, Morris JG. The Sydney multicenter study of Parkinson's disease: the inevitability of dementia at 20 years. *Mov Disord* 2008; 23: 837–44.
121. Nussbaum RL, Ellis CE. Alzheimer's disease and Parkinson's disease. *N Engl J Med* 2003; 348: 1356–64.
122. Jimenez-Escrig A, Rabano A, Guerrero C, et al. New V272A presenilin 1 mutation with very early onset subcortical dementia and parkinsonism. *Eur J Neurol* 2004; 11: 663–9.
123. Takao M, Ghetti B, Hayakawa I, et al. A novel mutation (G217D) in the Presenilin 1 gene (PSEN1) in a Japanese family: presenile dementia and parkinsonism are associated with cotton wool plaques in the cortex and striatum. *Acta Neuropathol* 2002; 104: 155–70.
124. Cruts M, Gijselinck I, van der Zee J, et al. Null mutations in progranulin cause ubiquitin-positive frontotemporal dementia linked to chromosome 17q21. *Nature* 2006; 442: 920–4.
125. Baker M, Mackenzie IR, Pickering-Brown SM, et al. Mutations in progranulin cause tau-negative frontotemporal dementia linked to chromosome 17. *Nature* 2006; 442: 916–19.
126. Yasuda M, Nakamura Y, Kawamata T, Kaneyuki H, Maeda K, Komure O. Phenotypic heterogeneity within a new family with the MAPT p301s mutation. *Ann Neurol* 2005; 58(6): 920–8.
127. Kelley BJ, Haidar W, Boeve BF, et al. Prominent phenotypic variability associated with mutations in progranulin. *Neurobiol Aging* 2009; 30: 739–51.
128. Farrer MJ, Williams LN, Algom AA, et al. Glucosidase-beta variations and Lewy body disorders. *Parkinsonism Relat Disord* 2009; 15: 414–16.
129. Wider C, Melquist S, Hauf M, et al. Study of a Swiss dopa-responsive dystonia family with a deletion in GCH1: redefining DYT14 as DYT5. *Neurology* 2008; 70: 1377–83.
130. Prusiner SB. Prion diseases and the BSE crisis. *Science* 1997; 278: 245–51.
131. Iida T, Doh-ura K, Kawashima T, Abe H, Iwaki T. An atypical case of sporadic Creutzfeldt–Jakob disease with Parkinson's disease. *Neuropathology* 2001; 21: 294–7.
132. Bull PC, Thomas GR, Rommens JM, Forbes JR, Cox DW. The Wilson disease gene is a putative copper transporting P-type ATPase similar to the Menkes gene. *Nat Genet* 1993; 5: 327–37.
133. Walshe JM, Yealland M. Wilson's disease: the problem of delayed diagnosis. *J Neurol Neurosurg Psychiatry* 1992; 55: 692–6.
134. Johnson S. Is Parkinson's disease the heterozygote form of Wilson's disease: PD = 1/2 WD? *Med Hypotheses* 2001; 56: 171–3.
135. Sechi G, Antonio Cocco G, Errigo A, et al. Three sisters with very-late-onset major depression and parkinsonism. *Parkinsonism Relat Disord* 2007; 13: 122–5.
136. Zhou B, Westaway SK, Levinson B, Johnson MA, Gitschier J, Hayflick SJ. A novel pantothenate kinase gene (PANK2) is defective in Hallervorden–Spatz syndrome. *Nat Genet* 2001; 28: 345–9.
137. Pellecchia MT, Valente EM, Cif L, et al. The diverse phenotype and genotype of pantothenate kinase-associated neurodegeneration. *Neurology* 2005; 64: 1810–12.
138. Klopstock T, Elstner M, Lucking CB, et al. Mutations in the pantothenate kinase gene PANK2 are not associated with Parkinson disease. *Neurosci Lett* 2005; 379: 195–8.
139. Curtis AR, Fey C, Morris CM, et al. Mutation in the gene encoding ferritin light polypeptide causes dominant adult-onset basal ganglia disease. *Nat Genet* 2001; 28: 350–4.
140. Burn J, Chinnery PF. Neuroferritinopathy. *Semin Pediatr Neurol* 2006; 13: 176–81.
141. Kohno S, Miyajima H, Takahashi Y, Inoue Y. Aceruloplasminemia with a novel mutation associated with parkinsonism. *Neurogenetics* 2000; 2: 237–8.
142. Bruggemann N, Wuerfel J, Petersen D, Klein C, Hagenah J, Schneider SA. Idiopathic NBIA—clinical spectrum and transcranial sonography findings. *Eur J Neurol* 2011; 18: e58–9.
143. Aggarwal A, Schneider SA, Houlden H, et al. Indian-subcontinent NBIA: unusual phenotypes, novel PANK2 mutations, and undetermined genetic forms. *Mov Disord* 2010; 25: 1424–31.
144. Shojaee S, Sina F, Banihosseini SS, et al. Genome-wide linkage analysis of a Parkinsonian-pyramidal syndrome pedigree by 500 K SNP arrays. *Am J Hum Genet* 2008; 82: 1375–84.
145. Di Fonzo A, Dekker MC, Montagna P, et al. FBXO7 mutations cause autosomal recessive, early-onset parkinsonian–pyramidal syndrome. *Neurology* 2009; 72: 240–5.
146. Oliveira JR, Spiteri E, Sobrido MJ, et al. Genetic heterogeneity in familial idiopathic basal ganglia calcification (Fahr disease). *Neurology* 2004; 63: 2165–7.
147. Bruggemann N, Schneider SA, Sander T, Klein C, Hagenah J. Distinct basal ganglia hyperechogenicity in idiopathic basal ganglia calcification. *Mov Disord* 2010; 25: 2661–4.

148. Group HsDS. A novel gene containing a trinucleotide repeat that is expanded and unstable on Huntington's disease chromosomes. The Huntington's Disease Collaborative Research Group. *Cell* 1993; 72: 817–18.
149. Walker F. Huntington's disease. *Lancet* 2007; 369: 218–28.
150. Nance MA, Mathias-Hagen V, Breningstall G, Wick MJ, McGlennen RC. Analysis of a very large trinucleotide repeat in a patient with juvenile Huntington's disease. *Neurology* 1999; 52: 392–4.
151. Rasmussen A, Macias R, Yescas P, Ochoa A, Davila G, Alonso E. Huntington disease in children: genotype–phenotype correlation. *Neuropediatrics* 2000; 31: 190–4.
152. Wojaczynska-Stanek K, Adamek D, Marszal E, Hoffman-Zacharska D. Huntington disease in a 9-year-old boy: clinical course and neuropathologic examination. *J Child Neurol* 2006; 21: 1068–73.
153. Nance MA, Myers RH. Juvenile onset Huntington's disease—clinical and research perspectives. *Ment Retard Dev Disabil Res Rev* 2001; 7: 153–7.
154. Squitieri F, Berardelli A, Nargi E, et al. Atypical movement disorders in the early stages of Huntington's disease: clinical and genetic analysis. *Clin Genet* 2000; 58: 50–6.
155. Racette BA, Perlmutter JS. Levodopa responsive parkinsonism in an adult with Huntington's disease. *J Neurol Neurosurg Psychiatry* 1998; 65: 577–9.
156. Reuter I, Hu MT, Andrews TC, Brooks DJ, Clough C, Chaudhuri KR. Late onset levodopa responsive Huntington's disease with minimal chorea masquerading as Parkinson plus syndrome. *J Neurol Neurosurg Psychiatry* 2000; 68: 238–41.
157. Schneider SA, Walker RH, Bhatia KP. The Huntington's disease-like syndromes: what to consider in patients with a negative Huntington's disease gene test. *Nat Clin Pract Neurol* 2007; 3: 517–25.
158. Rampoldi L, Dobson-Stone C, Rubio JP, et al. A conserved sorting-associated protein is mutant in chorea-acanthocytosis. *Nat Genet* 2001; 28: 119–20.
159. Hardie RJ, Pullon HW, Harding AE, et al. Neuroacanthocytosis: a clinical, haematological and pathological study of 19 cases. *Brain* 1991; 114: 13–49.
160. Spitz MC, Jankovic J, Killian JM. Familial tic disorder, parkinsonism, motor neuron disease, and acanthocytosis: a new syndrome. *Neurology* 1985; 35: 366–70.
161. Rampoldi L, Danek A, Monaco AP. Clinical features and molecular bases of neuroacanthocytosis. *J Mol Med* 2002; 80: 475–91.
162. Bostantjopoulou S, Katsarou Z, Kazis A, Vadikolia C. Neuroacanthocytosis presenting as parkinsonism. *Mov Disord* 2000; 15: 1271–3.
163. Geser F, Tolnay M, Jung H. The neuropathology of McLeod syndrome. In: Walker RH, Saiki S, Danek A (eds) *Neuroacanthocytosis syndromes II*, pp. 197–204. New York: Springer, 2008.
164. Costello DJ, Walsh SL, Harrington HJ, Walsh CH. Concurrent hereditary haemochromatosis and idiopathic Parkinson's disease: a case report series. *J Neurol Neurosurg Psychiatry* 2004; 75: 631–3.
165. Schneider SA, Bhatia KP. Three faces of the same gene: FA2H links neurodegeneration with brain iron accumulation, leukodystrophies, and hereditary spastic paraplegias. *Ann Neurol* 2011; 68: 575–7.
166. Roze E, Cochen V, Sangla S, et al. Rett syndrome: an overlooked diagnosis in women with stereotypic hand movements, psychomotor retardation, Parkinsonism, and dystonia? *Mov Disord* 2007; 22: 387–9.
167. Papapetropoulos S, Friedman J, Blackstone C, Kleiner GI, Bowen BC, Singer C. A progressive, fatal dystonia–Parkinsonism syndrome in a patient with primary immunodeficiency receiving chronic IVIG therapy. *Mov Disord* 2007; 22: 1664–6.
168. Poorkaj P, Raskind WH, Leverenz JB, et al. A novel X-linked four-repeat tauopathy with Parkinsonism and spasticity. *Mov Disord*; 25: 1409–17.
169. Klein C, Schneider SA, Lang AE. Hereditary parkinsonism: Parkinson disease look-alikes—an algorithm for clinicians to 'PARK' genes and beyond. *Mov Disord* 2009; 24: 2042–58.

CHAPTER 13

Multiple System Atrophy (MSA)

Gregor K. Wenning and Florian Krismer

Summary

Multiple system atrophy (MSA) is an adult-onset atypical parkinsonian disorder (APD) characterized by either rapidly progressive levodopa-unresponsive parkinsonism or a cerebellar syndrome associated with early autonomic failure (1). According to current consensus criteria two motor subtypes can be distinguished clinically, namely a parkinsonian variant labelled MSA-P and a cerebellar variant labelled MSA-C (2). Abundant (oligodendro-) glial cytoplasmic inclusions (GCIs) represent the histopathological signature lesion that is accompanied by a selective neuronal multisystem degeneration (3). The principal component of GCIs is α-synuclein, a finding which firmly places MSA among other α-synucleinopathies such as Parkinson's disease (PD) and dementia with Lewy bodies (DLB) (4). Currently, the management of MSA patients is based on symptomatic treatment targeting parkinsonian and autonomic features. Although research into disease-modifying strategies has accelerated, effective neuroprotective treatments are still lacking (5).

Essential background

Epidemiology

MSA affects both sexes equally and the median age at disease onset is around 55 years. The patient's median survival is 9 years, with survival rates at 5 and 10 years of 83.5% and 39.9%, respectively (6–10). However, there is considerable variation in the rate of disease progression, with individual cases reported with survival for as long as 15 years. The annual incidence rate is 0.6 cases per 100 000 (11). MSA disease risk increases with age. In the age group above 50 years, the annual incidence rate is estimated to be 3 cases per 100 000 (11). The prevalence rate of MSA is estimated to be 4.4 per 100 000 (12).

Aetiology and genetics

There is little information on environmental and occupational risk factors in MSA. A North American case–control study reported increased frequencies of exposure to metal dusts and fumes, plastic monomers and additives, organic solvents, and pesticides in MSA patients compared with healthy controls (13). Another multicentre case–control study in Europe, of which only the methodology has been published (14), showed a significantly higher risk of developing MSA in subjects who had worked in agriculture (14). Smoking seems to be less frequent in MSA cases than in healthy controls (15). The fact that the inverse association with smoking found previously in PD is shared by MSA but not by progressive supranuclear palsy (PSP) lends epidemiological support to the notion that different smoking habits are associated with different groups of neurodegenerative disease (15). A French case–control study demonstrated that MSA was not associated with exposure to pesticides, solvents, and other occupational toxins. However, aspirin intake, alcohol consumption, and consumption of fish and seafood were more common in the control group (16).

MSA is generally considered to be a sporadic disease, but recent reports of familial clustering suggest the presence of monogenic MSA with autosomal inheritance (17–19). However, no MSA genes have been identified in these pedigrees so far. Intriguingly, two independent research groups have demonstrated an association of single-nucleotide polymorphisms within the α-synuclein gene (*SNCA*) and increased MSA disease risk (20, 21).

Pathophysiology

The underlying pathophysiology is not completely understood. According to the consensus criteria, widespread aggregates of misfolded proteins within oligodendroglial cells (GCI) are required for a definite diagnosis of MSA (2). These aggregates are composed of α-synuclein and an increasing number of other proteins (3). The origin of oligodendroglial α-synuclein remains to be determined as α-synuclein mRNA expression is absent in both healthy and MSA oligodendrocytes (22). Nonetheless, oligodendroglial dysfunction is regarded as a principal mechanism in MSA pathogenesis (23), and this has been further supported by the discovery of early phosphoprotein-25-alpha (p25α) accumulation in oligodendrocytes (23–25). p25α is a phosphoprotein functionally associated with myelination (26), but in MSA it appears to relocate within oligodendrocytes, shifting from the myelin sheath towards the cell bodies (25). Moreover, p25α has been shown to co-localize with α-synuclein-positive GCI in MSA brains, and *in vitro* data suggest that p25α favours the fibrillation of α-synuclein (25, 27). In summary, both the assumption that p25α misprocessing is the earliest detectable change in MSA and the observation that neuronal cells are relatively preserved when oligodendroglial involvement is present support the hypothesis that MSA is a primary oligodendrogliopathy followed by secondary neurodegeneration (23).

Clinical features

MSA is an adult-onset rapidly progressive disorder characterized clinically by two major motor features, namely parkinsonism and cerebellar ataxia. These motor features serve as the basis for labelling patients with predominant parkinsonism as MSA-P and those with cerebellar ataxia as MSA-C (2). In a prospective European patient registry analysis, almost 70% of cases were classified as MSA-P and autonomic failure was almost universally present in both variants (28). Intriguingly, MSA-C outnumbered MSA-P in a Japanese cohort (8). Autonomic failure in MSA includes urinary symptoms, such as urge incontinence and incomplete bladder emptying, and orthostatic hypotension (28).

Presenting symptoms

The most common initial motor disturbance in MSA is levodopa-refractory akinetic–rigid parkinsonism, which is present in 58% of cases (10). Nevertheless, in this series of pathologically confirmed MSA, 28% of patients had transient benefit from levodopa treatment (10). These effects lasted for a median duration of 3 years (28). In contrast with the post-mortem confirmed series, only a minority of MSA patients experienced levodopa-associated adverse effects such as dyskinesias (27% and 7% in the post-mortem confirmed and the prospective clinical series, respectively) and ON–OFF fluctuations (24% versus 3.5%) in a prospective clinical series (10, 28). The second most common initial motor disturbance was cerebellar ataxia, with 29% of MSA patients being affected (10). Unusual presenting symptoms in pathologically proven cases include stroke-like episodes evolving into parkinsonism and transient ischaemic attacks in the anterior or posterior circulation (29), as well as REM sleep behaviour disorder (30).

Established disease

Parkinsonism associated with MSA is characterized by bradykinesia, rigidity, postural tremor, and gait unsteadiness (28). Moreover, patients frequently exhibit orofacial dystonia associated with a characteristic quivering high-pitched dysarthria (31). Although postural instability is common in early stages of the disease course, recurrent falls at disease onset are unusual (32). It has been suggested that a symmetric atremulous picture might distinguish MSA-P from PD (33, 34). However, motor disturbance was asymmetric in 74% of patients in a clinical series, and unilateral symptoms at onset were present in 47% of literature cases (10). Furthermore, some sort of tremor was present in the majority of cases in a clinical series (10). Therefore the differential diagnosis of MSA-P and PD may be difficult in the early stages because of a number of overlapping features such as rest tremor or asymmetric akinesia and rigidity. Nevertheless, the characteristic clinical picture of MSA-P usually evolves within 5 years of disease onset, allowing a clinical diagnosis to be made with greater certainty during follow-up (6, 35).

The cerebellar disorder comprises gait ataxia, limb kinetic ataxia, and scanning dysarthria, as well as cerebellar oculomotor disturbances. Cerebellar signs, most commonly manifesting as a wide-based gait ataxia, developed in 34–64% of patients (9, 10, 28, 32). Sustained gaze-evoked nystagmus is detected in 23–35% of patients (9, 10, 28), and cerebellar scanning dysarthria may occur in up to 69% (28). The finding of a mixed dysarthria with combinations of hypokinetic, ataxic, and spastic components is consistent with both the overall clinical and the neuropathological changes in MSA (36). Cerebellar symptoms occur universally in MSA-C patients, and patients with MSA-P frequently also develop cerebellar ataxia. In an analysis of a European patient registry, cerebellar signs were observed in 47% of patients with MSA-P (28). On the other hand, patients with MSA-C commonly develop additional non-cerebellar symptoms and signs (28). Nevertheless, at early stages MSA-C patients may be indistinguishable from patients with related disorders, including idiopathic late-onset cerebellar ataxia (37).

Autonomic dysfunction comprising primarily urogenital and orthostatic dysfunction is almost universally present in the disease course of both MSA subtypes (28). However, a retrospective analysis of pathologically confirmed MSA cases suggests that early autonomic symptoms (within 2 years of disease onset) occur in more than half of the patients with MSA (6). In a clinical series urge incontinence was the most frequent symptom, followed by the appearance of incomplete bladder emptying in 73% and 48%, respectively, and both symptoms were present in a third of patients with MSA (28). These findings confirm previous studies which identified comparable frequencies (9, 10, 38–40). Overall, impairment of micturition in MSA occurs earlier, more frequently, and to a more severe degree than in PD (38). In a series of patients with probable MSA, 43 per cent of males had undergone futile prostatic or bladder neck surgery before the correct diagnosis was made, although more than half of them had neurological symptoms or signs at the time of the procedure (38). Stress incontinence occurred in 57% of the women, and half of these underwent pelvic surgery with disappointing results (38, 41). Early impotence is universally present in men with MSA. In a series of 62 MSA patients, impotence occurred in 96% of the men and was the first symptom in 37% (38). These results were underpinned by a recent prospective study observing erectile dysfunction in 84 per cent of male patients with MSA (28). Reduced genital sensitivity with or without impaired libido has been reported in the majority of female MSA patients (42).

Orthostatic dysregulation is the second most common feature of autonomic dysfunction in MSA. Consensus criteria require a systolic blood pressure drop of at least 30 mmHg or a fall in diastolic blood pressure of 15 mmHg for the diagnosis of MSA-associated orthostatic hypotension (2). Characteristic symptoms of orthostatic hypotension include light-headedness, visual blurring, dizziness, pre-syncope, and recurrent syncopal episodes. Intriguingly, recurrent syncope (more than three falls) was reported in only 15% of subjects, whereas postural faintness was present in up to 53% (9, 10, 40). These findings were confirmed in a recent clinical series estimating the frequency of orthostatic complaints and recurrent falls to be 60% and 20%, respectively (28). Orthostatic symptoms may be further aggravated by dopaminergic drugs, fluid depletion, extensive food ingestion, and general physical deconditioning. Indeed, patients with autonomic failure are susceptible to substantial drops in blood pressure after high carbohydrate intake and sufficient fluid intake may beneficially alter orthostatic dysregulation (43–45). In severe cardiovascular autonomic failure, the loss of baroreflexes may cause recumbent arterial hypertension (46). Finally, the emergence of early autonomic failure in MSA patients within 2.5 years after disease onset is an independent predictor of rapid disease progression and reduced survival (6, 47).

Anhidrosis or hypohidrosis occur frequently in patients with MSA (48). However, the underlying site of the lesion is not well established. Although postganglionic structures might be involved in MSA-associated sudomotor dysfunction, anhidrosis in patients with MSA is mainly caused by preganglionic impairment. A recent prospective study suggested that there was more severe and diffuse anhidrosis in MSA patients than in PD patients (49). Additionally, impaired sympathetic skin response, altered heat tolerance, and skin temperature dysregulation have been described in MSA (48, 50, 51). Finally, patients with MSA often present with cold dusky violaceous hands and poor circulatory return after blanching by pressure, suggestive of impairment in neurovascular control of the distal extremities ('cold blue hand sign') (52). This finding is a clinical 'red flag' that should raise the suspicion of MSA (53). In addition, some patients may also develop a Raynaud-like phenomenon (54).

Sialorrhoea is a frequent and disabling condition in patients with parkinsonian conditions, and is an expression of swallowing difficulties rather than excessive saliva production (55, 56). Furthermore, severe dysphagia, which can be found in a third of patients with MSA-P, is an additional clinical 'red flag', suggesting bulbar dysfunction (53).

Although the literature on MSA-associated constipation is limited, it is widely accepted that patients with MSA experience reduced bowel frequency (57, 58) and difficulties in evacuation (58). Indeed, in an analysis of the European MSA registry, a third of MSA patients complained of chronic constipation (28). The underlying mechanism involves the degeneration of sacral autonomic nuclei, particularly Onuf's nucleus (59).

Diagnosis

According to clinical consensus criteria, patients with MSA are classified into two subtypes according to the predominant motor presentation. Patients with parkinsonism are designated MSA-P, and if cerebellar ataxia predominates the label MSA-C is recommended (2). However, many patients presenting with parkinsonism show ataxia during the disease course, and vice versa. Hence, the designation MSA-P or MSA-C refers to the predominant feature at the time the patient is evaluated, and the predominant feature can change with time. Nevertheless, in the western hemisphere MSA-P is more common (68% of cases) (28), whereas in a Japanese study MSA-C was observed more frequently (70% of cases) (8). In addition, autonomic failure is observed universally in both motor presentations.

The challenge of diagnosing MSA-P is aggravated by the fact that MSA and PD share not only parkinsonian features, but also numerous non-motor symptoms, as shown in several clinicopathological and prospective clinical studies. Indeed, in a clinicopathological study conducted by Litvan et al. (60), primary neurologists (who performed clinical follow-ups) identified only 25% of MSA patients correctly at the first visit (on average at 42 months after disease onset). Because of this overlap, MSA and PD are frequently indistinguishable in the early course of the disease, even when formal criteria are applied (61). Consistent with this observation, most of the MSA patients identified in the epidemiological survey by Schrag et al. (12) were diagnosed during the study period, emphasizing the fact that MSA is poorly recognized in clinical practice (35).

Clinical diagnostic criteria

The diagnosis of MSA is based on history and physical examination. The first set of diagnostic criteria for MSA was proposed by Quinn in 1989 (57), and slightly modified in 1994 (62). Optimized diagnostic criteria were developed during an International Consensus Conference held in 1998 (63). However, clinical advances in MSA required a revision of the consensus criteria (2). These criteria specify three levels of increasing certainty: possible, probable, and definite MSA. While definite MSA requires post-mortem confirmation of neuronal multisystem degeneration and the proof of abundant GCIs (3), the diagnosis of probable and possible MSA relies on clinical and neuroimaging features (2). Probable MSA requires clear evidence of autonomic failure, including orthostatic hypotension (i.e. decrease of blood pressure by at least 30 mmHg systolic or 15 mmHg diastolic within 3 min of standing) and urinary dysfunction (i.e. inability to control bladder emptying) in association with either levodopa-refractory parkinsonism or a cerebellar syndrome (Table 13.1) (2). Possible MSA is characterized as sporadic progressive adult-onset disease with either parkinsonism or a cerebellar syndrome associated with at least one feature suggesting autonomic failure and one additional feature suggestive of MSA according to consensus criteria (Table 13.2) (2). Disease onset is defined as the first occurrence of any motor symptom or the involvement of autonomic pathways determined by suggestive autonomic symptoms, with the exception of male erectile dysfunction (2). Table 13.3 lists the 'red flags' for MSA, which are features that support a diagnosis of MSA, and Table 13.4 lists the findings that do not support a diagnosis of MSA according to consensus criteria (2).

Management

Currently, disease-modifying medical treatments are lacking. Hence the management of MSA rests largely on the alleviation of parkinsonian and autonomic symptoms. Although autonomic failure is almost universally present in MSA, only a third of affected patients receive appropriate pharmacological treatment (28).

Neuroprotective strategies

Substantial progress towards underlying pathogenic mechanisms as well as the development of diagnostic consensus criteria and MSA-specific rating scales have allowed clinical investigators to conduct multisite randomized controlled trials to test the efficacy of

Table 13.1 Diagnostic criteria for probable MSA

A sporadic, progressive, adult (>30 y)–onset disease characterized by:

- Autonomic failure involving urinary incontinence (inability to control the release of urine from the bladder, with erectile dysfunction in males) or an orthostatic decrease of blood pressure within 3 min of standing by at least 30 mmHg systolic or 15 mmHg diastolic *AND*
- Poorly levodopa-responsive parkinsonism (bradykinesia with rigidity, tremor, or postural instability) *OR*
- A cerebellar syndrome (gait ataxia with cerebellar dysarthria, limb ataxia, or cerebellar oculomotor dysfunction)

Modified according to Gilman et al. (2) and reproduced from Wenning and Stefanova (106) (with kind permission of Springer Science+Business Media).

Table 13.2 Diagnostic criteria for possible MSA

A sporadic progressive adult-onset (>30 years) disease characterized by:
◆ Parkinsonism (bradykinesia with rigidity, tremor, or postural instability) *OR*
◆ A cerebellar syndrome (gait ataxia with cerebellar dysarthria, limb ataxia, or cerebellar oculomotor dysfunction) *AND*
◆ At least one feature suggesting autonomic dysfunction (otherwise unexplained urinary urgency, frequency, or incomplete bladder emptying, erectile dysfunction in males, or significant orthostatic blood pressure decline that does not meet the level required in probable MSA) *AND*
◆ At least one of the additional features:
◆ Possible MSA-P or MSA-C
• Babinski sign with hyperreflexia
• Stridor
◆ Possible MSA-P
• Rapidly progressive parkinsonism
• Poor response to levodopa
• Postural instability within 3 years of motor onset
• Gait ataxia, cerebellar dysarthria, limb ataxia, or cerebellar oculomotor dysfunction
• Dysphagia within 5 years of motor onset
• Atrophy on MRI of putamen, middle cerebellar peduncle, pons, or cerebellum
• Hypometabolism on FDG-PET in putamen, brainstem, or cerebellum
◆ Possible MSA-C
• Parkinsonism (bradykinesia and rigidity)
• Atrophy on MRI of putamen, middle cerebellar peduncle, or pons
• Hypometabolism on FDG-PET in putamen
• Presynaptic nigrostriatal dopaminergic denervation on SPECT or PET

Modified according to Gilman et al. (2) and reproduced from Wenning and Stefanova (106) (with kind permission of Springer Science+Business Media).

Table 13.3 Red flags for MSA

◆ Orofacial dystonia
◆ Disproportionate antecollis
◆ Camptocormia (severe anterior flexion of the spine) and/or Pisa syndrome (severe lateral flexion of the spine)
◆ Contractures of hands or feet
◆ Inspiratory sighs
◆ Severe dysphonia
◆ Severe dysarthria
◆ New or increased snoring
◆ Cold hands and feet
◆ Pathological laughter or crying
◆ Jerky myoclonic postural/action tremor

Modified according to Gilman et al. (2) and reproduced from Wenning and Stefanova (106) (with kind permission of Springer Science+Business Media).

Table 13.4 Non-supporting features of MSA

◆ Classic pill-rolling rest tremor
◆ Clinically significant neuropathy
◆ Onset after age of 75 years
◆ Family history of ataxia or parkinsonism
◆ Dementia (on DSM-IV)
◆ White matter lesions suggesting multiple sclerosis
◆ Hallucinations not induced by drugs

Modified according to Gilman et al. (2) and reproduced from Wenning and Stefanova (106) (with kind permission of Springer Science+Business Media).

candidate targets (5). Unfortunately, every multicentre randomized controlled trial so far has failed to confirm disease modification of candidate drugs. However, a placebo-controlled double-blind trial assessing the therapeutic value of recombinant human growth hormone (r-HGH) in patients with MSA revealed a trend towards reduction in progression of motor symptoms that failed to reach significance (64). After confirming the neuroprotective effects of minocycline in a pre-clinical MSA study (65) and in models of related neurodegenerative disorders (66, 67), this broad-spectrum tetracycline antibiotic was assessed in a phase II trial. This multisite trial conducted by the European MSA study group (EMSA-SG) (http: // www.emsa-sg.org) failed to show a clinical effect on symptom severity assessed by clinical motor function. Interestingly, data acquired by ^{11}C-(R)-PK11195 positron emission tomography (PET) suggested that minocycline may interfere with microglial activation (68). Another candidate drug which was assessed in a multisite setting was the antiglutamatergic agent riluzole (32). This study confirmed previous results obtained in a randomized controlled pilot trial proving riluzole to be ineffective. In contrast, a rather controversial trial was conducted by a South Korean research group which assessed efficacy and feasibility of autologous mesenchymal stem cell therapy. These stem cells appeared to delay the progression of neurological deficits in patients with MSA (69). Meanwhile, preclinical evidence supported a putative neuroprotective efficacy of these stem cells, suggesting trans-differentiation and the induction of non-specific immunological responses as underlying mechanisms (70).

Symptomatic treatment

Autonomic failure

Autonomic symptoms have a major impact on the quality of life, and therefore it is essential to treat autonomic failure thoroughly. Furthermore, because of the progressive course of MSA a regular treatment review is mandatory to adjust measures according to clinical needs.

A broad range of drugs have been used in the treatment of postural hypotension. Unfortunately, the benefits and side effects of many of these drugs have not been evaluated in MSA patients in randomized controlled trials. However, the concept of treatment of orthostatic hypotension is based on increasing intravascular volume and the prevention of blood pooling in lower body parts.

Non-pharmacological options include sufficient fluid intake, a high-salt diet, more frequent, but smaller, meals (spreading of total daily carbohydrate intake) to reduce postprandial hypotension, and custom-made elastic body garments. Head-up tilt during the night increases intravascular volume by up to 1 litre within a week, which is particularly helpful for improving early morning hypotension. The beneficial effects of this approach can be enhanced by the prescription of fludrocortisone, which further supports sodium retention (44).

Among the large number of vasoactive agents that have been evaluated in MSA, only one, the directly acting α-agonist midodrine, complies with the criteria of evidence based medicine (71, 72). Side effects are usually mild and rarely require withdrawal of treatment. The most frequent adverse effects are supine hypertension, urinary retention, goose bumps and paresthesias including troublesome scalp-tingling. Additionally, the parasympathomimetic and reversible cholinesterase inhibitor pyridostigmine provides a moderate but significant improvement in orthostatic hypotension via enhanced sympathetic activity (73).

Another promising drug appears to be the noradrenaline precursor L-threo-dihydroxy-phenylserine (L-threo DOPS, droxidopa), which is widely used in Japan and whose efficacy has been demonstrated in two double-blind placebo-controlled trials (74, 75).

Furthermore, octreotide, which is a somatostatin analogue, might alleviate postprandial hypotension without causing or increasing nocturnal hypertension (76). This effect is probably mediated by the inhibition of the release of vasodilatory gastrointestinal peptides (77). Additionally, the vasopressin analogue, desmopressin, which acts on renal tubular vasopressin-2 receptors, reduces nocturnal polyuria and improves early-morning postural hypotension (78). Sympathomimetics, such as ephedrine, have both direct and indirect effects which might be useful in central autonomic dysfunction. However, side effects arise with higher doses, including tremulousness, loss of appetite, and urinary retention, particularly in men.

The peptide erythropoietin may be beneficial in some patients, particularly in those with erythropoietin-associated normocytic normochromic anaemia. The substitution of erythropoietin increases red blood cell mass and subsequently improves cerebral oxygenation (79, 80). Interestingly, the neuroprotective effects of erythropoietin were demonstrated in a preclinical study of MSA (81).

With regard to neurogenic bladder dysfunction presenting with post-void residual volumes, clean intermittent catheterization three to four times per day is a widely accepted approach to prevent secondary consequences. If mechanical obstruction in the urethra or motor symptoms of MSA prevent uncomplicated catheterization, permanent transcutaneous suprapubic catheterization may become necessary (82).

Pharmacological options including anticholinergic, procholinergic, and adrenergic substances are not usually successful in adequately reducing post-void residual volume in MSA. However, anticholinergic agents, such as oxybutynin, can improve symptoms of detrusor hyperreflexia or sphincter–detrusor dyssynergia early in the course of the disease (38). Anticholinergic treatment might be dose limited by central nervous adverse effects. More recently, a peripherally acting anticholinergic agent, trospium chloride, has been shown to be equally effective in patients with detrusor hyperreflexia without causing central nervous adverse effects (83). Nevertheless, this drug has not yet been specifically investigated in MSA patients. Finally, α-adrenergic receptor antagonists (prazosin and moxisylyte) have been shown to improve voiding with reduction of residual volumes in MSA patients (84).

The necessity for specific treatment of sexual dysfunction needs to be evaluated individually in each patient. The phosphodiesterase type 5 inhibitor sildenafil improved male erectile function in a placebo-controlled double-blind study (85). However, sildenafil may only be prescribed after exclusion of severe postural hypotension, as this compound may unmask or worsen orthostatic hypotension. Furthermore, male impotence can be partially amended by the use of intracavernosal papaverine (86), apomorphine (87), prostaglandin E1, or penile implants (88). Finally, erectile failure in MSA may also be improved by oral yohimbine (38).

With regard to gastrointestinal symptoms, such as constipation, non-pharmacological treatment should be considered first. This includes daily exercise, high fluid and fibre intake, and the consumption of fruit juices. If laxative therapy becomes necessary, polycarbophil and mosapride citrate may relieve constipation symptoms, as suggested by two small open-label studies (89). An increase in intraluminal fluid, which can be achieved with a macrogol–water solution, may alleviate such symptoms as well (90).

Inspiratory stridor develops in about 30% of patients. Therapeutic approaches include the use of continuous positive airway pressure (CPAP), which may attenuate sleep apnoea and nocturnal stridor (91). However, in severe cases tracheostomy may be required.

Motor symptoms

General approach

Although some patients may benefit from drug treatment of MSA motor symptoms in the short term, the long-term results are generally considered to be poor. Therefore non-pharmacological therapies are even more important. Physiotherapy helps to maintain mobility and prevent contractures. Furthermore, speech therapy can not only improve speech and swallowing, but also provide communication aids. Severe dysphagia with pulmonary penetration of ingested food and fluids may require feeding by nasogastric tube or even percutaneous endoscopic gastrostomy (PEG). Occupational therapy with regular home visits may limit the burden resulting from the patient's disabilities. Provision of a four-wheel walker, and subsequently a wheelchair, is usually dictated by the liability of falls because of postural instability and gait ataxia, but not by akinesia and rigidity per se. Psychological support improves the quality of life for patients and their families.

Parkinsonism

Parkinsonism is the predominating motor symptom of MSA-P and therefore is a major target for symptomatic treatment. Despite the lack of randomized controlled trials, levodopa is the most frequently used antiparkinsonian agent in MSA. An analysis of a multisite patient registry revealed that up to 40% of MSA patients benefit from levodopa treatment (28). Unfortunately, this response is often transient, lasting for 3 years on average (92). Pre-existing orthostatic hypotension is often unmasked or exacerbated by levodopa treatment in patients with MSA. In contrast, psychiatric or toxic confusional states appear to be less common than in PD (9).

Treatment with dopamine agonists has been disappointing. Severe psychiatric side effects occurred in a double-blind crossover trial of six patients treated with lisuride, with nightmares, visual hallucinations, and toxic confusional states (93). Wenning et al. (9) reported a response to oral dopamine agonists in only four of forty-one patients; none of thirty patients receiving bromocriptine improved, but four of ten who received pergolide had some benefit. Twenty-two percent of the levodopa responders had good or excellent response to at least one dopamine agonist (9). Pathological hypersexuality, predominantly linked to adjuvant dopamine agonist treatment, has been reported in two MSA patients (94). Amantadine produced antiparkinsonian effects in four out of twenty-six MSA patients (9); however, there was no significant improvement in another open study of nine patients with atypical parkinsonian conditions, including five MSA patients (95). A more recent randomized placebo-controlled trial confirmed these observations by demonstrating amantadine to be ineffective in MSA patients (96). Interestingly, the selective serotonin-reuptake inhibitor paroxetine improved motor abilities of the upper limb and speech (97). In contrast with observations in PD, anticholinergics did not improve motor function in MSA; however, they may be helpful in alleviating severe and disturbing sialorrhoea.

Ten per cent of MSA patients show dystonia (28). Local botulinum toxin injections are effective in orofacial dystonia, including blepharospasm and limb dystonia (98). However, botulinum toxin injections should be avoided in the therapy of disproportionate antecollis as severe dysphagia resulting in the need for a nasogastric feeding tube has been reported (99).

Similarly to PD, sialorrhoea probably results from swallowing difficulty and may be substantially decreased by diminution of salivary production using botulinum toxin injections into the parotid and submandibular glands, as suggested by a double-blind placebo controlled trial (56).

Cerebellar ataxia

Cerebellar ataxia is the clinical hallmark of MSA-C and present in nearly two-thirds of MSA patients (28). Currently, there is no effective pharmacological treatment for MSA-associated cerebellar ataxia, although several case reports suggest beneficial effects mediated by a variety of compounds including cholinergics, NMDA receptor antagonists, derivatives of γ-aminobutyric acid, non-selective beta-blockers, 5-hydroxytryptophan, and isoniazid. However, none of these medications has been proved to be effective in larger patient series (31).

Key advances

Important advances in the understanding of MSA have been achieved in the last decade. Not only the revision of clinical consensus diagnostic criteria subdividing MSA according to the predominance of parkinsonism versus ataxia into MSA-P and MSA-C (2), but also the development and validation of clinical rating scales, including the unified MSA rating scale (UMSARS) (100) and MSA-QoL (101), will allow investigators to conduct multicentre clinical trials. Furthermore, research into functional and structural neuroimaging tools for early diagnosis and progression monitoring have provided surrogate markers which can be used in clinical trials (102). Finally, the development of animal models (103, 104) has permitted the testing of hypotheses regarding pathogenesis and accelerated preclinical research into disease-modifying drugs (5).

Future developments

In the forthcoming years, research into underlying pathogenic mechanisms of MSA will accelerate. Advances in the genetics and the molecular biology of this fatal disorder will permit researchers to develop novel interventional therapies targeting key pathogenic events. The early diagnosis of MSA will become even more important as disease-modifying therapies enter clinics. Therefore we will see an accelerated research into neuroimaging as well as into genomic and proteomic biomarkers. In preclinical research, we will see intensified efforts to develop additional animal models for thorough characterization of the effects and reversibility of α-synuclein-mediated toxicity.

Conclusion

The development of animal models replicating the human phenotype has led to substantial progress towards the understanding of underlying pathogenic mechanisms of MSA (5). At the same time, clinical consensus diagnostic criteria and specific rating scales assessing clinical symptoms and disability have greatly facilitated large multicentre trials (2, 100, 101). Finally, candidate SNP studies have identified variants of the α-synuclein gene with significantly increased disease risk (20, 21), reinforcing current basic research activities that address the role of α-synuclein toxicity in MSA pathogenesis (105). Unfortunately, we are not yet able to alter the course of MSA; however, recent progress will accelerate research into novel interventional therapies.

Top clinical tips

- MSA is an orphan disease with approximately 30 000 cases in EU countries.
- MSA is an atypical parkinsonian disorder with prominent autonomic failure and variably ataxia.
- MSA is an α-synucleinopathy associated with glial cytoplasmic inclusions and neuronal multisystem degeneration.
- Genetic vulnerability in MSA is reflected by association studies and familial MSA.
- Symptomatic therapy targets orthostatic hypertension, urogenital failure, and parkinsonism (levodopa response in 30%).
- Transgenic models of MSA are now available for target detection and drug development.
- There are now MSA research networks in Europe (http://www.emsa-sg.org), the USA, and Japan.

References

1. Wenning GK, Colosimo C, Geser F, Poewe W. Multiple system atrophy. *Lancet Neurol* 2004; 3: 93–103.
2. Gilman S, Wenning GK, Low PA, et al. Second consensus statement on the diagnosis of multiple system atrophy. *Neurology* 2008; 71: 670–6.
3. Trojanowski JQ, Revesz T. Proposed neuropathological criteria for the post mortem diagnosis of multiple system atrophy. *Neuropathol Appl Neurobiol* 2007; 33: 615–20.
4. Spillantini MG, Crowther RA, Jakes R, Cairns NJ, Lantos PL, Goedert M. Filamentous alpha-synuclein inclusions link multiple system atrophy with Parkinson's disease and dementia with Lewy bodies. *Neurosci Lett* 1998; 251: 205–8.
5. Stefanova N, Bucke P, Duerr S, Wenning GK. Multiple system atrophy: an update. *Lancet Neurol* 2009; 8: 1172–8.
6. O'Sullivan SS, Massey LA, Williams DR, et al. Clinical outcomes of progressive supranuclear palsy and multiple system atrophy. *Brain* 2008; 131: 1362–72.
7. Testa D, Filippini G, Farinotti M, Palazzini E, Caraceni T. Survival in multiple system atrophy: a study of prognostic factors in 59 cases. *J Neurol* 1996; 243: 401–4.
8. Watanabe H, Saito Y, Terao S, et al. Progression and prognosis in multiple system atrophy: an analysis of 230 Japanese patients. *Brain* 2002; 125: 1070–83.
9. Wenning GK, Ben Shlomo Y, Magalhaes M, Daniel SE, Quinn NP. Clinical features and natural history of multiple system atrophy. An analysis of 100 cases. *Brain* 1994; 117: 835–45.
10. Wenning GK, Tison F, Ben Shlomo Y, Daniel SE, Quinn NP. Multiple system atrophy: a review of 203 pathologically proven cases. *Mov Disord* 1997; 12: 133–47.
11. Bower JH, Maraganore DM, McDonnell SK, Rocca WA. Incidence of progressive supranuclear palsy and multiple system atrophy in Olmsted County, Minnesota, 1976 to 1990. *Neurology* 1997; 49: 1284–8.

12. Schrag A, Ben-Shlomo Y, Quinn NP. Prevalence of progressive supranuclear palsy and multiple system atrophy: a cross-sectional study. *Lancet* 1999; 354: 1771–5.
13. Nee LE, Gomez MR, Dambrosia J, Bale S, Eldridge R, Polinsky RJ. Environmental-occupational risk factors and familial associations in multiple system atrophy: a preliminary investigation. *Clin Auton Res* 1991; 1: 9–13.
14. Vanacore N, Bonifati V, Fabbrini G, et al. Epidemiology of multiple system atrophy. ESGAP Consortium. European Study Group on Atypical Parkinsonisms. *Neurol Sci* 2001; 22: 97–9.
15. Vanacore N, Bonifati V, Fabbrini G, et al. Smoking habits in multiple system atrophy and progressive supranuclear palsy. European Study Group on Atypical Parkinsonisms. *Neurology* 2000; 54: 114–19.
16. Vidal JS, Vidailhet M, Elbaz A, Derkinderen P, Tzourio C, Alperovitch A. Risk factors of multiple system atrophy: a case–control study in French patients. *Mov Disord* 2008; 23: 797–803.
17. Hara K, Momose Y, Tokiguchi S, et al. Multiplex families with multiple system atrophy. *Arch Neurol* 2007; 64: 545–51.
18. Wullner U, Abele M, Schmitz-Huebsch T, et al. Probable multiple system atrophy in a German family. *J Neurol Neurosurg Psychiatry* 2004; 75: 924–5.
19. Wullner U, Schmitz-Hubsch T, Abele M, Antony G, Bauer P, Eggert K. Features of probable multiple system atrophy patients identified among 4770 patients with parkinsonism enrolled in the multicentre registry of the German Competence Network on Parkinson's disease. *J Neural Transm* 2007; 114: 1161–5.
20. Al-Chalabi A, Durr A, Wood NW, et al. Genetic variants of the alpha-synuclein gene SNCA are associated with multiple system atrophy. *PLoS One* 2009; 4: e7114.
21. Scholz SW, Houlden H, Schulte C, et al. SNCA variants are associated with increased risk for multiple system atrophy. *Ann Neurol* 2009; 65: 610–14.
22. Miller DW, Johnson JM, Solano SM, Hollingsworth ZR, Standaert DG, Young AB. Absence of alpha-synuclein mRNA expression in normal and multiple system atrophy oligodendroglia. *J Neural Transm* 2005 Dec; 112: 1613–24.
23. Wenning GK, Stefanova N, Jellinger KA, Poewe W, Schlossmacher MG. Multiple system atrophy: a primary oligodendrogliopathy. *Ann Neurol* 2008; 64: 239–46.
24. Kovacs GG, Gelpi E, Lehotzky A, et al. The brain-specific protein TPPP/p25 in pathological protein deposits of neurodegenerative diseases. *Acta Neuropathol*; 113: 153–61.
25. Song YJ, Lundvig DM, Huang Y, et al. p25alpha relocalizes in oligodendroglia from myelin to cytoplasmic inclusions in multiple system atrophy. *Am J Pathol* 2007; 171: 1291–303.
26. Takahashi M, Tomizawa K, Ishiguro K, et al. A novel brain-specific 25 kDa protein (p25) is phosphorylated by a Ser/Thr-Pro kinase (TPK II) from tau protein kinase fractions. *FEBS Lett* 1991; 289: 37–43.
27. Lindersson E, Lundvig D, Petersen C, et al. p25alpha stimulates alpha-synuclein aggregation and is co-localized with aggregated alpha-synuclein in alpha-synucleinopathies. *J Biol Chem* 2005; 280: 5703–15.
28. Köllensperger M, Geser F, Ndayisaba JP, et al. Presentation, diagnosis, and management of multiple system atrophy in Europe: final analysis of the European multiple system atrophy registry. *Mov Disord* 2010; 25: 2604–12.
29. Klein C, Wenning GK, Quinn NP. [Pseudotransitory ischemic attacks as the initial symptom of multiple system atrophy.] *Nervenarzt* 1995; 66: 133–5.
30. Tison F, Wenning GK, Quinn NP, Smith SJ. REM sleep behaviour disorder as the presenting symptom of multiple system atrophy. *J Neurol Neurosurg Psychiatry* 1995; 58: 379–80.
31. Wenning GK, Geser F, Stampfer-Kountchev M, Tison F. Multiple system atrophy: an update. *Mov Disord* 2003; 18 (Suppl 6): S34–42.
32. Bensimon G, Ludolph A, Agid Y, Vidailhet M, Payan C, Leigh PN. Riluzole treatment, survival and diagnostic criteria in Parkinson plus disorders: the NNIPPS study. *Brain* 2009; 132: 156–71.
33. Albanese A, Colosimo C, Bentivoglio AR, et al. Multiple system atrophy presenting as parkinsonism: clinical features and diagnostic criteria. *J Neurol Neurosurg Psychiatry* 1995; 59: 144–51.
34. Fearnley JM, Lees AJ. Striatonigral degeneration: a clinicopathological study. *Brain* 1990; 113: 1823–42.
35. Wenning GK, Ben Shlomo Y, Hughes A, Daniel SE, Lees A, Quinn NP. What clinical features are most useful to distinguish definite multiple system atrophy from Parkinson's disease? *J Neurol Neurosurg Psychiatry* 2000; 68: 434–40.
36. Kluin KJ, Gilman S, Lohman M, Junck L. Characteristics of the dysarthria of multiple system atrophy. *Arch Neurol* 1996; 53: 545–8.
37. Abele M, Burk K, Schols L, et al. The aetiology of sporadic adult-onset ataxia. *Brain* 2002; 125: 961–8.
38. Beck RO, Betts CD, Fowler CJ. Genitourinary dysfunction in multiple system atrophy: clinical features and treatment in 62 cases. *J Urol* 1994; 151: 1336–41.
39. Sakakibara R, Hattori T, Uchiyama T, Kita K, Asahina M, Suzuki A, et al. Urinary dysfunction and orthostatic hypotension in multiple system atrophy: which is the more common and earlier manifestation? *J Neurol Neurosurg Psychiatry* 2000; 68: 65–9.
40. Wenning GK, Scherfler C, Granata R, et al. Time course of symptomatic orthostatic hypotension and urinary incontinence in patients with postmortem confirmed parkinsonian syndromes: a clinicopathological study. *J Neurol Neurosurg Psychiatry* 1999; 67: 620–3.
41. Chandiramani VA, Palace J, Fowler CJ. How to recognize patients with parkinsonism who should not have urological surgery. *Br J Urol* 1997; 80: 100–4.
42. Oertel WH, Wachter T, Quinn NP, Ulm G, Brandstadter D. Reduced genital sensitivity in female patients with multiple system atrophy of parkinsonian type. *Mov Disord* 2003; 18: 430–2.
43. Deguchi K, Ikeda K, Shimamura M, et al. Assessment of autonomic dysfunction of multiple system atrophy with laryngeal abductor paralysis as an early manifestation. *Clin Neurol Neurosurg* 2007; 109: 892–5.
44. Freeman R. Current pharmacologic treatment for orthostatic hypotension. *Clin Auton Res* 2008r; 18 (Suppl 1): 14–18.
45. Lipsitz LA, Ryan SM, Parker JA, Freeman R, Wei JY, Goldberger AL. Hemodynamic and autonomic nervous system responses to mixed meal ingestion in healthy young and old subjects and dysautonomic patients with postprandial hypotension. *Circulation* 1993; 87: 391–400.
46. Bannister R, Mathias CJ. Clinical features and evaluation of the primary chronic autonomic failure syndromes. In: Mathias CJ, Bannister R (eds) *Autonomic failure*, pp. 307–16. Oxford: Oxford University Press, 1999.
47. Tada M, Onodera O, Ozawa T, et al. Early development of autonomic dysfunction may predict poor prognosis in patients with multiple system atrophy. *Arch Neurol* 2007; 64: 256–60.
48. Cohen J, Low P, Fealey R, Sheps S, Jiang NS. Somatic and autonomic function in progressive autonomic failure and multiple system atrophy. *Ann Neurol* 1987; 22: 692–9.
49. Lipp A, Sandroni P, Ahlskog JE, et al. Prospective differentiation of multiple system atrophy from Parkinson disease, with and without autonomic failure. *Arch Neurol* 2009; 66: 742–50.
50. Sandroni P, Ahlskog JE, Fealey RD, Low PA. Autonomic involvement in extrapyramidal and cerebellar disorders. *Clin Auton Res* 1991; 1: 147–55.
51. Kihara M, Sugenoya J, Takahashi A. The assessment of sudomotor dysfunction in multiple system atrophy. *Clin Auton Res* 1991; 1: 297–302.
52. Klein C, Brown R, Wenning G, Quinn N. The 'cold hands sign' in multiple system atrophy. *Mov Disord* 1997; 12: 514–18.
53. Kollensperger M, Geser F, Seppi K, et al. Red flags for multiple system atrophy. *Mov Disord* 2008; 23: 1093–9.
54. Santens P, Crevits L, van der Linden C. Raynaud's phenomenon in a case of multiple system atrophy. *Mov Disord* 1996; 11: 586–8.
55. Friedman A, Potulska A. Quantitative assessment of parkinsonian sialorrhea and results of treatment with botulinum toxin. *Parkinsonism Relat Disord* 2001; 7: 329–32.

56. Mancini F, Zangaglia R, Cristina S, et al. Double-blind, placebo-controlled study to evaluate the efficacy and safety of botulinum toxin type A in the treatment of drooling in parkinsonism. *Mov Disord* 2003; 18: 685–8.
57. Quinn N. Multiple system atrophy—the nature of the beast. *J Neurol Neurosurg Psychiatry* 1989; 52 (Suppl): 78–89.
58. Sakakibara R, Odaka T, Uchiyama T, et al. Colonic transit time, sphincter EMG, and rectoanal videomanometry in multiple system atrophy. *Mov Disord* 2004; 19: 924–9.
59. Yamamoto T, Sakakibara R, Uchiyama T, et al. When is Onuf's nucleus involved in multiple system atrophy? A sphincter electromyography study. *J Neurol Neurosurg Psychiatry* 2005; 76: 1645–8.
60. Litvan I, Goetz CG, Jankovic J, et al. What is the accuracy of the clinical diagnosis of multiple system atrophy? A clinicopathologic study. *Arch Neurol* 1997; 54: 937–44.
61. Osaki Y, Ben-Shlomo Y, Lees AJ, Wenning GK, Quinn NP. A validation exercise on the new consensus criteria for multiple system atrophy. *Mov Disord* 2009; 24: 2272–6.
62. Quinn N, Wenning G. Multiple system atrophy. *Br J Hosp Med* 1994; 51: 492–4.
63. Gilman S, Low P, Quinn N, Albanese A, Ben-Shlomo Y, Fowler C, et al. Consensus statement on the diagnosis of multiple system atrophy. American Autonomic Society and American Academy of Neurology. *Clin Auton Res* 1998; 8: 359–62.
64. Holmberg B, Johansson JO, Poewe W, et al. Safety and tolerability of growth hormone therapy in multiple system atrophy: a double-blind, placebo-controlled study. *Mov Disord* 2007; 22: 1138–44.
65. Stefanova N, Reindl M, Neumann M, Kahle PJ, Poewe W, Wenning GK. Microglial activation mediates neurodegeneration related to oligodendroglial alpha-synucleinopathy: implications for multiple system atrophy. *Mov Disord* 2007; 22: 2196–203.
66. Zhu S, Stavrovskaya IG, Drozda M, et al. Minocycline inhibits cytochrome c release and delays progression of amyotrophic lateral sclerosis in mice. *Nature* 2002; 417: 74–8.
67. Casarejos MJ, Menendez J, Solano RM, Rodriguez-Navarro JA, Garcia de Yebenes J, Mena MA. Susceptibility to rotenone is increased in neurons from parkin null mice and is reduced by minocycline. *J Neurochem* 2006; 97: 934–46.
68. Dodel R, Spottke A, Gerhard A, et al. Minocycline 1-year therapy in multiple-system-atrophy: effect on clinical symptoms and [^{11}C](R)-PK11195 PET (MEMSA-trial). *Mov Disord* 2010; 25: 97–107.
69. Lee PH, Kim JW, Bang OY, Ahn YH, Joo IS, Huh K. Autologous mesenchymal stem cell therapy delays the progression of neurological deficits in patients with multiple system atrophy. *Clin Pharmacol Ther* 2008; 83: 723–30.
70. Park HJ, Bang G, Lee BR, Kim HO, Lee PH. Neuroprotective effect of human mesenchymal stem cells in an animal model of double toxin-induced multiple system atrophy-parkinsonism. *Cell Transplant* 2011; 20: 827–35.
71. Jankovic J, Gilden JL, Hiner BC, et al. Neurogenic orthostatic hypotension: a double-blind, placebo-controlled study with midodrine. *Am J Med* 1993; 95: 38–48.
72. Low PA, Gilden JL, Freeman R, Sheng KN, McElligott MA. Efficacy of midodrine vs placebo in neurogenic orthostatic hypotension: a randomized, double-blind multicenter study. Midodrine Study Group. *JAMA* 1997; 277: 1046–51.
73. Singer W, Sandroni P, Opfer-Gehrking TL, et al. Pyridostigmine treatment trial in neurogenic orthostatic hypotension. *Arch Neurol* 2006; 63: 513–18.
74. Kaufmann H. L-dihydroxyphenylserine (droxidopa): a new therapy for neurogenic orthostatic hypotension: the US experience. *Clin Auton Res* 2008; 18 (Suppl 1): 19–24.
75. Mathias CJ. L-dihydroxyphenylserine (droxidopa) in the treatment of orthostatic hypotension: the European experience. *Clin Auton Res* 2008; 18 (Suppl 1): 25–9.
76. Alam M, Smith G, Bleasdale-Barr K, Pavitt DV, Mathias CJ. Effects of the peptide release inhibitor, octreotide, on daytime hypotension and on nocturnal hypertension in primary autonomic failure. *J Hypertens* 1995; 13: 1664–9.
77. Raimbach SJ, Cortelli P, Kooner JS, Bannister R, Bloom SR, Mathias CJ. Prevention of glucose-induced hypotension by the somatostatin analogue octreotide (SMS 201–995) in chronic autonomic failure: haemodynamic and hormonal changes. *Clin Sci (Lond)* 1989; 77: 623–8.
78. Mathias CJ, Fosbraey P, da Costa DF, Thornley A, Bannister R. The effect of desmopressin on nocturnal polyuria, overnight weight loss, and morning postural hypotension in patients with autonomic failure. *Br Med J (Clin Res Ed)* 1986; 293: 353–4.
79. Perera R, Isola L, Kaufmann H. Effect of recombinant erythropoietin on anemia and orthostatic hypotension in primary autonomic failure. *Clin Auton Res* 1995; 5: 211–13.
80. Winkler AS, Marsden J, Parton M, Watkins PJ, Chaudhuri KR. Erythropoietin deficiency and anaemia in multiple system atrophy. *Mov Disord* 2001; 16: 233–9.
81. Köllensperger M, Krismer F, Pallua A, Stefanova N, Poewe W, Wenning GK. Erythropoietin is neuroprotective in a transgenic mouse model of multiple system atrophy. *Mov Disord* 2011; 26: 507–15.
82. Fowler CJ, O'Malley KJ. Investigation and management of neurogenic bladder dysfunction. *J Neurol Neurosurg Psychiatry* 2003; 74 (Suppl 4): iv27–31.
83. Halaska M, Ralph G, Wiedemann A, et al. Controlled, double-blind, multicentre clinical trial to investigate long-term tolerability and efficacy of trospium chloride in patients with detrusor instability. *World J Urol* 2003 May; 20: 392–9.
84. Sakakibara R, Hattori T, Uchiyama T, et al. Are alpha-blockers involved in lower urinary tract dysfunction in multiple system atrophy? A comparison of prazosin and moxisylyte. *J Auton Nerv Syst* 2000; 79: 191–5.
85. Hussain IF, Brady CM, Swinn MJ, Mathias CJ, Fowler CJ. Treatment of erectile dysfunction with sildenafil citrate (Viagra) in parkinsonism due to Parkinson's disease or multiple system atrophy with observations on orthostatic hypotension. *J Neurol Neurosurg Psychiatry* 2001; 71: 371–4.
86. Papatsoris AG, Papapetropoulos S, Singer C, Deliveliotis C. Urinary and erectile dysfunction in multiple system atrophy (MSA). *Neurourol Urodyn* 2008; 27: 22–7.
87. O'Sullivan JD. Apomorphine as an alternative to sildenafil in Parkinson's disease. *J Neurol Neurosurg Psychiatry* 2002; 72: 681.
88. Colosimo C, Pezzella FR. The symptomatic treatment of multiple system atrophy. *Eur J Neurol* 2002; 9: 195–9.
89. Sakakibara R, Yamaguchi T, Uchiyama T, et al. Calcium polycarbophil improves constipation in primary autonomic failure and multiple system atrophy subjects. *Mov Disord* 2007; 22: 1672–3.
90. Eichhorn TE, Oertel WH. Macrogol 3350/electrolyte improves constipation in Parkinson's disease and multiple system atrophy. *Mov Disord* 2001; 16: 1176–7.
91. Iranzo A, Santamaria J, Tolosa E, et al. Long-term effect of CPAP in the treatment of nocturnal stridor in multiple system atrophy. *Neurology* 2004; 63: 930–2.
92. Geser F, Wenning GK, Seppi K, et al. Progression of multiple system atrophy (MSA): a prospective natural history study by the European MSA Study Group (EMSA SG). *Mov Disord* 2006; 21: 179–86.
93. Lees AJ, Bannister R. The use of lisuride in the treatment of multiple system atrophy with autonomic failure (Shy–Drager syndrome). *J Neurol Neurosurg Psychiatry* 1981; 44: 347–51.
94. Klos KJ, Bower JH, Josephs KA, Matsumoto JY, Ahlskog JE. Pathological hypersexuality predominantly linked to adjuvant dopamine agonist therapy in Parkinson's disease and multiple system atrophy. *Parkinsonism Relat Disord* 2005; 11: 381–6.
95. Colosimo C, Merello M, Pontieri FE. Amantadine in parkinsonian patients unresponsive to levodopa: a pilot study. *J Neurol* 1996; 243: 422–5.

96. Wenning GK. Placebo-controlled trial of amantadine in multiple-system atrophy. *Clin Neuropharmacol* 2005; 28(5): 225–7.
97. Friess E, Kuempfel T, Modell S, et al. Paroxetine treatment improves motor symptoms in patients with multiple system atrophy. *Parkinsonism Relat Disord* 2006; 12: 432–7.
98. Muller J, Wenning GK, Wissel J, Seppi K, Poewe W. Botulinum toxin treatment in atypical parkinsonian disorders associated with disabling focal dystonia. *J Neurol* 2002; 249: 300–4.
99. Thobois S, Broussolle E, Toureille L, Vial C. Severe dysphagia after botulinum toxin injection for cervical dystonia in multiple system atrophy. *Mov Disord* 2001; 16: 764–5.
100. Wenning GK, Tison F, Seppi K, et al. Development and validation of the Unified Multiple System Atrophy Rating Scale (UMSARS). *Mov Disord* 2004; 19: 1391–402.
101. Schrag A, Selai C, Mathias C, et al. Measuring health-related quality of life in MSA: the MSA-QoL. *Mov Disord* 2007; 22: 2332–8.
102. Brooks DJ, Seppi K. Proposed neuroimaging criteria for the diagnosis of multiple system atrophy. *Mov Disord* 2009; 24: 949–64.
103. Stefanova N, Reindl M, Neumann M, et al. Oxidative stress in transgenic mice with oligodendroglial alpha-synuclein overexpression replicates the characteristic neuropathology of multiple system atrophy. *Am J Pathol* 2005; 166: 869–76.
104. Shults CW, Rockenstein E, Crews L, et al. Neurological and neurodegenerative alterations in a transgenic mouse model expressing human alpha-synuclein under oligodendrocyte promoter: implications for multiple system atrophy. *J Neurosci* 2005; 25: 10 689–99.
105. Wenning GK, Krismer F, Poewe W. New insights into atypical parkinsonism. *Curr Opin Neurol* 2011; 24: 331–8.
106. Wenning GK, Stefanova N. Recent developments in multiple system atrophy. *J Neurol* 2009; 256: 1791–808.

CHAPTER 14

Progressive Supranuclear Palsy and Corticobasal Degeneration

David R. Williams

Summary

Progressive supranuclear palsy (PSP) is the second most common form of neurodegenerative parkinsonism after idiopathic Parkinson's disease. Patients most often present with an insidious change in balance, personality, or cognitive function which characteristically leads to severe postural instability, vertical supranuclear gaze palsy, and death within 7–8 years; this classic clinical presentation is now know as Richardson syndrome (also Steele–Richardson–Olszewski syndrome). Less commonly, patients present with bradykinesia and rigidity (PSP–parkinsonism) which is only later followed by the emergence of falls, eye movement abnormalities, and cognitive impairment; others may present with pure akinesia and gait freezing (PSP–PAGF), corticobasal syndrome (PSP–CBS), or progressive non-fluent aphasia (PSP–PNFA). The characteristic neuropathological findings of abnormal accumulations of neurofibrillary tau protein in the subthalamic nucleus and other brainstem regions define the disease, and because of these findings PSP is included amongst the primary 'tauopathies' (1).

Corticobasal degeneration (CBD) is another, rarer tauopathy characterized by the accumulation of neurofibrillary and oligodendroglial tau in the cortex and basal ganglia. The classic 'motor' presentation of CBD is known as 'corticobasal syndrome': a combination of limb apraxia, cortical sensory loss, alien limb, focal myoclonus, limb dystonia, as well as rigidity and bradykinesia that do not respond to dopaminergic medications. Corticobasal syndrome is not specific to CBD and is also known to occur in other diseases such as PSP, Alzheimer's disease, and the frontotemporal dementias. The 'cognitive' presentation of CBD typically includes behavioural disturbance, including personality change and executive dysfunction, and progressive non-fluent aphasia.

There is some clinical and pathological overlap between these two conditions, and in both progressive decline over 6–12 years is usual. There are no disease-modifying therapies for PSP or CBD, and treatment is focused on optimizing independence, minimizing the complications of the advancing parkinsonism and supporting caregivers.

Essential background

Epidemiology

Community-based prevalence studies using operational diagnostic criteria suggest crude prevalence rates of between 3.2 and 6.5 per 100 000 and an age-adjusted prevalence of between 4.6 and 5.0 per 100 000 (2–4) which is about a factor of 25 less than the rates in PD (5). Estimating the true prevalence of PSP is problematic because of the difficulty in accurately diagnosing PSP and its different clinical phenotypes. The median age of onset for PSP is 65, and the median disease duration from disease onset to death ranges between 5 and 8 years (1). Patients who have PSP–parkinsonism (PSP–P) and PSP–PAGF appear to have a better prognosis, with median disease durations of between 8 and 11 years. The most common modes of death are aspiration pneumonia, primary neurogenic respiratory failure, and pulmonary emboli, regardless of clinical subtype (6). There are no reported gender differences. The epidemiology of CBD is more difficult to establish because of its rarity and difficulties in confirming the clinical diagnosis. It is probably about 10 times as rare as PSP, and appears to affect people at around the same age as PSP (7).

Aetiology and genetics

PSP and CBD are considered amongst the many different neurodegenerative diseases that are characterized and classified by deposition of insoluble proteins in the central nervous system (8). Thus both these diseases are defined by the characteristic post-mortem findings of accumulations of insoluble microtubule associated protein tau (MAPT, tau protein), hence their designation as 'tauopathies'. Tau protein is ubiquitous in the adult brain and its normal function is to assemble and stabilize microtubules, which are important structural elements in neuronal cells. Normal tau protein binds to microtubules in axons, but in PSP and CBD it is redistributed to the cell body where it accumulates to form insoluble fibrillary deposits (9).

Tau protein is the most abundant microtubule-associated protein in the brain. It was designated by the Greek letter T (τ, tau) because of its ability to induce tubule formation through assembly of tubulin (8). It exists in six isoforms, differing by the presence or absence of 29- or 59-amino-acid inserts located in the amino terminal end and a 31-amino-acid repeat in the microtubule-binding domain (Fig. 14.1). Depending on the presence or absence of the latter, the domain harbours either 3-repeat or 4-repeat sequences that are essential for microtubule binding. In normal adult brain there are similar levels of 3-repeat tau (3R) and 4-repeat tau (4R), but in neurodegeneration this ratio is often altered.

The gene encoding tau is on chromosome 17, and comprises 13 exons (Fig. 14.1). Exon 10 codes for the alternatively spliced amino acid repeat sequence in the binding domain, and mutations here cause disease by altering the ratio of 3R and 4R tau (10). Different mutations reduce the ability of tau to interact with microtubules (11), and others promote the assembly of tau into filaments associated with disease (Fig. 14.1) (10). A number of commonly occurring haplotypes of the *MAPT* gene are associated with the development of PSP and CBD, and although the precise mechanisms are yet to be determined the central importance of tau for these diseases is beyond doubt (12).

Pathophysiology

The neuronal degeneration and gliosis that occurs in these diseases is almost always most severe in regions of the basal ganglia, including the subthalamic nucleus and nigra (for PSP and CBD) and the striatum (for PSP), and, for patients with CBD, cortical atrophy centred on the peri-Rolandic posterior frontal and parietal cortex is conspicuous (13).

The pathological diagnosis of PSP relies on the identification of tau-positive neurofibrillary tangles and neuropil threads at high density in the pallidum, subthalamic nucleus, substantia nigra, or pons, and at a lower density in other subcortical structures (13). The pathological signature of PSP is the tufted astrocyte, which is rare in other tauopathies (Fig. 14.2) (14). CBD is defined pathologically by the presence of achromatic balloon-shaped neurons and prominent diffuse cortical glial tau pathology, including neuropil threads, coiled bodies, and astrocytic plaques (Fig. 14.2) (15).

The anatomical distribution of pathological changes, which include tau accumulation, neuronal loss, gliosis, and atrophy, is the most important factor that determines the clinical features that patients with PSP and CBD develop. To some extent this is independent of the nature of the tauopathy, and so there is variability and substantial overlap between the clinical 'expression' of PSP and CBD pathologies (1, 16, 17).

The substantia nigra pars compacta and ventrotegmental areas are affected more severely in Richardson's disease than in Parkinson's disease. These dopamine cell groups innervate motor and limbic cortical and thalamic regions, influencing motor, executive, and other cognitive and behavioural features, and their destruction is likely to contribute to the relative lack of levodopa responsiveness and frontostriatal cognitive dysfunction in PSP (18, 19).

Patients with PSP–P have less severe tau pathology than patients with Richardson's syndrome, although the pattern of distribution appears to be constant between the two, with the subthalamic nucleus and substantia nigra always the most severely affected regions (Fig. 14.3) (20, 21). The regions where the differences in pathological tau are greatest between Richardson's syndrome and PSP–P are the cerebral cortex, pons, caudate, cerebellar dentate nucleus, and cerebellar white matter (Fig. 14.3) (20–23). Atrophy of the pallidum, amygdala, thalamus, and frontal lobe (frontal pole, inferior gyrus) is also more severe in Richardson's syndrome than in PSP–P (23, 24). The tremor and moderate levodopa responsiveness that characterize PSP–P may be due to this less severe extra-nigral midbrain dopamine depletion (20, 21, 25).

Patients who present with PSP–PAGF have severe atrophy, neuronal loss, and gliosis in the globus pallidus, substantia nigra, and subthalamic nucleus, with less severe tau pathology in the motor cortex, striatum, pontine nuclei, and cerebellum (26, 27). Functional imaging studies reflect these pathological observations, with decreased glucose metabolism restricted to the midbrain in patients with PAGF and relative preservation of frontal metabolism (28).

Patients with PSP-tau pathology who present with progressive non-fluent aphasia have more severe pathology in the temporal cortex and superior frontal gyrus than patients with other subtypes of PSP, but less severe pathology in the brainstem and subcortical grey regions (29). Patients with PSP-tau pathology who present with corticobasal syndrome have a greater severity of tau pathology in the mid-frontal and inferior parietal cortices, but not the motor cortex, than patients with Richardson's syndrome (16). The

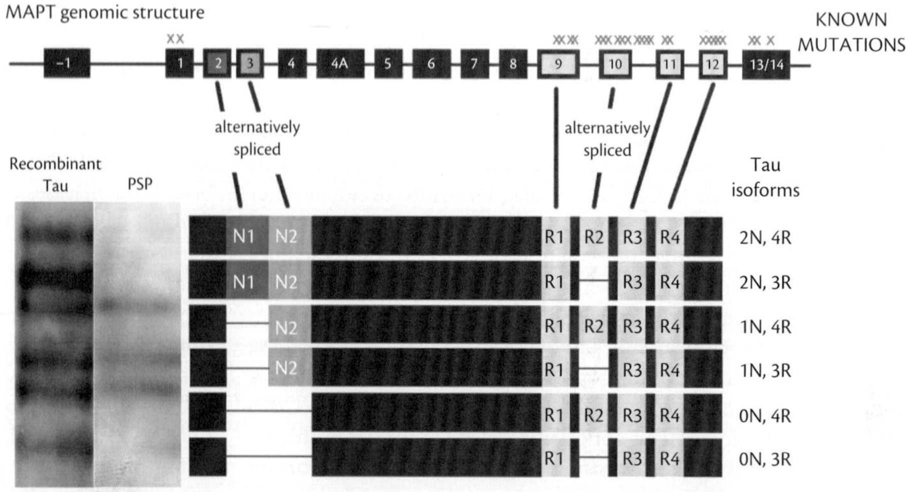

Fig. 14.1 MAPT genomic structure. (Reprinted with permission from Williams DR. Tauopathies: classification and clinical update on neurodegenerative diseases associated with microtubule-associated protein tau. *Intern Med J* 2006; 36: 652–60. © John Wiley & Sons Inc., 2006)

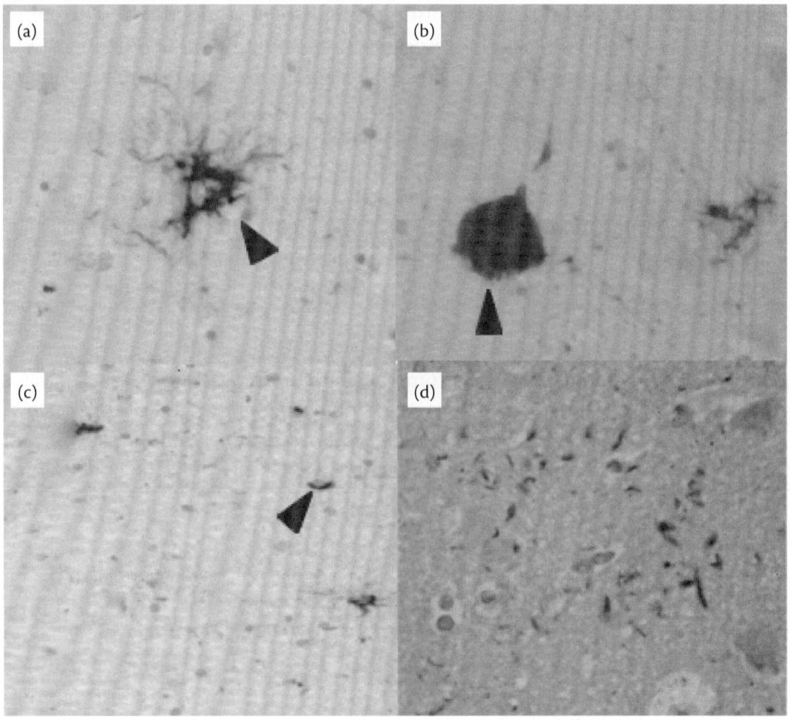

Fig. 14.2 Pathological characteristics of PSP-tau and CBD-tau pathology (AT8 anti-tau antibody): (a) tufted astrocyte (arrow head); (b) neurofibrillary tangle (arrow head); (c) glial pathology, coiled body (arrow head); (d) astrocytic plaque.

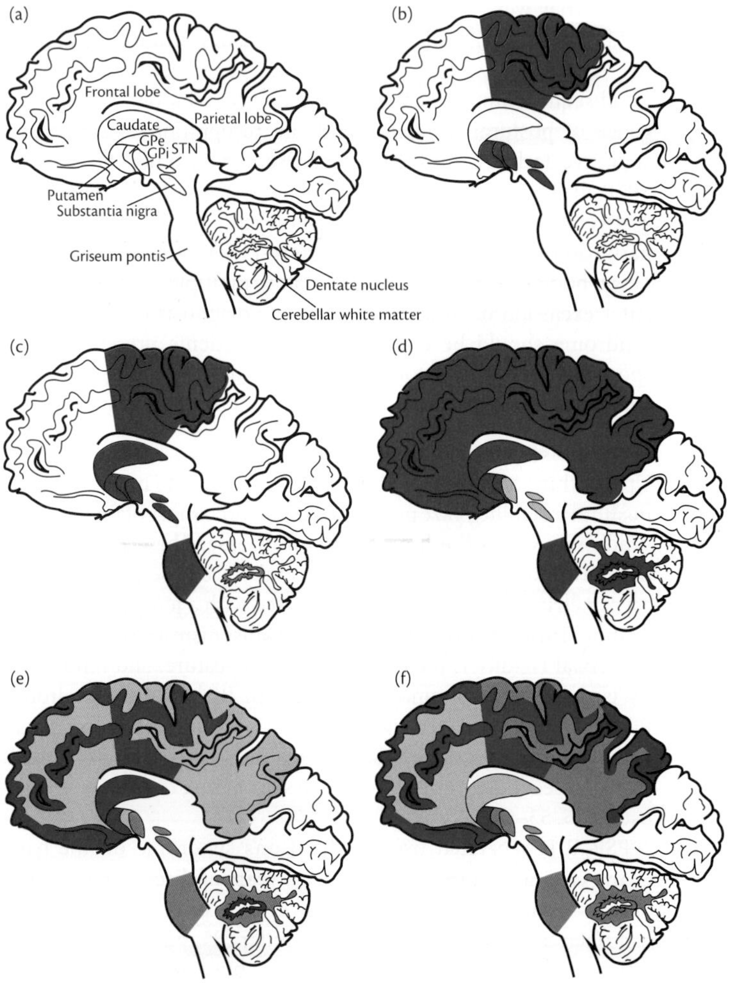

Fig. 14.3 The severity of PSP glial tau pathology varies according to distribution: grey, mild severity; light green, moderate severity; medium green, severe; dark green, very severe. PSP, progressive supranuclear palsy; PSP–P, PSP–parkinsonism; PAGF, pure akinesia with gait freezing; STN, subthalamic nucleus; GPi, globus pallidus internus; GPe, globus pallidus externus. (Reprinted from Williams DR, Holton J, Strand C, et al. Pathological tau burden and distribution distinguishes progressive supranuclear palsy–parkinsonism from Richardson's syndrome. *Brain* 2007; 130: 1566–76. © Oxford University Press, 2007)

distribution of the tau pathology in those patients is similar to that seen in CBD patients with corticobasal syndrome, suggesting that the topography and not the type of tau pathology influences the clinical picture (16).

Clinical features

The clinical manifestations of PSP-tau and CBD-tau pathology can be considered according to their syndromal associations. In this context the classic form of PSP is referred to as Richardson's syndrome (also known as Steele–Richardson–Olszewski syndrome) to differentiate it from the other clinical variants of PSP. They all share some clinical features and are linked by similar natural histories that lead to death usually within 6–12 years of diagnosis. The other variants include PSP–P (25), PSP–PAGF (27), PSP–CBS, and PSP–PNFA (16, 29).

The early features of all these clinical syndromes can be non-specific, and many PSP patients remain undiagnosed for up to 3 years (30). Nevertheless, symptom progression within these first few years of disease is most informative when it comes to prognosis and clinical characterization.

Clinical diagnosis of Richardson's syndrome

The earliest clinical features of Richardson's syndrome are often subtle, may be difficult to discern from other physical or psychological complaints, and often do not satisfy the operational clinical diagnostic criteria (see below) (31, 32). However, in most cases as the disease progresses the clinical diagnosis of Richardson's syndrome is evident within the first 2 years (25, 32, 33).

An unsteady gait and sudden unexplained falls is the most common presentation of PSP. Cognitive slowing occurs in the majority of patients within the first 2 years and may precede gait disturbance by many months (25, 34–36). PSP is the prototypic form of 'subcortical dementia', with reduced processing speed that can be demonstrated early at the bedside by testing verbal fluency, digit span, and alternating hand sequences, as well as demonstrating the applause sign.

The characteristic eye movement abnormality seen in patients with Richardson's syndrome develops over some time, often presenting initially as subtle diplopia. The first signs that emerge are failure of convergence and a slowing of vertical saccadic eye movements with hypometria (25, 35, 37–39). Increased frequency of macro-square wave jerks in the primary position of gaze is typical (40). Patients often report irritated reddened dry eyes with excessive tearing due to the reduced spontaneous blink rate. Eyelid abnormalities are common, and include spontaneous involuntary eyelid closure or apraxia of eyelid opening. Over time the range of spontaneous and target-directed eye movements becomes restricted, first in the vertical plane, and eventually the eyes become fixed. Characteristically, activation of the vestibulo-ocular reflex overcomes these limitations, indicating the 'supranuclear' lesion in PSP (38). However, in advanced disease this vestibulo-ocular reflex is diminished (39). Hypophonia may occasionally be prominent early but, typically, slow slurred growling speech and swallowing difficulties are common (25, 34, 35). Overactivity of the frontalis muscles with eyelid retraction and a staring gaze contribute to the characteristic surprised worried facial appearance (41).

Bradykinesia and extrapyramidal limb rigidity are often absent early, but may emerge as the disease advances (38). Axial (neck) rigidity is often most prominent. Ideomotor apraxia and limb dystonia contribute to impaired limb function in advanced disease. Patients often report insomnia and frequent nocturnal awakening, but REM behaviour disorder in not common. In distinction to PD, dementia with Lewy bodies, and multiple system atrophy, patients with Richardson's syndrome only rarely develop severe autonomic dysfunction (31). Cerebellar ataxia, as distinct from gait unsteadiness, is also unusual and is more common in MSA (31, 42, 43). Patients with PD are more likely to have severe hyposmia and visual hallucinations (44, 45). Rarely, patients with CBD-tau pathology present with Richardson's syndrome (CBD–RS), with early falls and vertical supranuclear gaze abnormalities (46). Patients with CBD–RS appear to have more frontal-type behavioural changes than patients with PSP–RS.

Patients usually become dependent on others for care 3–4 years after disease onset because of increasing motor and cognitive slowing (34, 47). Speech often becomes unintelligible and recurrent choking can lead to frequent episodes of aspiration pneumonia (34, 48).

Clinical diagnostic criteria

The National Institute of Neurological Disorders and Stroke and Society for Progressive Supranuclear Palsy (NINDS–SPSP) clinical diagnostic criteria (see Box 14.1) were developed to optimize diagnostic specificity and were developed after reviewing previously proposed criteria (49–52). These criteria allow a diagnosis of probable PSP in patients (1) older than 40 years of age, (2) with severe postural instability and falls within the first 12 months of disease, and (3) with vertical supranuclear gaze palsy or slowed vertical saccades. They were developed with research goals in mind, and may not be sensitive enough to define patients in routine clinical practice (32, 49, 50).

Subsequent amendments propose a 2-year window for the emergence of postural instability and the recognition of subcortical cognitive decline common in Richardson's syndrome. The NINDS–SPSP diagnostic criteria exclude patients with clinical signs suggestive of Alzheimer's disease, frontotemporal dementia, vascular parkinsonism, prion disease, Niemann–Pick type C, dementia with Lewy bodies, Parkinson's disease, and multiple system atrophy. After exclusion of these conditions, the diagnosis of Richardson's syndrome should be considered in all patients presenting with spontaneous falls, subcortical cognitive dysfunction, personality change, or vertical supranuclear ophthalmoplegia.

Clinical diagnosis of PSP–parkinsonism

Up to a third of patients with PSP-tau pathology do not develop the postural instability, gaze palsy, and cognitive changes of Richardson's syndrome within the first 2 years of disease. These patients may have bradykinesia and limb rigidity at disease onset, which can be asymmetric and in some cases associated with a jerky action or rest tremor. This is referred to as PSP–parkinsonism (PSP–P) (25, 35, 53). Axial rigidity is often a striking early feature, and limb rigidity is more common and severe than in Richardson's syndrome. Parkinsonism in this setting will often show a modest improvement with dopaminergic therapies, although the response is rarely 'excellent' and secondary unresponsiveness occurring over a few years is usual (25, 53–56).

PSP–P is separated from Richardson's syndrome on the basis of the clinical picture over the first 2 years of disease, but clinical overlap occurs and over 6 years of disease progression the clinical phenomenology may become similar (25, 53). Falls and cognitive dysfunction do eventually occur, but later in PSP–P than

Box 14.1 Diagnosing Richardson's syndrome

Within 2 years of presentation, patients over 40 develop two of:

(1) Progressive gait disturbance and spontaneous falls

(2) Loss of ocular vergence and hypometric vertical saccades (eventually leading to progressive vertical supranuclear ophthalmoplegia)

(3) Subcortical cognitive decline, including reduced verbal fluency

AND do not develop:

(4) Levodopa-responsive parkinsonism or rest tremor

(5) Cerebellar dysfunction

(6) More than one of:

 (a) REM behaviour disorder

 (b) Severe hyposmia

 (c) Visual hallucinations

 (d) Symptoms of generalized autonomic dysfunction (two of):

  (i) Chronic constipation
  (ii) Urinary urgency
  (iii) Postural hypotension

(7) Clinical features suggestive of:

 (a) Niemann–Pick type C

 (b) Prion disease

 (c) Alzheimer's disease

(8) MRI changes suggestive of:

 (a) Vascular parkinsonism

 (b) Frontotemporal lobar dementia

Box 14.2 Diagnosing PSP–parkinsonism

Within two years of presentation, patients over 40 develop:

(1) Progressive parkinsonism, including bradykinesia and extrapyramidal rigidity:

 (a) Parkinsonism will often have an axial predominance

 (b) Tremor is not an essential component, but may be present

 (c) Signs may initially be bilateral or unilateral

(2) At best a modest or good response to levodopa, with diminishing effect over time

AND do not have:

(3) Richardson's syndrome (by definition within the first 2 years of disease)

(4) An excellent sustained response to levodopa

(5) Evolving drug-induced dyskinesias

(6) Pyramidal signs

(7) Cerebellar signs

(8) More than one of:

 (a) REM behaviour disorder

 (b) Severe hyposmia

 (c) Visual hallucinations

 (d) Symptoms of generalized autonomic dysfunction:

  (i) Chronic constipation
  (ii) Urinary urgency
  (iii) Postural hypotension

(9) Radiological evidence of vascular disease affecting the basal ganglia

The diagnosis of PSP-P is supported by development of the following, after two years of disease:

(1) Severe postural instability and falls

(2) Loss of ocular vergence and hypometric vertical saccades (eventually leading to progressive vertical supranuclear ophthalmoplegia)

Richardson's syndrome and, perhaps as a consequence, disease duration to death is about 3 years longer in PSP–P (35, 53, 57). PSP–P is difficult to differentiate from PD in the earliest stages, but helpful pointers for PSP–P may include rapid progression, prominent axial symptomatology, and relatively poor response to levodopa despite typical clinical features of PD (25, 54, 56). Unlike in PD and multiple system atrophy, drug-induced dyskinesias are extremely unusual in PSP–P and autonomic dysfunction is not severe or widespread (54).

PSP–P should be considered in any patient over the age of 40 presenting with progressive parkinsonism, including those with rest tremor, bradykinesia, and extrapyramidal rigidity (see Box 14.2). Establishing the degree of response to dopaminergic medications and progression of disease over time are important elements in clarifying the diagnosis of PSP–P. The predominant differential diagnosis in this scenario will be PD, and it is likely that the final clinical designation can only be reached after a period of observation.

Clinical diagnosis of PSP–pure akinesia with gait freezing

In some patients with PSP-tau pathology the clinical presentation is almost entirely limited to bradykinesia predominantly affecting gait, and is referred to as PSP–pure akinesia with gait freezing (PSP–PAGF) (58). Patients report insidious gait difficulties and mild postural instability that may have been developing for months before they seek medical attention. This experience of unsteadiness may develop for up to 2 years before the emergence of freezing of gait and gait initiation failure (27). Phonation difficulties with hypophonia and slurred speech, facial immobility, and micrographia are additional early signs. Axial rigidity with marked neck stiffness in the absence of limb rigidity is a distinctive feature (27, 59). This clinical syndrome is highly suggestive of PSP-tau pathology (27, 60).

A supranuclear vertical gaze paresis and blepharospasm develop late in the majority, although careful evaluation of eye movements may reveal slow hypometric saccadic eye movements earlier in the disease (27, 39, 60). In contrast with Richardson's syndrome, cognitive deficits and bradyphrenia are not prominent, although they may occur late in the disease which has a median duration of more than 10 years (26, 27).

Box 14.3 Diagnosing PSP–PAGF

Patients over 40 develop:

(1) Progressive onset of gait disturbance, with start hesitation and subsequent freezing of gait

(2) Rapid micrographia or rapid hypophonia

AND do not have:

(3) Any measurable improvement following treatment with levodopa

(4) Limb rigidity

(5) Rest tremor

(6) Within the first five years of disease:

(a) Cognitive dysfunction

(b) Supranuclear gaze palsy

(7) Clinical or radiological evidence of lacunar infarcts and diffuse deep white matter ischaemia

The syndrome of PAGF should not be confused with isolated gait freezing where the associated neurological signs are not seen (27). Isolated gait freezing can be caused by a number of diseases, including subcortical white matter ischaemia (Binswanger leukoaraiosis). PD and dementia with Lewy bodies can also present in this way (61). The clinical syndrome of PAGF should be considered in any patient who presents with progressive gait disturbance, particularly if other signs of bradykinesia are present without limb rigidity (see Box 14.3). Establishing the degree of response to dopaminergic medications and progression of disease over time are important elements in clarifying the diagnosis of PAGF.

Clinical diagnosis of PSP and CBD with features of frontotemporal dementia

The behavioural variant of frontotemporal dementia (bvFTD) encompasses the clinical problem of progressive personality change including disinhibition, loss of empathy, change in eating patterns, ritualized or stereotypical behaviour, and apathy. These features may be the earliest signs of frontotemporal lobar degeneration due to CBD-tau or, more rarely, PSP-tau pathology (62, 63). In these cases clinical progression usually includes the emergence of motor symptoms of apraxia, dystonia, and parkinsonism (63). Pick disease and TDP-43 pathology are the most common causes of isolated bvFTD without parkinsonism or motor disturbances (62, 63).

Progressive non-fluent aphasia (PNFA) is a disorder of language characterized by non-fluent spontaneous speech, with hesitancy, agrammatism, and phonemic errors. Patients often require significant effort in speech production (64). It fits within the spectrum of a frontotemporal dementia syndrome and is most likely due to underlying Pick disease or CBD-tau neurodegeneration affecting the frontal lobes. It may be seen in association with CBS (63).

'Apraxia of speech' is one of several components of speech and language disturbance that make up PNFA, and it describes errors in timing, coordination, and initiation of speech secondary to disorders of motor command (65). Clinically this is evident when patients perform serial repetition and it usually accompanies agrammatism (29). When seen as an early and isolated feature, PSP-tau pathology is the most likely underlying pathology (PSP–PNFA), although CBD-tau pathology or Pick disease may also present in the same way (66). Patients who present in this way have a similar age of onset and disease duration as patients with Richardson syndrome (29, 66).

PSP-tau and CBD-tau pathology should be considered along with other primary tauopathies as a cause of isolated disturbances of language or bvFTD with associated motor disturbances. The clinical diagnosis of CBD-tau pathology in this setting is difficult and diagnostic accuracy is notoriously difficult, although radiological markers may be helpful (62, 67). In contrast, the rare presentation of patients with apraxia of speech appears to be highly suggestive of underlying PSP-tau pathology (66). A designation of PSP–PNFA should be reserved for patients who present with prominent (isolated) apraxia of speech that progresses slowly (see Box 14.4).

Clinical diagnosis of corticobasal syndrome

Corticobasal syndrome (CBS) is characterized by progressive asymmetric dyspraxia, cortical sensory loss including alien limb and jerky dystonia of the limb, and rigidity and bradykinesia that is unresponsive to levodopa (68). It was first described in patients with corticobasal degeneration (CBD); however, pathological series have indicated that only 50% of cases with CBS have CBD pathology (69). PSP, cerebrovascular disease, and Alzheimer's disease account for the majority of other cases (16, 70–73).

Approximately 25–50% of patients with post-mortem confirmed CBD-tau pathology develop CBS during life, and it appears to be an uncommon presentation of PSP-tau pathology, accounting for less than 5% of all pathologically diagnosed cases of PSP (67). PSP–CBS appears to run a less aggressive disease course, with a mean disease duration of 11 years compared with 6.9 years in PSP–RS (16). Patients with PSP–CBS develop postural instability or falls within the first year of disease; most eventually develop these features at a later stage (16, 71). Dysarthria, dysphagia, and axial rigidity are also absent in the early stages of PSP–CBS (16, 67, 71). The most common eye movement abnormality in PSP–CBS is an increase in latency to initiate saccadic eye movements, eventually with compensatory head tilts, and typically it is more marked on the side where apraxia predominates (67, 74).

Box 14.4 Diagnosing PSP–PNFA

Patients over 40 develop:

(1) A progressive language disorder characterized by early isolated apraxia of speech

AND do not have:

(2) Richardson's syndrome

(3) Corticobasal syndrome

The diagnosis of PSP–PNFA is supported by:

(1) Ideomotor limb apraxia

(2) After 2 years, the development of

(a) Loss of ocular vergence and hypometric vertical saccades (eventually leading to progressive vertical supranuclear ophthalmoplegia)

(b) Postural instability and falls

Box 14.5 Diagnosing corticobasal syndrome

Patients over 40 develop both:

(1) Progressive asymmetric onset of cortical dysfunction characterized by at least one of:
 (a) Apraxia
 (b) Cortical sensory loss
 (c) Alien limb

(2) Progressive asymmetric onset of at least one of:
 (a) Akinetic rigid syndrome that is levodopa resistant
 (b) Limb dystonia
 (c) Reflex or spontaneous positive myoclonus

Supportive investigations:

(1) Variable degrees of focal or lateralized cognitive dysfunction, with relative preservation of learning and memory on neuropsychometric testing

(2) Focal or asymmetric atrophy on CT or MRI imaging

(3) Focal or asymmetric hypoperfusion on SPECT or PET, typically maximal in parietofrontal cortex with or without basal ganglia involvement

Distinction of PSP–CBS from CBD–CBS on clinical grounds is difficult. While useful trends emerged from comparative studies, no clinical features, including vertical supranuclear gaze palsy, definitively distinguish PSP–CBS from CBD–CBS (16, 67, 75). Myoclonus seems to occur later and frontal release signs more frequently in PSP–CBS, while cortical sensory loss occurs more commonly in CBD–CBS (67, 75). Central to the established criteria of Richardson's syndrome, the occurrence of early falls and vertical supranuclear gaze palsy may be useful as a clue to distinguishing PSP–CBS from CBD–CBS (67). Substantial impairment of episodic memory on neuropsychology testing is a good predictor of underlying Alzheimer pathology in CBS (76).

The diagnosis of CBS should be considered in any patient who presents with progressive asymmetric apraxia, dystonia, and rigidity (see Box 14.5). However, predicting underlying pathology continues to be challenging (7). The terminology of 'corticobasal syndrome' is preferred to encompass all of these clinicopathological entities.

Diagnosis

Both PSP and CBD defy categorization as singular clinicopathological entities because of the substantially different modes of presentation seen in these conditions. Over the past two decades it has become increasingly apparent that pathological diagnoses are required to reach absolute diagnostic accuracy in these conditions. Ante-mortem diagnosis relies first upon the consideration of a clinical syndrome as being related to PSP-tau or CBD-tau pathology. Examination and observation of the patient over time is most helpful in establishing a diagnosis in patients with unclassifiable parkinsonism.

Clinical guidance is given by operational diagnostic criteria for PSP, which have been validated in a small selected group of patients with pathological diagnosis (50) and CBD on the basis of clinical observation and small clinicopathological cases series (7). The diagnosis of these conditions remains a clinical one, so guidelines such as those outlined in the previous section serve as a useful starting point.

Imaging modalities do not provide much useful diagnostic evidence early in the course of either PSP or CBD. In some cases the differential diagnosis includes vascular aetiologies which require MRI brain scanning for exclusion (77). Ventriculomegaly on imaging can lead to the radiological diagnosis of 'normal pressure hydrocephalus', but this does not exclude the possibility of an underlying tauopathy (78, 79). In the setting of an emerging behavioural variant of FTD, a relatively symmetric and predominantly extratemporal (frontal) pattern of atrophy is more suggestive of CBD pathology than of Pick's disease or TDP-43 pathology (62). In established disease, thinning of the superior cerebellar peduncle and midbrain atrophy are helpful diagnostic clues for a diagnosis of PSP (Fig. 14.4).

Biomarker studies, in particular cerebrospinal fluid (CSF) analysis of proteins related to the underlying neuropathology (80), hold some hope of improving clinical diagnostic accuracy. Direct measurement of CSF-tau levels has not proved sufficiently accurate in diagnostic studies, but exclusion of other pathologies, such as Parkinson's disease or Alzheimer's disease, using other biomarkers appears to be achievable (81, 82).

Management

There are currently no treatments that substantially alter the course of PSP or CBD, so it is important that diagnoses are delivered with compassion and reassurance. Patients and their carers should be informed that there are many options for optimizing independence, function, and care into the future. A management team which involves the primary caregiver, the neurologist, the primary care physician, and an allied health care team including a physiotherapist, an occupational therapist, and a speech therapist is important.

Medications

Dopaminergic medications

Levodopa may help up to 40% of PSP patients by modestly improving gait, rigidity, and swallowing function. Ocular motor dysfunction and dysarthria do not improve. Adverse effects are usually minimal. Patients with PSP–P are more likely to respond than those with the classic Richardson syndrome variant. A sensible practice is to prescribe levodopa–carbidopa for patients with PSP who have rigidity or bradykinesia causing disability. Treatment can begin at levodopa 100 mg (with peripheral decarboxylase inhibitor) once daily, increasing on a bid or tid schedule until efficacy, toxicity, or 1200 mg/day. If no benefit is seen after a month, the drug can be quickly tapered and discontinued.

Dopamine receptor agonists are only mildly beneficial in less than a quarter of patients. *Amantadine* has anticholinergic, antiglutamatergic, and modest dopaminergic properties and may help patients with PSP and CBD. In some patients (probably less than 10%) there may be a marked benefit in gait freezing, apraxia, speech, or swallowing. For that reason it should probably be tried in all patients with PSP, except those with severe constipation or dementia. If there is no benefit at 200–300 mg after four weeks, it should be tapered and discontinued.

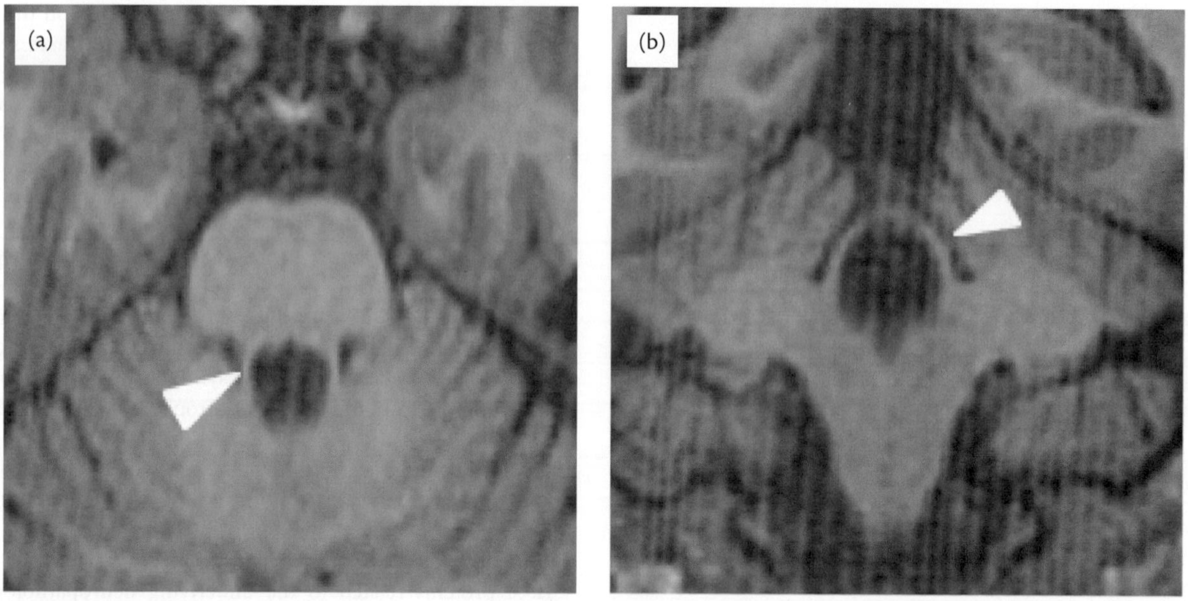

Fig. 14.4 MRI scan showing atrophy of the superior cerebral peduncles (arrow heads): (a) axial image; (b) coronal image. (Reprinted from Paviour DC, Price SL, Stevens JM, Lees AJ, Fox NC. Quantitative MRI measurement of superior cerebellar peduncle in progressive supranuclear palsy. *Neurology* 2005; 64: 675–9)

Antidepressants

Amitriptyline 10–50 mg may be of modest benefit, particularly for muscle pain, hypophonia, and dysphagia. *Selective serotonin-reuptake inhibitors* are commonly used for the depression and pseudobulbar affect of PSP, with very little literature to guide this choice.

Benzodiazepines and related drugs

Bedtime sedatives can be used for the sleep disturbances that are common in PSP. *Clonazepam* may be helpful for persistent and intrusive myoclonus in CBD. *Zolpidem* is also useful in many patients for sleep and may occasionally improve the motor features of PSP.

Others

The mitochondrial defect in PSP has prompted a trial of *co-enzyme Q-10* for neuroprotection in PSP. There is some emerging evidence of improvement compared with placebo and possibly of symptomatic benefit of doses up to 1200 mg/day (83). *Botulinum toxin injections* for disabling blepharospasm, painful cervical dystonia, or limb dystonia, when skin integrity and hygiene are compromised, are often helpful in well-selected patients with CBD or PSP. Care must be taken not to exacerbate dysphagia when injecting even small doses in the neck muscles.

Surgical approaches

There are no established targets for deep brain stimulation or lesional therapy in PSP. Pedunculopontine nucleus stimulation may improve gait freezing in patients with pure akinesia.

Physical therapies and strategies

Postural instability/physical therapy

The frontal disinhibition in PSP causes many patients to suddenly rise from a chair, only to fall on attempting to walk. Strategy training may be of benefit for some patients, and ongoing physiotherapy is important to maintain range of motion and ensure that optimal gait aids are prescribed.

Dysphagia and dysarthrophonia

A swallowing evaluation should be performed in response to the first evidence of dysphagia, which usually affects fluids before solids. The evaluation should usually include a modified barium swallow and may result in recommendations to alter feeding habits or food texture. Thickeners for thin fluids are available. The issue of tube feeding is often difficult to discuss with patients and caregivers, and it is important to guide the patient and family according to their cultural beliefs. Tube feeding can be helpful in maintaining weight when oral intake is poor, but may not necessarily improve quality of life. Potential abdominal complications should be considered. Dysarthrophonia is a common problem that may require use of communication aids.

Gaze paresis in PSP

Prisms for the downgaze palsy are rarely successful. However, a single lens prism may help the dysconjugate gaze that is common in PSP. Practical measures to compensate for gaze paresis include elevating reading material and placing food more horizontal to the eye level.

Other physical therapies

Acupuncture, massage, and gentle passive stretching exercises can be applied to alleviate symptoms of discomfort throughout the disease. Enrolment with a support group can be helpful for patients and their caregivers, and information booklets published for care-givers provide helpful advice for home care. Occupational therapy helps to limit the handicap resulting from the patient's disabilities and should include a home visit. Provision of a wheelchair is usually dictated by the likelihood of falls because of postural instability and gait ataxia, but not by akinesia and rigidity per se. Psychological support for patients and partners is also of great importance.

Key advances

The increasing recognition and clarification of clinical variants associated with PSP-tau and CBD-tau pathology have been important in understanding these broader clinicopathological entities. This is most likely to impact on the diagnosis of patients with 'unclassifiable parkinsonism' (84) and will lead to patients and their care-givers having a clearer understanding of the disease and prognosis when faced with the rarer presentations of these diseases (1). It has become clear that experiments involving patients with PSP and CBD need to address the clinical presentation of those studied, as the severity and distribution of tau-pathology varies and is likely to affect the interpretation of results of clinical and pathological studies as well as the analysis of environmental and genetic risk factors.

The improved understanding of regional vulnerability to tau-pathology in this context has led to interesting hypotheses about the 'cause' of this tau-neurodegeneration. Chen and colleagues suggest that the distribution of PSP-tau pathology may be related to neural systems that have evolved to promote erect bipedal locomotion in *Homo sapiens* and the visual needs consequent on freedom to independently use the upper limbs (39). The suggestion that this recently evolved neural system is vulnerable to PSP-tau neurodegeneration has resonance with other tauopathies (Alzheimer's disease and CBD-tau pathology) and their regions of selective vulnerability that affect cognition, language and the ability to learn motor tasks which all involve functions characteristic of human evolution.

One of the enduring challenges in treating patients with these diseases is providing accurate early diagnosis. This will be most important when disease-modifying therapies become available. There are no radiological features that absolutely separate these pathological entities from other causes of progressive parkinsonism, but taken in the context of the clinical presentation a number of imaging techniques show some promise. Using MRI measures of midbrain and pons areas, as well as superior and middle cerebellar peduncle widths, it may be possible to separate patients with PSP-tau pathology from PD (85).

The understanding and identification of genetic factors involved in PSP and CBD have opened up new lines of investigation in the aetiopathogenesis of these disorders. It is of great interest that a genetic variation of a Mendelian gene (*MAPT*) predisposes patients to a sporadic disease, and identification of the risk allele is a key advance in our understanding of this process (12, 86). The recent identification of families with 'inherited PSP' has confirmed the genetic link to this classically sporadic disorder, and provides further lines of enquiry aimed at understanding the biology of this disorder (10).

Future developments

Future developments in the understanding and treatment of PSP- and CBD-tau pathology are likely to follow several paths.

Molecular studies of these tauopathies will continue to unravel the nature of the pathological lesion and the relationship between tau-protein accumulation and neuronal and glial dysfunction. This will further inform strategies for combating cell death. A number of clinical trials using different compounds with the putative action of reducing the accumulation of hyperphosphorylated tau *in vivo* have already started. These studies necessarily rely on measures to assess clinical progression of disease, and the most widely used measure relies on a clinical rating scale that requires further validation (87). It is likely that imaging (62, 85, 88), electrophysiological (89, 90), and biochemical (80) studies will yield more reliable measures of disease progression that will improve future clinical trial design. The development of these biomarkers is likely to lead to improved strategies for diagnosing PSP and CBD, which in turn will clarify the epidemiology and clinical characteristics of these diseases.

Conclusion

PSP and CBD are tauopathies that are related by their clinical and pathological overlap. Both conditions rely on refined clinical skills and consideration of a broad range of clinical features for diagnosis and categorization. The inevitable progression of these forms of neurodegenerative parkinsonism challenges the scientist and physician to develop strategies that decrease or cure the cell loss that is so prominent at post-mortem. While the future holds hope for compounds that directly reduce tau-protein toxicity, there are a number of current strategies that can be employed to reduce suffering and improve symptoms in patients with these conditions.

Key points

- PSP and CBD are related, but distinct, forms of neurodegenerative parkinsonism associated with the accumulation of hyperphosphorylated tau protein in the basal ganglia and cortex. They are considered amongst the 'tauopathies'.
- The clinical presentation of these conditions can be variable, and it is best to consider a number of different clinical variants of both PSP and CBD.
- PSP-tau pathology most commonly causes progressive postural instability, falls, subcortical cognitive slowing, and vertical supranuclear gaze palsy (Richardson's syndrome). Other variants include progressive parkinsonism with diminishing response to levodopa (PSP–P), gait disturbance with micrographia, hypophonia, and eventually gait freezing (PSP–PAGF), corticobasal syndrome (PSP–CBS), and progressive non-fluent aphasia characterized by apraxia of speech (PSP–PNFA).
- CBD-tau pathology classically presents with a corticobasal syndrome (CBD–CBS), but may also present with a behavioural variant of frontotemporal dementia, progressive non-fluent aphasia, or rarely Richardson's syndrome.
- Brain imaging is not sufficiently sensitive or specific to be useful in diagnosing these conditions, but the presence of the 'hummingbird' sign and atrophy of the superior cerebellar peduncle are suggestive of underlying PSP-tau pathology. Asymmetric frontal (>temporal) atrophy is more suggestive of underlying CBD-tau pathology.
- Treatment strategies that include optimization of function and support for caregivers are an important aspect of managing these diseases. Involvement of a multidisciplinary care team is essential for achieving these goals.
- Drugs aimed at reducing tau-neurotoxicity hold some hope for future treatment.

References

1. Williams DR, Lees AJ. Progressive supranuclear palsy: clinicopathological concepts and diagnostic challenges. *Lancet Neurol* 2009; 8: 270–9.
2. Schrag A, Ben-Shlomo Y, Quinn NP. Prevalence of progressive supranuclear palsy and multiple system atrophy: a cross-sectional study. *Lancet* 1999; 354: 1771–5.
3. Nath U, Ben-Shlomo Y, Thomson RG, et al. The prevalence of progressive supranuclear palsy (Steele–Richardson–Olszewski syndrome) in the UK. *Brain* 2001; 124: 1438–49.

4. Kawashima M, Miyake M, Kusumi M, Adachi Y, Nakashima K. Prevalence of progressive supranuclear palsy in Yonago, Japan. *Mov Disord* 2004; 19: 1239–40.
5. Porter B, Macfarlane R, Unwin N, Walker R. The prevalence of Parkinson's disease in an area of North Tyneside in the North-East of England. *Neuroepidemiology* 2006; 26: 156–61.
6. Nath U, Thomson R, Wood R, et al. Population based mortality and quality of death certification in progressive supranuclear palsy (Steele–Richardson–Olszewski syndrome). *J Neurol Neurosurg Psychiatry* 2005; 76: 498–502.
7. Mahapatra RK, Edwards MJ, Schott JM, Bhatia KP. Corticobasal degeneration. *Lancet Neurol* 2004; 3: 736–43.
8. Williams DR. Tauopathies: classification and clinical update on neurodegenerative diseases associated with microtubule-associated protein tau. *Intern Med J* 2006; 36: 652–60.
9. Goedert M. Tau protein and neurodegeneration. *Semin Cell Dev Biol* 2004; 15: 45–9.
10. Pittman A, Silva RD, Lees AJ, Wood NW. Genetics of progressive supranuclear palsy. *Handb Clin Neurol* 2008: 89; 475–85.
11. Hasegawa M, Smith MJ, Goedert M. Tau proteins with FTDP-17 mutations have a reduced ability to promote microtubule assembly. *FEBS Lett* 1998; 437: 207–10.
12. Pittman AM, Myers AJ, Abou-Sleiman P, et al. Linkage disequilibrium fine mapping and haplotype association analysis of the tau gene in progressive supranuclear palsy and corticobasal degeneration. *J Med Genet* 2005; 42: 837–46.
13. Dickson DW. Neuropathologic differentiation of progressive supranuclear palsy and corticobasal degeneration. *J Neurol* 1999; 246 (Suppl 2): II6–15.
14. Litvan I, Hauw JJ, Bartko JJ, et al. Validity and reliability of the preliminary NINDS neuropathologic criteria for progressive supranuclear palsy and related disorders. *J Neuropathol Exp Neurol* 1996; 55: 97–105.
15. Komori T. Tau-positive glial inclusions in progressive supranuclear palsy, corticobasal degeneration and Pick's disease. *Brain Pathol* 1999; 9: 663–79.
16. Tsuboi Y, Josephs KA, Boeve BF, et al. Increased tau burden in the cortices of progressive supranuclear palsy presenting with corticobasal syndrome. *Mov Disord* 2005; 20: 982–8.
17. Cordato NJ, Duggins AJ, Halliday GM, Morris JG, Pantelis C. Clinical deficits correlate with regional cerebral atrophy in progressive supranuclear palsy. *Brain* 2005; 128: 1259–66.
18. Halliday GM, Macdonald V, Henderson JM. A comparison of degeneration in motor thalamus and cortex between progressive supranuclear palsy and Parkinson's disease. *Brain* 2005; 128: 2272–80.
19. Murphy KE, Karaconji T, Hardman CD, Halliday GM. Excessive dopamine neuron loss in progressive supranuclear palsy. *Mov Disord* 2008; 23: 607–10.
20. Williams DR, Holton J, Strand C, et al. Pathological tau burden and distribution distinguishes progressive supranuclear palsy–parkinsonism from Richardson's syndrome. *Brain* 2007; 130: 1566–76.
21. Jellinger KA. Different tau pathology pattern in two clinical phenotypes of progressive supranuclear palsy. *Neurodegener Dis* 2008: 5: 339–46.
22. Schofield EC, Hodges JR, Bak TH, Xuereb JH, Halliday GM. The relationship between clinical and pathological variables in Richardson's syndrome. *J Neurol* 2012; 259: 482–90.
23. Agosta F, Kostic VS, Galantucci S, et al. The in *vivo* distribution of brain tissue loss in Richardson's syndrome and PSP–parkinsonism: a VBM-DARTEL study. *Eur J Neurosci* 2010; 32: 640–7.
24. Schofield EC, Hodges JR, Macdonald V, Cordato NJ, Kril JJ, Halliday GM. Cortical atrophy differentiates Richardson's syndrome from the parkinsonian form of progressive supranuclear palsy. *Mov Disord* 2011; 26: 256–63.
25. Williams DR, de Silva R, Paviour DC, et al. Characteristics of two distinct clinical phenotypes in pathologically proven progressive supranuclear palsy: Richardson's syndrome and PSP–parkinsonism. *Brain* 2005; 128: 1247–58.
26. Ahmed Z, Josephs KA, Gonzalez J, DelleDonne A, Dickson DW. Clinical and neuropathologic features of progressive supranuclear palsy with severe pallido-nigro-luysial degeneration and axonal dystrophy. *Brain* 2008; 131: 460–72.
27. Williams DR, Holton JL, Strand K, Revesz T, Lees AJ. Pure akinesia with gait freezing: a third clinical phenotype of progressive supranuclear palsy. *Mov Disord* 2007; 22: 2235–41.
28. Park HK, Kim JS, Im KC, et al. Functional brain imaging in pure akinesia with gait freezing: [^{18}F] FDG PET and [^{18}F] FP-CIT PET analyses. *Mov Disord* 2008; 24: 237–45.
29. Josephs KA, Boeve BF, Duffy JR, et al. Atypical progressive supranuclear palsy underlying progressive apraxia of speech and nonfluent aphasia. *Neurocase* 2005; 11: 283–96.
30. Litvan I, Bhatia KP, Burn DJ, et al. Movement Disorders Society Scientific Issues Committee report: SIC Task Force appraisal of clinical diagnostic criteria for Parkinsonian disorders. *Mov Disord* 2003; 18: 467–86.
31. Williams DR, Lees AJ. How do patients with parkinsonism present? A clinicopathological study. *Int Med J* 2009; 39: 7–12.
32. Osaki Y, Ben-Shlomo Y, Lees AJ, et al. Accuracy of clinical diagnosis of progressive supranuclear palsy. *Mov Disord* 2004; 19: 181–9.
33. Santacruz P, Uttl B, Litvan I, Grafman J. Progressive supranuclear palsy: a survey of the disease course. *Neurology* 1998; 50: 1637–47.
34. Nath U, Ben-Shlomo Y, Thomson RG, Lees AJ, Burn DJ. Clinical features and natural history of progressive supranuclear palsy: a clinical cohort study. *Neurology* 2003; 60: 910–16.
35. Kaat LD, Boon AJ, Kamphorst W, Ravid R, Duivenvoorden HJ, van Swieten JC. Frontal presentation in progressive supranuclear palsy. *Neurology* 2007; 69: 723–9.
36. Richardson JC, Steele JC, Olszewski J. Supranuclear ophthalmoplegia, pseudobulbar palsy, nuchal dystonia and dementia. *Trans Am Neurol Assoc* 1963; 8: 25–9.
37. Rottach KG, Riley DE, DiScenna AO, Zivotofsky AZ, Leigh RJ. Dynamic properties of horizontal and vertical eye movements in parkinsonian syndromes. *Ann Neurol* 1996; 39: 368–77.
38. Steele JC, Richardson JC, Olszewski J. Progressive supranuclear palsy: a heterogeneous degeneration involving the brain stem, basal ganglia and cerebellum with vertical supranuclear gaze and pseudobulbar palsy, nuchal dystonia and dementia. *Arch Neurol* 1964; 10: 333–59.
39. Chen AL, Riley DE, King SA, et al. The disturbance of gaze in progressive supranuclear palsy: implications for pathogenesis. *Front Neurol* 2010; 1: 1–19.
40. Otero-Millan J, Serra A, Leigh RJ, Troncoso XG, Macknik SL, Martinez-Conde S. Distinctive features of saccadic intrusions and microsaccades in progressive supranuclear palsy. *J Neurosci* 2011; (31): 4379–87.
41. Romano S, Colosimo C. Procerus sign in progressive supranuclear palsy. *Neurology* 2001; 57: 1928.
42. Kanazawa M, Shimohata T, Toyoshima Y, et al. Cerebellar involvement in progressive supranuclear palsy: a clinicopathological study. *Mov Disord* 2009; 24: 1312–18.
43. de Bruin VM, Lees AJ. The clinical features of 67 patients with clinically definite Steele–Richardson–Olszewski syndrome. *Behav Neurol* 1992; 5: 229–32.
44. Silveira-Moriyama L, Hughes G, Church A, et al. Hyposmia in progressive supranuclear palsy. *Mov Disord* 2010; 25: 570–7.
45. Williams DR, Warren JD, Lees AJ. Using the presence of visual hallucinations to differentiate Parkinson's disease from atypical Parkinsonism. *J Neurol Neurosurg Psychiatry* 2008; 79: 652–5.
46. Kouri N, Murray ME, Hassan A, et al. Neuropathological features of corticobasal degeneration presenting as corticobasal syndrome or Richardson syndrome. *Brain* 2011; 134: 3264–75.
47. O'Sullivan SS, Massey LA, Williams DR, et al. Clinical outcomes of progressive supranuclear palsy and multiple system atrophy. *Brain* 2008; 131: 1362–72.

48. Goetz CG, Leurgans S, Lang AE, Litvan I. Progression of gait, speech and swallowing deficits in progressive supranuclear palsy. *Neurology* 2003; 60: 917–22.
49. Litvan I, Agid Y, Calne D, et al. Clinical research criteria for the diagnosis of progressive supranuclear palsy (Steele–Richardson–Olszewski syndrome): report of the NINDS–SPSP international workshop. *Neurology* 1996; 47: 1–9.
50. Litvan I, Agid Y, Jankovic J, et al. Accuracy of clinical criteria for the diagnosis of progressive supranuclear palsy (Steele–Richardson–Olszewski syndrome). *Neurology* 1996; 46: 922–30.
51. Lees AJ. The Steele–Richardson–Olszewski syndrome (progressive upranuclear palsy). In: Marsden CD, Fahn S (eds) *Movement Disorders 2*, pp. 272–87. London: Butterworths, 1987.
52. Blin J, Baron JC, Dubois B, et al. Positron emission tomography study in progressive supranuclear palsy: brain hypometabolic pattern and clinicometabolic correlations. *Arch Neurol* 1990; 47: 747–52.
53. Srulijes K, Mallien G, Bauer S, et al. *In vivo* comparison of Richardson's syndrome and progressive supranuclear palsy-parkinsonism. *J Neural Transm* 2011; 118: 1191–7.
54. Williams DR, Lees AJ. What features improve the accuracy of the clinical diagnosis of progressive supranuclear palsy-parkinsonism (PSP–P)? *Mov Disord* 2010; 25: 357–62.
55. Maher ER, Lees AJ. The clinical features and natural history of the Steele–Richardson–Olszewski syndrome (progressive supranuclear palsy). *Neurology* 1986; 36: 1005–8.
56. Birdi S, Rajput AH, Fenton M, et al. Progressive supranuclear palsy diagnosis and confounding features: report on 16 autopsied cases. *Mov Disord* 2002; 17: 1255–64.
57. Williams DR, Watt HC, Lees AJ. Predictors of falls and fractures in bradykinetic rigid syndromes: a retrospective study. *J Neurol Neurosurg Psychiatry* 2006; 77: 468–73.
58. Imai H, Narabayashi H. Akinesia—concerning 2 cases of pure akinesia. *Adv Neurol Sci (Tokyo)* 1974; 18: 787–94.
59. Mizusawa H, Mochizuki A, Ohkoshi N, Yoshizawa K, Kanazawa I, Imai H. Progressive supranuclear palsy presenting with pure akinesia. *Adv Neurol* 1993; 60: 618–21.
60. Riley DE, Fogt N, Leigh RJ. The syndrome of 'pure akinesia' and its relationship to progressive supranuclear palsy. *Neurology* 1994; 44: 1025–9.
61. Factor SA, Higgins DS, Qian J. Primary progressive freezing gait: a syndrome with many causes. *Neurology* 2006; 66: 411–14.
62. Rohrer JD, Lashley T, Schott JM, et al. Clinical and neuroanatomical signatures of tissue pathology in frontotemporal lobar degeneration. *Brain* 2011; 134: 2565–81.
63. Hodges JR, Davies RR, Xuereb JH, et al. Clinicopathological correlates in frontotemporal dementia. *Ann Neurol* 2004; 56: 399–406.
64. Neary D, Snowden JS, Gustafson L, et al. Frontotemporal lobar degeneration: a consensus on clinical diagnostic criteria. *Neurology* 1998; 51: 1546–54.
65. Duffy JR. *Motor speech disorders: substrates, differential diagnosis, and management.* St Louis, MO: CV Mosby, 1995.
66. Josephs KA, Duffy JR, Strand EA, et al. Clinicopathological and imaging correlates of progressive aphasia and apraxia of speech. *Brain* 2006; 129: 1385–98.
67. Ling H, O'Sullivan SS, Holton JL, et al. Does corticobasal degeneration exist? A clinicopathological re-evaluation. *Brain* 2010; 133: 2045–57.
68. Cordato NJ, Halliday GM, McCann H, et al. Corticobasal syndrome with tau pathology. *Mov Disord* 2001; 16: 656–67.
69. Rebeiz JJ, Kolodny EH, Richardson EP, Jr. Corticodentatonigral degeneration with neuronal achromasia: a progressive disorder of late adult life. *Trans Am Neurol Assoc* 1967; 92: 23–6.
70. Josephs KA, Petersen RC, Knopman DS, et al. Clinicopathologic analysis of frontotemporal and corticobasal degenerations and PSP. *Neurology* 2006; 66: 41–8.
71. Wakabayashi K, Takahashi H. Pathological heterogeneity in progressive supranuclear palsy and corticobasal degeneration. *Neuropathology* 2004; 24: 79–86.
72. Boeve BF, Maraganore DM, Parisi JE, et al. Pathologic heterogeneity in clinically diagnosed corticobasal degeneration. *Neurology* 1999; 53: 795–800.
73. Motoi Y, Takanashi M, Itaya M, Ikeda K, Mizuno Y, Mori H. Glial localization of four-repeat tau in atypical progressive supranuclear palsy. *Neuropathology* 2004; 24: 60–5.
74. Rivaud-Pechoux S, Vidailhet M, Gallouedec G, Litvan I, Gaymard B, Pierrot-Deseilligny C. Longitudinal ocular motor study in corticobasal degeneration and progressive supranuclear palsy. *Neurology* 2000; 54: 1029–32.
75. Whitwell JL, Jack CR, Jr, Boeve BF, et al. Imaging correlates of pathology in corticobasal syndrome. *Neurology* 2010; 75: 1879–87.
76. Shelley BP, Hodges JR, Kipps CM, Xuereb JH, Bak TH. Is the pathology of corticobasal syndrome predictable in life? *Mov Disord* 2009; 24: 1593–9.
77. Winikates J, Jankovic J. Clinical correlates of vascular parkinsonism. *Arch Neurol* 1999; 56: 98–102.
78. Klassen BT, Ahlskog JE. Normal pressure hydrocephalus. How often does the diagnosis hold water? *Neurology* 2011; 77: 1119–25.
79. Schott JM, Williams DR, Butterworth RJ, et al. Shunt responsive progressive supranuclear palsy? *Mov Disord* 2007; 22: 902–3.
80. Eller M, Williams DR. Biological fluid biomarkers in neurodegenerative parkinsonism. *Nat Rev Neurol* 2009; 5: 561–70.
81. Eller M, Williams DR. Alpha-synuclein in Parkinson disease and other neurodegenerative disorders. *Clin Chem Lab Med* 2010; 49: 403–8.
82. Mollenhauer B, Locascio JJ, Schulz-Schaeffer W, Sixel-Doring F, Trenkwalder C, Schlossmacher MG. Alpha-synuclein and tau concentrations in cerebrospinal fluid of patients presenting with parkinsonism: a cohort study. *Lancet Neurol* 2011; 10: 230–40.
83. Stamelou M, Reuss A, Pilatus U, et al. Short-term effects of coenzyme Q10 in progressive supranuclear palsy: a randomized, placebo-controlled trial. *Mov Disord* 2008; 23: 942–9.
84. Katzenschlager R, Cardozo A, Avila Cobo MR, Tolosa E, Lees AJ. Unclassifiable parkinsonism in two European tertiary referral centres for movement disorders. *Mov Disord* 2003; 18: 1123–31.
85. Longoni G, Agosta F, Kostic VS, et al. MRI measurements of brainstem structures in patients with Richardson's syndrome, progressive supranuclear palsy-parkinsonism, and Parkinson's disease. *Mov Disord* 2011; 26: 247–55.
86. Myers AJ, Pittman AM, Zhao AS, et al. The MAPT H1c risk haplotype is associated with increased expression of tau and especially of 4 repeat containing transcripts. *Neurobiol Dis* 2007; 25: 561–70.
87. Golbe LI, Ohman-Strickland PA. A clinical rating scale for progressive supranuclear palsy. *Brain* 2007; 130: 1552–65.
88. Zwergal A, la Fougere C, Lorenzl S et al. Postural imbalance and falls in PSP correlate with functional pathology of the thalamus. *Neurology* 2011; 77: 101–9.
89. Conte A, Belvisi D, Bologna M, et al. Abnormal cortical synaptic plasticity in primary motor area in progressive supranuclear palsy. *Cereb Cortex* 2012; 22: 693–700.
90. Bologna M, Agostino R, Gregori B, et al. Voluntary, spontaneous and reflex blinking in patients with clinically probable progressive supranuclear palsy. *Brain* 2009; 132: 502–10.

CHAPTER 15

Primary Dementia Syndromes and Parkinsonism

A.W. Lemstra, H. Seelaar, and J.C. van Swieten

Summary

This chapter addresses neurodegenerative diseases that are primarily dementia syndromes but are frequently, or by definition, accompanied by parkinsonism. In many neurodegenerative diseases cognitive dysfunction and extrapyramidal signs occur during the course of the disease. This chapter is limited to those diseases in which dementia is a core feature and parkinsonism is mostly present early in the disease. We will discuss dementia with Lewy bodies (DLB) and frontotemporal lobar degeneration (FTLD), syndromes which present with parkinsonism. DLB is part of the spectrum of Parkinson's disease and is clinically challenging from the diagnostic and management perspective. Recent advances in genetic and molecular research have greatly improved insight into disease mechanisms in FTLD, with mutations in two MAPT and *GRN* genes on chromosome 17. We will discuss the clinical and pathological overlap between FTDP-17 and other parkinsonian syndromes. The combination of cognitive dysfunction and extrapyramidal symptoms in corticobasal degeneration and progressive supranuclear palsy may overlap with FTLD, but these diseases are not considered primary dementia syndromes and are addressed in Chapter 14.

Dementia with Lewy bodies

The term dementia with Lewy bodies (DLB) was coined in 1996; before this the disease was known by various names such as diffuse Lewy body disease, Lewy body dementia, the Lewy body variant of Alzheimer's disease, senile dementia of Lewy body type, and dementia associated with Lewy bodies.

DLB has been reported as the second most common form of dementia after Alzheimer's disease (AD), but epidemiological studies of this disorder are lacking. Its estimated prevalence ranges from zero to 5% in the general population and from zero to 30.5% in dementia cases. The mean age of onset in DLB is 75 years, with a range from 50 to 80 years, and there is a slight male predominance (1). The current knowledge of genetics in Lewy body disorders is described in more detail elsewhere in this book. Familial aggregation in DLB supports the idea of genetic risk factors, and a novel locus on chromosome 2 was found in a Belgian family, although a pathogenic mutation has not been found (2). There is evidence for overlap in genetic determinants for PD based on mutations found in some patients with DLB (3).

Pathophysiology

Deposits of the synaptic protein α-synuclein are the pathological substrate of the diseases known as synucleinopathies which include DLB, Parkinson's disease, multiple system atrophy, and some other rarer clinical conditions. Alpha-synuclein is an abundant brain protein whose precise function remains to be elucidated, but it is probably involved in vesicular processes. Conformational changes convert α-synuclein from an α-helical structure into a β-sheet-rich insoluble state which oligomerizes and aggregates into fibrillary structures (4). These aggregates are found in intracytoplasmic inclusion bodies, termed Lewy bodies, which are the hallmark pathological lesion of DLB. These aggregates are found more abundantly in dystrophic neurites, termed Lewy neurites (LNs). The exact mechanism of the pathogenic pathway remains to be elucidated. It is not clear which species of α-synuclein are toxic, but there is growing evidence in favour of the soluble α-synuclein oligomers (4, 5). The presence of LNs and the successive extensive loss of dendritic spines in postsynaptic areas are probably closely related to the clinical symptomatology (6, 7).

All autopsy studies show a considerable variability in the burden and distribution of Lewy-related pathology in different regions of the nervous system. This probably accounts for the heterogeneity of the clinical phenotype. Braak and colleagues described the pathological progression of Lewy-related pathology in both DLB and PD as occurring via caudorostral propagation (8). Although this has been confirmed in several studies, a substantial portion of subjects do not match this paradigm, and more research is needed to fully validate the pathological progression of the disease (9). The consensus pathological guidelines, which also take AD pathology into account, distinguish three phenotypes: brainstem, transitory/limbic, and diffuse cortical (9, 10). The diagnosis of DLB is based on the severity of the LB/LN pathology present in the brainstem, basal forebrain/limbic system, and cortical areas as detected by immunohistochemical staining for α-synuclein. DLB is frequently associated to a variable extent with AD pathology, specifically amyloid plaques and neurofibrillary tangles, especially in older patients. Guidelines for the pathological assessment of DLB recommend taking into account both the extent of Lewy-related pathology and the concomitant AD pathology (11). In patients with severe AD pathology (Braak stage V–VI) in combination with Lewy-related pathology, the probability that neuropathological findings are associated with the DLB clinical syndrome is considered to be low. DLB cannot be clearly differentiated pathologically from Parkinson's disease dementia (PDD), as they both result in endstage diffuse brain pathology and similar clinical phenotypes. Some subtle pathological differences have been described. In DLB, Lewy-related pathology is more extensive in the striatum than it is in PDD. Neuronal loss in the substantia nigra is greater in PDD, while β-amyloid plaques are more frequent in DLB (7).

Cortical LB density does not always correlate well with cognitive dysfunction. Lewy neurites and neurotransmitter deficiencies may be more closely related to clinical symptoms (1).

A profound loss of cholinergic neurons in the basal forebrain, the basal ganglia, and the pedunculopontine pathway is found in DLB. The cholinergic system is a major modulating system of the neocortex and is involved in attentional processes. Cholinergic deficiency is probably related to clinical symptoms in DLB, such as attentional deficits, cognitive fluctuations, and hallucinations. The cholinergic deficiency in DLB is more extensive than in AD, but postsynaptic muscarinic receptors are relatively preserved. This could partly explain why DLB patients can benefit more from cholinesterase inhibitor drugs (12). Other neurotransmitter systems are also affected in DLB. The dopaminergic deficits, although less prominent than in classic PD, are related to parkinsonian signs. Marked reduction of serotonin levels has been reported, but the association with clinical symptoms is not yet fully elucidated (12).

Clinical presentation

The central feature of DLB is dementia, which is defined as a progressive cognitive decline leading to functional impairment. Patients with DLB show a wide spectrum of cognitive symptoms, with an emphasis on attentional deficits, frontal executive disorder, and decline of visuospatial and constructional abilities (Fig. 15.1). Memory functions are usually relatively preserved early in the disease course, which can help to differentiate DLB from AD. Patients with AD perform worse in naming and memory tests than patients with DLB, but the latter have more visuospatial difficulties. The cognitive profiles of AD and DLB show greater overlap in more advanced stages of the diseases. Fluctuations in cognitive functioning occur in more than 50% of DLB patients; they can occur over minutes, hours, or days, and are associated with episodes of disturbed consciousness and reduced attention and alertness (1). Identification and assessment of cognitive fluctuations is challenging as the operationalization of the term remains elusive. A few validated scales for assessing fluctuations are available, but inter-rater reliability is poor and the literature on the diagnostic utility of these scales is scarce (13).

Visual hallucinations are a prominent psychiatric feature of DLB. These hallucinations can be very vivid images of people or animals, which cause great distress to patients and caregivers. Other frequently occurring neuropsychiatric symptoms are delusions, depression, and hallucinations in other modalities.

Compared with classic Parkinson's disease, motor dysfunction may be less prominent at onset. Based on information from autopsy-confirmed DLB cases, in some cases parkinsonism may not develop at all during the disease course. The most common parkinsonian phenotype is that of symmetric hypokinetic rigidity. Postural instability and gait abnormalities are frequently present. Tremor is less common in DLB, but both action and resting tremor have been described (1).

REM sleep behaviour disorder (RBD) is a supportive feature for the diagnosis of DLB. RBD is common in synucleinopathies and can precede other symptoms by several years. The muscle atonia that usually occurs during REM sleep—the dream phase of sleep—is absent. Patients start acting out their dreams with abnormal behaviours that can range from simple twitches to complex integrated movements like kicking and punching, but also screaming and leaving the bed. These behaviours can cause injury and may sometimes be dangerous to the patient and their bed partner (14).

Autonomic failure is regularly encountered in DLB patients. The most common features are orthostatic hypotension, leading to dizziness and syncope, and micturition problems.

Diagnosis

The first diagnostic criteria for DLB were published in 1996. These criteria were subsequently revised at the third international workshop of the DLB consortium in 2005 (see Table 15.1) (10, 11). The central feature is progressive dementia, defined as in the previous section. Core features are hallucinations, fluctuation in cognition, and parkinsonism. *Probable* DLB can be diagnosed if two of these three core features are present with the dementia. If only one core feature is present, *possible* DLB is suggested. Additional symptoms suggestive of DLB are RBD, neuroleptic sensitivity, and low dopamine transporter uptake on SPECT/PET imaging. Possible DLB becomes probable DLB when a suggestive symptom is present.

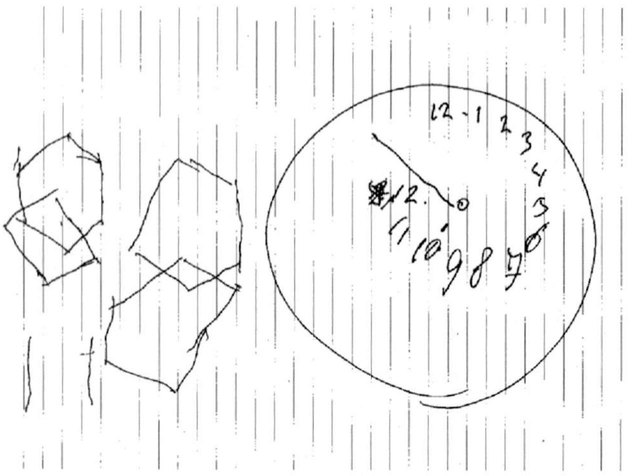

Fig. 15.1 Example of visuoconstructional dysfunction in a DLB patient. The patient was asked to copy pentagons from the MMSE and draw a clock in which the hands indicated ten past eleven.

A range of supportive *phenomena*, including autonomic dysfunction and EEG characteristics, are listed in the diagnostic criteria (see Table 15.1). The presence of these phenomena is not essential to make the diagnosis of DLB.

DLB and PDD share many features and are considered by many investigators as opposite ends of a spectrum due to the same underlying neuropathology. These two entities are separated by consensus using a so-called 'one-year rule': if dementia and parkinsonism appear within less than a year of each other, the clinical diagnosis should be DLB. However, it has been widely acknowledged that the one-year cut-off is a rather arbitrary time frame and should be used for research settings only. In clinical practice, PDD is diagnosed in cases of dementia that occur in the context of well-established Parkinson's disease, while DLB should be diagnosed when dementia occurs before or concurrently with parkinsonism (10).

The diagnosis of DLB is predominantly based on clinical features, and some expertise in cognitive neurology is needed to understand this complex disease. The most important differential diagnosis is probably AD. The use of additional investigations to support the diagnosis of DLB is limited. Structural imaging studies have shown varying results. MRI scans usually show diffuse cortical and subcortical atrophy with no specific distribution. Substantial medial temporal lobe atrophy has been described in DLB, but is more indicative of AD (15). Nuclear imaging has been shown to be helpful in differentiating DLB from healthy controls and AD. Reduced occipital lobe blood flow or metabolism on SPECT or PET has been reported in DLB but not in AD patients. Dopamine transporter (DAT) imaging with ^{123}I-FP-CIT SPECT assesses the presynaptic dopaminergic system. A large multicentre study showed that abnormal DAT scans have a high overall diagnostic accuracy of 85.7%, with a sensitivity of 77.7% and a specificity of 90.4%, in differentiating probable DLB from AD (Fig. 15.2). A DAT scan result is now included in the diagnostic criteria (16, 17).

A small Australian study found relative preservation of the mid or posterior cingulate gyrus with ^{18}F-fluorodeoxyglucose (FDG) PET scanning in DLB patients. This 'cingulate island sign' had a 73% sensitivity and 100% specificity for DLB when compared with AD patients (18) (Fig. 15.3). These findings need replication in a larger cohort.

Amyloid PET imaging with Pittsburgh Compound B (PiB) does not differentiate AD from DLB since amyloid deposition is found

Table 15.1 Diagnostic criteria for DLB

◆ Central feature (essential for possible or probable DLB): ◆ dementia—commonly deficits in attention, executive functions, and visuospatial abilities
◆ Core features (at least two for probable DLB; at least one for possible DLB)*: ◆ visual hallucinations ◆ fluctuations in cognition ◆ parkinsonism
◆ Suggestive features*: ◆ REM sleep behaviour disorder ◆ Neuroleptic sensitivity ◆ Low dopamine transporter uptake (SPECT/PET)
◆ Supportive features (not proven diagnostic specificity): ◆ repeated falls and syncope ◆ transient unexplained loss of consciousness ◆ severe autonomic dysfunction ◆ hallucinations in other modalities ◆ systematized delusions ◆ depression ◆ relative preservation of temporal lobe structures on CT/MRI ◆ generalized low uptake on SPECT/PET perfusion scans with reduced occipital activity ◆ abnormal MIBG myocardial scintigraphy ◆ prominent slow wave activity on EEG with temporal lobe transient sharp waves
◆ A diagnosis of DLB is less likely: ◆ in the presence of cerebrovascular disease ◆ in the presence of another illness sufficient to account for the clinical picture ◆ if parkinsonism appears for the first time only in the stage of severe dementia
◆ Temporal sequence of symptoms: DLB should be diagnosed when dementia occurs before or concurrently with parkinsonism (if present)

* Probable DLB: dementia plus two core features or dementia plus one core feature and one suggestive feature.

Possible DLB: dementia plus one core feature or dementia plus one or more suggestive features.

Adapted from McKeith et al. (10).

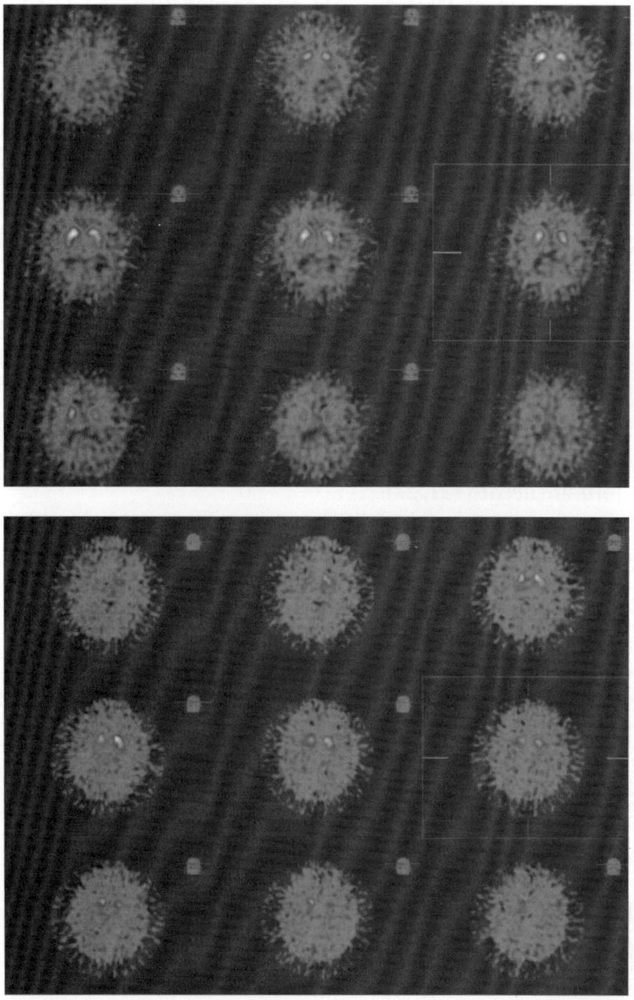

Fig. 15.2 ^{123}I-FP-CIT SPECT scan in AD and DLB patients. Normal DAT scan in the AD patient (upper panel) and abnormal DAT scan showing reduced dopamine transporter uptake in the striatum in the DLB patient (lower panel).

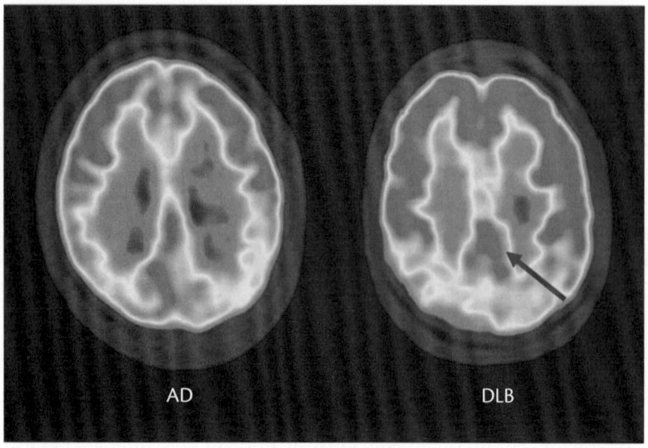

Fig. 15.3 Cingulate island sign [^{18}F]-FDG PET. In AD there is biparietal hypometabolism on FDG PET with involvement of the posterior cingulate. In DLB there is hypometabolism in the occipital lobe with relative sparing of the posterior cingulate.

in both diseases, compatible with the pathological findings mentioned above (19, 20).

Cerebrospinal fluid (CSF) markers are less useful in the diagnostic work-up of DLB. For AD, the combination of low CSF amyloid-beta 42 and elevated concentration of tau and phosphorylated tau have been shown to increase diagnostic certainty. Because of the concomitant Alzheimer pathology in DLB, these CSF markers can also be abnormal in DLB patients and do not necessarily differentiate AD and DLB. Specific CSF markers for DLB have not been found to date. Several investigators have studied the value of CSF α-synuclein in differentiating dementia disorders. Although some of these studies showed a remarkable positive predictive value for lower CSF α-synuclein concentration, others could not reproduce these findings. These differences could have been caused by methodological and technical variations. Other biological features of CSF α-synuclein, such as low concentrations in CSF and great inter-individual variability, could hamper the use of this protein as a viable biomarker. More studies of the optimal operational procedures and prospective validation of previous findings in large cohorts are needed (21, 22).

Electroencephalography (EEG) shows slowing of the EEG rhythm in DLB. There is little published evidence of the ability of EEG to discriminate DLB from other dementias. There are several reports of frontal intermittent rhythmic delta activity (FIRDA) as a specific feature of DLB compared with AD, but test characteristics are lacking.

Although the consensus criteria for the diagnosis of DLB reach a high specificity of around 90%, sensitivity varies among studies (22–83%, mean 63%), depending on patient selection and clinical settings. This implies that the criteria are of limited value for screening DLB cases in a demented population and stresses the need for robust biomarkers.

Management

Managing DLB can be a challenge since the disease displays a wide array of symptoms. As with most neurodegenerative disease, there is no curative treatment for DLB. After establishing the diagnosis, the clinician sets out the symptoms and needs with the patient and carer. Different problems can be targeted, and one has to bear in mind that treating one feature can be at the expense of worsening others. Treatment goals are reduced cognitive dysfunction, extrapyramidal motor symptoms, neuropsychiatric features, sleep disturbances, and autonomic dysfunction. Pharmacological symptomatic treatment is limited (10). Cholinesterase inhibitors can be prescribed to treat cognitive decline and neuropsychiatric symptoms, based on three randomized controlled trials and a few open-label studies which support this strategy (23–25). Hallucinations and attentional deficits, in particular, can show a favourable response to cholinergic treatment. Cholinesterase inhibitors can be administered orally or via transdermal patches. Doses should be increased gradually to decrease the occurrence of side effects, which commonly include gastrointestinal problems. Worsening of motor symptoms (tremor, postural instability) and hypersalivation have been reported in some DLB patients. Treatment with the NMDA receptor antagonist memantine has been studied in mild to moderate DLB and PDD patients (26). There was a mild beneficial effect on clinical global impression and improvement of neuropsychiatric features. However, the evidence is limited and the exact role of memantine in the symptomatic treatment of DLB has still to be established.

Since up to 50% of DLB patients have neuroleptic sensitivity, antipsychotic drugs should be administered with a great deal of caution. Classic neuroleptic drugs with strong D2-receptor antagonistic activity should be avoided completely. Neuroleptic sensitivity greatly increases mortality. Atypical neuroleptic drugs such as clozapine and quetiapine can be effective in treating severe psychiatric disturbances, but should be started at a low dose and closely monitored since sensitivity reactions have also been described with these agents (10).

Although there is limited evidence that dopaminergic agents can improve motor symptoms in DLB, treatment of significant parkinsonian features with low-dose levodopa is commonly accepted. Response to dopaminergic medication is believed to be limited because postsynaptic striatal pathology has been described in DLB. However, lack of response could be due to failure to treat because of fear of side effects, and reasonable results have been achieved in individual patients.

There are limited pharmacological options for treating autonomic dysfunction such as micturition disturbances and postural hypotension. Proper education and instructions help patients and their carers to deal with these often (socially) disabling symptoms. Antispasmodics should be avoided in the treatment of urinary incontinence since these agents have an anticholinergic action and can worsen DLB symptoms via variable penetration of the blood–brain barrier.

Treatment of RBD should be considered when there is sleep disruption, anxiety, and risk of injury. The treatment of first choice is normally clonazepam, but this is relatively contraindicated in demented inattentive patients with postural instability. A few small case series have suggested a beneficial effect for cholinesterase inhibitors. Non-pharmacological interventions have not been systematically studied, but should include providing information to the patient and family on the various aspects of DLB and assessment of special needs to provide comfort and safety in the patient's environment. Physiotherapy can be helpful to address fitness, walking, and balance difficulties.

Key advances

Since the first publication of diagnostic criteria for DLB by McKeith and colleagues in 1996 (11), awareness of this disease entity has steadily increased, much to the benefit of patients and their relatives. DLB is now considered the second most common type of degenerative dementia in older people. With the advent of cholinesterase inhibitors, symptomatic treatment has become available and the cognitive and neuropsychiatric features of DLB can be improved, at least temporarily, in many of these patients. Accurate diagnosis and heightened awareness of specific features of DLB, such as RBD and neuroleptic sensitivity, have improved management. The discovery of α-synuclein as the pathological substrate in disorders with Lewy body pathology has further increased knowledge of disease processes and aetiological factors. It is now commonly believed that PD, PDD, and DLB are part of a spectrum with different phenotypes, although there is still controversy on the progression of α-synuclein pathology. The mechanisms that underlie the conformational changes of α-synuclein and how this leads to neurodegeneration remain to be clarified, but potential links to genetic and metabolic defects are suggested by recent research.

Future directions

In the last decade much has been achieved in the recognition of DLB as a disease entity. It is now recognized as a synucleinopathy in a spectrum with PD and PDD. Future clinicopathological studies in well-defined prospective autopsy cohorts should further identify mechanisms that are responsible for the variability of Lewy-related pathology and the subsequent phenotypes in this spectrum. Understanding the pathology of DLB and Lewy body disorders in general will probably have implications for the current classification system. Another remaining question is the co-localization of pathologies. Currently, it is not clear what the exact relationship is between these misfolded proteins (i.e. α-synuclein, amyloid-beta and tau), how they interact, and if they share common molecular processes. The biggest issue is how these pathological processes are related to clinical symptoms.

At present only symptomatic treatment can be offered to patients suffering from DLB. Novel treatment strategies should be directed at the α-synuclein pathology. In order to find a rational target for future drug development it is necessary to elucidate the toxic species of α-synuclein that are responsible for disease pathogenesis. More research is needed to find reliable biomarkers to identify patients as early as possible, ideally even in a prodromal or preclinical phase. Similar extensive research has already taken place in AD, including clinical trials with potential disease-modifying drugs. There are many lessons to be learned, and this could probably speed up progress to find effective treatments in the synucleinopathies.

Top clinical tips

- Diagnosing DLB can be challenging; recognition of the key symptoms in patients with dementia in combination with SPECT-imaging can increase diagnostic accuracy.
- Patients with DLB benefit from cholinesterase inhibitors with regard to cognitive decline and neuropsychiatric problems; parkinsonism can be treated with dopaminergic drugs titrated up to levels that are tolerated in the individual patient.
- Do not administer classic neuroleptics to treat neuropsychiatric features in DLB; about 50% of patients with DLB experience severe neuroleptic sensitivity reaction.
- Address the clinical phenotype for the purposes of patient management instead of trying to artificially distinguish between DLB and PDD.

Frontotemporal dementia with parkinsonism

Frontotemporal dementia (FTD) is the clinical term covering a range of clinical syndromes associated with selective atrophy of the frontal and temporal lobes with relative preservation of the more posterior cortices. FTD is a predominantly presenile dementia, characterized by behavioural changes (disinhibition, apathy, loss of empathy) and cognitive impairment comprising language and executive dysfunction.

The disease that used to be known as Pick's disease was considered very rare. In the last two decades major advances have been made in the field of FTDs. The prevalence is now estimated at about 10–15 per 100 000 habitants in the age group 45–65 years, and FTD is considered the second most common type of presenile dementia. The incidence in the age group 45–64 years is around four cases per 100 000 person-years. Most cases of FTD are sporadic, but hereditary forms are found in 20–30% (27).

FTD is a clinical syndrome with distinct subtypes. The underlying pathological syndrome of FTD is known as frontotemporal lobe degeneration (FTLD), and it can be divided into two major neuropathological subtypes depending on the presence or absence of specific protein accumulations in neurons and/or glial cells: FTLD with tau-positive inclusions (FTLD-tau), and FTLD with ubiquitin-positive and TDP-43-positive inclusions (FTLD-TDP). A third minor neuropathological subtype of FTLD has ubiquitin-positive, TDP-43 negative pathology, but has shown immunoreactivity with a fused in sarcoma (FUS) antibody.

Additionally, several genetic defects have been identified in some forms of hereditary FTD, which have led to growing insight into disease mechanisms. Different clinical variants (behavioural, aphasic, and motor neuron disease variants) are now recognized as being part of the clinical spectrum of FTD (28). The most common form of FTD is the behavioural variant in which changes in behaviour and executive dysfunction define the clinical picture. In this chapter we will focus on the variants of FTD that are accompanied by parkinsonism. Most of these syndromes are linked to genetic mutations, especially on chromosome 17 (FTDP-17).

Microtubule associated protein tau (MAPT)

Around 30% of cases of familial FTD are caused by mutations in the microtubule associated protein tau (MAPT) gene on chromosome 17. FTD caused by MAPT mutation is an autosomal dominantly inherited disease, although recessive forms have been described. Incomplete penetrance is extremely rare in MAPT mutations, which may help to discriminate it from progranulin (PGRN) mutations in genetic counselling (29).

Hyperphosphorylated tau in neurons and/or glial cells is the pathological hallmark of MAPT mutations. Tau stabilizes microtubules (MTs) and promotes tubulin assembly into microtubules. In the human brain, alternate mRNA splicing of exons 2, 3, and 10 of the MAPT gene leads to the production of six tau isoforms. They differ by the presence of three or four repeats, which constitute the MT-binding domains of tau. More than 40 mutations in tau have been identified to date (30).

Mutations in MAPT exert their pathogenic effects through several different actions. Missense mutations in exons 9–13 impair the normal function of tau binding and stabilization of MT and promotion of tau filament formation, while intronic mutations and some coding mutations disturb alternate splicing and isoform expression. These mechanisms promote hyperphosphorylation and tau filament formation. MAPT mutations are associated with different types of neuronal tau inclusions; these include diffuse or punctate staining, Pick bodies (intraneuronal argyrophilic inclusions, consisting of abnormal three repeat tau protein), neurofibrillary tangles, and pre-tangles. Histopathological examination reveals severe frontotemporal atrophy with neuronal loss, gliosis, and spongiform changes in layer 2. Involvement of medial temporal lobe structures (e.g. entorhinal cortex, hippocampus, and amygdala) is more variable. Degeneration of substantia nigra and basal ganglia is common. Tau-positive inclusions are most often found in frontotemporal cortex and subcortical nuclei, but can also occur in midbrain, brainstem, cerebellum, and spinal cord. Tau-positive inclusions usually reflect the severity of neuronal loss, but can also be prominent in regions with less severe nerve cell loss. Glial tangles and coiled bodies are found in white matter, and these consist mainly of four repeat tau isoforms. Glial tau pathology can be more severe than neuronal pathology (30).

Filamentous tau inclusions are the pathological hallmark of a number of neurodegenerative disorders, of which AD is the most common, as well as progressive supranuclear palsy (PSP), corticobasal degeneration (CBD), Pick's disease, and argyrophilic grain disease (AGD).

Clinical presentation

The age at onset is usually between 45 and 65 years, although there may be some variation according to type or location of mutation within tau. The disease can present after 65 years of age, but is unusual after the age of 70. In some mutations clinical symptoms can develop before 40 years of age, and even in the mid-twenties (Fig. 15.4). The mean disease duration is on average 9 years after presentation of the first symptoms. An exception is mutation R406W, which is characterized by a slow rate of disease progression lasting up to 25 years. An early age at onset is often associated with a more rapid disease progression, leading to death within 5 years.

Two major clinical subtypes can be distinguished in patients with MAPT mutations: dementia-predominant and parkinsonism-predominant (Table 15.2). Both subtypes can occur in patients with the same mutation and even within the same family. The dementia phenotype is usually associated with mutations G272V and P301L. Cognitive dysfunction differs from that seen in patients with AD. Episodic memory, orientation, and visuoconstructive functions are relatively intact. There is prominent frontal dysfunction, expressed as impairment in verbal fluency, abstract thinking, and executive functions, causing difficulties with planning and mental set-shifting. Impaired judgement and loss of insight affect social and professional lives. Attention and concentration are decreased and often influence neuropsychological testing. Personality changes

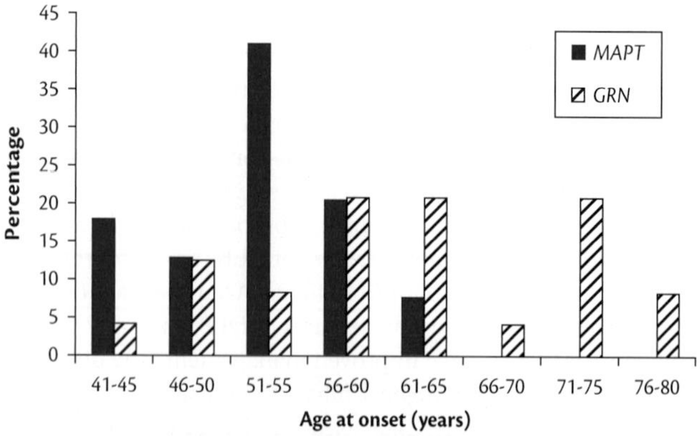

Fig. 15.4 Variability in age at onset between patients with MAPT and *GRN* gene mutations. (Reproduced with permission from Seelaar H, Kamphorst W, Rosso SM, et al. Distinct genetic forms of frontotemporal dementia. *Neurology* 2008; 71: 1220–6).

are characteristic. Disinhibition gives way to impulsive reactions, such as hyper-orality, jocularity, and emotional insensitivity. Poor social conduct leads to embarrassment and upset for those close to these patients. Apathy and loss of initiative are prominent when the disease manifests. Some patients present with distinct psychiatric features such as obsessive–compulsive behaviours or paranoid delusions and hallucinations, initially suggesting a psychiatric disorder.

Patients may develop language difficulties, consisting of inefficient word retrieval, anomia, and stereotypical language use. Mildly impaired comprehension can be present. Reduced spontaneous speech results in mutism within 5 years in all patients, although relative preservation of language abilities has been described in some mutations. The pattern of cognitive dysfunction is similar for all individuals with MAPT gene mutations. Cognitive function may be impaired decades before the presentation of dementia, and asymptomatic mutation carriers have reduced verbal fluency, attention, and motor speed, and set-shifting in their twenties and early thirties.

Epilepsy, both partial and generalized epileptic seizures, has been reported in some mutations.

In the parkinsonism-predominant type characteristic features include resting tremor, rigidity, bradykinesia, postural instability, and gait impairment. There is usually no or only a transient benefit from levodopa treatment. Vertical gaze palsy, saccadic pursuit eye movements, and axial rigidity can develop even at onset in some mutations. Corticospinal tract signs have been reported in some cases. In some families, patients presented with a corticobasal syndrome with unilateral rigidity, dystonia, and contractures, in combination with impaired eye movement. These observations indicate that there is a clinical overlap between FTDP-17, PSP, and CBD (27, 29, 31).

Progranulin

A substantial proportion (20–40%) of hereditary FTD cases do not have MAPT mutations. Some of these families are histopathologically characterized by ubiquitin-positive but tau-negative inclusions and show linkage to chromosome 17q21–22. It is now known that they have mutations in the progranulin (PGRN) gene (32, 33). More than 60 mutations in the PGRN gene on chromosome 17 have been identified. The frequency of PGRN mutations is similar to

Table 15.2 Clinical and pathological features of FTDP

	Mean age at onset (years)	Mean duration (years)	Clinical presentation	Behavioural presentation	Language features	Pathology
MAPT	55 (40–65)	9 (5–20)	BvFTD PSP-like CBS	Disinhibition Obsessive–compulsive	Impaired comprehension	Neuronal and glial tau-positive inclusions
PGRN	60 (35–89)	8 (3–22)	BvFTD PNFA aMCI CBS	Apathy Social withdrawal	Non-fluent speech	Ubiquitin- and TDP-43-positive NCI, NII, DN
C9orf72	55 (34–76)	8 (1–22)*	BvFTD MND PPA aMCI	Apathy Social withdrawal	Non-fluent speech	Ubiquitin- and TDP-43-positive NCI, NII, DN P62-positive TDP-43-negative inclusions cerebellar

aMCI, amnestic MCI; NCI, neuronal cytoplasmic inclusions; NII, neuronal intranuclear inclusions; DN, dystrophic neurites; CBS, corticobasal syndrome; MND, motor neuron disease; BvFTD, behavioural variant of FTD.

*FTD patients with MND have a significant shorter survival than FTD patients without MND.

that of MAPT gene mutations in hereditary FTD. PGRN mutations have been reported in a few sporadic cases of FTD. This apparently non-Mendelian form of the disease might be due to incomplete penetrance, *de novo* mutations, or non-paternity (34).

Little is known about the function of the progranulin protein that is expressed in specific neuronal subsets. PGRN mutations result in a loss of protein, whereas the tau mutations result in a toxic gain of function. The characteristic feature in FTLD with PGRN mutations is the presence of abundant ubiquitin-positive neuronal cytoplasmic inclusions (NCI), neuronal intranuclear inclusions (NII), and irregular dystrophic neurites in the neocortex and subcortical nuclei. The major protein in the ubiquitin-positive inclusions is the hyperphosphorylated TAR DNA-binding protein (TDP-43) (35, 36) (Fig. 15.5). It is not yet known how PGRN mutations are involved in the accumulation of TDP-43 protein.

PGRN mutations invariably lead to severe frontal cortical atrophy, and to a lesser extent temporal, perisylvian, and parietal atrophy, often with an asymmetric pattern (Fig. 15.6). This can distinguish PGRN mutations from MAPT mutations, where a more symmetrical atrophy is seen without parietal involvement. Subcortical structures are frequently affected, with marked atrophy of the caudate nucleus and depigmentation of the substantia nigra. Occasionally, atrophy of cortex and subcortical nuclei may be very mild. Hippocampal atrophy has been reported in some cases (34).

Histopathological examination exhibits very similar findings in different PGRN mutations. There is moderate to severe neuronal

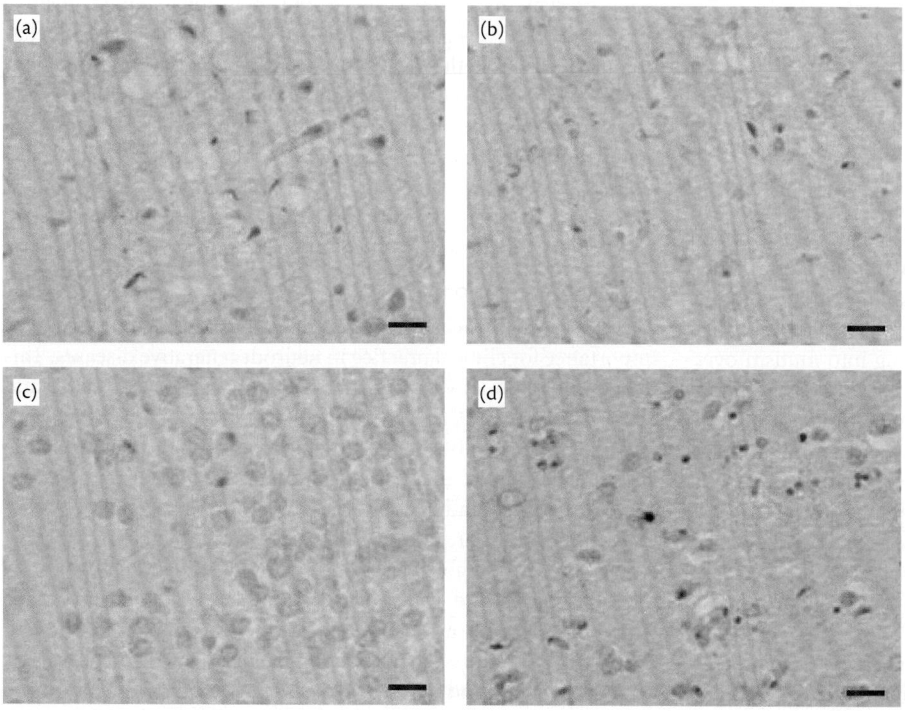

Fig. 15.5 Pathology of an FTD patient with PGRN gene mutation: (a) TDP-43-positive dystrophic neurites in the frontal cortex; (b) a TDP-43-positive neuronal intranuclear inclusion in the parietal cortex; TDP-43-positive neuronal cytoplasmic inclusions in (c) the hippocampus and (d) the caudate nucleus and putamen. Scale bar, 20°μm. (Reproduced with permission from Dopper EG, Seelaar H, Chiu WZ, et al. Symmetrical corticobasal syndrome caused by a novel C.314dup progranulin mutation. *J Mol Neurosci* 2011; 45: 354–8. ©Authors, 2011)

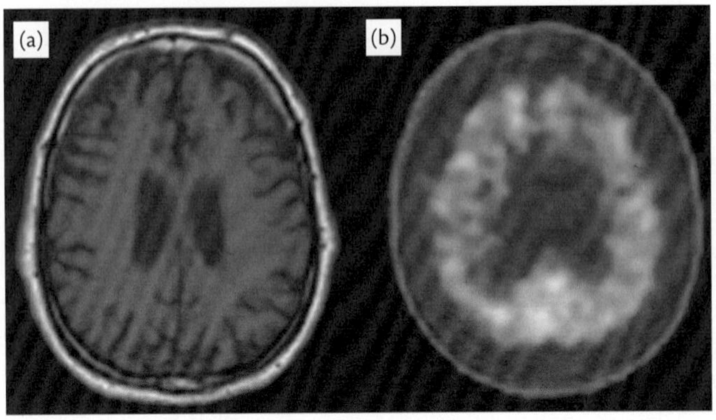

Fig. 15.6 Structural MRI and SPECT in FTD with PGRN gene mutation: (a) mild symmetric frontoparietal atrophy on MRI scan; (b) symmetric parietal hypoperfusion on SPECT scan. (Reproduced with permission from Dopper EG, Seelaar H, Chiu WZ, et al. Symmetrical corticobasal syndrome caused by a novel C.314dup progranulin mutation. *J Mol Neurosci* 2011; 45: 354–8. ©Authors, 2011)

loss in combination with spongiosis in the frontal and temporal cortex (orbital and insular). White matter is frequently affected in PGRN mutations, showing extensive astrocytic gliosis and myelin, and hippocampal sclerosis with severe neuronal loss and gliosis in CA1 and subiculum.

Clinical presentation

The mean age of onset of FTD with PGRN mutations is 60 years, ranging from 35 to 89 years. Even within families there is considerable variation in age of onset with a tendency to present at an earlier age (up to 10–20 years) in consecutive generations. The mean duration of disease from presentation is about 8 years, but again this can vary substantially from 3 to 22 years where a higher age of onset is associated with a shorter disease duration. The penetrance is 90% by the age of 70 years (see Fig. 15.4). Sex or type of mutation do not affect age of onset. The variation in age at onset can cause failure to recognize an autosomal dominant inheritance pattern in small families with only a few relatives (34).

PGRN mutations are characterized by heterogeneous symptomatology with cognitive decline, behavioural disturbances, neuropsychiatric features, and movement disorders (see Table 15.2). Clinical presentation can vary within families, with a parkinsonian phenotype in one affected relative and dementia phenotype in another. Patients with PGRN mutations have a positive family history for dementia or parkinsonism in 70–90% of cases. Behavioural changes are the most common clinical presentation, with apathy and social withdrawal as prominent features. Language abilities are frequently affected, comprising reduced spontaneous speech, word-finding difficulties, and phonemic paraphasias evolving into mutism over the course of the disease. In 20–25% of patients with PGRN mutations language dysfunction presents early and in relative isolation over a considerable period of time, consistent with the diagnosis of progressive non-fluent aphasia (37).

Impaired comprehension and semantic paraphasias have occasionally been described. Cognitive decline is usually revealed by frontal lobe deficits such as executive dysfunction and reduced verbal fluency. Patients can erroneously be diagnosed with the amnestic type of mild cognitive impairment (aMCI) or AD as episodic memory deficits occur in the initial stage in 10–30%. The fact that apraxia and dyscalculia are frequently encountered as a reflection of the involvement of the parietal cortex amplifies the confusion with AD. Visuospatial deficits are uncommon, although they are reported in a few cases. Hallucinations and delusions are reported in up to 25%. Extrapyramidal signs occur throughout the course of the disease in many patients with FTD as a result of PGRN. Bradykinesia and asymmetric rigidity may occur early in the disease, sometimes with resting tremor and dystonia resembling Parkinson's disease. Treatment with levodopa usually has no or only a modest benefit on the parkinsonian features. A corticobasal syndrome with limb apraxia, asymmetric parkinsonism, and dystonia of the upper extremity can occur, but usually in combination with considerable cognitive deficits compared with non-carriers. Pyramidal signs and primitive reflexes may be seen in advanced endstage cases (34, 38, 39).

C9orf72

After the identification of PGRN, there remained a number of families, in particular familial FTD-MND, that were linked to chromosome 9p. Very recently, hexanucleotide repeat expansions in the chromosome 9 open-reading frame 72 (C9orf72) have been described in families with FTD with or without amyotrophic lateral sclerosis (ALS) (40, 41). The expansion is located in a non-coding region. The exact cut-off indicating a pathological repeat expansion is still unknown. Quantitative messenger RNA analysis has shown that the presence of the expanded repeats leads to reduced expression of one of the transcripts of C9orf72 encoding a protein with an unknown function, suggesting a (partial) loss-of-function disease mechanism (40). However, a toxic gain-of-function of abnormal messenger RNA has also been hypothesized based on the discovery, using fluorescence *in situ* hybridization experiments with a probe targeting the GGGGCC repeat, of multiple nuclear RNA foci in brain tissue from patients carrying the expanded repeats (40).

Histopathological examination shows that ubiquitin- and TDP-43 positive neuronal cytoplasmic inclusions and dystrophic neurites are present in all cases, with neuronal intranuclear inclusions present in several cases. Some inclusions stained positive for p62, but were negative for TDP-43, in particular in cerebellar granular cells. Together with the extensive ubiquitin pathology in the hippocampal molecular layer and CA regions found in C9orf72 cases, this may neuropathologically differentiate, although not completely, FTD and ALS cases with and without repeat expansions (42–44). How the repeat expansions lead to accumulation of TDP-43 in the brain, and why some inclusions are TDP-43 negative has yet to be elucidated.

Clinical presentation

The discovery of the C9orf72 repeat expansion has extraordinary importance for clinical practice in neurodegenerative diseases. This is due in part to its very high frequency, varying between 10 and 30% of familial FTD, and between 20 and 50% of familial ALS, and its broad range of clinical manifestations, including an anterograde amnestic dementia, easily misdiagnosed as AD, and its apparent occurrence in sporadic cases. These and other aspects of C9orf72 expansion repeats are emphasized in two studies (45, 46).

There is considerable variation in age at onset and clinical presentation among and within families with C9orf72 repeat expansions (45–47) with a mean age of 55 years, ranging from 34 to 76 years. For cohorts of pure ALS patients, a younger onset age, co-morbid FTD, and apathy or dysexecutive behaviour are more common in carriers with expanded repeats (48). Motor neuron disease occurs in approximately 20–40% of FTD cases with expanded repeats. The behavioural variant, predominantly with apathy and loss of initiative, is the most common clinical manifestation of FTD (45, 46). The occurrence of psychotic symptoms has been reported. Delusions are more common than hallucinations, and sometimes lead to an initial psychiatric diagnosis (44). Primary progressive aphasia (PPA) may occur as the presenting clinical manifestation of C9orf72 repeat expansion (44, 49, 50). Parkinsonism and akinetic–rigid syndromes without resting tremor frequently occur, but are rarely the dominant presentation in patients with C9orf72 repeat expansions (49, 51).

Another possible distinctive feature may be the pattern of cerebral atrophy on MRI in patients with C9orf72 repeat expansions. FTD patients with expansions showed more parietal and bilateral thalamic atrophy than those without expansions. Apart from frontal, anterior temporal, and parietal atrophy, cerebellar atrophy and changes in diffusivity and fractional anisotropy in thalamic radiations have been reported (49, 51). However, the value of these distinct anatomic profiles must be interpreted cautiously in what have been only small studies to date.

Diagnosis

The clinical diagnosis of FTD is based on criteria proposed by the Work Group on Frontotemporal Dementia and Pick's Disease in 2000 (52). Recently revised diagnostic criteria for the behavioural variant of FTD have been published in which patients are classified as possible, probable, or definite bvFTD. The most important revisions are the incorporation of neuropsychological, neuroimaging, genetic, and pathological findings within the criteria and the expansion of the role of supportive behavioural features for the diagnosis of bvFTD (28). FTD can be diagnosed when there are clear behavioural or cognitive deficits which interfere with social and occupational functioning. These deficits are manifested by either early and progressive change in personality, characterized by difficulty in modulating behaviour, often resulting in inappropriate responses or activities, or by early and progressive change in language. Other features are prominent in FTDP-17, but there are no standardized clinical criteria in which these FTD variants are included.

A clinical diagnosis of FTDP-17 can be supported by neuroimaging. Frontotemporal lobar atrophy is the most common neuroradiological feature. Atrophy patterns can vary among MAPT mutations. Predominant, often asymmetric, temporal atrophy, sometimes with additional hippocampal atrophy, has been described. Other patients have a more diffuse cerebral atrophy, especially those with intronic mutations (29).

In PGRN mutations MRI may occasionally be normal, even a few years after onset. The cerebral atrophy of the anterior regions frequently extends more posteriorly into the parietal lobe. The cerebral atrophy often has an asymmetric pattern. The ventricles are usually enlarged. Sometimes the cortical atrophy has a more diffuse pattern, or it may be accompanied by cerebellar atrophy. Subcortical hyperintensities on T_2-weighted MR images may be seen in areas of severe cortical involvement (34).

Early in the disease, even before morphological changes occur, hypoperfusion and reduced glucose metabolism can be observed in the frontal and temporal lobe on SPECT and PET, respectively. Hypoperfusion of the hippocampus and cingulate gyrus in patients with PGRN mutations reflects the involvement of these regions in the pathogenesis (37).

In patients with parkinsonism, SPECT with the radioligand ^{123}I-FP-CIT shows a severe symmetrical decrease of presynaptic dopamine transporter binding in the striatum in individuals with some mutations. This technique has probably no added value in the diagnostic work-up of FTD. EEG tends to be normal in FTD, as opposed to AD and DLB. Interictal epileptic discharges have been described in some MAPT mutations. CSF levels of total and hyperphosphorylated tau are usually normal in FTD with tau pathology, in contrast with elevated levels of CSF-tau in AD and PSP (53).

Management

No clear risk factors are known in FTD. Supportive care is essential to manage the behavioural symptoms for the patients, and also for the family and caregivers. Important non-pharmacological options are offering regularity and structure, often in a formal setting such as day-care centres or nursing homes. Curative pharmacological options are not available. There have been no large double-blind placebo-controlled trials performed in FTD. A small double-blind controlled trial with trazodone in 26 FTD patients showed that 150 mg twice daily had a favourable effect on the behavioural problems in FTD, especially irritability, agitation, depression, and eating disorders (54).

The only double-blind randomized trial with an SSRI (paroxetine) showed no positive behavioural changes in FTD (55). Acetylcholinesterase inhibitors and glutamate blockers (memantine) are not currently indicated for FTD. Patients with FTD–MND with difficulty in swallowing are often started on riluzole or amitriptyline (personal experience), with generally good response (56).

Genetic counselling can be advised in patients with a hereditary form of FTD. The benefit of genetic screening depends on the strength of the family history and the clinical subtype. Both MAPT and PGRN gene defects are most often found in patients with an autosomal dominant form of bvFTD. Screening in sporadic patients will be of little value, as a very few mutations have been found in sporadic cases except for those with a concealed or incomplete family history.

Presymptomatic screening for MAPT or PGRN gene mutations is possible. The motivation to perform presymptomatic screening is often based on life decisions, for example the children's wishes. Therefore support by a clinical geneticist and psychologist is indicated in presymptomatic screening. It must be realized that the age of onset varies widely within families, especially in PGRN families with a range from 35 to 89 years.

Key advances

Over the past years three major breakthroughs have been achieved. One of them is the discovery of mutations in the PGRN gene in hereditary FTD. The second major breakthrough was the identification of TDP-43 as major constituent of ubiquitin-positive inclusions. These inclusions were found in patients with ALS, indicating that these two distinct clinical disorders belong to the same clinicopathological spectrum. All patients with PGRN gene mutations have TDP-43 pathology. It remains unclear how mutations in the PGRN gene lead to accumulation of TDP-43 in the brain. The third important finding has been the recent identification of repeats in C9orf72 in a number of FTD and ALS patients.

Future developments

Important advances over the last decade have led to an impressive change in the clinical recognition of this disease. Future scientific efforts should focus on three major goals:

- improving the early detection of the disease;
- developing reliable markers for predicting the underlying pathology;
- unravelling the pathophysiology in order to develop therapeutic strategies which will prevent or delay the disease process.

FTD is a clinically, genetically, and pathologically heterogeneous disorder. To conduct future clinical trials, it will be important to determine the underlying pathology (tau, TDP-43, FUS) in the early stages of the disease. Further development of biomarkers, using CSF, plasma, serum, or neuroimaging are of major interest for clinicians and will hopefully be implemented in the diagnostic work-up of FTD in the near future.

The identification of tau, TDP-43, and FUS protein as pathological components in FTD emphasizes the existence of different pathways and will contribute to the further understanding of the underlying pathophysiology. Unravelling the pathophysiology should finally lead to the development of therapeutic interventions for FTD (27).

Conclusions

This chapter has highlighted DLB and FTDP as important primary dementia syndromes that are accompanied by parkinsonism. Parkinsonism is not uncommon in other types of dementia, such as AD and vascular dementia, but parkinsonism usually occurs relatively late in the course of these diseases. DLB and FTD are both challenging neurodegenerative disease entities in terms of diagnosis and management. There is no cure, but symptomatic treatment is available, especially for DLB, albeit with limited effectiveness, and long-term efficacy needs to be established. DLB shares many features with PD/PDD and future clinical research will probably be directed towards the whole spectrum of disorders with Lewy-related pathology.

FTD is a clinically, genetically, and pathologically heterogeneous disorder. The recent advances in unravelling the genetic and pathological mechanisms in FTD have greatly improved insight into these devastating diseases and will guide future research towards better treatment of patients with FTD.

Top clinical tips

- Frontotemporal dementia (FTD) is hereditary in 20–30% of patients in whom MAPT or PGRN gene mutations or hexanucleotide repeat expansions in C9orf72 can be found.
- To determine the family history, ask about the presence of FTD or dementia, Parkinson's disease or parkinsonism, and motor neuron disease in all first- *and* second-degree relatives.
- Functional imaging using PET or SPECT may reveal hypometabolism or hypoperfusion before structural changes on MRI are detectable.
- Genetic counselling is possible in patients with hereditary FTD.
- The underlying pathology in FTD can be tau, TDP-43, or FUS.

References

1. McKeith I, Mintzer J, Aarsland D, et al. Dementia with Lewy bodies. *Lancet Neurol* 2004; 3: 19–28.
2. Bogaerts V, Engelborghs S, Kumar-Singh S, et al. A novel locus for dementia with Lewy bodies: a clinically and genetically heterogeneous disorder. *Brain* 2007; 130: 2277–91.
3. Bonifati V. Recent advances in the genetics of dementia with Lewy bodies. *Curr Neurol Neurosci Rep* 2008; 8: 187–9.
4. Vekrellis K, Xilouri M, Emmanouilidou E, Rideout HJ, Stefanis L. Pathological roles of alpha-synuclein in neurological disorders. *Lancet Neurol* 2011; 10: 1015–25.
5. Halliday GM, Holton JL, Revesz T, Dickson DW. Neuropathology underlying clinical variability in patients with synucleinopathies. *Acta Neuropathol* 2011; 122: 187–204.
6. Kramer ML, Schulz-Schaeffer WJ. Presynaptic alpha-synuclein aggregates, not Lewy bodies, cause neurodegeneration in dementia with Lewy bodies. *J Neurosci* 2007; 27: 1405–10.
7. Lippa CF, Duda JE, Grossman M, et al. DLB and PDD boundary issues: diagnosis, treatment, molecular pathology, and biomarkers. *Neurology* 2007; 68: 812–19.
8. Braak H, Del TK, Rub U, de Vos RA, Jansen Steur EN, Braak E. Staging of brain pathology related to sporadic Parkinson's disease. *Neurobiol Aging* 2003; 24: 197–211.
9. Jellinger KA. A critical evaluation of current staging of alpha-synuclein pathology in Lewy body disorders. *Biochim Biophys Acta* 2009; 1792: 730–40.
10. McKeith IG, Dickson DW, Lowe J, et al. Diagnosis and management of dementia with Lewy bodies: third report of the DLB Consortium. *Neurology* 2005; 65: 1863–72.
11. McKeith IG, Galasko D, Kosaka K, et al. Consensus guidelines for the clinical and pathologic diagnosis of dementia with Lewy bodies (DLB): report of the consortium on DLB international workshop. *Neurology* 1996; 47: 1113–24.
12. Francis PT. Biochemical and pathological correlates of cognitive and behavioural change in DLB/PDD. *J Neurol* 2009; 256 (Suppl 3): 280–5.
13. Lee DR, Taylor JP, Thomas AJ. Assessment of cognitive fluctuation in dementia: a systematic review of the literature. *Int J Geriatr Psychiatry* 2012; 27: 989–98.
14. Trotti LM. REM sleep behaviour disorder in older individuals: epidemiology, pathophysiology and management. *Drugs Aging* 2010; 27: 457–70.
15. Watson R, Blamire AM, O'Brien JT. Magnetic resonance imaging in Lewy body dementias. *Dement Geriatr Cogn Disord* 2009; 28: 493–506.
16. McKeith I, O'Brien J, Walker Z, Tatsch K, Booij J, et al. Sensitivity and specificity of dopamine transporter imaging with 123I-FP-CIT SPECT in dementia with Lewy bodies: a phase III, multicentre study. *Lancet Neurol* 2007; 6(4): 305–13.
17. Walker Z, Costa DC, Walker RW, Shaw K, Gacinovic S, et al. http://www.ncbi.nlm.nih.gov/pubmed/12122169 Differentiation of dementia with Lewy bodies from Alzheimer's disease using a dopaminergic presynaptic ligand. *J Neurol Neurosurg Psychiatry* 2002; 73(2): 134–40.
18. Lim SM, Katsifis A, Villemagne VL, et al. The ^{18}F-FDG PET cingulate island sign and comparison to ^{123}I-beta-CIT SPECT for diagnosis of dementia with Lewy bodies. *J Nucl Med* 2009; 50: 1638–45.
19. Brooks DJ. Imaging amyloid in Parkinson's disease dementia and dementia with Lewy bodies with positron emission tomography. *Mov Disord* 2009; 24 (Suppl 2): S742–7.
20. Villemagne VL, Okamura N, Pejoska S, et al. Differential diagnosis in Alzheimer's disease and dementia with Lewy bodies via VMAT2 and amyloid imaging. *Neurodegener Dis* 2012; 10: 161–5.
21. Johansen KK, White LR, Sando SB, Aasly JO. Biomarkers: Parkinson disease with dementia and dementia with Lewy bodies. *Parkinsonism Relat Disord* 2010; 16: 307–15.
22. Mollenhauer B, Locascio JJ, Schulz-Schaeffer W, Sixel-Doring F, Trenkwalder C, Schlossmacher MG. Alpha-synuclein and tau concentrations in cerebrospinal fluid of patients presenting with parkinsonism: a cohort study. *Lancet Neurol* 2011; 10: 230–40.

23. Aarsland D, Laake K, Larsen JP, Janvin C. Donepezil for cognitive impairment in Parkinson's disease: a randomised controlled study. *J Neurol Neurosurg Psychiatry* 2002; 72: 708–12.
24. Emre M, Aarsland D, Albanese A, et al. Rivastigmine for dementia associated with Parkinson's disease. *N Engl J Med* 2004; 351: 2509–18.
25. McKeith I, Del ST, Spano P, et al. Efficacy of rivastigmine in dementia with Lewy bodies: a randomised, double-blind, placebo-controlled international study. *Lancet* 2000; 356: 2031–6.
26. Emre M, Tsolaki M, Bonuccelli U, et al. Memantine for patients with Parkinson's disease dementia or dementia with Lewy bodies: a randomised, double-blind, placebo-controlled trial. *Lancet Neurol* 2010; 9: 969–77.
27. Seelaar H, Rohrer JD, Pijnenburg YA, Fox NC, van Swieten JC. Clinical, genetic and pathological heterogeneity of frontotemporal dementia: a review. *J Neurol Neurosurg Psychiatry* 2011; 82: 476–86.
28. Rascovsky K, Hodges JR, Knopman D, et al. Sensitivity of revised diagnostic criteria for the behavioural variant of frontotemporal dementia. *Brain* 2011; 134: 2456–77.
29. van Swieten J, Spillantini MG. Hereditary frontotemporal dementia caused by Tau gene mutations. *Brain Pathol* 2007; 17: 63–73.
30. Spillantini MG, Goedert M. Tau protein pathology in neurodegenerative diseases. *Trends Neurosci* 1998; 21: 428–33.
31. Boeve BF, Hutton M. Refining frontotemporal dementia with parkinsonism linked to chromosome 17: introducing FTDP-17 (MAPT) and FTDP-17 (PGRN). *Arch Neurol* 2008; 65: 460–4.
32. Cruts M, Gijselinck I, van der Zee J, et al. Null mutations in progranulin cause ubiquitin-positive frontotemporal dementia linked to chromosome 17q21. *Nature* 2006; 442: 920–4.
33. Baker M, Mackenzie IR, Pickering-Brown SM, et al. Mutations in progranulin cause tau-negative frontotemporal dementia linked to chromosome 17. *Nature* 2006; 442: 916–19.
34. van Swieten JC, Heutink P. Mutations in progranulin (GRN) within the spectrum of clinical and pathological phenotypes of frontotemporal dementia. *Lancet Neurol* 2008; 7: 965–74.
35. Cairns NJ, Neumann M, Bigio EH, et al. TDP-43 in familial and sporadic frontotemporal lobar degeneration with ubiquitin inclusions. *Am J Pathol* 2007; 171: 227–40.
36. Neumann M, Sampathu DM, Kwong LK, et al. Ubiquitinated TDP-43 in frontotemporal lobar degeneration and amyotrophic lateral sclerosis. *Science* 2006; 314: 130–3.
37. Le Ber I, Camuzat A, Hannequin D, et al. Phenotype variability in progranulin mutation carriers: a clinical, neuropsychological, imaging and genetic study. *Brain* 2008; 131: 732–46.
38. Rademakers R, Baker M, Gass J, et al. Phenotypic variability associated with progranulin haploinsufficiency in patients with the common 1477C→T (Arg493X) mutation: an international initiative. *Lancet Neurol* 2007; 6: 857–68.
39. Rohrer JD, Warren JD, Omar R, et al. Parietal lobe deficits in frontotemporal lobar degeneration caused by a mutation in the progranulin gene. *Arch Neurol* 2008; 65: 506–13.
40. Jesus-Hernandez M, Mackenzie IR, Boeve BF, et al. Expanded GGGGCC hexanucleotide repeat in noncoding region of C9ORF72 causes chromosome 9p-linked FTD and ALS. *Neuron* 2011; 72: 245–56.
41. Renton AE, Majounie E, Waite A, et al. A hexanucleotide repeat expansion in C9ORF72 is the cause of chromosome 9p21-linked ALS-FTD. *Neuron* 2011; 72: 257–68.
42. Brettschneider J, van Deerlin, VM, Robinson JL, et al. Pattern of ubiquitin pathology in ALS and FTLD indicates presence of C9ORF72 hexanucleotide expansion. *Acta Neuropathol* 2012; 123: 825–39.
43. Cooper-Knock J, Hewitt C, Highley JR, et al. Clinico-pathological features in amyotrophic lateral sclerosis with expansions in C9ORF72. *Brain* 2012; 135: 751–64.
44. Snowden JS, Rollinson S, Thompson JC, et al. Distinct clinical and pathological characteristics of frontotemporal dementia associated with C9ORF72 mutations. *Brain* 2012; 135: 693–708.
45. Dobson-Stone C, Hallupp M, Bartley L, Shepherd CE, Halliday GM, Schofield PR. C9orf72 repeat expansion in clinical and neuropathological dementia cohorts. *Neurology* 2012; 79: 995–1001.
46. Sha SJ, Takada LT, Rankin KP, Yokoyama JS, Rutherford NJ, Fong JC. Frontotemporal dementia due to C9orf72 mutations: clinical and imaging features. *Neurology* 2012; 1002–11.
47. Mahoney CJ, Beck J, Rohrer JD, Lashley T, Mok K, Shakespeare T, et al. Frontotemporal dementia with the C9ORF72 hexanucleotide repeat expansion: clinical, neuroanatomical and neuropathological features. *Brain* 2012; 135 (Pt 3): 736–50.
48. Whitwell JL, Weigand SD, Boeve BF, et al. Neuroimaging signatures of frontotemporal dementia genetics: C9ORF72, tau, progranulin and sporadics. *Brain* 2012; 135: 794–806.
49. Boeve BF, Boylan KB, Graff-Radford NR, et al. Characterization of frontotemporal dementia and/or amyotrophic lateral sclerosis associated with the GGGGCC repeat expansion in C9ORF72. *Brain* 2012; 135: 765–83.
50. Simon-Sanchez J, Dopper EG, Cohn-Hokke PE, et al. The clinical and pathological phenotype of C9ORF72 hexanucleotide repeat expansions. *Brain* 2012; 135: 723–35.
51. Mahoney CJ, Beck J, Rohrer JD, et al. Frontotemporal dementia with the C9ORF72 hexanucleotide repeat expansion: clinical, neuroanatomical and neuropathological features. *Brain* 2012; 135: 736–50.
52. McKhann GM, Albert MS, Grossman M, Miller B, Dickson D, Trojanowski JQ. Clinical and pathological diagnosis of frontotemporal dementia: report of the Work Group on Frontotemporal Dementia and Pick's Disease. *Arch Neurol* 2001; 58: 1803–9.
53. Pijnenburg YA, Schoonenboom NS, Rosso SM, et al. CSF tau and Abeta42 are not useful in the diagnosis of frontotemporal lobar degeneration. *Neurology* 2004; 62: 1649.
54. Lebert F, Stekke W, Hasenbroekx C, Pasquier F. Frontotemporal dementia: a randomised, controlled trial with trazodone. *Dement Geriatr Cogn Disord* 2004; 17: 355–9.
55. Deakin JB, Rahman S, Nestor PJ, Hodges JR, Sahakian BJ. Paroxetine does not improve symptoms and impairs cognition in frontotemporal dementia: a double-blind randomized controlled trial. *Psychopharmacology* 2004; 172: 400–8.
56. Miller RG, Mitchell JD, Moore DH. Riluzole for amyotrophic lateral sclerosis (ALS)/motor neuron disease (MND). *Cochrane Database Syst Rev* 2012; 3: CD001447.

CHAPTER 16

Essential Tremor and Other Tremors

Steffen Paschen and Günther Deuschl

Essential tremor

Epidemiology

Essential tremor (ET) is the second most common movement disorder and the most frequent tremor type (1). A recent meta-analysis of 28 studies found the overall prevalence to be 0.4–0.9% and the prevalence in people aged 60 and above to be 4.6% (1). However, prevalence estimates vary between 0.008 and 22%, and increase with age. A third of published studies show a gender difference, with males generally being affected more often (1). Most people with ET have only a mild tremor and have not consulted a physician about their problem (2, 3). In a recent population-based study of subjects aged over 50, the prevalence of any kind of tremor was 14.5%, with 3.05% suffering from ET, 9.52% from exaggerated physiological tremor, 2.75% from parkinsonian tremor, and fewer than 0.2% from other tremors (4). Most patients with ET do not receive a diagnosis and therefore are never treated (3).

Aetiology and genetics

Twin studies have shown a high heritability of ET of up to 99% (5), and therefore genetic factors play a major role in pathogenesis of the condition. Moreover, 80% of young patients with early-onset ET have a positive family history (6). Genetic analysis has so far revealed three chromosomal loci: 3q13 (ETM1) (7), 2p22–25 (ETM2) (8), and 6p23 (ETM3) (9), but attempts to find the responsible genes in these loci (e.g. dopamine D3 receptor or heat shock 1 protein) have been unsuccessful (10). A genome-wide association study demonstrated an association of ET with the protein LINGO1 (7), and this was subsequently confirmed in independent cohorts (10–15). LINGO1 has different functions and is involved in myelination of the central nervous system (CNS). Regarding environmental factors, harmaline, a beta-carboline which produces tremor in animals and intoxication in humans, has also been shown to produce an action tremor in humans (16). Beta-carbolines have been found to be elevated in the blood of ET patients compared with controls (17).

There is an ongoing discussion about ET as a risk factor for developing Parkinson's disease. This notion is supported by epidemiological studies which have recently been summarized (18), but the overwhelming epidemiological, genetic, pathological, and clinical information does not support it (19). Thus the relationship is unclear and needs further study, but in practice we do not explain this possible risk to our patients.

Pathology of ET

Routine post-mortem studies have not shown a consistent pathology (20, 21). However, two pathological variants have recently been proposed in a group of 33 patients (22–31): a cerebellar variant in 75% of the patients with Purkinje cell loss, axonal torpedoes, and basket cell changes, and a Lewy body variant in about 25% with increased numbers of brainstem Lewy bodies. So far these findings have not been reproduced. One group found no increase in Lewy bodies, but observed some cases with cerebellar pathology (32), and another group did not find a higher Purkinje cell loss in ET patients compared with controls (33). Incidental neuropathology and the clinical diagnosis of the patient may compromise the results and therefore more studies are needed.

Pathophysiology and pathogenesis

Physiological mechanisms generating tremor

Almost all pathological tremors, particularly ET, emerge from networks within the central nervous system. ET and parkinsonian tremor are the most common examples. Damped mechanical oscillations and reflex contributions may also contribute to the expression of tremor (34), but they play a minor role.

Coherence analysis of tremor signals and simultaneous electroencephalography (EEG) or magnetoencephalography (MEG) have revealed involvement of the ipsilateral cerebellum and contralateral thalamus and sensorimotor cortex in ET (35, 36). Therefore, it is believed that these structures are involved in the genesis of essential tremor. For many reasons it is assumed that the olivocerebellothalamic nuclei play a pacemaker role in ET, but this has not yet been proved. Coherence analysis has also been used to study the relation between rhythms in the muscles of different extremities. There is often strong coherence between the muscles of one extremity, little or no coherence between the muscles of the ipsilateral arm and leg, and no coherence between extremities on different sides of the body (37, 38). It is believed that rhythmically firing thalamic neurons have variable coherence with ET recorded from various muscles. Thus, the 'central oscillator' in these disorders may be a network of many variably coupled oscillators.

General concepts on the genesis of ET

Overall, two pathophysiological hypotheses for the development of ET are currently accepted (39). In the first, ET is thought to be a disorder which is primarily limited to the release of tremorgenic neuronal oscillations in the central nervous system which is caused by both genetic abnormalities and non-genetic factors (39, 40). Such neuronal oscillations could be generated by, for example, altered ion channels or altered receptors for neurotransmitters. This would fit with the overall benign course apart from tremor, the lack of consistent pathology, and the potential reversibility. The other hypothesis assumes that genetic factors together with putative non-genetic factors might lead to neurodegeneration, which consequently causes the tremor syndrome and other disturbances of neurological function (27). In this sense, it is proposed that ET is a neurodegenerative disease. The evidence for this hypothesis is relatively weak, given the benign course of the disease and the inconsistent pathological data.

Diagnosis

Since no specific biomarker or diagnostic test is available, the diagnosis of ET is mainly based on clinical examination and the patient's history. The published clinical criteria for the diagnosis in ET differ slightly. An ad hoc group of the Movement Disorder Society (MDS) agreed on the following definition of classic ET in a consensus statement (41) (Table 16.1).

The criteria of the Tremor Investigation Group (TRIG) are similar, but they exclude isolated head tremor in the absence of dystonic posturing as a variant of ET and suggest a 5-year history of hand tremor without any signs of other disease for the diagnosis of definite ET (41). However, the presenting symptom of ET is always tremor. Finally, particularly for epidemiological studies, research criteria have been defined which request that, in addition, the tremor has an amplitude of at least 2 cm (42).

Table 16.1 Diagnostic criteria for essential tremor (41)

Inclusion criteria
1. Bilateral, largely symmetric postural or kinetic tremor involving hands and forearms that is visible and persistent
2. Additional or isolated tremor of the head may occur but in the absence of abnormal posturing
Exclusion criteria
1. Other abnormal neurological signs, especially dystonia, in addition to the cogwheel sign and a mild gait impairment
2. The presence of known causes of enhanced physiological tremor, including current or recent exposure to tremorgenic drugs or the presence of a drug withdrawal state
3. Further exclusion criteria: evidence for psychogenic tremor, primary orthostatic tremor, isolated voice tremor, isolated position-specific or task-specific tremors (primary writing tremor), other isolated tremors (tongue, chin, leg)
Supportive criteria
1. Tremor duration of >3 years
2. Positive family history
3. Reduction of tremor by alcohol (in 50–90% of patients with ET)

The sensitivity and specificity of the supportive criteria are unknown. It is assumed that any other cause of tremor should become obvious after a period of 3 years. A family history of tremor is usually assumed if patients report more than two relatives with an obvious postural tremor. Alcohol sensitivity is not pathognomonic for ET as it can also be found in other conditions (43), such as myoclonic dystonia, although it is probably more frequently found in ET even though many patients are not aware of this effect.

Clinical features of ET

The topographical distribution of ET differs from other tremors. A meta-analysis of 1569 patients illustrated that the tremor in ET has a typical topographical distribution, with the hands affected in 94% (80–100%), the head in 33% (20–41%), the voice in 16% (9–20%), the chin in 8% (0–9%), the face in 3%, and the trunk in 2.5% (0–3%) (44, 45). Alcohol leads to a reduction of the tremor in two out of every three patients. Moreover, there are no significant differences in clinical features between patients with a positive family history and sporadic cases.

The main characteristic of ET is the bilateral visible postural and kinetic tremor of the forearms. In advanced ET, which is more common at older ages, a subgroup of 50–60% of patients develop a severe intention tremor of the hands which is found in cerebellar disease. Intention tremor is a characteristic hallmark of a cerebellar syndrome and may be seen in advanced essential tremor syndrome (46), but clinically visible cerebellar symptoms are generally unusual in ET, except for impaired tandem gait. Tremor at rest occurs in 10–15% (47, 48). Sometimes slight postural abnormalities may be observed, such as flexion of the hands during postural tasks in the context of upper limb tremor or slight deviations of the head in cases of head tremor. These signs have been interpreted as evidence of dystonic tremor (49) but they could also be a postural adaptation to minimize tremor amplitude.

The condition may begin in childhood, but the incidence increases above age 40 years, with a mean onset at 35–45 years (50, 51). At older ages the incidence increases, but most cases seem to be sporadic and there is almost complete penetrance for familial cases by the age of 65 (5, 52). Currently, few data on progression of the condition are available, but they have shown a decrease in tremor frequency and a tendency to develop larger amplitudes (53). Intention tremor develops between 3 and 30 years after the onset of postural tremor (46).

Disease-related disability varies significantly and depends on the severity of intention tremor (2). Disability and handicap vary among patients. Notably, studies with community-based cohorts show less severe tremor compared with outpatient cohorts. Fine motor control of the hands is most affected, leading to impairments in activities of daily living (ADL) such as eating, drinking, and writing. In severe cases the patients are unable to drink and eat independently. Head and voice tremor may cause separate disabilities, including handicaps in communication. Tremor severity has been classified on the basis of the ability to drink from a glass (54). Most patients suffer from a significant disability (55). Up to 25% of patients seeking medical attention have to change jobs or retire from work (56, 57). A third to two-thirds of outpatient cohorts have reduced working abilities or retire prematurely (3, 58). On a generic quality of life (QoL) questionnaire ET patients had reduced scores in all eight domains of the SF-36. Tremor severity correlated with some of the physical domains, as well as with social function in the mental domains (48).

Tremor severity is measured clinically using the Fahn–Tolosa–Marin scale (59), which has been validated. An ET-specific QoL questionnaire has recently been validated (60).

Additional symptoms

Patients with ET may also suffer from a mild ataxic gait disorder which can be detected on tandem gait testing (61), particularly in those with a visible intention tremor of the hands. Furthermore, patients with ET have minor changes in oculomotor function which can be detected using formal oculographic measurements, again pointing to subtle but definite cerebellar dysfunction (62). The cerebellar disturbance of ET does not worsen with small amounts of alcohol, as would be expected in most cerebellar disease (63). Furthermore, a frontal dysexecutive syndrome and mild personality changes have been described in ET (64, 65). More recently, an increased frequency of dementia (66, 67), hearing deficits (68), and deficits of olfaction (69) have been described, although these findings need independent confirmation.

Differential diagnosis and ancillary tests

Neurophysiological tests can be used in clinical practice. Tremor can be measured with accelerometry and electromyography, which give the power, frequency, and additional characteristics of the tremor. There are proposals to define essential tremor on the basis of such measurements (70). These criteria are as follows (70, 71):

- rhythmic bursts of postural tremor on EMG;
- tremor frequency greater than or equal to 4 Hz;
- absence of latency of tremor recurrence when the hands are moving from rest into postural position;
- changes of the dominant frequency peak less than or equal to 1 Hz after the weight load test (Fig. 16.1);
- no changes in tremor amplitude after mental concentration.

The major significance of these criteria may be to assist in the differentiation of ET from other tremors, although further validation is necessary (70, 72).

The most frequent differential diagnostic considerations are enhanced physiological, parkinsonian, dystonic, and psychogenic tremors.

Enhanced or exaggerated physiological tremor is probably the most important differential diagnosis as it is even more common than essential tremor. Enhanced physiological tremor is a reversible tremor with mainly postural and action tremor of the hands (41). It may occur as a side effect of medication, or as a symptom of other disease. Electrophysiological tests may help to separate ET from enhanced physiological tremor (Fig. 16.1). A detailed medical history with a particular focus on medication (see Table 16.3) and laboratory diagnostics (see Table 16.4) should be conducted.

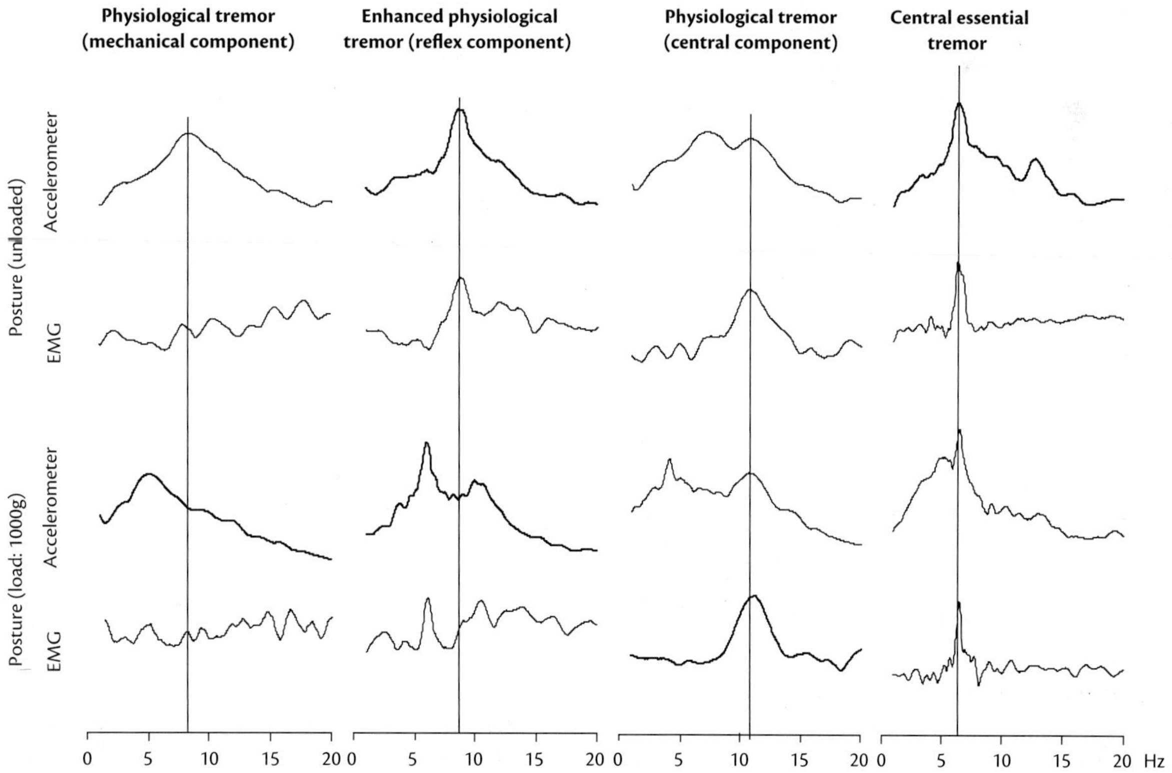

Fig. 16.1 Frequency analysis of hand accelerometry and wrist extensor electromyogram. The first column shows a mechanical tremor in the upper row and the EMG signal which is flat. Loading of the hand with 1000 g shows a decrease of the mechanical frequency without synchronization of the EMG. The second column shows a reduction of both accelerometry and EMG signal during loading which indicates a reflex origin of tremor. The third column shows a central component in physiological tremor which is typically invariant to loading of the hand and is only rarely found in normal subjects. The last column shows the findings in essential tremor. (Modified from Deuschl G, Raethjen J, Lindemann M, Krack P. The pathophysiology of tremor. *Muscle Nerve* 2001; 24: 716–35)

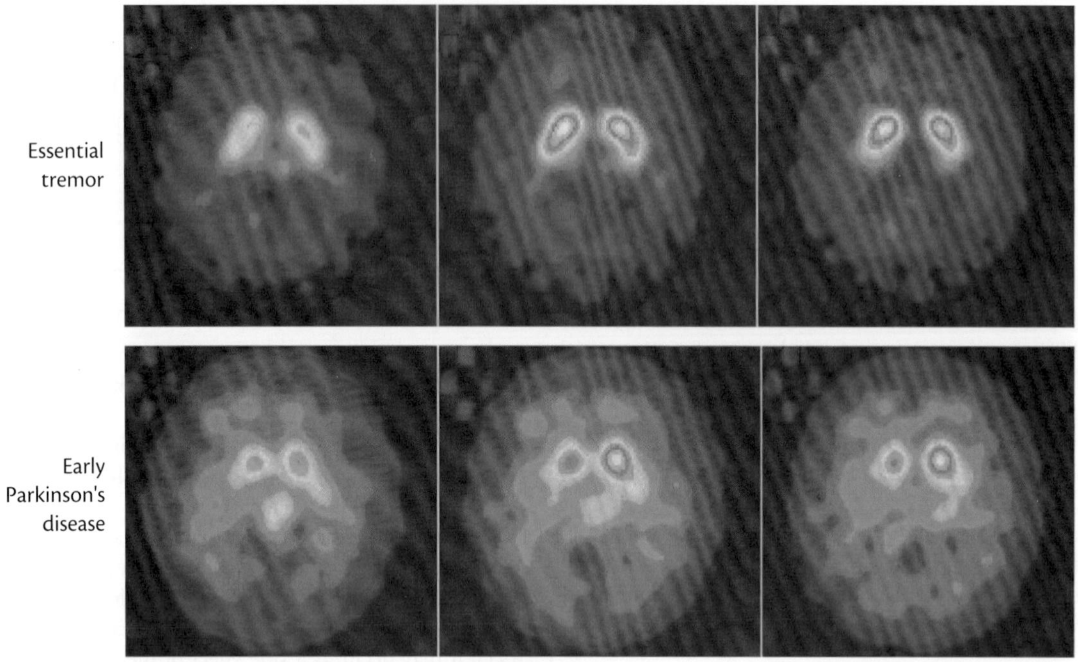

Fig. 16.2 Dopamine transporter imaging with SPECT in a patient with essential tremor and a patient with very early Parkinson's disease. Unilateral reduction of dopamine transporter binding can be seen in the PD patient, but the pattern is symmetric in the ET patient. Detailed quantitative assessment demonstrates bilateral reduction in the PD patient. (Courtesy of Dr Lürcken, Dr Luetzen, and Professor Henze, Department of Nuclear Medicine, Kiel University)

Parkinsonian and essential tremor can often be separated on clinical grounds as most PD patients suffer from tremor at rest, have a cessation of tremor when voluntary movements are initiated, and display additional symptoms such as akinesia, rigidity, and postural disturbances. However, early PD can easily be misinterpreted as ET, and vice versa. Electrophysiological criteria may be useful, and advanced methods of accelerometry and EMG analysis seem to separate the two conditions with high accuracy (72). Dopamine transporter SPECT or PET imaging of the dopaminergic system is currently the most sensitive test for the differential diagnosis of parkinsonian tremor, as the depletion of dopamine within the striatum is considered a hallmark of Parkinson's disease (Fig. 16.2). The sensitivity and specificity of these imaging tests are high, but the costs are considerable and their availability is limited.

Dystonic tremor usually starts with a focal distribution and may have additional clear-cut dystonic features. The separation of ET from psychogenic tremor is generally possible on clinical grounds. The co-contraction sign and the entrainment effect of psychogenic tremor are the most useful clinical tests.

The management of patients with ET

Therapeutic principles

Since the cause of essential tremor is still unknown, no curative therapies are available. In the long-term management of ET patients the first step is always to make a proper diagnosis and to counsel the patient that the condition is usually slowly progressive and not a sign of a life-threatening disease. Most patients worry that this tremor is the first sign of PD. Treatment needs to be as individualized as possible. The indication for starting treatment for a particular patient is mainly determined by the impairment, which depends on the severity of tremor, the objective needs for improving tremor severity, the psychosocial handicap, and the individual coping strategies. The same objective severity of tremor may or may not lead to initiation of treatment in different patients.

Pharmacotherapy

All interventions for the treatment of ET have been discovered by chance. The exact mechanisms of action of drugs, deep brain stimulation (DBS), and lesioning are unclear. Presumably, drugs used in ET interfere with the widespread pathological oscillations which occur throughout the motor system in the disorder (73). Surgical lesioning and DBS are thought to disrupt these oscillations, leading to reduced tremor amplitude. All drugs recommended in this chapter have other approved clinical indications. Using them for treatment of ET might be off-label in some countries. In order to improve compliance, the patient should be informed that pharmacotherapy cannot entirely suppress tremor.

Treatment effects can be quantified with rating scales or accelerometry, and the relation between these measures is well known (74). This was used in a recent review (73) to calculate the percentage improvement found for the different interventions and these values are reported here (Table 16.2).

Treatment attempts will be reported for hands, head, and voice separately. First-line pharmacotherapy for hand tremor has remained unchanged during the last three decades; several controlled trials have shown that non-selective beta-blockers, especially propranolol, and the anti-epileptic drug primidone are able to reduce tremor amplitude by approximately 50–60% (75, 76). Primidone is usually preferred in older patients with a possible risk of a concomitant cardiac and/or pulmonary disease. Side effects of primidone (e.g. drowsiness, dizziness, and

Table 16.2 Recommended drugs for the treatment of essential hand tremor (73)

Recommendation	Drug and dosage	Improvement	Treatment recommendation
First-line	*Propranolol* Dosage: 3× 20 to 3× 40 mg/day, maximum dosage 320 mg/day	~55%	A
	Primidone Dosage: 62.5–250 mg in evening, maximum dosage 750 mg/day	~60%	A
Second-line	*Topiramate* Increase dosage weekly by 25–50 mg, standard dosage 2× 50 to 2× 250 mg, maximum dose 400 mg/day	~40%	B
	Gabapentin Increase dosage every 3–5 days by 300 mg, standard dosage 3× 300 to 3× 600 mg, maximum dose 2400 mg/day	~40%	B
Third-line	*Clonazepam* Start with 3× 0.5 mg, increase dosage by 0.5 mg every 2 days, standard dosage 3× 0.5 to 3× 2 mg	–	C (intention tremor)
	Alprazolam Start with 3× 0.25–0.5 mg, increase dosage every 3 days by 0.25–0.5 mg, standard dose 3× 0.5 to 3× 1 mg	~50%	C (risk of addiction)
	Botulinum toxin Symmetric injections in cervical muscles; recommended dosages: see cervical dystonia	– –	C (hand tremor) B (head tremor)

disequilibrium) are common when treatment is started. Therefore a starting dose of 62.5 mg or less in the evening is recommended. Fatigue is a common and sometimes dose-limiting side effect of primidone.

Propranolol is usually favoured over primidone in young patients without any evidence of heart disease or bronchial asthma. Side effects such as bradycardia, syncope, fatigue, and erectile dysfunction may be dose-limiting. Treatment should start with 20–60 mg/day, and the dose should be increased gradually. Total daily doses of 60–240 mg are adequate in most responders (73). If one of the first-line drugs does not sufficiently improve tremor it should be increased to the maximally tolerated dosage. The two drugs can be combined if required.

Second-line drugs (Table 16.2) include topiramate and gabapentin (73). Alprazolam showed comparable effects to first-line medication in less rigorous trials, but as it is a benzodiazepine it is not recommended for long-term treatment because of its addictive potential. Studies with selective beta-blockers (e.g. atenolol, sotalol) have shown less beneficial effects than the non-selective beta-blocker propranolol (73). Injection of botulinum toxin in hand muscles has been successfully used for hand tremor, but symptomatic hand weakness in 30–70% of patients limits its use (77). In patients with advanced ET, intention tremor can cause serious disability. Thompson and co-workers (78) showed that clonazepam can specifically improve action tremor compared with propranolol.

Head and voice tremor are usually less suppressed than hand tremor with drug therapy (73). Improvements of 30–50% in head tremor with propranolol and primidone have been reported in several studies (79, 80). For severe head tremors, particularly when an intention tremor is present, patients may require bilateral DBS which can reduce head tremor by up to 75% (81–86).

Treatment of voice tremor with propranolol and methazolamide did not show a positive effect (87). Results for laryngeal botulinum toxin injections for voice tremor are conflicting. Typical side effects are a weak voice, coughing, and dysphagia (88, 89).

Deep brain stimulation

Destructive therapies like thermocoagulation have been largely abandoned since the discovery of DBS. DBS of the nucleus ventrointermedius of the thalamus (Vim) (90) is an efficient treatment in patients who are unresponsive to medical therapy, although controlled studies are not yet available. Improvements are of the order of 90%, superior to any pharmacological intervention reported so far (73). Long-term follow-up suggests a loss of tremor control for various reasons (83). Stimulation-induced side effects (e.g. dysarthria, paraesthesias, dystonia, balance disturbances, ataxia, and limb weakness) can usually be reduced by adjusting stimulation parameters. Hardware complications may occur in up to 25% of patients (e.g. lead fracture, infections, connection cable malfunction). The risk of a perioperative complication, including intracerebral haemorrhage, ischaemic stroke, or infection is less than 2% (91). The optimum stereotactic target of Vim stimulation is considered below the Vim in the radiation pre-lemniscalis and the caudal zona incerta (92) (Fig. 16.3). Other targets like the zona incerta and the subthalamic nucleus have been proposed, but have not yet been adequately studied (73).

Other tremors

Enhanced physiological tremor

The term enhanced physiological tremor (EPT) refers to a tremor with the frequency and activation characteristics of normal physiological tremor but with a larger amplitude when all other causes of tremor are excluded. It is a visible postural and action tremor which can be troublesome, particularly on action. There are many causes for the enhancement of tremor (Table 16.3), among which drugs are the most common (Table 16.4). The exclusion of other neurological symptoms or diseases that could cause tremor is mandatory for the diagnosis (41). For tremors of unknown origin, the laboratory tests summarized in Table 16.5 may be considered. Moreover, in the case

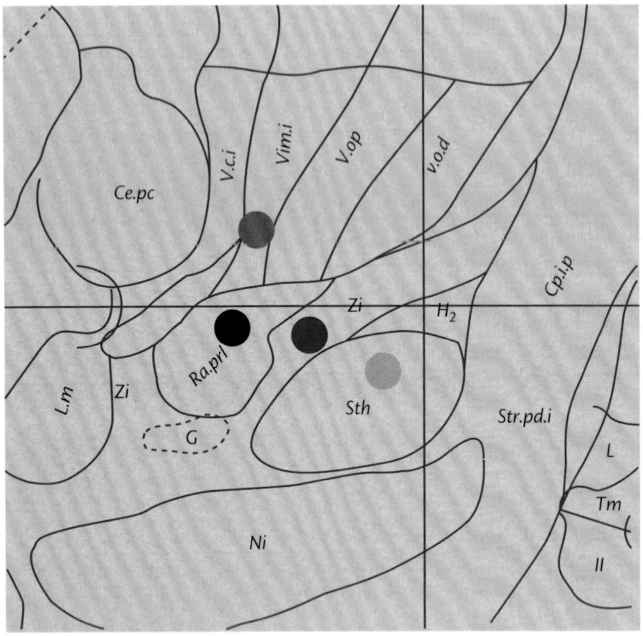

Fig. 16.3 Targets for the standard treatment of tremor (73). The standard target is the nucleus ventrointermedius of the thalamus (Vim, grey dot) and the region below the Vim, the radiation pre-lemniscalis (Ra.prl, black dot). Less established targets are the caudal zona incerta (Zi, dark green dot) and the subthalamic nucleus (Sth, light green dot). Sth is the standard target for Parkinson's disease. Sth, corpus subthalamicum; Ra.prl, radiatio pre-lemniscalis; H_2, ampus forelii, pars H_2; V.o.d, nucleus ventro-oralis dorsalis; V.op, nucleus ventro-oralis posterior; Vim.i, nucleus ventrointermedius internus; V.c.i, nucleus ventrocaudalis internus; Ce.pc, nucleus centralis parvocellularis; Cp.i.p, capsula interna crus posterior; Str.pd.i, striae pedunculi interni; Tm, nucleus tuberomammillaris; L, lemniscus; L.m, lemniscus medialis; Ni, nucleus niger; Zi, zona incerta; G, fasciculus gracilis; II, opticus.

Table 16.3 Causes of enhanced physiological tremor

Drugs	Neuroleptics, metoclopramide, antidepressants (tricyclics), lithium, cocaine, alcohol, sympathomimetics, steroids, valproate, anti-arrhythmics (amiodarone), thyroid hormones, cytostatics, immunodepressants
Toxins	Mercury, lead, manganese, alcohol, DDT, lindan
Metabolic disturbances	Hyperthyroidism, hyperparathyroidism, hypoglycaemia, hepatic encephalopathy, magnesium deficiency, hypocalcaemia, hyponatraemia
Others	Anxiety, fatigue, sympathetic reflex dystrophy, withdrawal of alcohol or drugs

of an undiagnosed, new onset tremor syndrome without discernible cause, a brain MRI scan is recommended if the symptoms are unilateral, since focal lesions can produce tremor.

A recent study found the prevalence of EPT to be 9.5% in subjects over 50 years of age. EPT was much more common than ET (3.06%), parkinsonian tremor (2.05%) or Parkinson's disease (4.49%) (4). There are no studies available on the natural history of the condition. The pathophysiological mechanism may be either activation of the reflex loops (e.g. hyperthyroidism) or activation of a central oscillator which is related to physiological tremor (93) caused, for example, by drugs.

The causes of an enhancement of one or both of the physiological tremor components are diverse. Trembling with excitement, fear, or

Table 16.4 Drugs with tremor as a possible side effect

Group	Example
Beta-adrenergic drugs	Fenoterol, salbutamol
Phosphodiesterase inhibitors	Theophylline, caffeine
Anti-arrhythmic drugs	Amiodarone, mexiletine, procainamide
Calcium-channel inhibitors	Nifedipine, amlodipine
Immunotherapy	Ciclosporin, tacrolimus, interferon
Antidepressants	Tricyclic antidepressants, SSRIs
Lithium	
Neuroleptics, antidopaminergics	Haloperidol, metoclopramide
Antiepileptics	Valproate, lamotrigine
Anti-infective agents	Co-trimoxazole, amphotericin B, vidarabine
Hormone therapy	Thyroxine, calcitonin, progesterone, corticosteroids

Table 16.5 Recommended laboratory tests for postural and action tremors of unknown origin

Laboratory value	Question
Thyroid (T_3, T_4, TSH)	Hyperthyroidism
Electrolytes (Na^+, K^+, Ca^{2+}, Cl^-)	Hypocalcaemia, hypokalaemia, metabolic alteration
Liver enzymes (GGT, GOT, GPT, CE)	Alcoholic disease, Wilson disease (hepatocerebral degeneration)
Glucose	Hypoglycaemia
Immuno-electrophoresis	Neuropathy in paraproteinaemia, neuropathic tremor
If clinically suspected	
Serum ceruloplasmin, copper in 24 hour urine	Wilson disease
Toxicological diagnostics	Arsenic, bismuth, mercury, lead poisoning, alcohol-related, medication withdrawal

anxiety is common and may be problematic for performing artists or people who need a high accuracy of dexterity, such as surgeons. It is thought to be mediated via increased sympathetic tone which results in a beta-adrenergically driven sensitization of the muscle spindles, increasing the gain in the reflex loops (94). A similar origin via the sympathetic nervous system has been proposed for the tremor in reflex sympathetic dystrophy. Metabolic abnormalities, drugs and toxins, or withdrawal from such substances are common causes of EPT. The pathophysiology may be peripheral or central, depending on the cause.

As both EPT and early ET are unaccompanied by other obvious neurological symptoms, they are difficult to distinguish. The positive family history in ET, its chronic course, and the lack of an overt cause for the tremor are important clues. Sometimes the diagnosis can only be made after having observed the patient for an extended time period. EPT is usually bilateral and thus any tremor presenting unilaterally, even with a high frequency and a pure postural component, must be suspected to be a symptomatic tremor. Spectral analysis of accelerometry and EMG signal data can be helpful in demonstrating a centrally driven component in ET (95). A frequency below 8 Hz, which can be seen in the very early stage of ET, favours ET rather than EPT (96).

Treatment

Depending on the aetiology of EPT, addressing the potential underlying cause is always the first step. There are only a few studies that have reported on symptomatic treatment of EPT. Treatment of thyrotoxic tremor is recommended with propranolol (<160 mg daily) but other beta-blockers, namely atenolol (<200 mg daily), metoprolol (<200 mg daily), acebutolol (<400 mg daily), oxprenolol (<160 mg daily), nadolol (<80 mg daily, and molol (<20 mg daily), have similar effects (97). Other treatment recommendations are based solely on expert opinion. A single dose of a beta-blocking agent (e.g. propranolol 10–60 mg) 30 minutes before a stressful situation is recommended to suppress transient tremor that is known to interfere with important (e.g. professional) activities in a predisposed subject.

Parkinsonian tremor

The most common and classic parkinsonian tremor is a rest tremor or a combination of a rest and a postural/kinetic tremor with the same frequency (type I PD tremor) (41). The tremor frequency is mostly above 4 Hz. Higher frequencies (of up to 9 Hz) can occur in early PD. The asymmetric rest tremor is suppressed during movement and recurs in some posture conditions. Clinically this type I tremor affects the upper and lower limbs and the face. Occasionally the tremor can start in the lower extremities.

In some patients the posture/kinetic tremor has a higher frequency (>1.5 Hz) that is non-harmonically related to the rest tremor (type II PD tremor) (41), if this is present. It is unknown whether the postural tremor is part of a co-existing essential tremor or a specific feature of PD tremor. An isolated postural and kinetic tremor with a frequency of 4–9 Hz may be seen (type III PD tremor), particularly in PD subjects with predominant akinesia and rigidity (41). This has been related to rigidity (98) and can be demonstrated particularly during finger movements (99). The majority of patients with PD have the classic parkinsonian rest tremor (type I PD tremor).

Treatment

Studies with PD tremor as the main outcome measure are rare, but the tremor items of the Unified Parkinson's Disease Rating Scale provide an estimate of the anti-tremor effect of these interventions.

Levodopa is an efficient drug against parkinsonian tremor. This has recently been confirmed in the ELLDOPA trial (100). All dopamine agonists have a significant anti-tremor effect, and a specific study addressed this issue for pramipexole, but there is no compelling evidence that any dopamine agonist has a better anti-tremor effect than the others (101–103).

Anticholinergic drugs can improve rest tremor, but cognitive adverse effects limit their use, especially in older patients. A small pathological series (104) which has yet to be confirmed suggested that patients with previous anticholinergic therapy showed more tau pathology. The clinical side effects of anticholinergic treatment are considered to be reversible. Clozapine is effective against PD tremor (105), but is mainly used for otherwise drug-resistant tremors, especially when those patients have concomitant hallucinations. Amantadine is a poorly studied second-line drug for tremor with limited efficacy. Budipine is well studied and effective (106), but may cause cardiac arrhythmias and is available only in some European countries. In cases with a significant postural/kinetic tremor (type II PD tremor) propranolol (107, 108) and primidone (107) are an option if dopaminergic therapy is not sufficiently effective. Dosing of all drugs is summarized in Table 16.6.

Table 16.6 Treatment of parkinsonian tremor

1. Dopaminergic therapy Levodopa, dopamine agonists at dosages used for the treatment of akinesia and rigidity
2. Anticholinergics Bornaprine 3× 2 mg to 3× 4 mg Biperidine 3× 2 mg to 3× 4 mg Trihexyphenidyl 3× 2 mg to 3× 4 mg Metixene 3× 5 mg to 3× 10 mg Benztropine 3× 2 mg Procyclidine 3× 5 to 3× 10 mg
3. Propranolol/primidone Propranolol 3× 20 to 3× 60 mg Primidone 62.5–750 mg
4. Amantadine 3× 100 to 3× 150 mg
5. Clozapine <12.5 mg to 3× 25 mg
6. Bilateral DBS of the STN or GPi (for selected cases Vim)

Stereotactic surgery can be considered in patients with a disabling tremor. All three targets of deep brain stimulation for PD (subthalamic nucleus (STN), globus pallidus internus (GPi), and ventrointermedius nucleus of the thalamus (Vim)) are efficacious (109–112). STN and GPi stimulation also improve akinesia and rigidity, but Vim stimulation only improves tremor. Therefore Vim stimulation is reserved for selected cases only, mainly elderly patients with a stable course of tremor-dominant PD.

For pragmatic therapy, the first decision is to determine clinically if the PD tremor syndrome has a higher-frequency postural component (type II PD tremor). In this case, non-dopaminergic treatment with propranolol or primidone is recommended. Two standard situations of complicated PD tremor will be considered: the *de novo* patient and the advanced patient with drug-resistant tremor.

In the *de novo* patient tremor may need more time to improve during the dosing-in period than akinesia and rigidity. Therefore the amount of dopaminergic treatment should be geared to address akinesia and rigidity. When akinesia and rigidity are adequately treated with a dopamine agonist or levodopa, it is advisable to wait for another 2 months before specifically targeting the tremor because this symptom can improve further with time. If a significant tremor is still present, anticholinergic treatment is an option for the younger patient or an increase in dopaminergic treatment for the elderly. Amantadine is mostly ineffective, but can be tried. Clozapine in low dose (6.75–7.5 mg) may be considered, with adequate monitoring for potential side effects (particularly agranulocytosis). If this is not effective, very high doses of levodopa can be tried, but otherwise DBS is the next option to be considered.

In the advanced patient treatment-refractory tremor may occur in the OFF period and may require further smoothing of dopaminergic treatment with levodopa, dopamine agonists and/or COMT inhibitors. If tremor continues to be a problem, despite otherwise treated OFF periods, the first step is usually to increase the total dose of dopaminergic treatment. This is often limited by dyskinesias; tremor may abate, but at the expense of severe dykinesias.

In this situation anticholinergic treatment is almost never used but clozapine may be considered. STN or GPi DBS may be a very worthwhile option in selected cases.

Dystonic tremor

Dystonic tremor is an entity which is under debate and different definitions have been proposed (113, 114). Its pathophysiology is largely unknown (115). Typical dystonic tremor occurs in a body region affected by dystonia. It is defined (115) as a postural/kinetic tremor not usually seen during complete rest. At onset, and sometimes during the course of the disease, dystonic tremor is focal and limited to one or a few extremities, with irregular amplitude and variable frequencies (mostly below 7 Hz). However, some patients exhibit focal tremors even without overt signs of dystonia. They have been included as dystonic tremor (116) because some later develop evidence of dystonia. Special forms of dystonic tremor are task-specific in nature, such as dystonic voice tremor (117) or dystonic writing tremor (118, 119). Jaw tremor and dystonia has been proposed as a specific entity (120).

The prevalence of dystonic tremor is unknown. In one cross-sectional study 20% of patients with primary or secondary dystonia (121) suffered from tremor. Tremor is more common in cervical dystonia (122).

Antagonistic gestures can lead to a reduction of the tremor amplitude in patients with dystonic tremor. This is frequently seen in dystonic head tremor or tremulous spasmodic torticollis (123). As this sign is absent in essential head tremor it can be an important differential diagnostic clue for head tremors in which the dystonic posture is not immediately obvious. Other important, but less specific, differential diagnostic clues are the focal nature and relatively low frequency of dystonic tremor. The tremor associated with dystonia is more difficult to separate from ET, especially when the accompanying dystonia has not evolved completely. Dopamine transporter imaging may be necessary to separate parkinsonian tremor from dystonic tremor (124).

Treatment

No controlled study of oral medication is available. A positive effect of propranolol or anticholinergics has been reported in case series of dystonic head tremor. The efficacy of botulinum toxin for dystonic head tremor and tremulous spasmodic dysphonia is well documented (51). A double-blind study has also documented the efficacy of botulinum toxin for hand tremor (77), but the use of this agent for this indication is limited because of associated paresis. Dystonic tremor in the setting of segmental or generalized dystonia has been successfully treated with DBS of the pallidum in a controlled study (125). Stimulation of the ventrolateral thalamus can also alleviate the tremor, but may occasionally lead to worsening of the dystonia. Tremor associated with dystonia may respond to medication used for classic ET.

Task-specific tremor

Task-specific tremor (TST) is a form of action tremor that occurs when a person performs a specific task, for example writing, speaking, or playing an instrument (41, 126). TST often occurs with dystonia and may share common pathophysiological mechanisms.

TST is labelled as uncomplicated if tremor occurs only during the task, and complicated if it has a tendency to generalize to other tasks. Primary writing tremor (PWT) is the most common form of task-specific tremor. It has a frequency of 5–7 Hz and can be subdivided into type A (task-induced tremor) and type B (positionally sensitive tremor) (119). The pathophysiology is unknown. Highly skilled and over-learned tasks, in combination with an individual's disposition, may lead to a task-specific tremor (119). There is controversy as to whether PWT is a variant of essential tremor, a focal dystonia, or a separate nosological entity (41, 119, 127).

Other task-specific tremors include highly trained tasks, typically in musicians and athletes. Alcohol reduces the tremor in some patients.

Treatment

Controlled studies are not available. The treatment is escalated according to the specific needs of the patient. Pharmacotherapy with propranolol or primidone has been recommended. Other therapeutic options include sensory and motor training (128–130) as well as personalized tools like special writing pencils (131). In 50% of patients injections of botulinum toxin can reduce the tremor significantly (132, 133). Vim DBS for task-specific tremor is experimental (134).

Cerebellar tremor syndromes

Cerebellar tremor is a symptomatic tremor with an intention component as the most prominent sign. For diagnosis of a cerebellar tremor, the following conditions have to be satisfied (41):

- pure or dominant intention tremor (unilateral or bilateral);
- tremor frequency mainly below 5 Hz;
- postural tremor may be present, but no rest tremor.

Titubation is another tremulous manifestation of cerebellar disease, and is a low-frequency oscillation (around 3 Hz) of the head and trunk depending on postural innervation (135).

Depending on the aetiology a full spectrum of cerebellar symptoms and signs may be present. Cerebellar tremor syndromes are most frequently caused by multiple sclerosis (136). Other causes include chronic alcohol toxicity, trauma, or degenerative cerebellar disorder (e.g. spinocerebellar ataxias). Tremor in fragile X-associated tremor–ataxia syndrome (FXTAS) is mostly a postural and intention tremor, and gait ataxia is usually present in these patients (137).

Treatment

Pharmacotherapy of cerebellar tremor is often disappointing. Studies with cholinomimetic compounds (e.g. physostigmine, lecithin) have shown improvement in some patients, but failed to demonstrate benefit in the majority. Isoniazid failed to show significant results (138). 5-Hydroxytryptophan (5-HTP) has been found to be effective in some patients (139, 140). Open-label studies or single-case observations have shown favourable results with amantadine, propranolol, clonazepam, carbamazepine, tetrahydrocannabiol, and trihexyphenidyl. Levetiracetam (50 mg/kg/day) was beneficial in a pilot trial (141). Cannabis is not effective (142). Probably the greatest symptomatic improvement is obtained with either DBS of the thalamus or thalamotomy (143–145) but the functional benefit can worsen over time, particularly in patients with multiple sclerosis (146).

Orthostatic tremor

Orthostatic tremor (OT) is a rare tremor characterized by an unsteady stance because of a high-frequency tremor of the legs

(147, 148). OT usually begins after the fourth decade, and women (50 years) seem to be affected earlier than men (60 years). In most cases the origin is unknown or idiopathic, although some patients have been reported with a positive family history. So far no candidate genes have been identified. Some authors have reported OT in advanced Parkinson's disease (149, 150).

Clinical features of patients with OT include unsteadiness on standing, which rarely may cause falls. A mild gait ataxia in older patients has been described. Sitting and walking are unaffected. Patients try to avoid standing still. No obvious tremor is seen on visual inspection, but tremor can be palpated or auscultated in leg muscles. OT must be separated from the stance tremors of ET, PD, or cerebellar tremors.

OT is diagnosed by electromyography of the quadriceps muscle, with surface electrodes showing the pathognomonic 13–18 Hz burst discharges while standing, which mostly cease when sitting (151, 152). An extremely rare variant of slow orthostatic tremor has been described (153, 154).

Treatment

Therapy of OT is often challenging. First-line therapy includes gabapentin (1200–2400 mg/day) and clonazepam (1.5–6 mg/day) (155, 156). Alternatively, primidone (62.5–500 mg/day) may be used. Although a mild dopaminergic deficit has been found in some patients, levodopa does not seem to be an effective therapy (157). Bilateral Vim DBS has been described in single-case reports with OT (158, 159), and spinal stimulation has also been successful in some patients (160). Both treatments need further evaluation.

Holmes tremor and thalamic tremor

Holmes tremor is a combination of rest, postural, and intention tremors with a low frequency (<4 Hz) (41, 161, 162). It is a symptomatic tremor, typically developing after a lesion in the brainstem. Different names have been used in the past (rubral tremor, midbrain tremor, Benedikt's syndrome). Such a lesion may be due to stroke, neoplasm, cystic degeneration, operative lesion, or cavernoma. The pathophysiology is explained by a 'double-hit' disruption of both nigrostriatal dopaminergic and cerebellothalamic systems (163, 164), causing the combination of a parkinsonian rest tremor and a cerebellar intention tremor. Some patients with Holmes tremor may have additional dystonia.

Thalamic tremor is an entity which can present with the same symptoms of rest and intention tremor as a Holmes tremor. However, additional symptoms, such as dystonia, jerky movements, or a sensory disturbance, are also found. The cause is a lesion of the lateral thalamus, which is most often ischaemic.

Treatment

No controlled trials are available. Levodopa and dopamine agonists are helpful in some patients (164). Anticholinergics, propranolol, clonazepam, primidone, and levetiracetam have also been described as being efficacious (165–168). Some patients may benefit from Vim DBS (169).

Palatal tremor syndromes

Palatal tremors are rare tremor syndromes and can be separated into two forms (170, 171).

Symptomatic palatal tremor (SPT) is characterized by rhythmic movements of the soft palate (levator veli palatini), clinically visible as a rhythmic movement of the edge of the palate. Other brainstem-innervated muscles (leading to oscillopsia in case of eye muscle involvement) or extremity muscles can also be affected (172). SPT typically follows a brainstem or cerebellar lesion after a variable delay (173, 174) and is often associated with a cerebellar syndrome (175).

Essential palatal tremor (EPaT) occurs without any overt central nervous pathology and is characterized by rhythmic movements of the soft palate (tensor veli palatini), usually with an associated ear click. The tensor contraction is visible as a movement of the roof of the palate. Extremity or eye muscles are not involved.

The pathophysiology of SPT is considered to be abnormal discharges of the inferior olive. The pathophysiology of EPaT is unknown.

Treatment

The disability of patients with SPT is mostly due to other clinical symptoms related to the underlying cerebellar lesion. The rhythmic palatal movement in SPT does not cause discomfort or disability for the patient, except when the eyes are involved or when there is an extremity tremor. Oscillopsia is a difficult complaint to treat. Single cases have been described with a favourable response to clonazepam. Other oral drugs which have been proposed are trihexyphenidyl and valproate. Botulinum toxin has been used to treat oscillopsia. The toxin can either be injected into the retrobulbar fat tissue or individual eye muscles can be targeted selectively (176, 177). No controlled studies are available. We have found that this treatment is helpful for some patients, but is not always acceptable for long-term use because of its limited effect. In the treatment of extremity tremors, single cases have been reported to respond to clonazepam (178) or trihexiphenidyl (179).

The only complaint by patients with EPaT is the ear click. A number of medications have been reported to be successful—valproate (180), trihexyphenidyl (179), and flunarizine (181). Recently, sumatriptan has been found to be effective in a few patients (182, 183) but was unsuccessful in others (184). The most established current therapy is injection of botulinum toxin into the tensor veli palatini muscle (185).

Tremor syndromes in peripheral neuropathy

Several peripheral neuropathies may present with tremor. The tremors are mostly postural and action in nature. The frequency in hand muscles can be lower than in proximal arm muscles. Dysgammaglobulinaemia and chronic inflammatory demyelinating neuropathy are the acquired neuropathies presenting most frequently with tremor (186). A similar type of tremor can be observed in around 40% of patients with hereditary motor and sensory neuropathy (HMSN) (187).

Treatment

No specific therapies have been reported to be beneficial for this type of tremor. Successful treatment of the underlying neuropathy can improve the tremor in some patients (186). We have found propranolol and primidone at similar dosages as used in essential tremor to be helpful for some patients. Some patients have been successfully implanted with DBS electrodes (188).

Psychogenic tremors

Psychogenic tremors have diverse clinical presentations and are a specific variant of psychogenic movement disorders (see Chapter 31).

Most of them are action tremors, but they often show very unusual combinations of rest/postural and intention tremors (189). Sudden onset and sometimes spontaneous remission are often reported. On clinical examination the 'entrainment manoeuvre' (i.e. changes of amplitude and frequency of the trembling limb) is observed when an external rhythm is imitated by the patient with the other arm. Some patients have a positive 'co-activation sign' which is evaluated like rigidity testing at the wrist. Variable voluntary-like force exertion can be felt in both movement directions (41). Some patients have a history of somatization or additional unrelated (psychogenic) neurological symptoms and signs (41).

Among psychogenic movement disorders, tremor is the most common diagnosis (50%) (190). Electrophysiological tests can help in the differential diagnosis (see Chapter 5 for more details) (191–193).

Treatment

Studies of treatment of psychogenic tremor are rare (194). Antidepressants may be helpful (195). Psychotherapy is helpful in only a minority of patients. We recommend physiotherapy, aiming to avoid co-contraction of the muscles during voluntary movement. In addition, propranolol may be administered at medium or high dosages to desensitize the muscle spindles which are necessary to maintain the clonus mechanism in these patients. Conclusive data on the prognosis and long-term outcome in these patients are lacking, but the prognosis is generally believed to be poor (196).

References

1. Louis ED, Ferreira JJ. How common is the most common adult movement disorder? Update on the worldwide prevalence of essential tremor. *Mov Disord* 2010; 25: 534–41.
2. Louis ED, Ford B, Wendt KJ, Cameron G. Clinical characteristics of essential tremor: data from a community-based study. *Mov Disord* 1998; 13: 803–8.
3. Lorenz D, Poremba C, Papengut F, Schreiber S, Deuschl G. The psychosocial burden of essential tremor in an outpatient- and a community-based cohort. *Eur J Neurol* 2011; 18: 972–9.
4. Wenning GK, Kiechl S, Seppi K, et al. Prevalence of movement disorders in men and women aged 50–89 years (Bruneck Study cohort): a population-based study. *Lancet Neurol* 2005; 4: 815–20.
5. Lorenz D, Frederiksen H, Moises H, Kopper F, Deuschl G, Christensen K. High concordance for essential tremor in monozygotic twins of old age. *Neurology* 2004; 62: 208–11.
6. Raethjen J, Deuschl G. Tremor. *Curr Opin Neurol* 2009; 22: 400–5.
7. Stefansson H, Steinberg S, Petursson H, et al. Variant in the sequence of the LINGO1 gene confers risk of essential tremor. *Nat Genet* 2009; 41: 277–9.
8. Higgins JJ, Pho LT, Nee LE. A gene (ETM) for essential tremor maps to chromosome 2p22-p25. *Mov Disord* 1997; 12: 859–64.
9. Shatunov A, Sambuughin N, Jankovic J, et al. Genomewide scans in North American families reveal genetic linkage of essential tremor to a region on chromosome 6p23. *Brain* 2006; 129: 2318–31.
10. Tan EK. LINGO1 and essential tremor: linking the shakes. Linking LINGO1 to essential tremor. *Eur J Hum Genet* 2010; 18: 739–40.
11. Thier S, Lorenz D, Nothnagel M, et al. LINGO1 polymorphisms are associated with essential tremor in Europeans. *Mov Disord* 2010; 25: 709–15.
12. Tan EK, Teo YY, Prakash KM, et al. LINGO1 variant increases risk of familial essential tremor. *Neurology* 2009; 73: 1161–2.
13. Vilarino-Guell C, Wider C, Ross OA, et al. LINGO1 and LINGO2 variants are associated with essential tremor and Parkinson disease. *Neurogenetics* 2010; 11: 401–8.
14. Vilarino-Guell C, Ross OA, Wider C, et al. LINGO1 rs9652490 is associated with essential tremor and Parkinson disease. *Parkinsonism Relat Disord* 2010; 16: 109–11.
15. Clark LN, Park N, Kisselev S, Rios E, Lee JH, Louis ED. Replication of the LINGO1 gene association with essential tremor in a North American population. *Eur J Hum Genet* 2010; 18: 838–43.
16. Wilms H, Sievers J, Deuschl G. Animal models of tremor. *Mov Disord* 1999; 14: 557–71.
17. Louis ED, Zheng W, Jurewicz EC, et al. Elevation of blood beta-carboline alkaloids in essential tremor. *Neurology* 2002; 59: 1940–4.
18. Fekete R, Jankovic J. Revisiting the relationship between essential tremor and Parkinson's disease. *Mov Disord* 2011; 26: 391–8.
19. Adler CH, Shill HA, Beach TG. Essential tremor and Parkinson's disease: lack of a link. *Mov Disord* 2011; 26: 372–7.
20. Rajput AH, Rozdilsky B, Ang L, Rajput A. Clinicopathologic observations in essential tremor: report of six cases. *Neurology* 1991; 41: 1422–4.
21. Rajput A, Robinson CA, Rajput AH. Essential tremor course and disability: a clinicopathologic study of 20 cases. *Neurology* 2004; 62: 932–6.
22. Louis ED. Essential tremor: evolving clinicopathological concepts in an era of intensive post-mortem enquiry. *Lancet Neurol* 2010; 9: 613–22.
23. Erickson-Davis CR, Faust PL, Vonsattel JP, Gupta S, Honig LS, Louis ED. 'Hairy baskets' associated with degenerative Purkinje cell changes in essential tremor. *J Neuropathol Exp Neurol* 2010; 69: 262–71.
24. Louis ED, Yi H, Erickson-Davis C, Vonsattel JP, Faust PL. Structural study of Purkinje cell axonal torpedoes in essential tremor. *Neurosci Lett* 2009; 450: 287–91.
25. Louis ED, Faust PL, Vonsattel JP, et al. Torpedoes in Parkinson's disease, Alzheimer's disease, essential tremor, and control brains. *Mov Disord* 2009; 24: 1600–5.
26. Louis ED. Essential tremors: a family of neurodegenerative disorders? *Arch Neurol* 2009; 66: 1202–8.
27. Louis ED, Vonsattel JP. The emerging neuropathology of essential tremor. *Mov Disord* 2008; 23: 174–82.
28. Axelrad JE, Louis ED, Honig LS, et al. Reduced Purkinje cell number in essential tremor: a postmortem study. *Arch Neurol* 2008; 65: 101–7.
29. Louis ED, Faust PL, Vonsattel JP, et al. Neuropathological changes in essential tremor: 33 cases compared with 21 controls. *Brain* 2007; 130: 3297–307.
30. Louis ED, Vonsattel JP, Honig LS, Ross GW, Lyons KE, Pahwa R. Neuropathologic findings in essential tremor. *Neurology* 2006; 66: 1756–9.
31. Louis ED, Honig LS, Vonsattel JP, Maraganore DM, Borden S, Moskowitz CB. Essential tremor associated with focal nonnigral Lewy bodies: a clinicopathologic study. *Arch Neurol* 2005; 62: 1004–7.
32. Shill HA, Adler CH, Sabbagh MN, et al. Pathologic findings in prospectively ascertained essential tremor subjects. *Neurology* 2008; 70: 1452–5.
33. Rajput AH, Robinson CA, Rajput ML, Rajput A. Cerebellar Purkinje cell loss is not pathognomonic of essential tremor. *Parkinsonism Relat Disord* 2011; 17: 16–21.
34. Elble RJ. Animal models of action tremor. *Mov Disord* 1998; 13 (Suppl 3): 35–9.
35. Schnitzler A, Munks C, Butz M, Timmermann L, Gross J. Synchronized brain network associated with essential tremor as revealed by magnetoencephalography. *Mov Disord* 2009; 24: 1629–35.
36. Hellwig B, Haussler S, Schelter B, et al. Tremor-correlated cortical activity in essential tremor. *Lancet* 2001; 357: 519–23.
37. Hurtado JM, Lachaux JP, Beckley DJ, Gray CM, Sigvardt KA. Inter- and intralimb oscillator coupling in parkinsonian tremor. *Mov Disord* 2000; 15: 683–91.
38. Raethjen J, Lindemann M, Schmaljohann H, Wenzelburger R, Pfister G, Deuschl G. Multiple oscillators are causing parkinsonian and essential tremor. *Mov Disord* 2000; 15: 84–94.
39. Deuschl G, Elble R. Essential tremor—neurodegenerative or nondegenerative disease. Towards a working definition of ET. *Mov Disord* 2009; 24: 2033–41.

40. Jankovic J, Noebels JL. Genetic mouse models of essential tremor. Are they essential? *J Clin Invest* 2005; 115: 584–6.
41. Deuschl G, Bain P, Brin M. Consensus statement of the Movement Disorder Society on Tremor. Ad Hoc Scientific Committee. *Mov Disord* 1998; 13 (Suppl 3): 2–23.
42. Louis ED, Ottman R, Ford B, et al. The Washington Heights–Inwood Genetic Study of Essential Tremor: methodologic issues in essential-tremor research. *Neuroepidemiology* 1997; 16: 124–33.
43. Mostile G, Jankovic J. Alcohol in essential tremor and other movement disorders. *Mov Disord* 2010; 25: 2274–84.
44. Elble RJ. Diagnostic criteria for essential tremor and differential diagnosis. *Neurology* 2000; 54: S2–6.
45. Whaley NR, Putzke JD, Baba Y, Wszolek ZK, Uitti RJ. Essential tremor: phenotypic expression in a clinical cohort. *Parkinsonism Relat Disord* 2007; 13: 333–9.
46. Deuschl G, Wenzelburger R, Loffler K, Raethjen J, Stolze H. Essential tremor and cerebellar dysfunction: clinical and kinematic analysis of intention tremor. *Brain* 2000; 123: 1568–80.
47. Cohen O, Pullman S, Jurewicz E, Watner D, Louis ED. Rest tremor in patients with essential tremor: prevalence, clinical correlates, and electrophysiologic characteristics. *Arch Neurol* 2003; 60: 405–10.
48. Lorenz D, Schwieger D, Moises H, Deuschl G. Quality of life and personality in essential tremor patients. *Mov Disord* 2006; 21: 1114–18.
49. Quinn NP, Schneider SA, Schwingenschuh P, Bhatia KP. Tremor—some controversial aspects. *Mov Disord* 2011; 26: 18–23.
50. Bain PG, Findley LJ, Thompson PD, et al. A study of hereditary essential tremor. *Brain* 1994; 117: 805–24.
51. Lou JS, Jankovic J. Essential tremor: clinical correlates in 350 patients. *Neurology* 1991; 41: 234–8.
52. Tanner CM, Goldman SM, Lyons KE, et al. Essential tremor in twins: an assessment of genetic vs environmental determinants of etiology. *Neurology* 2001; 57: 1389–91.
53. Elble RJ. Essential tremor frequency decreases with time. *Neurology* 2000; 55: 1547–51.
54. Gironell A, Martinez-Corral M, Pagonabarraga J, Kulisevsky J. The Glass scale: a simple tool to determine severity in essential tremor. *Parkinsonism Relat Disord* 2010; 16: 412–14.
55. Auff E, Doppelbauer A, Fertl E. Essential tremor: functional disability vs. subjective impairment. *J Neural Transm* 1991; 33: 105–10.
56. Busenbark KL, Nash J, Nash S, Hubble JP, Koller WC. Is essential tremor benign? *Neurology* 1991; 41: 1982–3.
57. Louis ED, Levy G, Cote LJ, Mejia H, Fahn S, Marder K. Clinical correlates of action tremor in Parkinson disease. *Arch Neurol* 2001; 58: 1630–4.
58. Louis ED, Barnes L, Albert SM, et al. Correlates of functional disability in essential tremor. *Mov Disord* 2001; 16: 914–20.
59. Fahn S, Tolosa E, Marin C. Clinical rating scale for tremor. In: Jankovic J, Tolosa E (eds) *Parkinson's disease and movement disorders*, pp. 271–80. Baltimore, MD: Williams & Wilkins, 1993.
60. Troster AI, Pahwa R, Fields JA, Tanner CM, Lyons KE. Quality of life in Essential Tremor Questionnaire (QUEST): development and initial validation. *Parkinsonism Relat Disord* 2005; 11: 367–73.
61. Stolze H, Petersen G, Raethjen J, Wenzelburger R, Deuschl G. The gait disorder of advanced essential tremor. *Brain* 2001; 124: 2278–86.
62. Helmchen C, Hagenow A, Miesner J, et al. Eye movement abnormalities in essential tremor may indicate cerebellar dysfunction. *Brain* 2003; 126: 1319–32.
63. Klebe S, Stolze H, Grensing K, Volkmann J, Wenzelburger R, Deuschl G. Influence of alcohol on gait in patients with essential tremor. *Neurology* 2005; 65: 96–101.
64. Duane DD, Vermilion KJ. Cognitive deficits in patients with essential tremor. *Neurology* 2002; 58: 1706.
65. Lombardi WJ, Woolston DJ, Roberts JW, Gross RE. Cognitive deficits in patients with essential tremor. *Neurology* 2001; 57: 785–90.
66. Louis ED, Benito-Leon J, Vega-Quiroga S, Bermejo-Pareja F. Faster rate of cognitive decline in essential tremor cases than controls: a prospective study. *Eur J Neurol* 2010; 17: 1291–7.
67. Benito-León J, Louis ED, Bermejo-Pareja F. Risk of incident Parkinson's disease and parkinsonism in essential tremor: a population based study. *J Neurol Neurosurg Psychiatry* 2009; 80: 423–5.
68. Ondo WG, Sutton L, Dat Vuong K, Lai D, Jankovic J. Hearing impairment in essential tremor. *Neurology* 2003; 61: 1093–7.
69. Hawkes C, Shah M, Findley L. Olfactory function in essential tremor: a deficit unrelated to disease duration or severity. *Neurology* 2003; 61: 871–2.
70. Gironell A, Kulisevsky J, Pascual-Sedano B, Barbanoj M. Routine neurophysiologic tremor analysis as a diagnostic tool for essential tremor: a prospective study. *J Clin Neurophysiol* 2004; 21: 446–50.
71. Deuschl G, Krack P, Lauk M, Timmer J. Clinical neurophysiology of tremor. *J Clin Neurophysiol* 1996; 13: 110–21.
72. Muthuraman M, Hossen A, Heute U, Deuschl G, Raethjen J. A new diagnostic test to distinguish tremulous Parkinson's disease from advanced essential tremor. *Mov Disord* 2011; 26: 1548–52.
73. Deuschl G, Raethjen J, Hellriegel H, Elble R. Treatment of patients with essential tremor. *Lancet Neurol* 2011; 10: 148–61.
74. Elble RJ, Pullman SL, Matsumoto JY, Raethjen J, Deuschl G, Tintner R. Tremor amplitude is logarithmically related to 4- and 5-point tremor rating scales. *Brain* 2006; 129: 2660–6.
75. Sasso E, Perucca E, Calzetti S. Double-blind comparison of primidone and phenobarbital in essential tremor. *Neurology* 1988; 38: 808–10.
76. Findley LJ, Cleeves L, Calzetti S. Primidone in essential tremor of the hands and head: a double blind controlled clinical study. *J Neurol Neurosurg Psychiatry* 1985; 48: 911–15.
77. Brin MF, Lyons KE, Doucette J, et al. A randomized, double masked, controlled trial of botulinum toxin type A in essential hand tremor. *Neurology* 2001; 56: 1523–8.
78. Thompson C, Lang A, Parkes JD, Marsden CD. A double-blind trial of clonazepam in benign essential tremor. *Clin Neuropharmacol* 1984; 7: 83–8.
79. Wissel J, Masuhr F, Schelosky L, Ebersbach G, Poewe W. Quantitative assessment of botulinum toxin treatment in 43 patients with head tremor. *Mov Disord* 1997; 12: 722–6.
80. Pahwa R, Busenbark K, Swanson-Hyland EF, et al. Botulinum toxin treatment of essential head tremor. *Neurology* 1995; 45: 822–4.
81. Blomstedt P, Sandvik U, Tisch S. Deep brain stimulation in the posterior subthalamic area in the treatment of essential tremor. *Mov Disord* 2010; 25: 1350–6.
82. Hariz MI, Krack P, Alesch F, et al. Multicentre European study of thalamic stimulation for parkinsonian tremor: a 6 year follow-up. *J Neurol Neurosurg Psychiatry* 2008; 79: 694–9.
83. Blomstedt P, Hariz GM, Hariz MI, Koskinen LO. Thalamic deep brain stimulation in the treatment of essential tremor: a long-term follow-up. *Br J Neurosurg* 2007; 21: 504–9.
84. Sydow O, Thobois S, Alesch F, Speelman JD. Multicentre European study of thalamic stimulation in essential tremor: a six year follow up. *J Neurol Neurosurg Psychiatry* 2003; 74: 1387–91.
85. Lyons KE, Koller WC, Wilkinson SB, Pahwa R. Long term safety and efficacy of unilateral deep brain stimulation of the thalamus for parkinsonian tremor. *J Neurol Neurosurg Psychiatry* 2001; 71: 682–4.
86. Limousin P, Speelman JD, Gielen F, Janssens M. Multicentre European study of thalamic stimulation in parkinsonian and essential tremor. *J Neurol Neurosurg Psychiatry* 1999; 66: 289–96.
87. Koller W, Graner D, Mlcoch A. Essential voice tremor: treatment with propranolol. *Neurology* 1985; 35: 106–8.
88. Warrick P, Dromey C, Irish J, Durkin L. The treatment of essential voice tremor with botulinum toxin A: a longitudinal case report. *J Voice* 2000; 14: 410–21.

89. Warrick P, Dromey C, Irish JC, Durkin L, Pakiam A, Lang A. Botulinum toxin for essential tremor of the voice with multiple anatomical sites of tremor: a crossover design study of unilateral versus bilateral injection. *Laryngoscope* 2000; 110: 1366–74.
90. Hassler R, Mundinger F, Riechert T. *Stereotaxis in Parkinson syndrome: clinical-anatomical contributions to its physiology, with an atlas of the basal ganglia in parkinsonism.* Berlin: Springer Verlag, 1979.
91. Voges J, Hilker R, Botzel K, et al. Thirty days complication rate following surgery performed for deep-brain-stimulation. *Mov Disord* 2007; 22: 1486–9.
92. Plaha P, Ben-Shlomo Y, Patel NK, Gill SS. Stimulation of the caudal zona incerta is superior to stimulation of the subthalamic nucleus in improving contralateral parkinsonism. *Brain* 2006; 129: 1732–47.
93. Raethjen J, Lemke MR, Lindemann M, Wenzelburger R, Krack P, Deuschl G. Amitriptyline enhances the central component of physiological tremor. *J Neurol Neurosurg Psychiatry* 2001; 70: 78–82.
94. Marsden CD, Meadows JC. The effect of adrenaline on the contraction of human muscle: one mechanism whereby adrenaline increases the amplitude of physiological tremor. *J Physiol* 1968; 194: 70–1P.
95. Raethjen J, Lauk M, Koster B, et al. Tremor analysis in two normal cohorts. *Clin Neurophysiol* 2004; 115: 2151–6.
96. Elble RJ, Higgins C, Elble S. Electrophysiologic transition from physiologic tremor to essential tremor. *Mov Disord* 2005; 20: 1038–42.
97. Feely J, Peden N. Use of beta-adrenoceptor blocking drugs in hyperthyroidism. *Drugs* 1984; 27: 425–46.
98. Findley LJ, Gresty MA, Halmagyi GM. Tremor, the cogwheel phenomenon and clonus in Parkinson's disease. *J Neurol Neurosurg Psychiatry* 1981; 44: 534–46.
99. Raethjen J, Pohle S, Govindan RB, Morsnowski A, Wenzelburger R, Deuschl G. Parkinsonian action tremor: interference with object manipulation and lacking levodopa response. *Exp Neurol* 2005; 194: 151–60.
100. Fahn S, Oakes D, Shoulson I, et al. Levodopa and the progression of Parkinson's disease. *N Engl J Med* 2004; 351: 2498–508.
101. Navan P, Findley LJ, Undy MB, Pearce RK, Bain PG. A randomly assigned double-blind cross-over study examining the relative anti-parkinsonian tremor effects of pramipexole and pergolide. *Eur J Neurol* 2005; 12: 1–8.
102. Pogarell O, Gasser T, van Hilten JJ, et al. Pramipexole in patients with Parkinson's disease and marked drug resistant tremor: a randomised, double blind, placebo controlled multicentre study. *J Neurol Neurosurg Psychiatry* 2002; 72: 713–20.
103. Schrag A, Keens J, Warner J. Ropinirole for the treatment of tremor in early Parkinson's disease. *Eur J Neurol* 2002; 9: 253–7.
104. Perry EK, Kilford L, Lees AJ, Burn DJ, Perry RH. Increased Alzheimer pathology in Parkinson's disease related to antimuscarinic drugs. *Ann Neurol* 2003; 54: 235–8.
105. Bonuccelli U, Ceravolo R, Salvetti S, et al. Clozapine in Parkinson's disease tremor. Effects of acute and chronic administration. *Neurology* 1997; 49: 1587–90.
106. Spieker S, Eisebitt R, Breit S, et al. Tremorlytic activity of budipine in Parkinson's disease. *Clin Neuropharmacol* 1999; 22: 115–19.
107. Koller WC, Herbster G. Adjuvant therapy of parkinsonian tremor. *Arch Neurol* 1987; 44: 921–3.
108. Rajput AH, Jamieson H, Hirsh S, Quraishi A. Relative efficacy of alcohol and propranolol in action tremor. *Can J Neurol Sci* 1975; 2: 31–5.
109. Deuschl G, Schade-Brittinger C, Krack P, et al. A randomized trial of deep-brain stimulation for Parkinson's disease. *N Engl J Med* 2006; 355: 896–908.
110. Krack P, Benazzouz A, Pollak P, et al. Treatment of tremor in Parkinson's disease by subthalamic nucleus stimulation. *Mov Disord* 1998; 13: 907–14.
111. Weaver FM, Follett K, Stern M, et al. Bilateral deep brain stimulation vs best medical therapy for patients with advanced Parkinson disease: a randomized controlled trial. *JAMA* 2009; 301: 63–73.
112. Williams A, Gill S, Varma T, et al. Deep brain stimulation plus best medical therapy versus best medical therapy alone for advanced Parkinson's disease (PD SURG trial): a randomised, open-label trial. *Lancet Neurol* 2010; 9: 581–91.
113. Jedynak CP, Bonnet AM, Agid Y. Tremor and idiopathic dystonia. *Mov Disord* 1991; 6: 230–6.
114. Vidailhet M, Jedynak CP, Pollak P, Agid Y. Pathology of symptomatic tremors. *Mov Disord* 1998; 13 (Suppl 3): 49–54.
115. Deuschl G. Dystonic tremor. *Rev Neurol (Paris)* 2003; 159: 900–5.
116. Rivest J, Marsden CD. Trunk and head tremor as isolated manifestations of dystonia. *Mov Disord* 1990; 5: 60–5.
117. Koda J, Ludlow CL. An evaluation of laryngeal muscle activation in patients with voice tremor. *Otolaryngol Head Neck Surg* 1992; 107: 684–96.
118. Elble RJ, Moody C, Higgins C. Primary writing tremor. A form of focal dystonia? *Mov Disord* 1990; 5: 118–26.
119. Bain PG, Findley LJ, Britton TC, et al. Primary writing tremor. *Brain* 1995; 116: 203–9.
120. Schneider SA, Bhatia KP. The entity of jaw tremor and dystonia. *Mov Disord* 2007; 22: 1491–5.
121. Ferraz HB, De Andrade LA, Silva SM, Borges V, Rocha MS. [Postural tremor and dystonia. Clinical aspects and physiopathological considerations.] *Arq Neuropsiquiatr* 1994; 52: 466–70.
122. Bartolome FM, Fanjul S, Cantarero S, Hernandez J, Garcia Ruiz PJ. [Primary focal dystonia: descriptive study of 205 patients.] *Neurologia* 2003; 18: 59–65.
123. Masuhr F, Wissel J, Muller J, Scholz U, Poewe W. Quantification of sensory trick impact on tremor amplitude and frequency in 60 patients with head tremor. *Mov Disord* 2000; 15: 960–4.
124. Schwingenschuh P, Ruge D, Edwards MJ, et al. Distinguishing SWEDDs patients with asymmetric resting tremor from Parkinson's disease: a clinical and electrophysiological study. *Mov Disord* 2011; 25: 560–9.
125. Kupsch A, Benecke R, Muller J, et al. Pallidal deep-brain stimulation in primary generalized or segmental dystonia. *N Engl J Med* 2006; 355: 1978–90.
126. Elble RJ. Origins of tremor [comment]. *Lancet* 2000; 355: 1113–14.
127. Ljubisavljevic M, Kacar A, Milanovic S, Svetel M, Kostic VS. Changes in cortical inhibition during task-specific contractions in primary writing tremor patients. *Mov Disord* 2006; 21: 855–9.
128. Zeuner KE, Peller M, Knutzen A, Hallett M, Deuschl G, Siebner HR. Motor re-training does not need to be task specific to improve writer's cramp. *Mov Disord* 2008; 23: 2319–27.
129. Zeuner KE, Shill HA, Sohn YH, et al. Motor training as treatment in focal hand dystonia. *Mov Disord* 2005; 20: 335–41.
130. Zeuner KE, Bara-Jimenez W, Noguchi PS, Goldstein SR, Dambrosia JM, Hallett M. Sensory training for patients with focal hand dystonia. *Ann Neurol* 2002; 51: 593–8.
131. Espay AJ, Hung SW, Sanger TD, Moro E, Fox SH, Lang AE. A writing device improves writing in primary writing tremor. *Neurology* 2005; 64: 1648–50.
132. Papapetropoulos S, Singer C. Treatment of primary writing tremor with botulinum toxin type a injections: report of a case series. *Clin Neuropharmacol* 2006; 29: 364–7.
133. Lungu C, Karp BI, Alter K, Zolbrod R, Hallett M. Long-term follow-up of botulinum toxin therapy for focal hand dystonia: outcome at 10 years or more. *Mov Disord* 2011; 26: 750–3.
134. Blomstedt P, Fytagoridis A, Tisch S. Deep brain stimulation of the posterior subthalamic area in the treatment of tremor. *Acta Neurochir (Wien)* 2009; 151: 31–6.
135. Findley L, Capildeo R. *Movement disorders: tremor*. London: Macmillan, 1984.
136. Alusi SH, Glickman S, Aziz TZ, Bain PG. Tremor in multiple sclerosis. *J Neurol Neurosurg Psychiatry* 1999; 66: 131–4.
137. Baba Y, Uitti RJ. Fragile X-associated tremor/ataxia syndrome and movements disorders. *Curr Opin Neurol* 2005; 18: 393–8.

138. Hallett M, Berardelli A, Matheson J, Rothwell J, Marsden CD. Physiological analysis of simple rapid movements in patients with cerebellar deficits. *J Neurol Neurosurg Psychiatry* 1991; 54: 124–33.
139. Rascol A, Clanet M, Montastruc JL, Delage W, Guiraud-Chaumeil B. L5H tryptophan in the cerebellar syndrome treatment. *Biomedicine* 1981; 35: 112–13.
140. Trouillas P, Serratrice G, Laplane D, et al. Levorotatory form of 5-hydroxytryptophan in Friedreich's ataxia: results of a double-blind drug-placebo cooperative study. *Arch Neurol* 1995; 52: 456–60.
141. Striano P, Coppola A, Vacca G, et al. Levetiracetam for cerebellar tremor in multiple sclerosis: an open-label pilot tolerability and efficacy study. *J Neurol* 2006; 253: 762–6.
142. Fox P, Bain PG, Glickman S, Carroll C, Zajicek J. The effect of cannabis on tremor in patients with multiple sclerosis. *Neurology* 2004; 62: 1105–9.
143. Alusi SH, Aziz TZ, Glickman S, Jahanshahi M, Stein JF, Bain PG. Stereotactic lesional surgery for the treatment of tremor in multiple sclerosis: a prospective case-controlled study. *Brain* 2001; 124: 1576–89.
144. Lozano AM. Vim thalamic stimulation for tremor. *Arch Med Res* 2000; 31: 266–9.
145. Schuurman PR, Bosch DA, Bossuyt PM, et al. A comparison of continuous thalamic stimulation and thalamotomy for suppression of severe tremor. *N Engl J Med* 2000; 342: 461–8.
146. Herzog J, Hamel W, Wenzelburger R, et al. Kinematic analysis of thalamic versus subthalamic neurostimulation in postural and intention tremor. *Brain* 2007; 130: 1608–25.
147. Heilman KM. Orthostatic tremor. *Arch Neurol* 1984; 41: 880–1.
148. Thompson PD, Rothwell JC, Day BL, et al. The physiology of orthostatic tremor. *Arch Neurol* 1986; 43: 584–7.
149. Aguilar D, Sigford KE, Soontarapornchai K, et al. A quantitative assessment of tremor and ataxia in FMR1 premutation carriers using CATSYS. *Am J Med Genet A* 2008; 146: 629–35.
150. Apartis E, Tison F, Arne P, Jedynak CP, Vidailhet M. Fast orthostatic tremor in Parkinson's disease mimicking primary orthostatic tremor. *Mov Disord* 2001; 16: 1133–6.
151. McManis PG, Sharbrough FW. Orthostatic tremor: clinical and electrophysiologic characteristics. *Muscle Nerve* 1993; 16: 1254–60.
152. Britton TC, Thompson PD. Primary orthostatic tremor. *BMJ* 1995; 310: 143–4.
153. Leu-Semenescu S, Roze E, Vidailhet M, et al. Myoclonus or tremor in orthostatism: an under-recognized cause of unsteadiness in Parkinson's disease. *Mov Disord* 2007; 22: 2063–9.
154. Williams ER, Jones RE, Baker SN, Baker MR. Slow orthostatic tremor can persist when walking backward. *Mov Disord* 2011; 25: 788–90.
155. Rodrigues JP, Edwards DJ, Walters SE, et al. Gabapentin can improve postural stability and quality of life in primary orthostatic tremor. *Mov Disord* 2005; 20: 865–70.
156. Poersch M. Orthostatic tremor: combined treatment with primidone and clonazepam. *Mov Disord* 1994; 9: 467.
157. Katzenschlager R, Costa D, Gerschlager W, et al. [^{123}I]-FP-CIT-SPECT demonstrates dopaminergic deficit in orthostatic tremor. *Ann Neurol* 2003; 53: 489–96.
158. Espay AJ, Duker AP, Chen R, et al. Deep brain stimulation of the ventral intermediate nucleus of the thalamus in medically refractory orthostatic tremor: preliminary observations. *Mov Disord* 2008; 23: 2357–62.
159. Guridi J, Rodriguez-Oroz MC, Arbizu J, et al. Successful thalamic deep brain stimulation for orthostatic tremor. *Mov Disord* 2008; 23: 1808–11.
160. Krauss JK, Weigel R, Blahak C, et al. Chronic spinal cord stimulation in medically intractable orthostatic tremor. *J Neurol Neurosurg Psychiatry* 2006; 77: 1013–16.
161. Miwa H, Hatori K, Kondo T, Imai H, Mizuno Y. Thalamic tremor: case reports and implications of the tremor-generating mechanism. *Neurology* 1996; 46: 75–9.
162. Holmes G. On certain tremors in organic cerebral lesions. *Brain* 1904; 27: 327–75.
163. Krack P, Deuschl G, Kaps M, Warnke P, Schneider S, Traupe H. Delayed onset of 'rubral tremor' 23 years after brainstem trauma. *Mov Disord* 1994; 9: 240–2.
164. Remy P, de Recondo A, Defer G, et al. Peduncular 'rubral' tremor and dopaminergic denervation: a PET study. *Neurology* 1995; 45: 472–7.
165. Samie MR, Selhorst JB, Koller WC. Post-traumatic midbrain tremors. *Neurology* 1990; 40: 62–6.
166. Biary N, Cleeves L, Findley L, Koller W. Post-traumatic tremor. *Neurology* 1989; 39: 103–6.
167. Ferlazzo E, Morgante F, Rizzo V, et al. Successful treatment of Holmes tremor by levetiracetam. *Mov Disord* 2008; 23: 2101–3.
168. Striano P, Elefante A, Coppola A, et al. Dramatic response to levetiracetam in post-ischaemic Holmes' tremor. *J Neurol Neurosurg Psychiatry* 2007; 78: 438–9.
169. Acar G, Acar F, Bir LS, Kizilay Z, Cirak B. Vim stimulation in Holmes' tremor secondary to subarachnoid hemorrhage. *Neurol Res* 2010; 32: 992–4.
170. Deuschl G, Mischke G, Schenck E, Schulte-Monting J, Lucking CH. Symptomatic and essential rhythmic palatal myoclonus. *Brain* 1990; 113: 1645–72.
171. Deuschl G, Toro C, Valls-Sole J, Zeffiro T, Zee DS, Hallett M. Symptomatic and essential palatal tremor. 1: Clinical, physiological and MRI analysis. *Brain* 1994; 117: 775–88.
172. Masucci EF, Kurtzke JF, Saini N. Myorhythmia: a widespread movement disorder. Clinicopathological correlations. *Brain* 1984; 107: 53–79.
173. Deuschl G, Wilms H. Clinical spectrum and physiology of palatal tremor. *Mov Disord* 2002; 17 (Suppl 2): S63–6.
174. Samuel M, Torun N, Tuite PJ, Sharpe JA, Lang AE. Progressive ataxia and palatal tremor (PAPT): clinical and MRI assessment with review of palatal tremors. *Brain* 2004; 127: 1252–68.
175. Deuschl G, Jost S, Schumacher M. Symptomatic palatal tremor is associated with signs of cerebellar dysfunction. *J Neurol* 1996; 243: 553–6.
176. Leigh RJ, Averbuch-Heller L, Tomsak RL, Remler BF, Yaniglos SS, Dell'Osso LF. Treatment of abnormal eye movements that impair vision: strategies based on current concepts of physiology and pharmacology. *Ann Neurol* 1994; 36: 129–41.
177. Repka MX, Savino PJ, Reinecke RD. Treatment of acquired nystagmus with botulinum neurotoxin A. *Arch Ophthalmol* 1994; 112: 1320–4.
178. Bakheit AM, Behan PO. Palatal myoclonus successfully treated with clonazepam. *J Neurol Neurosurg Psychiatry* 1990; 53: 806.
179. Erickson JC, Carrasco H, Grimes JB, Jabbari B, Cannard KR. Palatal tremor and myorhythmia in Hashimoto's encephalopathy. *Neurology* 2002; 58: 504–5.
180. Borggreve F, Hageman G. A case of idiopathic palatal myoclonus: treatment with sodium valproate. *Eur Neurol* 1991; 31: 403–4.
181. Cakmur R, Idiman E, Idiman F, Baklan B, Ozkiziltan S. Essential palatal tremor successfully treated with flunarizine. *Eur Neurol* 1997; 38: 133–4.
182. Gambardella A, Quattrone A. Treatment of palatal myoclonus with sumatriptan. *Mov Disord* 1998; 13: 195.
183. Scott BL, Evans RW, Jankovic J. Treatment of palatal myoclonus with sumatriptan. *Mov Disord* 1996; 11: 748–51.
184. Pakiam AS, Lang AE. Essential palatal tremor: evidence of heterogeneity based on clinical features and response to sumatriptan. *Mov Disord* 1999; 14: 179–80.
185. Deuschl G, Lohle E, Heinen F, Lucking C. Ear click in palatal tremor: its origin and treatment with botulinum toxin. *Neurology* 1991; 41: 1677–9.
186. Dalakas MC, Teravainen H, Engel WK. Tremor as a feature of chronic relapsing and dysgammaglobulinemic polyneuropathies: incidence and management. *Arch Neurol* 1984; 41: 711–14.
187. Cardoso FE, Jankovic J. Hereditary motor-sensory neuropathy and movement disorders. *Muscle Nerve* 1993; 16: 904–10.

188. Ruzicka E, Jech R, Zarubova K, Roth J, Urgosik D. VIM thalamic stimulation for tremor in a patient with IgM paraproteinaemic demyelinating neuropathy. *Mov Disord* 2003; 18: 1192–5.
189. Kim YJ, Pakiam AS, Lang AE. Historical and clinical features of psychogenic tremor: a review of 70 cases. *Can J Neurol Sci* 1999; 26: 190–5.
190. Factor SA, Podskalny GD, Molho ES. Psychogenic movement disorders: frequency, clinical profile, and characteristics. *J Neurol Neurosurg Psychiatry* 1995; 59: 406–12.
191. Raethjen J, Kopper F, Govindan RB, Volkmann J, Deuschl G. Two different pathogenetic mechanisms in psychogenic tremor. *Neurology* 2004; 63: 812–15.
192. McAuley J, Rothwell J. Identification of psychogenic, dystonic, and other organic tremors by a coherence entrainment test. *Mov Disord* 2004; 19: 253–67.
193. Zeuner KE, Shoge RO, Goldstein SR, Dambrosia JM, Hallett M. Accelerometry to distinguish psychogenic from essential or parkinsonian tremor. *Neurology* 2003; 61: 548–50.
194. Koller W, Lang A, Vetere-Overfield B, et al. Psychogenic tremors. *Neurology* 1989; 39: 1094–9.
195. Voon V, Lang AE. Antidepressant treatment outcomes of psychogenic movement disorder. *J Clin Psychiatry* 2005; 66: 1529–34.
196. Feinstein A, Stergiopoulos V, Fine J, Lang AE. Psychiatric outcome in patients with a psychogenic movement disorder: a prospective study. *Neuropsychiatry Neuropsychol Behav Neurol* 2001; 14: 169–76.

CHAPTER 17

Dystonia: An Overview

K.P. Bhatia, M. Stamelou, and S. Bressman

Definition

Dystonia is a movement disorder characterized by sustained muscle contractions, frequently causing twisting and repetitive movements or abnormal postures (1). The abnormal postures are typically not fixed, are caused by co-contraction of agonist and antagonist muscles, and tend to be repetitive or patterned, consistently involving the same muscle groups. Slow writhing movements can occur (athetosis), where the dominant muscle activity switches from agonist to antagonist and vice versa. Tremor occurs commonly with dystonia and either involves the affected body part (dystonic tremor) or another body part not affected by dystonia (tremor associated with dystonia). Dystonic tremor is jerky, irregular, and variable in amplitude, and typically worsens in particular positions of the affected body part.

Dystonia is often aggravated by voluntary movement. In action dystonia, the dystonic movements are elicited only with voluntary movement. When dystonia is evinced only with particular actions, it is called task-specific dystonia; examples include writer's cramp and the embouchure dystonia of woodwind and brass musicians. Activation of dystonic movements by actions in remote parts of the body is called overflow; examples include leg dystonia while writing or axial dystonia with talking. Factors that tend to exacerbate dystonia include fatigue and emotional stress, whereas the movements usually decrease with relaxation or sleep. Dystonia can often improve by tactile or proprioceptive sensory tricks (*geste antagoniste*). Often a patient will be able to improve the abnormal posture to some degree by touching, or even sometimes thinking about touching, the affected body part (2–6).

Despite the 'motor' definition of primary dystonia, there are other, non-motor, features in many patients with primary dystonia, but these are less studied in secondary/heredodegenerative dystonias (7, 8). Disease-related pain occurs in 30–70% of patients, and mild sensory symptoms such as discomfort in the neck, irritation of the eyes or throat before the development of cervical dystonia, blepharospasm, and spasmodic dysphonia, respectively, are common (9, 10). Depressive disorders and a family history of depression are more frequent in adult-onset focal dystonia (11–14) and in manifesting and non-manifesting DYT1 mutation carriers (15). These non-motor symptoms are clinically relevant, since they may impair quality of life equally to the motor symptoms (10, 16, 17).

Classification

Dystonia can be classified in three parallel ways: by anatomical distribution, age of onset, and aetiology (1). *Anatomical distribution* is subclassified into focal, segmental, multifocal, hemidystonia, and generalized dystonia. In focal dystonia, the abnormal movements involve a single body region only (e.g. hand). In segmental dystonia, abnormal movements affect two or more contiguous body regions (e.g. arm and neck). When dystonia is multifocal, two or more non-contiguous body areas are involved (e.g. right arm, left leg). Hemidystonia affects one side of the body, while generalized dystonia includes both legs or one leg and the trunk (i.e. crural dystonia) plus at least one other body region (usually one or both arms). *Age at onset* is divided into young-onset (<20–30 years) and adult-onset dystonia. *Aetiology* is usually divided into four groups: primary, dystonia-plus, secondary (or acquired), and heredodegenerative. In the primary group dystonia is the only sign (although most allow tremor to be present as well) and there is no secondary cause or neurodegeneration; in dystonia-plus syndromes, which are similar to primary dystonia, there is no evidence of a secondary cause or neurodegeneration, but signs other than dystonia (e.g. parkinsonism, myoclonus) are present; in secondary dystonia a clear acquired or exogenous cause is present (e.g. brain injury, drug exposure); and in heredodegenerative dystonia, dystonia is part of a neurodegenerative syndrome that is often inherited (e.g. Wilson disease). The European Federation of Neurological Societies (EFNS) has proposed including dystonia-plus syndromes and paroxysmal dystonias under the primary dystonias (Table 17.1). The three different ways of classifying dystonia occur in parallel in clinical practice and are essential for diagnosis, prognosis, guiding therapy, and genetic counselling. Psychogenic dystonia is not described in the classification of dystonia. It occurs as part of a conversion disorder, tends to be fixed, and is accompanied by other signs suggestive of a conversion disorder (18–21).

Genetic classification of dystonia

The DYT loci represent a clinically heterogeneous group of disorders including primary dystonia (DYT1, 2, 4, 6, 7, 13, 17, 21), dystonia-plus (DYT3, 5/14, 11, 12, 15, 16), and paroxysmal dystonias (DYT8, 9, 10, 18, 19, 20) (Table 17.2). Therefore a genetic classification of dystonia is not clinically useful. With regard to

Table 17.1 Classifications of dystonia

	Fahn et al. 1998 (22)	Fahn et al. 2011 (23)	EFNS guidelines 2011 (24)
Age at onset	1. Childhood 2. Adolescence 3. Adulthood	1. Young-onset (<26) 2. Adult-onset (>26)	1. Early-onset (variably defined as <20–30 years) 2. Late-onset
Distribution	Focal Segmental Multifocal Generalized hemidystonia	Focal Segmental Multifocal Generalized hemidystonia	Focal Segmental Multifocal Generalized hemidystonia
Aetiology	Primary (a) Familial (b) Sporadic	Primary	Primary (a) Primary pure (e.g. DYT1, 6) (a) Primary paroxysmal (e.g. DYT8, 10, 18)
	Dystonia-plus	Dystonia-plus	(c) Primary-plus (former dystonia-plus syndromes, e.g. DYT5,11)
	Secondary	Secondary	Secondary
	Heredodegenerative	Heredodegenerative Feature of another neurological disease (e.g. dystonic tics, paroxysmal dyskinesias, PD, PSP, etc.)	Heredodegenerative

Table 17.2 The DYT genes, phenotype, and transmission

Primary dystonia	Gene or locus	Phenotype	Transmission
DYT1	*TOR1A*	Generalized early-limb-onset dystonia	AD
DYT2	None	Early-onset generalized dystonia	AR
DYT4	None	Whispering dysphonia	AD
DYT6	*THAP1*	Craniocervical and limb dystonia	AD
DYT7	18p	Adult-onset cervical dystonia	AD
DYT13	1p36.13–36.32	Craniocervical, laryngeal, and limb dystonia	AD
DYT17	20p11.2-q13.12	Segmental or generalized dystonia, severe dysphonia	AR
DYT21	2q14.3-q21.3	Adult-onset generalized or multifocal dystonia, starting with blepharospasm	AD
Dystonia-plus syndromes			
DYT3	*TAF1*	Dystonia–parkinsonism (neurodegeneration)	XR
DYT5a	*GTPCH1*	Dopa-responsive dystonia	AD
DYT5b	*TH*	Dopa-responsive dystonia	AR
DYT11	*SGCE*	Myoclonus–dystonia	AD
DYT12	*ATP1A3*	Rapid-onset dystonia–parkinsonism	AD
DYT15	18p11	Myoclonus–dystonia	AD
DYT16	*PRKRA*	Early-onset dystonia–parkinsonism	AR
Paroxysmal dystonias			
DYT8	*MR1*	Paroxysmal non-kinesigenic dyskinesia	AD
DYT9/DYT18	*SLC2A1* (GLUT1)	Paroxysmal exercise-induced dystonia with wide phenotypical spectrum (e.g. spasticity, ataxia, seizures)	AD
DYT10	*PRRT2*	Paroxysmal kinesigenic dyskinesia	AD
DYT19	16q	Paroxysmal kinesigenic dyskinesia 2	AD
DYT20	2q	Paroxysmal non-kinesigenic dyskinesia 2	AD

genetic causes of heredodegenerative dystonias, many genes have been identified (Table 17.3).

Primary dystonia

The phenotypic spectrum of primary dystonia is wide, ranging from young-onset generalized to adult-onset focal dystonia (25, 26). As per the definition, there are no additional signs and the disorder usually plateaus 5–10 years after onset. Prevalence reports of primary dystonia vary widely from 3 to over 7000 per million depending on dystonia subtype (e.g. focal vs generalized), ethnicity, and ascertainment methodology; most point to an estimated crude prevalence of about 300–500 per million with focal dystonias being about seven to ten times more common than generalized dystonia (27–29). However, the prevalence of primary dystonia is thought to be underestimated (29).

Young-onset primary dystonia

Age at onset is usually in childhood or adolescence. Limb onset is typical, with spread of symptoms over some years which then plateaus, often resulting in generalized dystonia. However, some patients may only develop focal or segmental dystonia. Young-onset primary dystonia does not usually involve cranial or bulbar structures.

DYT1 dystonia (Oppenheim dystonia, dystonia musculorum deformans), a major cause of young-onset primary dystonia, is an autosomal dominant condition with reduced penetrance (30%). It is caused by a heterozygous GAG deletion mutation of the *TOR1A* (TorsinA) gene located on the long arm of chromosome 9. *TOR1A* codes for torsinA, an AAA+ superfamily of molecular chaperones (30). The GAG deletion in *TOR1A* accounts for about 80% of young-onset primary dystonia in the Ashkenazi Jewish population because of the founder mutation, but less than 50% in the non-Jewish population (31–35). Two missense mutations in the *TOR1A* gene have been described, each in a single case (36). A third missense variant, D216H, is protective against penetrance of the GAG deletion when inherited in *trans* (37, 38). The typical clinical phenotype associated with DYT1 dystonia is characterized by young onset (mean age 13 years), starting in a limb (arm or leg is affected first in 90% of cases) and progressing to generalized/multifocal (65%) involvement; spread to cranial structures is less common (15–20%) (31, 35). However, there is a wide phenotypic and intrafamilial variability, from severe dystonic storm to mild writer's cramp, as well as various atypical phenotypes (39, 40).

Another cause of young-onset primary dystonia is DYT6 dystonia due to heterozygous mutations in the gene *THAP1* (thanatos-associated protein domain-containing apoptosis-associated protein 1), initially described in three Amish-Mennonite families (41, 42). *THAP1* is a transcription factor whose function in the brain remains unknown. More than 45 heterozygous mutations have been reported in *THAP1* (43–47). Recently, *THAP1* has been shown to bind to the *TOR1A* promoter, repressing its expression, which links the molecular pathways underlying DYT1 and DYT6 dystonia (48). The typical DYT6 phenotype is characterized by young onset (mean 13 years, range 2–62 years), most often in an arm (47%) followed by cranial muscles (25%) or the neck (23%) but, in contrast with DYT1, rarely in the leg (5%), with spread to a generalized or multifocal distribution in over half and prominent speech involvement in more than 60% of cases (44–47). However, about 10–18% of cases have only focal dystonia, and in screening studies of adult-onset focal cases a low frequency (>1%) of *THAP1* mutations has been reported (45).

DYT2 is an autosomal recessive primary dystonia reported in consanguineous families of Spanish gypsy (49), Sephardic Jewish (50), and Arab descent (51). The phenotype is similar to DYT1 dystonia with young-onset limb dystonia followed by generalization. DYT4 is an autosomal dominant primary dystonia, reported in a single large Australian family, with prominent whispering dysphonia that begins in the second decade in most family members (52, 53). No chromosomal location or gene has been identified for either disorder.

DYT13 is an autosomal dominant disorder with reduced penetrance, mapped to chromosome 1p36 in an Italian family, with adolescence onset, mainly segmental, dystonia, and prominent craniocervical involvement (54).

DYT17 is autosomal recessive and was mapped to chromosome 20 in a consanguineous Lebanese family with cervical dystonia and progression to segmental dystonia in two siblings and generalized dystonia in a third sibling who also featured severe dysphonia and dysarthria (55).

Adult-onset primary dystonia (APD)

The onset of APD is in adulthood, and the muscles affected depend on the age at onset. Focal dystonia is more common, but can become segmental, with spread of symptoms over some years, especially with blepharospasm (56, 57). Lower limb APD is very unusual for primary dystonia and is usually due to secondary/heredodegenerative causes.

Clinical phenotypes

Among adult-onset cranial and cervical dystonias, *cervical dystonia* is the most common. Typical age at onset is around 40 years (56, 58), and women are more often affected than men. It may start with gradual onset of discomfort or pain in the neck, followed by involuntary pulling of the head in a particular direction because of contraction of certain neck and shoulder muscles. Various combinations of neck muscles may be involved to produce abnormal head positions, including horizontal turning (torticollis), tilting (laterocollis), flexion (anterocollis), or extension (retrocollis). Jerky tremor, which worsens when turning the head towards the normal position, is very common and can be the predominant feature. Patients may have a *geste antagoniste,* where they can partially relieve their spasm by touching the chin or part of their face. Symptoms usually progress over 6–12 months and then plateau. Remission can occur in 10–15% of the patients, especially those with younger onset, and may be sustained.

Blepharospasm causes contraction of the orbicularis oculi muscles; it tends to start later than other craniocervical dystonias, with mean age at onset around 55 years (58, 59). Women are more commonly affected than men. An uncomfortable feeling around the eyes, dry eyes, and photophobia may precede the spasm. Mild cases are characterized by increased blink rate with flurries of blinking, whereas more severely affected patients have visual impairment due to sustained forceful eye closure. In some patients there is an inability to activate the levator palpebri, so that the eyelid cannot open; this is called levator inhibition. About two-thirds of patients are significantly disabled and 12–36% are considered functionally blind (60).

Spasmodic dysphonia (SD) results from dystonia of the vocal cords and has a similar age at onset and sex ratio to cervical dystonia. Compared with other forms of cranial dystonia, it occurs less often in conjunction with other cranial dystonias (57). It is estimated that the majority of patients have isolated SD, about 10–15% progress to another cranial region, and about 5% progress to extracranial sites (61, 62). In adductor dysphonia (the most common form), which involves the thyroarytenoid muscles, there is excessive glottal closure in a rigid fashion, preventing air flow and causing a strained, strangled voice. Abductor dysphonia (much less common) involves the posterior cricoarytenoid muscles; it is characterized by open glottal configuration and a paucity of vocal cord vibration so that the voice sounds whispering and breathy.

In *oromandibular dystonia* (OMD) there is abnormal activity in lower facial, tongue, jaw, and pharyngeal muscles. It has a similar age at onset to blepharospasm, and women are more commonly affected than men. Jaw-closing dystonia has been considered to be the most common form, while simultaneous movements of jaw openers (lateral pterygoids, digastric muscles) and closers (medial pterygoids, masseter and temporalis muscles) may result in jaw tremor (63). OMD may cause pain and difficulty in speaking, chewing, and swallowing. Sensory tricks such as putting a finger in the mouth, chewing gum, or placing a toothpick in the mouth can partially help to reduce the symptoms (64). An important differential diagnosis is OMD caused by neuroleptic drugs, since this presents with a similar clinical picture. A combination of blepharospasm and OMD is called *Meige's syndrome*.

Primary *lingual dystonia* is rare and may or may not be associated with OMD. Although severe tongue protrusion dystonia is more frequent in heredodegenerative disorders (65), it has also been described in APD (66). Tongue movements may be repetitive or protrusion may be sustained. Movements are often action-induced, commonly by speaking (67), and the tongue may also curl instead of protruding (68).

The most common adult-onset *limb dystonia* is writer's cramp, where the patient shows abnormal postures affecting the hand when writing, but not while performing other tasks. Age at onset is around 25–35 years and men are more commonly affected than women. The unaffected hand may show mirror movements when the patient is writing with the affected hand. Other adult-onset limb dystonias include task-specific dystonias like musicians', typists', or golfers' dystonia. Adult-onset leg dystonia is very rarely reported as a primary phenomenon and is almost always due to a secondary/heredodegenerative cause. Adult-onset primary *truncal dystonia* is also reported. The mean age of onset is 41 and men seem to be slightly more commonly affected than women. It tends to remain focal, although there may be an initial contiguous spread, sometimes beginning in the craniocervical region and spreading axially or, rarely, vice versa (69).

Genetics of APD

APD is complex, with family studies suggesting autosomal dominant inheritance but with very low penetrance (about 12–15% compared with 30% for early-onset dystonia) (70, 71). The role of specific genes in the aetiology of APD is not fully elucidated. There are some descriptions of large families with highly penetrant autosomal dominant APD (72–74) which have resulted in the mapping of two genes for APD: *DYT7* (75) and *DYT21* (76) (see Table 17.2). *DYT7* is mapped to chromosome 18p in a German family with adult-onset cervical dystonia (mean 43 years), some of whom also had brachial and cranial involvement (75). *DYT21*was linked to a region on chromosome 2q14.3-q21.3 in a Swedish family (76) phenotypically characterized by later-onset (mean 27 years) mainly generalized or multifocal dystonia with onset in the craniocervical muscles in most and the hands in about 25%. *DYT6* has been associated with adult-onset focal dystonia (45), and cervical dystonia as well as writer's cramp cases with *DYT1* mutations (77–79). Reports with regard to an association of torticollis and blepharospasm with a polymorphism in the dopamine D5 receptor (*DRD5*) gene are contradictory (77, 80–83).

Dystonia-plus syndromes

Within the dystonia-plus syndromes there are two forms that have predominantly myoclonus in addition to dystonia (DYT11, 15) and four forms that have predominantly parkinsonism but also other features as part of their phenotype (DYT3, 5/14, 12, 16).

Myoclonus–dystonia

DYT11 myoclonus–dystonia (MD) is an autosomal dominant condition with reduced penetrance due to maternal imprinting, i.e. the selective silencing of the maternal allele, so that almost all affected individuals inherit a mutation from their father (84, 85). It is due to mutations in the *SGCE* (epsilon sarcoglycan) gene. SGCE function in the brain is largely unknown, but experimental studies expressing pathogenic missense mutations show impaired trafficking of the mutant protein to the plasma membrane and degradation by the proteasome, which is enhanced by an interaction with torsinA (the protein encoded by *TOR1A*/DYT1). DYT11 MD is characterized typically by brief lightning-like myoclonic jerks and dystonia, and usually begins in childhood. Myoclonus is usually the presenting symptom and most often affects the neck, trunk, and upper limbs, with the legs affected less prominently. The myoclonic jerks show a dramatic response to alcohol in many patients (86, 87) and they are not stimulus-sensitive, indicating a subcortical origin. About two-thirds of patients with DYT11 have dystonia, mostly cervical or writer's cramp, which tends to remain mild. Psychiatric manifestations including depression, anxiety, panic attacks, and obsessive–compulsive disorder (OCD) have been reported, and, in particular, OCD has been found in those not affected with motor signs, suggesting that it is related to the genetic defect (88–90). Exonic deletion mutations and other larger deletions result in more complex manifestations, including skeletal abnormalities, facial dysmorphism, developmental delay, or cavernous cerebral malformations (91).

Although the *SGCE* gene appears to be a major locus for MD, sporadic and familial cases without mutations in *SGCE* have been reported (92, 93), suggesting genetic heterogeneity. One of these families, with autosomal dominant inheritance and reduced penetrance, was used to map a second locus for MD to chromosome 18p (*DYT15*). The average age at onset is 9.6 years (range 7–15 years) and the MD phenotype is alcohol responsive (94).

Dystonia–parkinsonism

DYT3 is the only form of dystonia that is inherited as an X-linked trait. The disease originated on the island of Panay in the Philippines due to a founder mutation in the *TAF1* (TATA-binding protein-associated factor 1) gene and primarily affects males, although a few females have been reported (95–98). Disease onset occurs in the mid-thirties (range 12–52 years) with complete penetrance by the end of the fifth decade. The symptoms start as focal dystonia in almost any part of the body and progress to multifocal or generalized dystonia, in most cases within 5 years. Parkinsonism evolves later in the disease in about 50% of patients (99, 100). However, DYT3 dystonia is unique among the DYT loci in that neuronal degeneration, consisting mainly of neuronal loss and a multifocal mosaic pattern of astrocytosis restricted to the caudate and lateral putamen, has been noted on post-mortem analysis (95, 96, 98).

DYT5 was initially described by Segawa in 1976 (101), and later by Nygaard and colleagues as dopa-responsive dystonia (DRD) because of the dramatic and sustained response to a low dose of levodopa (102). The disease is inherited as an autosomal dominant trait with reduced penetrance that appears to be gender dependent, with females expressing symptoms more frequently. It is caused by mutations in the *GTPCH1* (GTP cyclohydrolase 1) gene (103). GTPCH1 is the rate-limiting enzyme in the synthesis of tetrahydrobiopterin, an essential co-factor for tyrosine hydroxylase (TH) which, in turn, is needed to synthesize dopamine (Fig. 17.1). Comprehensive screening of the *GTPCH1* gene identifies mutations in approximately 80% of 'typical' DRD patients (103, 104), and comprehensive molecular testing is available. The typical phenotype includes childhood (average 6 years) limb onset dystonia with diurnal variation (i.e. worsening of symptoms as the day progresses), improvement after sleep, and dramatic response to levodopa. With identification of the causative gene, the clinical spectrum of DRD has expanded to include oromandibular dystonia, spasticity with developmental delay mimicking cerebral palsy, psychiatric abnormalities, and generalized hypotonia with proximal weakness (105, 106).

In a minority of cases DRD can also be inherited as an autosomal recessive disorder with mutations in the genes coding for other enzymes involved in dopamine synthesis, including TH (often referred to as DYT5b) (106, 107) and sepiapterin reductase (SR) (Fig. 17.1) (108). The clinical manifestations are often more severe and can include mental retardation, oculogyria, hypotonia, severe bradykinesia, ptosis, and seizures.

A further dystonia–parkinsonism syndrome, which has been designated the *DYT12* locus, was mapped to chromosome 19q13. The disease is inherited as an autosomal dominant trait with reduced penetrance. Six heterozygous missense mutations have been identified in the Na^+, K^+-ATPase *ATP1A3* (alpha 3 subunit) gene, and all are shown to impair cell viability in cell culture experiments (109). A total of ten novel mutations in 17 families, and eight *de novo* cases have been reported (110, 111). The disease phenotype is designated rapid-onset dystonia–parkinsonism because key clinical features include abrupt onset, within hours to weeks, of dystonia with signs of parkinsonism usually triggered by physical or emotional stress (fever, childbirth, running, alcohol bingeing). The age of onset varies from 4 to 58 years, but typically presents in the teens or early twenties, and the distribution follows a rostrocaudal (face > arm > leg) gradient with prominent bulbar involvement.

An autosomal recessive form of dystonia-parkinsonism, DYT16, was assigned to chromosome 2q31 and the same homozygous missense mutation (P222L) was identified in the *PRKRA* (protein kinase, interferon-inducible double-stranded RNA-dependent activator) gene in the six affected family members as well as in one sporadic case (112). The phenotype in these patients is characterized by early (2–18 years) limb onset, with progression to generalized dystonia including prominent bulbar involvement with spasmodic dysphonia, dysarthria, and even dysphagia. Some affected members also had parkinsonism. A heterozygous frameshift mutation leading to a protein truncation was identified in a sporadic German case with early-onset dystonia (113, 114).

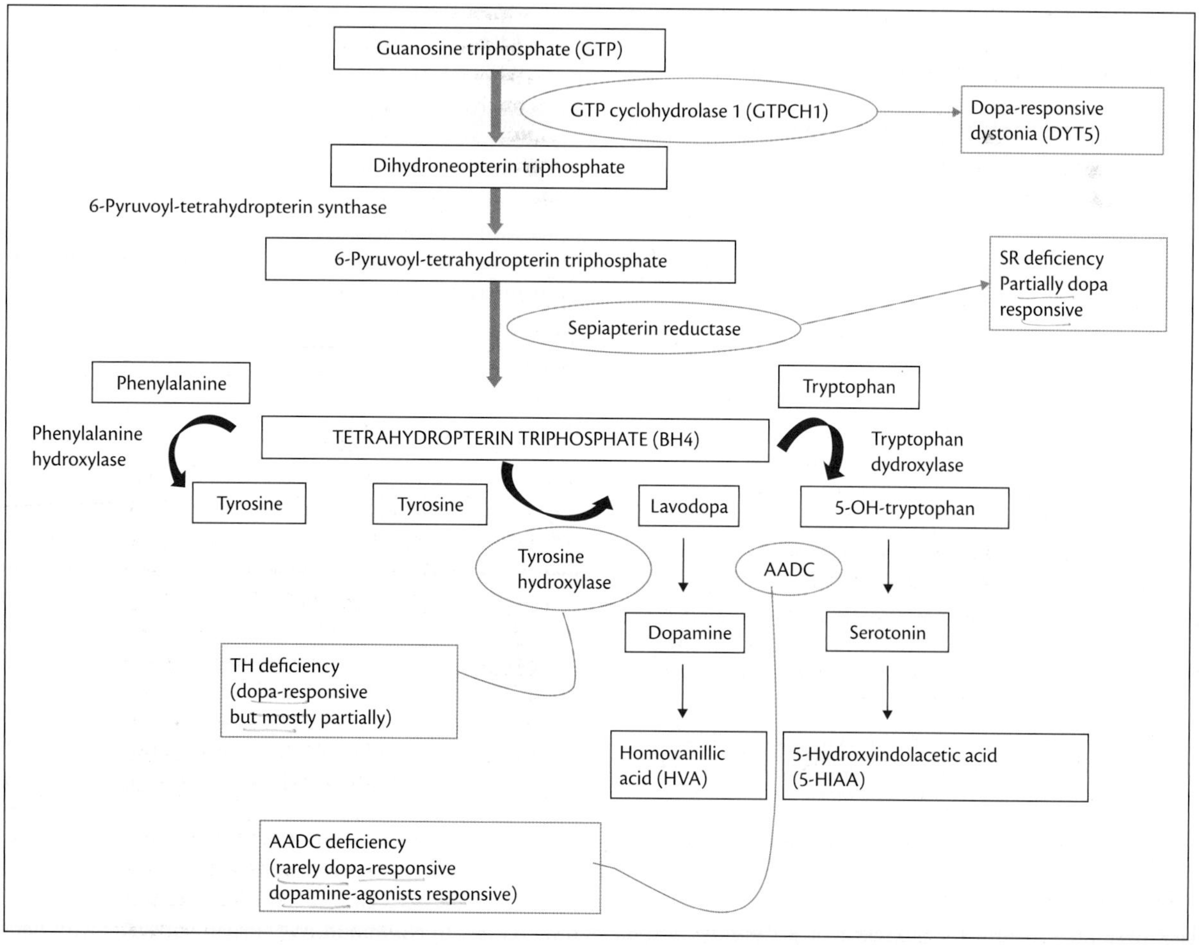

Fig. 17.1 Dopamine, tyrosine, and serotonin metabolic synthesis pathway and enzyme deficiencies with corresponding disorders.

Paroxysmal dystonia

This is a heterogeneous group of disorders characterized by paroxysmal attacks of involuntary movements. They are subdivided into kinesigenic (PKD) (DYT10, 19), non-kinesigenic (PNKD) (DYT8, 20), and exercise-induced forms (PED) (DYT9, 18).

Paroxysmal non-kinesigenic dyskinesia (PNKD) is characterized by attacks of dystonia, chorea, ballism, or athetosis, often provoked by alcohol or caffeine. The episodes last from minutes to hours, with a frequency ranging from once per day to one or two per year. The age of onset is typically in childhood or adolescents, but can be as late as 50 years (115). *DYT8* (PNKD1) is inherited as an autosomal dominant trait with high penetrance. The locus was localized to chromosome 2q33–36 (116–118) and mutations were identified in the *MR1* (myofibrillogenesis regulator 1) gene (119–121). The *DYT20* (PNKD2) locus designates a second form of paroxysmal non-kinesigenic dyskinesia, which was described in a single Canadian family, in which linkage analysis assigned the locus to chromosome 2q31 with no mutations in the *MR1* gene (122). The clinical symptoms in this family are very similar to those described in the DYT8 families.

Paroxysmal kinesigenic dyskinesia (PKD) is characterized by short (seconds to minutes) frequent (up to 100 times per day) attacks of dystonic or choreiform movements precipitated by sudden movements. Age of onset is usually during childhood or adolescence, but symptoms can resolve in adulthood. PKD is inherited as an autosomal dominant trait. The *DYT10* locus was mapped to chromosome 16p11.2-q12.1 (123, 124) and mutations have been identified in the *PRRT2* (proline-rich transmembrane protein 2) gene (125, 126). A second locus for PKD, designated *DYT19*, maps to an overlapping region and thus could represent the same locus (127). Another PKD pedigree has been excluded from linkage analysis to chromosome 16 and thus most likely represents a different PKD locus (128).

Paroxysmal exercise-induced dyskinesia (PED) is characterized by exercise-induced attacks of dystonic, choreoathetotic, and ballistic movements affecting the exercised limbs which last from a few minutes to an hour. The disease usually has its onset in childhood, and can have other disease manifestations including epilepsy, migraine, developmental delay, and haemolytic anemia. It shows an autosomal dominant inheritance pattern with slightly reduced penetrance. The locus is designated *DYT18* (129, 130) and mutations in the *SLC2A1* gene encoding glucose transporter 1 (GLUT1) have been identified (129). Mutations in *SLC2A1* have also been found in sporadic cases of PED (131) and in a family with dystonic tremor as the presenting feature (132). *SLC2A1*/GLUT1 is the main glucose transporter in the brain. PED is thought to be caused by reduced glucose transport into the brain, particularly when energy demand is high after prolonged exercise. Paroxysmal choreoathetosis/spasticity (DYT9), originally described in a large German pedigree with autosomal dominant inheritance, was linked to chromosome 1p. Recently, re-examination of this family revealed a causative mutation in *SLC2A1*; thus DYT9 and DYT18 are allelic disorders (133).

Secondary/heredodegenerative dystonia

Secondary dystonia

Secondary dystonias require the presence of a causative lesion, exposure, or event, such as an abscess, dopamine blocking agents, or stroke. In cases of a precipitating event dystonia may sometimes develop some time after the event. Secondary dystonia is typically not progressive; however, it could be that there is an initial worsening of symptoms after the event for up to some years before the condition becomes static. Continuous progression should raise suspicion of a heredodegenerative cause of dystonia (134, 135). Past medical history, abnormalities in the neurological examination, neuroimaging, or laboratory evaluation, distribution (e.g. hemidystonia), age at onset, and distribution which is unusual for primary dystonia, such as young-onset cranial dystonia or late-onset lower limb dystonia, are clues for the diagnosis of secondary dystonia.

One major cause of secondary dystonia is *brain injury or infection* (e.g. perinatal injury, stroke, head trauma or peripheral trauma, brain tumour, exposure to neurotoxic agents, Japanese B encephalitis, encephalitis lethargica, brain abscesses) especially involving the basal ganglia (mostly putamen), cerebellum, and thalamus (136). Perinatal hypoxic injury often leads to severe generalized dystonia, with or without spasticity. This is often called athetoid cerebral palsy and should be differentiated from DRDs (106, 137, 138).

Exposure to *dopamine-receptor-blocking drugs* (DRBs) or other agents (amine depleters, serotonin-reuptake inhibitors, monoamine oxidase inhibitors, calcium antagonists, benzodiazepines, general anaesthetic agents, carbamazepine, phenytoin, triptans, ranitidine, cocaine, ecstasy) is a common cause of secondary dystonia. *Acute dystonic reactions* may occur in up to 2% of patients beginning treatment with DRBs. Time to onset is variable, but 50% will develop dystonia within 1–2 days and 90% within 5 days. Common presentations are OMD, oculogyric crisis, cervical dystonia, and laryngeal dystonic spasm. *Tardive dystonia* is caused by chronic exposure to DRBs. All neuroleptic drugs including so-called atypical agents, with the exception of clozapine, can cause tardive dystonia (139). In contrast with acute dystonic reactions, amine depleters (e.g. tetrabenazine) do not cause tardive syndromes. Clinically, the dystonia is characterized by axial dystonia with hyperextension of the spine and retrocollis. The mean time from exposure to onset is around 6 years, but the shortest exposure time to onset reported is 4 days. Around 10% of patients show spontaneous remission, while the prognosis of the others depends on the prompt discontinuation of the DRB and the total duration of the exposure (139).

Heredodegenerative dystonia

Inherited degenerative diseases that can cause dystonia include many autosomal dominant and autosomal recessive conditions, X-linked dominant and recessive conditions, and mitochondrial defects. As per the definition, there are other symptoms and signs, and dystonia occurs as part of neurodegeneration. The most important conditions, along with the responsible genes, are given in Table 17.3. A logical approach in these patients is to look for syndromic associations that help to narrow down the differential diagnosis (Table 17.3). Of particular note is *Wilson disease* (WD), because it is treatable. It is caused by mutations in the *ATP7B* (ATPase, Cu^{2+} transporting, beta polypeptide) gene on chromosome 13, which produce a defect in copper metabolism, leading to the insidious development of neurological, psychiatric, or hepatic dysfunction. Inheritance is autosomal recessive; more than 200 different mutations have been reported, making genetic testing impractical. In childhood, WD usually presents with hepatic dysfunction, while neurological presentation is typical in adult-onset

Table 17.3 Syndromic associations in diagnosing some of the most important heredodegenerative dystonias

Syndrome	Disorder	Gene	Transmission
Dystonia–parkinsonism	Parkinson's disease (PD)	esp. *PRKN* (PARK2), *DJ-1* (PARK7)	AR
	Sporadic PD, CBD, PSP, MSA	–	
	Wilson disease	*ATP7B*	AR
	Neurodegeneration with brain iron accumulation (NBIA)	*PANK2*	AR
		PLA2G6 (PARK14)	AR
		Kufor–Rakeb (PARK9) *ATP13A2*	AR
		FA2H	AR
		Aceruloplasminaemia (*ceruloplasmin* gene)	AR
		Neuroferritinopathy (*FTL*)	AR
	Huntington's disease	*IT-15*	AD
	Spinocerebellar ataxia	SCA2 (*ATXN2*), SCA3 (*ATXN3*)	AD
	GM1 gangliosidosis	*LacZ*	AR
	Mitochondrial	*POLG*	AD, AR
Dystonia–ataxia	MSA	–	
	Spinocerebellar ataxia	SCA2 (*ATXN2*), SCA3 (*ATXN3*)	AD
	Wilson disease	*ATP7B*	AR
	Neuroacanthocytosis	*VPS13A*	AD
	Huntington's disease	*IT-15*	AD
	Dentatorubral-pallidoluysian atrophy (DRPLA)	*ATN1*	AR
	GM2 gangliosidosis	*HEXB3*	AR
Dystonia–eye movement disorder	Ataxia telangiectasia	*ATM*	AR
	Ataxia oculomotor apraxia 1,2	*APTX, SETX*	AR
	Niemann–Pick C	*NPC1, NPC2*	AD
	Kufor–Rakeb disease	*ATP13A2*	AD
	Spinocerebellar ataxia	SCA2 (*ATXN2*)	AR
	Huntington's disease	*IT-15*	AR
	PSP	–	
Dystonia–bulbar involvement	NBIA Neuroacanthocytosis Wilson disease	See above	
Dystonia–peripheral neuropathy	Spinocerebellar ataxia Neuroacanthocytosis GM2 gangliosidosis	See above	
	Metachromatic leucodystrophy	*ARSA*	AR

disease (see Chapter 23 for more details). Dystonia can be generalized, segmental, or multifocal, but cranial involvement is characteristic; other common signs include a 'sardonic' smile, wing-beating tremor, dysarthria, dysphagia, drooling, ataxia, and dementia. In addition to brain and liver involvement (cirrhosis, acute hepatitis), systemic findings can involve the eye (Keyser–Fleischer rings), heart, kidney, bones, joints, glands, and muscles.

Pathophysiology of dystonia

The pathophysiology of dystonia is unknown. Most research has focused on the primary dystonias and the role of genetic susceptibility in disease mechanisms. Imaging and neurophysiological abnormalities have been identified in unaffected DYT1 mutation carriers. These endophenotypic traits may require additional genetic or environmental factors to become fully penetrant, or they may simply reflect stochastic expression of the mutant protein. Examples include impaired temporal discrimination threshold in DYT1 manifesting and non-manifesting mutation carriers (140) and higher temporal and spatial discrimination threshold in adult-onset primary focal dystonia (141–143), also in unaffected body regions (141, 142, 144) and in patients' unaffected first- and second-degree relatives (145–147), suggesting a primary endophenotypic deficit rather than a deficit secondary to the presence of dystonic contractions. Kinaesthesia and vibration-induced illusion of movement have been found to be impaired in patients with APD in the affected and unaffected body regions (148–151) and in asymptomatic first-degree relatives, again indicating the probable primary origin of this feature. Mental rotation of corporeal objects, reflecting mental simulation of movements, is abnormal in both focal hand dystonia and cervical dystonia (152). This suggests that, apart from the motor deficit, there is also a primary deficit in sensory processing in primary dystonia (7).

Motor, sensory, and sensorimotor integration abnormalities are thought to derive from two clear abnormalities that have been repeatedly demonstrated across different forms of the disorder using electrophysiological and neuroimaging studies. The first is that mechanisms that usually produce inhibition within the motor system are underfunctioning; this has been demonstrated at a cortical, brainstem, and spinal cord level (153). Increased motor cortical excitability then causes the excessive and inappropriate muscle contraction that occurs during motor tasks. However, such abnormalities can be present in clinically unaffected body parts and in non-manifesting DYT1 gene carriers, indicating that additional factors are necessary to produce the clinical symptoms of dystonia (154). The second abnormality is that there is an excessive response to experimental protocols that produce plastic changes within the motor system (155–157). Again, such abnormalities are present in clinically unaffected body parts, but importantly are not present in non-manifesting DYT1 gene carriers (158), where a subnormal response to plasticity protocols is seen. This suggests that abnormal brain plasticity may be an essential component of the clinical manifestation of dystonia.

One pathophysiological hypothesis for these abnormalities is that altered basal ganglia input to the motor cortex causes reduced excitability of cortical inhibitory circuits. Evidence from DBS experience in primary dystonia patients and DYT1 animal findings points to dysfunction in the globus pallidus internus (GPi) which may be related to abnormal striatal dopaminergic signalling and increased cholinergic tone; this dysfunction leads to abnormal synchronization of the basal ganglia output to the thalamus and sensory feedback misprocessing. Together they have the effect of increasing striatal, brainstem, and cortical plasticity, and producing, over time, neural reorganization and overt dystonia. D2 receptors are deficient in the putamen in focal dystonia, and this could cause a decrease in D2-dependent inhibition of GABA transmission and subsequently a loss of inhibition in the basal ganglia. This abnormality in D2-receptor function has also been found in clinically unaffected DYT1 gene carriers (159), suggesting that D2-receptor dysfunction represents a feature of the non-manifesting carrier state.

In summary, genetic susceptibility could lead to a neurochemical and functional imbalance in the basal ganglia (but possibly even more widespread) that subsequently may lead to a widespread loss of inhibition and increased plasticity, which could explain a number of motor and non-motor features seen in unaffected relatives of patients with primary dystonia and unaffected mutation carriers. The presence of other genetic or environmental factors, such as repetitive activity, trauma, or emotional arousal and stress, could lead to a breakdown of compensatory mechanisms and ultimately to the motor manifestation of dystonia.

Differential diagnosis of dystonia

A variety of central and peripheral nervous system disorders, as well as non-neurological conditions, such as neuromyotonia, myotonic disorders, inflammatory myopathies, and glycogen storage diseases, can be associated with abnormal postures that resemble dystonia. Stiff person syndrome causes contraction of axial and proximal limb muscles. Carpopedal spasms of tetany can be the manifestation of hypocalcaemia, hypomagnesaemia, or alkalosis. Orthopaedic and rheumatological processes involving bones, ligaments, or joints can result in abnormal postures. In Sandifer syndrome, patients (typically young boys) with hiatus hernia develop head tilt in association with gastro-oesophageal reflux.

Once the presence of dystonia is established, the next diagnostic step is to differentiate between primary and secondary/heredodegenerative dystonia. Distribution and age at onset provide important clues for this differential. Primary dystonia has an anatomical distribution which depends on age at onset. Young-onset primary dystonia tends to be generalized or multifocal, with onset of dystonia typically in a limb (typically lower), sparing cranial muscles. Adult-onset dystonia is more commonly focal or segmental and often in an upper limb (such as task-specific writer's cramp), or it may affect the neck and head, while legs are almost never affected. Therefore an unusual pattern (e.g. adult-onset lower limb dystonia) is a clue pointing to secondary/heredodegenerative dystonia.

If dystonia is primary, genetic testing for DYT1 dystonia is indicated for patients with onset of dystonia before 26 years of age, as well as for patients with later onset who have a relative with young-onset dystonia. Data to guide DYT6 testing are insufficient at present, but may be indicated in DYT1-negative individuals with early-onset arm, cranial, or cervical involvement. Most patients with clinically typical DRD will have identified mutations in *GTPCH1* if comprehensive analysis is performed, including testing for deletions. Genetic testing for myoclonus–dystonia is available, although many sporadic cases do not harbour *SGCE* mutations. Evaluation of secondary/heredodegenerative dystonia is dictated by clues provided by the history and examination. Routine blood tests, kidney, liver, thyroid function, iron, ferritin, copper, ceruloplasmin, white cell enzymes, acanthocytes, lactate, pyruvate, creatine kinase, and antinuclear antibody screen may be indicated. Specific clinical findings or laboratory abnormalities may dictate further investigations, including electrophysiological studies, lumbar puncture, muscle or skin biopsy, metabolic studies of blood, urine, or cerebrospinal fluid, MRI brain imaging with sequences to detect iron, and dopamine transporter imaging. Genetic testing is also available for many of the heredodegenerative dystonias (see Table 17.3). Lastly, one should keep in mind the possibility of psychogenic dystonia which could be diagnosed based on established clinical criteria (20).

Treatment of dystonia

A comprehensive algorithm for the treatment of dystonia is given in Fig. 17.2.

Primary dystonia and dystonia-plus syndromes

Young-onset primary dystonia

A trial of levodopa is recommended for all patients with early onset of symptoms to exclude DRD. Although a daily dose of 600 mg levodopa is sometimes required, failure to respond to a dose of 300 mg/day usually excludes the diagnosis of DRD. Once DRD is excluded, anticholinergic agents such as trihexyphenidyl are usually tried. Use is often limited by peripheral anticholinergic adverse effects, including blurred vision, dry mouth, urinary retention, sedation, and confusion, and doses should be titrated slowly. Anticholinergic medications can be used singly or in combination with other drugs, including baclofen, clonazepam,

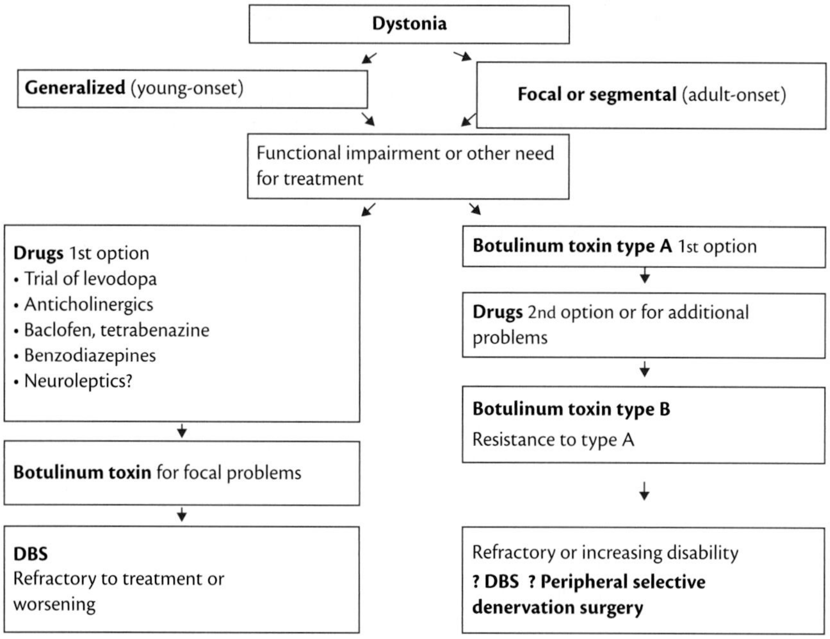

Fig. 17.2 Algorithm for the treatment of dystonia.

or tetrabenazine. Botulinum toxin (BoNT) injections have a limited role in generalized dystonia but can be helpful in focal or segmental dystonia. Deep brain stimulation (DBS) of the internal segment of the GPi can be of remarkable benefit. DYT1 dystonia was shown to improve by 40–90% (160–164) and efficacy is sustained after more than 5 years of follow-up (165, 166). Improvement frequently follows a particular pattern, with phasic, myoclonic, and tremulous elements improving earlier than tonic elements, the latter often with a delay of weeks or months (160, 161, 167).

Adult-onset primary dystonia

BoNT injections are the first-line treatment option for cervical dystonia and are also efficacious for blepharospasm, focal upper extremity dystonia, adductor laryngeal dystonia, and focal lower limb dystonia (61, 168, 169). Side effects can arise from unintended weakness in nearby muscles due to diffusion of toxin. Antibodies to BoNT can develop with repeated injections, resulting in loss of therapeutic effect. The use of oral drugs (anticholinergics) is less effective than in young-onset dystonia, although large controlled studies are lacking. Long-term GPi DBS is effective for various types of adult-onset primary dystonia. In patients with cervical dystonia, GPi DBS has been used primarily in those who were thought not to be ideal candidates for peripheral denervation, including patients with head tremor and myoclonus, or marked phasic dystonic movements. Indications have been widened in the past few years (170–172).

Paroxysmal dystonia

For PNKDs, avoiding the precipitants helps but oral treatments are largely inadequate. There may be a limited response to phenytoin, acetazolamide, benzodiazepines, and levodopa (173, 174). PKDs show a typically excellent response to carbamazepine (100–200 mg/day), and other treatment options include phenytoin and acetazolamide (173, 174). For PEDs prolonged exercise should be avoided. There is evidence that patients with *SLC2A1*/GLUT1 mutation may improve by following a ketogenic diet (175).

Secondary/heredodegenerative dystonia

When dystonia is secondary, treatment of the underlying condition may produce improvement in the dystonia. Structural lesions may be amenable to surgical correction.

Treatment of a drug-induced acute dystonic reaction may be an emergency because of possible respiratory compromise. It comprises stopping the offending drug, monitoring basic functions, and use of anticholinergic drugs (benzatropine, procyclidine intravenously). Anticholinergic drugs such as trihexyphenidyl, benzodiazepines, baclofen, and tetrabenazine, and also BoNT, are used for treatment of tardive dystonia. Tardive dystonia appears also to be a good indication for GPi DBS with benefits similar to those seen in primary dystonia (176). Patients with cerebral palsy may achieve a 10–40% benefit in motor scores (177).

With to regard to heredodegenerative dystonia, treatment depends on the underlying condition. Management of Wilson disease consists of copper chelation therapy (usually with penicillamine as a first-line agent) and oral zinc, which induces copper-binding metallothionein in enterocytes. Some inborn errors of metabolism may respond to dietary restriction or supplementation. There is some preliminary evidence of benefit from GPi DBS, but further studies are needed (178, 179).

Supportive treatment

Because patients with dystonia often have associated co-morbidities, consultation with specialists, including orthopaedic surgeons and psychiatrists, can be useful. Many patients derive benefit from physical, occupational, and speech therapy. Various devices have been developed that provide sensory input via the affected body part, simulating a sensory trick. Alternative and complementary modalities such as acupuncture, biofeedback, massage, and relaxation techniques may be helpful.

A rehabilitative programme with BoNT injections in patients with cervical dystonia can provide more marked improvement and a longer duration effect than BoNT injections alone (180).

References

1. Fahn S, Marsden CD, Calne DB. Classification and investigation of dystonia. In: Marsden CD, Fahm S (eds) *Movement disorders 2*, pp. 332–58. London: Butterworths, 1987.
2. Gomez-Wong E, Marti MJ, Cossu G, Fabregat N, Tolosa ES, Valls-Sole J. The 'geste antagonistique' induces transient modulation of the blink reflex in human patients with blepharospasm. *Neurosci Lett* 1998; 251: 125–8.
3. Jankovic J, Leder S, Warner D, Schwartz K. Cervical dystonia: clinical findings and associated movement disorders. *Neurology* 1991; 41: 1088–91.
4. Naumann M, Magyar-Lehmann S, Reiners K, Erbguth F, Leenders KL. Sensory tricks in cervical dystonia: perceptual dysbalance of parietal cortex modulates frontal motor programming. *Ann Neurol* 2000; 47: 322–8.
5. Schramm A, Classen J, Reiners K, Naumann M. Characteristics of sensory trick-like manoeuvres in jaw-opening dystonia. *Mov Disord* 2007; 22: 430–3.
6. Schramm A, Reiners K, Naumann M. Complex mechanisms of sensory tricks in cervical dystonia. *Mov Disord* 2004; 19: 452–8.
7. Stamelou M, Edwards MJ, Hallett M, Bhatia KP. The non-motor syndrome of primary dystonia: clinical and pathophysiological implications. *Brain* 2012; 135: 1668–81.
8. Kuyper DJ, Parra V, Aerts S, Okun MS, Kluger BM. Nonmotor manifestations of dystonia: a systematic review. *Mov Disord* 2011; 26: 1206–17.
9. Ghika J, Regli F, Growdon JH. Sensory symptoms in cranial dystonia: a potential role in the etiology? *J Neurol Sci* 1993; 116: 142–7.
10. Pekmezovic T, Svetel M, Ivanovic N, et al. Quality of life in patients with focal dystonia. *Clin Neurol Neurosurg* 2009; 111: 161–4.
11. Gundel H, Busch R, Ceballos-Baumann A, Seifert E. Psychiatric comorbidity in patients with spasmodic dysphonia: a controlled study. *J Neurol Neurosurg Psychiatry* 2007; 78: 1398–400.
12. Gundel H, Wolf A, Xidara V, Busch R, Ceballos-Baumann AO. Social phobia in spasmodic torticollis. *J Neurol Neurosurg Psychiatry* 2001; 71: 499–504.
13. Gundel H, Wolf A, Xidara V, et al. High psychiatric comorbidity in spasmodic torticollis: a controlled study. *J Nerv Ment Dis* 2003; 191: 465–73.
14. Voon V, Butler TR, Ekanayake V, et al. Psychiatric symptoms associated with focal hand dystonia. *Mov Disord* 2010; 25: 2249–52.
15. Heiman GA, Ottman R, Saunders-Pullman RJ, Ozelius LJ, Risch NJ, Bressman SB. Increased risk for recurrent major depression in DYT1 dystonia mutation carriers. *Neurology* 2004; 63: 631–7.
16. Cano SJ, Hobart JC, Edwards M, et al. CDIP-58 can measure the impact of botulinum toxin treatment in cervical dystonia. *Neurology* 2006; 67: 2230–2.
17. Soeder A, Kluger BM, Okun MS, et al. Mood and energy determinants of quality of life in dystonia. *J Neurol* 2009; 256: 996–1001.
18. Edwards MJ, Bhatia KP, Cordivari C. Immediate response to botulinum toxin injections in patients with fixed dystonia. *Mov Disord* 2011; 26: 917–18.
19. Katschnig P, Edwards MJ, Schwingenschuh P, et al. Mental rotation of body parts and sensory temporal discrimination in fixed dystonia. *Mov Disord* 2010; 25: 1061–7.
20. Fahn S, Williams DT. Psychogenic dystonia. *Adv Neurol* 1988; 50: 431–55.
21. Schrag A, Trimble M, Quinn N, Bhatia K. The syndrome of fixed dystonia: an evaluation of 103 patients. *Brain* 2004; 127: 2360–72.
22. Fahn S, Bressman SB, Marsden CD. Classification of dystonia. *Adv Neurol* 1998; 78: 1–10.
23. Fahn S, Jankovic J, Hallett M. *Principles and Practice of Movement Disorders* (2nd edn). Philadelphia, PA: Saunders, 2011.
24. Albanese A, Asmus F, Bhatia KP, et al. EFNS guidelines on diagnosis and treatment of primary dystonias. *Eur J Neurol* 2011; 18: 5–18.
25. Fuchs T, Gavarini S, Saunders-Pullman R, et al. Mutations in the THAP1 gene are responsible for DYT6 primary torsion dystonia. *Nat Genet* 2009; 41: 286–8.
26. Ozelius LJ, Bressman SB. Genetic and clinical features of primary torsion dystonia. *Neurobiol Dis* 2011; 42: 127–35.
27. Defazio G, Abbruzzese G, Livrea P, Berardelli A. Epidemiology of primary dystonia. *Lancet Neurol* 2004; 3: 673–8.
28. Muller J, Kiechl S, Wenning GK, et al. The prevalence of primary dystonia in the general community. *Neurology* 2002; 59: 941–3.
29. Defazio G. The epidemiology of primary dystonia: current evidence and perspectives. *Eur J Neurol* 2010; 17 (Suppl 1): 9–14.
30. Neuwald AF, Aravind L, Spouge JL, Koonin EV. AAA+: A class of chaperone-like ATPases associated with the assembly, operation, and disassembly of protein complexes. *Genome Res* 1999; 9: 27–43.
31. Valente EM, Warner TT, Jarman PR, et al. The role of DYT1 in primary torsion dystonia in Europe. *Brain* 1998; 121: 2335–9.
32. Lebre AS, Durr A, Jedynak P, et al. DYT1 mutation in French families with idiopathic torsion dystonia. *Brain* 1999; 122: 41–5.
33. Slominsky PA, Markova ED, Shadrina MI, et al. A common 3-bp deletion in the DYT1 gene in Russian families with early-onset torsion dystonia. *Hum Mutat* 1999; 14: 269.
34. Brassat D, Camuzat A, Vidailhet M, et al. Frequency of the DYT1 mutation in primary torsion dystonia without family history. *Arch Neurol* 2000; 57: 333–5.
35. Bressman SB, Sabatti C, Raymond D, et al. The DYT1 phenotype and guidelines for diagnostic testing. *Neurology* 2000; 54: 1746–52.
36. Calakos N, Patel VD, Gottron M, et al. Functional evidence implicating a novel TOR1A mutation in idiopathic, late-onset focal dystonia. *J Med Genet* 2010; 47: 646–50.
37. Risch NJ, Bressman SB, Senthil G, Ozelius LJ. Intragenic Cis and Trans modification of genetic susceptibility in DYT1 torsion dystonia. *Am J Hum Genet* 2007; 80: 1188–93.
38. Kamm C, Fischer H, Garavaglia B, et al. Susceptibility to DYT1 dystonia in European patients is modified by the D216H polymorphism. *Neurology* 2008; 70: 2261–2.
39. Gambarin M, Valente EM, Liberini P, et al. Atypical phenotypes and clinical variability in a large Italian family with DYT1-primary torsion dystonia. *Mov Disord* 2006; 21: 1782–4.
40. Edwards M, Wood N, Bhatia K. Unusual phenotypes in DYT1 dystonia: a report of five cases and a review of the literature. *Mov Disord* 2003; 18: 706–11.
41. Almasy L, Bressman SB, Raymond D, et al. Idiopathic torsion dystonia linked to chromosome 8 in two Mennonite families. *Ann Neurol* 1997; 42: 670–3.
42. Saunders-Pullman R, Raymond D, Senthil G, et al. Narrowing the DYT6 dystonia region and evidence for locus heterogeneity in the Amish-Mennonites. *Am J Med Genet A* 2007; 143A: 2098–105.
43. Bonetti M, Barzaghi C, Brancati F, et al. Mutation screening of the DYT6/THAP1 gene in Italy. *Mov Disord* 2009; 24: 2424–7.
44. Bressman SB, Raymond D, Fuchs T, Heiman GA, Ozelius LJ, Saunders-Pullman R. Mutations in THAP1 (DYT6) in early-onset dystonia: a genetic screening study. *Lancet Neurol* 2009; 8: 441–6.
45. Houlden H, Schneider SA, Paudel R, et al. THAP1 mutations (DYT6) are an additional cause of early-onset dystonia. *Neurology* 2010; 74: 846–50.
46. Schneider SA, Ramirez A, Shafiee K, et al. Homozygous THAP1 mutations as cause of early-onset generalized dystonia. *Mov Disord* 2011; 26: 858–61.
47. Clot F, Grabli D, Burbaud P, et al. Screening of the THAP1 gene in patients with early-onset dystonia: myoclonic jerks are part of the dystonia 6 phenotype. *Neurogenetics* 2011; 12: 87–9.

48. Gavarini S, Cayrol C, Fuchs T, et al. Direct interaction between causative genes of DYT1 and DYT6 primary dystonia. *Ann Neurol* 2010; 68: 549–53.
49. Gimenez-Roldan S, Delgado G, Marin M, Villanueva JA, Mateo D. Hereditary torsion dystonia in gypsies. *Adv Neurol* 1988; 50: 73–81.
50. Khan NL, Wood NW, Bhatia KP. Autosomal recessive, DYT2-like primary torsion dystonia: a new family. *Neurology* 2003; 61: 1801–3.
51. Moretti P, Hedera P, Wald J, Fink J. Autosomal recessive primary generalized dystonia in two siblings from a consanguineous family. *Mov Disord* 2005; 20: 245–7.
52. Parker N. Hereditary whispering dysphonia. *J Neurol Neurosurg Psychiatry* 1985; 48: 218–24.
53. Ahmad F, Davis MB, Waddy HM, Oley CA, Marsden CD, Harding AE. Evidence for locus heterogeneity in autosomal dominant torsion dystonia. *Genomics* 1993; 15: 9–12.
54. Bentivoglio AR, Ialongo T, Contarino MF, Valente EM, Albanese A. Phenotypic characterization of DYT13 primary torsion dystonia. *Mov Disord* 2004; 19: 200–6.
55. Chouery E, Kfoury J, Delague V, et al. A novel locus for autosomal recessive primary torsion dystonia (DYT17) maps to 20p11.22-q13.12. *Neurogenetics* 2008; 9: 287–93.
56. Svetel M, Pekmezovic T, Jovic J, et al. Spread of primary dystonia in relation to initially affected region. *J Neurol* 2007; 254: 879–83.
57. Weiss EM, Hershey T, Karimi M, et al. Relative risk of spread of symptoms among the focal onset primary dystonias. *Mov Disord* 2006; 21: 1175–81.
58. O'Riordan S, Raymond D, Lynch T, et al. Age at onset as a factor in determining the phenotype of primary torsion dystonia. *Neurology* 2004; 63: 1423–6.
59. Peckham EL, Lopez G, Shamim EA, et al. Clinical features of patients with blepharospasm: a report of 240 patients. *Eur J Neurol* 2011; 18: 382–6.
60. Jankovic J, Ford J. Blepharospasm and orofacial-cervical dystonia: clinical and pharmacological findings in 100 patients. *Ann Neurol* 1983; 13: 402–11.
61. Hallett M, Benecke R, Blitzer A, Comella CL. Treatment of focal dystonias with botulinum neurotoxin. *Toxicon* 2009; 54: 628–33.
62. Blitzer A, Brin MF, Stewart CF. Botulinum toxin management of spasmodic dysphonia (laryngeal dystonia): a 12-year experience in more than 900 patients. *Laryngoscope* 1998; 108: 1435–41.
63. Schneider SA, Bhatia KP. The entity of jaw tremor and dystonia. *Mov Disord* 2007; 22: 1491–5.
64. Lo SE, Frucht SJ. Is focal task-specific dystonia limited to the hand and face? *Mov Disord* 2007; 22: 1009–11.
65. Schneider SA, Aggarwal A, Bhatt M, et al. Severe tongue protrusion dystonia: clinical syndromes and possible treatment. *Neurology* 2006; 67: 940–3.
66. Esper CD, Freeman A, Factor SA. Lingual protrusion dystonia: frequency, etiology and botulinum toxin therapy. *Parkinsonism Relat Disord* 2010; 16: 438–41.
67. Baik JS, Park JH, Kim JY. Primary lingual dystonia induced by speaking. *Mov Disord* 2004; 19: 1251–2.
68. Papapetropoulos S, Singer C. Primary focal lingual dystonia. *Mov Disord* 2006; 21: 429–30.
69. Bhatia KP, Quinn NP, Marsden CD. Clinical features and natural history of axial predominant adult onset primary dystonia. *J Neurol Neurosurg Psychiatry* 1997; 63: 788–91.
70. Waddy HM, Fletcher NA, Harding AE, Marsden CD. A genetic study of idiopathic focal dystonias. *Ann Neurol* 1991; 29: 320–4.
71. Defazio G, Livrea P, Guanti G, Lepore V, Ferrari E. Genetic contribution to idiopathic adult-onset blepharospasm and cranial-cervical dystonia. *Eur Neurol* 1993; 33: 345–50.
72. Uitti RJ, Maraganore DM. Adult onset familial cervical dystonia: report of a family including monozygotic twins. *Mov Disord* 1993; 8: 489–94.
73. Bressman SB, Warner TT, Almasy L, et al. Exclusion of the DYT1 locus in familial torticollis. *Ann Neurol* 1996; 40: 681–4.
74. Munchau A, Valente EM, Davis MB, et al. A Yorkshire family with adult-onset cranio-cervical primary torsion dystonia. *Mov Disord* 2000; 15: 954–9.
75. Leube B, Rudnicki D, Ratzlaff T, Kessler KR, Benecke R, Auburger G. Idiopathic torsion dystonia: assignment of a gene to chromosome 18p in a German family with adult onset, autosomal dominant inheritance and purely focal distribution. *Hum Mol Genet* 1996; 5: 1673–7.
76. Norgren N, Mattson E, Forsgren L, Holmberg M. A high-penetrance form of late-onset torsion dystonia maps to a novel locus (DYT21) on chromosome 2q14.3-q21.3. *Neurogenetics* 2011; 12: 137–43.
77. Sibbing D, Trender-Gerhardt I, Wood NW, Oertel WH, Bhatia KP, Bandmann O. The promoter region of the Menkes gene ATP7A is not altered in focal or generalized dystonia. *Ann Neurol* 2003; 53: 278–80.
78. Sharma N, Franco RA, Jr, Kuster JK, et al. Genetic evidence for an association of the TOR1A locus with segmental/focal dystonia. *Mov Disord* 2010; 25: 2183–7.
79. Hague S, Klaffke S, Clarimon J, et al. Lack of association with TorsinA haplotype in German patients with sporadic dystonia. *Neurology* 2006; 66: 951–2.
80. Placzek MR, Misbahuddin A, Chaudhuri KR, Wood NW, Bhatia KP, Warner TT. Cervical dystonia is associated with a polymorphism in the dopamine (D5) receptor gene. *J Neurol Neurosurg Psychiatry* 2001; 71: 262–4.
81. Brancati F, Valente EM, Castori M, et al. Role of the dopamine D5 receptor (DRD5) as a susceptibility gene for cervical dystonia. *J Neurol Neurosurg Psychiatry* 2003; 74: 665–6.
82. Misbahuddin A, Placzek MR, Chaudhuri KR, Wood NW, Bhatia KP, Warner TT. A polymorphism in the dopamine receptor DRD5 is associated with blepharospasm. *Neurology* 2002; 58: 124–6.
83. Clarimon J, Brancati F, Peckham E, et al. Assessing the role of DRD5 and DYT1 in two different case-control series with primary blepharospasm. *Mov Disord* 2007; 22: 162–6.
84. Grabowski M, Zimprich A, Lorenz-Depiereux B, et al. The epsilon-sarcoglycan gene (SGCE), mutated in myoclonus-dystonia syndrome, is maternally imprinted. *Eur J Hum Genet* 2003; 11: 138–44.
85. Muller B, Hedrich K, Kock N, et al. Evidence that paternal expression of the epsilon-sarcoglycan gene accounts for reduced penetrance in myoclonus–dystonia. *Am J Hum Genet* 2002; 71: 1303–11.
86. Quinn NP. Essential myoclonus and myoclonic dystonia. *Mov Disord* 1996; 11: 119–24.
87. Kyllerman M, Forsgren L, Sanner G, Holmgren G, Wahlstrom J, Drugge U. Alcohol-responsive myoclonic dystonia in a large family: dominant inheritance and phenotypic variation. *Mov Disord* 1990; 5: 270–9.
88. Saunders-Pullman R, Shriberg J, Heiman G, et al. Myoclonus dystonia: possible association with obsessive-compulsive disorder and alcohol dependence. *Neurology* 2002; 58: 242–5.
89. Hess CW, Raymond D, Aguiar P de C, et al. Myoclonus–dystonia, obsessive–compulsive disorder, and alcohol dependence in SGCE mutation carriers. *Neurology* 2007; 68: 522–4.
90. Foncke EM, Cath D, Zwinderman K, Smit J, Schmand B, Tijssen M. Is psychopathology part of the phenotypic spectrum of myoclonus-dystonia?: a study of a large Dutch M-D family. *Cogn Behav Neurol* 2009; 22: 127–33.
91. Bonnet C, Gregoire MJ, Vibert M, Raffo E, Leheup B, Jonveaux P. Cryptic 7q21 and 9p23 deletions in a patient with apparently balanced *de novo* reciprocal translocation t(7; 9)(q21; p23) associated with a dystonia-plus syndrome: paternal deletion of the epsilon-sarcoglycan (SGCE) gene. *J Hum Genet* 2008; 53: 876–85.
92. Ritz K, Gerrits MC, Foncke EM, et al. Myoclonus–dystonia: clinical and genetic evaluation of a large cohort. *J Neurol Neurosurg Psychiatry* 2009; 80: 653–8.
93. Tezenas du Montcel S, Clot F, Vidailhet M, et al. Epsilon sarcoglycan mutations and phenotype in French patients with myoclonic syndromes. *J Med Genet* 2006; 43: 394–400.

94. Han F, Racacho L, Lang AE, Bulman DE, Grimes DA. Refinement of the DYT15 locus in myoclonus dystonia. *Mov Disord* 2007; 22: 888–92.
95. Waters CH, Faust PL, Powers J, et al. Neuropathology of lubag (X-linked dystonia parkinsonism). *Mov Disord* 1993; 8: 387–90.
96. Waters CH, Takahashi H, Wilhelmsen KC, et al. Phenotypic expression of X-linked dystonia-parkinsonism (lubag) in two women. *Neurology* 1993; 43: 1555–8.
97. Evidente VG, Advincula J, Esteban R, et al. Phenomenology of 'lubag' or X-linked dystonia-parkinsonism. *Mov Disord* 2002; 17: 1271–7.
98. Evidente VG, Nolte D, Niemann S, et al. Phenotypic and molecular analyses of X-linked dystonia-parkinsonism ('lubag') in women. *Arch Neurol* 2004; 61: 1956–9.
99. Lee LV, Maranon E, Demaisip C, et al. The natural history of sex-linked recessive dystonia parkinsonism of Panay, Philippines (XDP). *Parkinsonism Relat Disord* 2002; 9: 29–38.
100. Lee LV, Rivera C, Teleg RA, et al. The unique phenomenology of sex-linked dystonia parkinsonism (XDP, DYT3, 'lubag'). *Int J Neurosci* 2011; 121 (Suppl 1): 3–11.
101. Segawa M, Hosaka A, Miyagawa F, Nomura Y, Imai H. Hereditary progressive dystonia with marked diurnal fluctuation. *Adv Neurol* 1976; 14: 215–33.
102. Nygaard TG, Marsden CD, Duvoisin RC. Dopa-responsive dystonia. *Adv Neurol* 1988; 50: 377–84.
103. Ichinose H, Ohye T, Takahashi E, et al. Hereditary progressive dystonia with marked diurnal fluctuation caused by mutations in the GTP cyclohydrolase I gene. *Nat Genet* 1994; 8: 236–42.
104. Hagenah J, Saunders-Pullman R, Hedrich K, et al. High mutation rate in dopa-responsive dystonia: detection with comprehensive GCHI screening. *Neurology* 2005; 64: 908–11.
105. Steinberger D, Weber Y, Korinthenberg R, et al. High penetrance and pronounced variation in expressivity of GCH1 mutations in five families with dopa-responsive dystonia. *Ann Neurol* 1998; 43: 634–9.
106. Furukawa Y, Graf WD, Wong H, Shimadzu M, Kish SJ. Dopa-responsive dystonia simulating spastic paraplegia due to tyrosine hydroxylase (TH) gene mutations. *Neurology* 2001; 56: 260–3.
107. Ludecke B, Dworniczak B, Bartholome K. A point mutation in the tyrosine hydroxylase gene associated with Segawa's syndrome. *Hum Genet* 1995; 95: 123–5.
108. Abeling NG, Duran M, Bakker HD, et al. Sepiapterin reductase deficiency: an autosomal recessive DOPA-responsive dystonia. *Mol Genet Metab* 2006; 89: 116–20.
109. de Carvalho Aguiar P, Sweadner KJ, Penniston JT, et al. Mutations in the Na^+/K^+-ATPase alpha3 gene ATP1A3 are associated with rapid-onset dystonia parkinsonism. *Neuron* 2004; 43: 169–75.
110. Lee JY, Gollamudi S, Ozelius LJ, Kim JY, Jeon BS. ATP1A3 mutation in the first Asian case of rapid-onset dystonia-parkinsonism. *Mov Disord* 2007; 22: 1808–9.
111. Brashear A, Dobyns WB, de Carvalho Aguiar P, et al. The phenotypic spectrum of rapid-onset dystonia-parkinsonism (RDP) and mutations in the ATP1A3 gene. *Brain* 2007; 130: 828–35.
112. Camargos S, Scholz S, Simon-Sanchez J, et al. DYT16, a novel young-onset dystonia-parkinsonism disorder: identification of a segregating mutation in the stress-response protein PRKRA. *Lancet Neurol* 2008; 7: 207–15.
113. Seibler P, Djarmati A, Langpap B, et al. A heterozygous frameshift mutation in PRKRA (DYT16) associated with generalised dystonia in a German patient. *Lancet Neurol* 2008; 7: 380–1.
114. Klein C. DYT16: a new twist to familial dystonia. *Lancet Neurol* 2008; 7: 192–3.
115. Demirkiran M, Jankovic J. Paroxysmal dyskinesias: clinical features and classification. *Ann Neurol* 1995; 38: 571–9.
116. Fouad GT, Servidei S, Durcan S, Bertini E, Ptacek LJ. A gene for familial paroxysmal dyskinesia (FPD1) maps to chromosome 2q. *Am J Hum Genet* 1996; 59: 135–9.
117. Fink JK, Rainer S, Wilkowski J, et al. Paroxysmal dystonic choreoathetosis: tight linkage to chromosome 2q. *Am J Hum Genet* 1996; 59: 140–5.
118. Raskind WH, Bolin T, Wolff J, et al. Further localization of a gene for paroxysmal dystonic choreoathetosis to a 5-cM region on chromosome 2q34. *Hum Genet* 1998; 102: 93–7.
119. Rainier S, Thomas D, Tokarz D, et al. Myofibrillogenesis regulator 1 gene mutations cause paroxysmal dystonic choreoathetosis. *Arch Neurol* 2004; 61: 1025–9.
120. Lee HY, Xu Y, Huang Y, et al. The gene for paroxysmal non-kinesigenic dyskinesia encodes an enzyme in a stress response pathway. *Hum Mol Genet* 2004; 13: 3161–70.
121. Hempelmann A, Kumar S, Muralitharan S, Sander T. Myofibrillogenesis regulator 1 gene (MR-1) mutation in an Omani family with paroxysmal nonkinesigenic dyskinesia. *Neurosci Lett* 2006; 402: 118–20.
122. Spacey SD, Adams PJ, Lam PC, et al. Genetic heterogeneity in paroxysmal nonkinesigenic dyskinesia. *Neurology* 2006; 66: 1588–90.
123. Tomita H, Nagamitsu S, Wakui K, et al. Paroxysmal kinesigenic choreoathetosis locus maps to chromosome 16p11.2-q12.1. *Am J Hum Genet* 1999; 65: 1688–97.
124. Kikuchi T, Nomura M, Tomita H, et al. Paroxysmal kinesigenic choreoathetosis (PKC): confirmation of linkage to 16p11-q21, but unsuccessful detection of mutations among 157 genes at the PKC-critical region in seven PKC families. *J Hum Genet* 2007; 52: 334–41.
125. Cheng FB, Wan XH, Feng JC, Wang L, Yang YM, Cui LY. Clinical and genetic evaluation of DYT1 and DYT6 primary dystonia in China. *Eur J Neurol* 2011; 18: 497–503.
126. Wang JL, Cao L, Li XH, et al. Identification of PRRT2 as the causative gene of paroxysmal kinesigenic dyskinesias. *Brain* 2011; 134: 3493–501.
127. Valente EM, Spacey SD, Wali GM, et al. A second paroxysmal kinesigenic choreoathetosis locus (EKD2) mapping on 16q13-q22.1 indicates a family of genes which give rise to paroxysmal disorders on human chromosome 16. *Brain* 2000; 123: 2040–5.
128. Spacey SD, Valente EM, Wali GM, et al. Genetic and clinical heterogeneity in paroxysmal kinesigenic dyskinesia: evidence for a third EKD gene. *Mov Disord* 2002; 17: 717–25.
129. Weber YG, Storch A, Wuttke TV, et al. GLUT1 mutations are a cause of paroxysmal exertion-induced dyskinesias and induce hemolytic anemia by a cation leak. *J Clin Invest* 2008; 118: 2157–68.
130. Suls A, Dedeken P, Goffin K, et al. Paroxysmal exercise-induced dyskinesia and epilepsy is due to mutations in SLC2A1, encoding the glucose transporter GLUT1. *Brain* 2008; 131: 1831–44.
131. Schneider SA, Paisan-Ruiz C, Garcia-Gorostiaga I, et al. GLUT1 gene mutations cause sporadic paroxysmal exercise-induced dyskinesias. *Mov Disord* 2009; 24: 1684–8.
132. Roubergue A, Apartis E, Mesnage V, et al. Dystonic tremor caused by mutation of the glucose transporter gene GLUT1. *J Inherit Metab Dis* 2011; 34: 483–8.
133. Weber YG, Kamm C, Suls A, et al. Paroxysmal choreoathetosis/spasticity (DYT9) is caused by a GLUT1 defect. *Neurology* 2011; 77: 959–64.
134. Kojovic M, Kuoppamaki M, Quinn N, Bhatia KP. 'Progressive delayed-onset postanoxic dystonia' diagnosed with PANK2 mutations 26 years after onset—an update. *Mov Disord* 2010; 25: 2889–91.
135. Kuoppamaki M, Bhatia KP, Quinn N. Progressive delayed-onset dystonia after cerebral anoxic insult in adults. *Mov Disord* 2002; 17: 1345–9.
136. Bhatia KP, Marsden CD. The behavioural and motor consequences of focal lesions of the basal ganglia in man. *Brain* 1994; 117: 859–76.
137. Lee JH, Ki CS, Kim DS, Cho JW, Park KP, Kim S. Dopa-responsive dystonia with a novel initiation codon mutation in the GCH1 gene misdiagnosed as cerebral palsy. *J Korean Med Sci* 2011; 26: 1244–6.
138. Slawek J, Friedman A, Bogucki A, Budrewicz S, Banach M. Dopa-responsive dystonia (Segawa variant): clinical analysis of 7 cases with delayed diagnosis. *Neurol Neurochir Pol* 2003; 37 (Suppl 5): 117–26.

139. Kiriakakis V, Bhatia KP, Quinn NP, Marsden CD. The natural history of tardive dystonia: a long-term follow-up study of 107 cases. *Brain* 1998; 121: 2053–66.
140. Fiorio M, Gambarin M, Valente EM, et al. Defective temporal processing of sensory stimuli in DYT1 mutation carriers: a new endophenotype of dystonia? *Brain* 2007; 130: 134–42.
141. Bara-Jimenez W, Shelton P, Hallett M. Spatial discrimination is abnormal in focal hand dystonia. *Neurology* 2000; 55: 1869–73.
142. Sanger TD, Tarsy D, Pascual-Leone A. Abnormalities of spatial and temporal sensory discrimination in writer's cramp. *Mov Disord* 2001; 16: 94–9.
143. Tinazzi M, Fiaschi A, Frasson E, Fiorio M, Cortese F, Aglioti SM. Deficits of temporal discrimination in dystonia are independent from the spatial distance between the loci of tactile stimulation. *Mov Disord* 2002; 17: 333–8.
144. Scontrini A, Conte A, Fabbrini G, et al. Somatosensory temporal discrimination tested in patients receiving botulinum toxin injection for cervical dystonia. *Mov Disord* 2011; 26: 742–6.
145. Bradley D, Whelan R, Kimmich O, et al. Temporal discrimination thresholds in adult-onset primary torsion dystonia: an analysis by task type and by dystonia phenotype. *J Neurol* 2012; 259: 77–82.
146. Bradley D, Whelan R, Walsh R, et al. Comparing endophenotypes in adult-onset primary torsion dystonia. *Mov Disord* 2010; 25: 84–90.
147. Bradley D, Whelan R, Walsh R, et al. Temporal discrimination threshold: VBM evidence for an endophenotype in adult onset primary torsion dystonia. *Brain* 2009; 132: 2327–35.
148. Frima N, Nasir J, Grunewald RA. Abnormal vibration-induced illusion of movement in idiopathic focal dystonia: an endophenotypic marker? *Mov Disord* 2008; 23: 373–7.
149. Frima N, Rome SM, Grunewald RA. The effect of fatigue on abnormal vibration induced illusion of movement in idiopathic focal dystonia. *J Neurol Neurosurg Psychiatry* 2003; 74: 1154–6.
150. Grunewald RA, Yoneda Y, Shipman JM, Sagar HJ. Idiopathic focal dystonia: a disorder of muscle spindle afferent processing? *Brain* 1997; 120: 2179–85.
151. Rome S, Grunewald RA. Abnormal perception of vibration-induced illusion of movement in dystonia. *Neurology* 1999; 53: 1794–800.
152. Fiorio M, Tinazzi M, Aglioti SM. Selective impairment of hand mental rotation in patients with focal hand dystonia. *Brain* 2006; 129: 47–54.
153. Hallett M. Neurophysiology of dystonia: the role of inhibition. *Neurobiol Dis* 2011; 42: 177–84.
154. Edwards MJ, Huang YZ, Wood NW, Rothwell JC, Bhatia KP. Different patterns of electrophysiological deficits in manifesting and non-manifesting carriers of the DYT1 gene mutation. *Brain* 2003; 126: 2074–80.
155. Quartarone A, Bagnato S, Rizzo V, et al. Abnormal associative plasticity of the human motor cortex in writer's cramp. *Brain* 2003; 126: 2586–96.
156. Quartarone A, Morgante F, Sant'angelo A, et al. Abnormal plasticity of sensorimotor circuits extends beyond the affected body part in focal dystonia. *J Neurol Neurosurg Psychiatry* 2008; 79: 985–90.
157. Quartarone A, Pisani A. Abnormal plasticity in dystonia: disruption of synaptic homeostasis. *Neurobiol Dis* 2011; 42: 162–70.
158. Edwards MJ, Huang YZ, Mir P, Rothwell JC, Bhatia KP. Abnormalities in motor cortical plasticity differentiate manifesting and nonmanifesting DYT1 carriers. *Mov Disord* 2006; 21: 2181–6.
159. Augood SJ, Hollingsworth Z, Albers DS, et al. Dopamine transmission in DYT1 dystonia: a biochemical and autoradiographical study. *Neurology* 2002; 59: 445–8.
160. Coubes P, Cif L, El Fertit H, et al. Electrical stimulation of the globus pallidus internus in patients with primary generalized dystonia: long-term results. *J Neurosurg* 2004; 101: 189–94.
161. Coubes P, Roubertie A, Vayssiere N, Hemm S, Echenne B. Treatment of DYT1-generalised dystonia by stimulation of the internal globus pallidus. *Lancet* 2000; 355: 2220–1.
162. Egidi M, Franzini A, Marras C, et al. A survey of Italian cases of dystonia treated by deep brain stimulation. *J Neurosurg Sci* 2007; 51: 153–8.
163. Borggraefe I, Boetzel K, Boehmer J, et al. Return to participation—significant improvement after bilateral pallidal stimulation in rapidly progressive DYT-1 dystonia. *Neuropediatrics* 2008; 39: 239–42.
164. Borggraefe I, Mehrkens JH, Telegravciska M, Berweck S, Botzel K, Heinen F. Bilateral pallidal stimulation in children and adolescents with primary generalized dystonia—report of six patients and literature-based analysis of predictive outcomes variables. *Brain Dev* 2010; 32: 223–8.
165. Isaias IU, Alterman RL, Tagliati M. Deep brain stimulation for primary generalized dystonia: long-term outcomes. *Arch Neurol* 2009; 66: 465–70.
166. Isaias IU, Alterman RL, Tagliati M. Outcome predictors of pallidal stimulation in patients with primary dystonia: the role of disease duration. *Brain* 2008; 131: 1895–902.
167. Loher TJ, Capelle HH, Kaelin-Lang A, et al. Deep brain stimulation for dystonia: outcome at long-term follow-up. *J Neurol* 2008; 255: 881–4.
168. Benecke R, Jost WH, Kanovsky P, Ruzicka E, Comes G, Grafe S. A new botulinum toxin type A free of complexing proteins for treatment of cervical dystonia. *Neurology* 2005; 64: 1949–51.
169. Comella CL, Jankovic J, Shannon KM, et al. Comparison of botulinum toxin serotypes A and B for the treatment of cervical dystonia. *Neurology* 2005; 65: 1423–9.
170. Krauss JK, Pohle T, Weber S, Ozdoba C, Burgunder JM. Bilateral stimulation of globus pallidus internus for treatment of cervical dystonia. *Lancet* 1999; 354: 837–8.
171. Krauss JK, Yianni J, Loher TJ, Aziz TZ. Deep brain stimulation for dystonia. *J Clin Neurophysiol* 2004; 21: 18–30.
172. Eltahawy HA, Saint-Cyr J, Poon YY, Moro E, Lang AE, Lozano AM. Pallidal deep brain stimulation in cervical dystonia: clinical outcome in four cases. Can *J Neurol Sci* 2004; 31: 328–32.
173. Bhatia KP. Familial (idiopathic) paroxysmal dyskinesias: an update. *Semin Neurol* 2001; 21: 69–74.
174. Bhatia KP. The paroxysmal dyskinesias. *J Neurol* 1999; 246: 149–55.
175. Klepper J. Glucose transporter deficiency syndrome (GLUT1DS) and the ketogenic diet. *Epilepsia* 2008; 49 (Suppl 8): 46–9.
176. Damier P, Thobois S, Witjas T, et al. Bilateral deep brain stimulation of the globus pallidus to treat tardive dyskinesia. *Arch Gen Psychiatry* 2007; 64: 170–6.
177. Vidailhet M, Yelnik J, Lagrange C, et al. Bilateral pallidal deep brain stimulation for the treatment of patients with dystonia–choreoathetosis cerebral palsy: a prospective pilot study. *Lancet Neurol* 2009; 8: 709–17.
178. Ruiz PJ, Ayerbe J, Bader B, et al. Deep brain stimulation in chorea acanthocytosis. *Mov Disord* 2009; 24: 1546–7.
179. Grandas F, Fernandez-Carballal C, Guzman-de-Villoria J, Ampuero I. Treatment of a dystonic storm with pallidal stimulation in a patient with PANK2 mutation. *Mov Disord* 2011; 26: 921–2.
180. Tassorelli C, Mancini F, Balloni L, et al. Botulinum toxin and neuromotor rehabilitation: an integrated approach to idiopathic cervical dystonia. *Mov Disord* 2006; 21: 2240–3.

CHAPTER 18

Primary Dystonia

Antonio A. Elia and Alberto Albanese

Definition and classification

The term dystonia was introduced to describe patients with severe generalized abnormal movements and postures, who were believed to have an alteration of muscle tone (hence the word 'dystonia') (1). The phenomenological description coincided with the generalized phenotype for many decades. In June 1975, an international conference chaired by Stanley Fahn in New York recognized the clinical features of focal forms of dystonia (2). Later, David Marsden proposed gathering together under the heading of dystonia nosologic entities that were previously considered independent forms (e.g. blepharospasm, torticollis, 'spastic' dysphonia, writer's cramp) (3–5). Finally, in 1984, an ad hoc committee of the Dystonia Medical Research Foundation documented the occurrence in all forms of dystonia 'of sustained muscle contractions, frequently causing twisting and repetitive movements, or abnormal postures' (6). Later, the basic clinical features (dystonic movements and postures) and additional clinical features (activation/deactivation) of dystonia were described (7, 8).

Classification of dystonia syndromes has changed over time. Fahn and Eldridge (2) first distinguished primary dystonia (with or without hereditary pattern), secondary dystonia (with other hereditary neurological syndromes or due to known environmental cause), and psychological forms of dystonia. Later, Fahn, Marsden, and Calne proposed a classification of dystonia based on three axes, describing for each patient the age at disease onset (early vs adult), distribution of involved body sites (from focal to generalized), and aetiology (differentiating idiopathic dystonia syndromes, sporadic or familial, from symptomatic ones) (6, 9). The first two axes have remained unchanged over years, whereas the aetiological classification has been expanded to include four subgroups of dystonia syndromes: primary, dystonia-plus (i.e. dystonia with parkinsonism or myoclonic jerks), secondary, and heredodegenerative (10).

The recently published European dystonia guidelines (11) refine the aetiological axis distinguishing primary (or idiopathic) syndromes, heredodegenerative (where dystonia is a feature of a genetic disorder characterized by neurodegeneration) and secondary (or symptomatic) syndromes (Table 18.1). Based on the phenotype, primary dystonias are further subdivided into primary pure (with dystonia only), primary-plus (with other associated movement disorders), and primary paroxysmal (characterized by intermittent symptoms). This classification has recently been revised by an ad hoc committee which convened in Grottaferrata, Rome, in May 2011 (consensus not yet published).

Phenomenology of primary dystonia

Dystonia can occur at rest, during voluntary movement, or in paroxysmal form, following a specific trigger. These features must be appreciated by expert clinical examination and are best observed in primary dystonia forms. The clinical picture becomes more complex when dystonia features are combined or intermixed with other movement disorders in dystonia-plus syndromes.

Cardinal features

Following Marsden's seminal observation (12), it is commonly accepted that dystonia encompasses a combination of movements and postures to generate sustained muscle contractions, repetitive twisting movements, and abnormal postures (torsion dystonia). Dystonic postures can precede the occurrence of dystonic movements, and in rare cases can persist without appearance of the latter (fixed dystonia) (7). Dystonic movements have specific features that can be recognized by clinical examination: speed of contractions may be slow or rapid, but at the peak of movement it is sustained; movements almost always have a consistent directional or posture-assuming character. Dystonic movements and postures are commonly aggravated during voluntary motion, and in milder forms they may only occur during some specific voluntary actions (task-specific dystonia).

Dystonic movements may be regular, appearing as tremor (dystonic tremor (13)). When they are fast and jerky, they may resemble myoclonus. Dystonic tremor may precede clear abnormal posturing, and its occurrence in isolation may lead to the diagnosis of dystonia being missed (7). A tremor similar to essential tremor may occur in dystonia and can be mistaken for non-dystonic tremor, particularly when isolated (14). The diagnosis of dystonia can be missed or delayed in a number of patients with task- and position-specific tremors, particularly primary writing tremor, occupational tremors, or isolated voice tremor, as typical features of dystonia may not develop until many years after onset. Head or voice tremors observed in tremulous forms of cervical dystonia can be very hard to distinguish from essential tremor. In some cases, only family history orientates in favour of the correct diagnosis, particularly if family members are ascertained to have dystonia.

Table 18.1 Aetiological classification of dystonia (11)

- *Primary pure dystonia* Dystonia is the only clinical sign (apart from tremor) and there is no identifiable exogenous cause or other inherited or degenerative disease. Examples are DYT1 and DYT6 dystonias.
- *Primary dystonia-plus* Dystonia is a prominent sign, but is associated with another movement disorder (e.g. myoclonus or parkinsonism). There is no evidence of neurodegeneration. Examples are levodopa-responsive dystonia (DYT5) and myoclonus–dystonia (DYT11).
- *Primary paroxysmal* Dystonia occurs in brief episodes with normality in between. These disorders are classified as idiopathic (often familial, although sporadic cases also occur) and symptomatic due to a variety of causes. Three main forms are known depending on the triggering factor. In paroxysmal kinesigenic dyskinesia (PKD, DYT9) attacks are induced by sudden movement; in paroxysmal exercise-induced dystonia (PED) attacks are induced by exercise such as walking or swimming; and in the non-kinesigenic form (PNKD, DYT8) attacks are induced by alcohol, coffee, tea, etc. A complicated familial form with PNKD and spasticity (DYT10) has also been described.
- *Heredodegenerative* Dystonia is a feature, among other neurological signs, of a heredodegenerative disorder. An example is Wilson disease.
- *Secondary* Dystonia is a symptom of an identified neurological condition, such as a focal brain lesion, or exposure to drugs or chemicals. Examples are dystonia due to a brain tumour, OFF-period dystonia in Parkinson's disease.

Associated features

Dystonia has some unique activation/deactivation features that can be recognized if appropriately looked for and serve as a basis for the diagnosis: *geste antagoniste* (or sensory tricks), mirroring, and overflow. Criteria for identifying these features, when present, have recently been published (8).

Geste antagoniste has been described in patients with different forms of focal dystonia, who reduce or even abolish dystonic postures while making some specific voluntary movements. For example, cranial dystonia patients can apply pressure to the eyebrows or touch the skin beside the eyes to relief blepharospasm; cervical dystonia patients can place a hand on the side of the face, the chin, or the back of the head, or touch these areas with one or more fingers, to reduce neck contractions; writer's cramp patients can touch the affected arm with the opposite hand. In contrast with the cardinal signs of dystonia, the *geste* is never forceful, but is natural and elegant (8). The mechanism of action of the *geste* is debated; its action is not associated with mechanical correction by counter-pressure (15). A *geste* does not improve non-dystonic essential head tremor, it is uncommon in early post-traumatic dystonia, and it has atypical phenomenology in patients with psychogenic dystonia (8). *Geste* efficacy may diminish as the disease progresses.

Overflow and mirroring are two related clinical phenomena that reveal or enhance dystonia and prove particularly helpful in cases with mild or inconstant phenomenology. Overflow is an unintentional contraction of muscles not primarily involved by dystonia, usually located in neighbouring body sites, which are activated at the peak of dystonic movements (16). For example, a patient with cervical dystonia may have involvement of the unaffected upper limb by occasional spread of dystonia activity. Mirror dystonia occurs on the affected body side when a specific task is performed by the homologous opposite unaffected body part. Usually specific tasks elicit mirror dystonia; they must be identified in order to appreciate this feature. For example, patients with writer's cramp may present mirror dystonia of the dominant hand while writing with the non-dominant unaffected hand (17). Overflow and mirroring are considered a clinical expression of lack of inhibition occurring in dystonia (8).

Diagnostic algorithm

A diagnostic algorithm for identifying the features of primary dystonia has recently been proposed (8). According to this schema, when all the cardinal features of dystonia are observed, the clinical diagnosis is clearly evidenced by physical examination. Otherwise, at least two associated features must be observed to reach a clinical diagnosis. EMG observation of features associated with dystonia is helpful when physical observation is insufficient (Fig. 18.1).

Epidemiology

The prevalence of primary dystonia is difficult to ascertain, ranging from 2 to 50 cases per million for early-onset primary dystonia, and from 30 to 7320 cases per million for late-onset dystonia. On the basis of the best available prevalence studies, primary dystonia may account for 11.1 per 100 000 early-onset cases in Ashkenazi Jews from the New York area, 60 per 100 000 late-onset cases in Northern England, and 300 per 100 000 late-onset cases in the Italian population aged over 50 (18).

For a number of reasons, the true prevalence of dystonia is probably underestimated. Patients with mild phenotypes (so-called *formes frustes* (19)) may not seek medical advice; those in whom the clinical diagnosis is missed require expert evaluation to resolve diagnostic uncertainty. Conditions that are more common or better known than dystonia often include other movement disorders, such as Parkinson's disease, essential tremor, myoclonus, tics, and psychogenic forms (14).

Aetiology

A genetic predisposition and environmental factors both play a significant role in the aetiology of primary dystonia. Genetic defects are known for only a minority of cases presenting with a pure dystonia phenotype (20). In contrast, dystonia-plus syndromes are better classified genetically (Table 18.2). We describe here only the primary pure dystonia syndromes. Dystonia-plus and paroxysmal dystonias are dealt with in Chapters 19 and 26.

DYT1 dystonia

A common cause of generalized primary pure dystonia is the GAG deletion in the *DYT1* gene encoding the protein TorsinA (21). The disease was originally described among Ashkenazi Jews as having a relatively homogeneous phenotype characterized by early limb-onset generalized dystonia (22). It was later reported that, particularly in Caucasian patients (23), the DYT1 phenotype is broader than originally thought. The 'classical' DYT1 phenotype is characterized by early onset in a limb, and generalization without spread to the craniocervical region (23). In a series of patients with early-onset

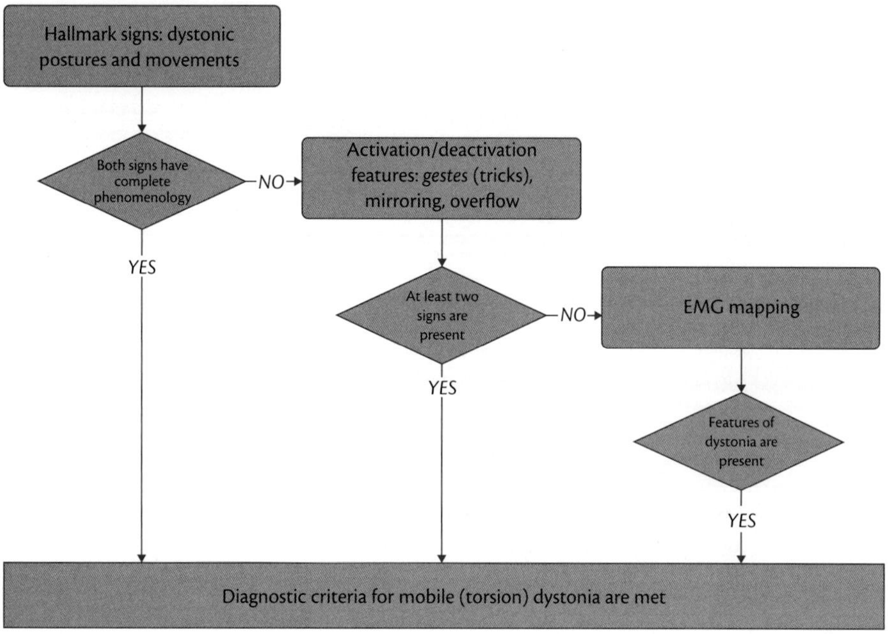

Fig. 18.1 Flowchart for the diagnosis of mobile (torsion) dystonia. This stepped approach allows a clinical diagnostic level to be reached based on objective clinical criteria. (Reproduced with permission from Albanese A, Lalli S. Is this dystonia? *Mov Disord* 2009; 24: 1725–31)

primary dystonia, it has been confirmed that dystonia never starts in the craniocervical region in *DYT1* carriers, although craniocervical sites can be involved at later stages (24). It is remarkable that DYT1 patients who develop severe generalized involvement can carry out their daily activities with significant adaptation in many cases. Extreme cases have also been observed, ranging from asymptomatic status to craniocervical involvement or even status dystonicus (25–28).

Owing to phenotypic heterogeneity, it is not possible to identify DYT1 patients based only on their clinical presentation. Five other phenotypes have been described in addition to the classic limb-onset presentation (24, 29): generalized dystonia with craniocervical involvement, more frequent in Europe than in North America (30), generalized myoclonus–dystonia, with a phenotype more severe than observed in DYT11 myoclonus–dystonia (31), focal dystonia with slow progression and occasional later spread even several years after onset (32, 33); late-onset DYT1 forms (25), and rarer cases of DYT1 dystonia with non-limb presentation which may have cervical, laryngeal, or trunk onset (34, 35).

Gene penetrance is believed to be around 30% (21, 27), meaning that the proportion of asymptomatic mutation carriers is higher than that of manifesting patients. This has prompted the search for potential endophenotypes to help identify manifesting as well as non-manifesting DYT1 carriers. Two potential endophenotypes have emerged: reduction of striatal D2 receptor binding shown by PET studies (36), and higher tactile and visuotactile temporal discrimination thresholds or temporal order judgements (37). These findings need to be confirmed and have not been integrated into a coherent diagnostic protocol.

The DYT1 gene is named *TOR1A* (21). The disease is caused by a unique mutation that deletes one of a pair of GAG triplets from the carboxyl terminal in TorsinA. This unique DYT1 haplotype, originally found in Ashkenazi Jews, has also been observed in non-Jewish patients (38) and represents the only pathogenic disease mutation identified in *TOR1A*. An 18 bp deletion has also been found in families with primary dystonia and myoclonus, but its pathogenicity has not been ascertained (39). TorsinA is a heat-shock and ATP-binding protein and a member of the AAA+ superfamily. The normal protein is widely distributed in many species and is located in the endoplasmic reticulum (40, 41). Immunohistochemical studies have revealed that TorsinA is a constituent of Lewy bodies (42).

DYT6 dystonia

The DYT6 locus was originally mapped in two Mennonite families with primary pure dystonia and autosomal dominant transmission (43). Mutations in the *THAP1* (Thanatos-associated-domain containing apoptosis-associated protein 1) gene have been found to be responsible for DYT6 dystonia with an estimated penetrance of approximately 60% (44). In an American series, *THAP1* heterozygous mutations were identified in nine out of thirty-six (25%) DYT1-negative families with early-onset non-focal primary dystonia (45). European series have reported a lower mutation frequency with an overall prevalence of 1–2.5% in primary dystonia cohorts from all over Europe (46, 47). The spectrum of THAP1 mutations includes missense, nonsense, and frame-shift mutations of all three exons.

The *THAP1* phenotype typically presents with early-onset dystonia (age range, 9–49 years) and frequent involvement of the craniocervical area. The motor features often appear in adolescence and may progress rapidly. Speech is commonly affected because of oromandibular or laryngeal involvement (or both). Interestingly, *THAP1* mutations have been recently found in cases with much later onset (fifth or sixth decade) and focal or segmental phenomenology involving the cervical or laryngeal areas (46, 47). This suggests that the gene may also play a pathogenic role in late-onset, focal, or segmental PD.

THAP1 is a member of the family of sequence-specific DNA-binding factors. Its function is still poorly understood; recent studies provided evidence that *THAP1* and *TOR1A* are interconnected in a common pathway (48), because wild-type *THAP1* represses the expression of *TOR1A* (49).

Table 18.2 DYT genotypes associated with dystonias*

Disease (OMIM)	Map position	Gene	Transmission	Phenotype
Pure dystonia				
DYT1 (128100)	9q34	*TOR1A*	AD	Generalized early-limb-onset dystonia
DYT2 (224500)			AR	Early-onset generalized dystonia with prominent craniocervical involvement
DYT4 (128101)			AD	Whispering dysphonia
DYT6 (602629)	8p11. 21	*THAP1*	AD	Mixed-type dystonia, early-onset generalized with craniocervical involvement
DYT7 (602124)	18p		AD	Mixed-type dystonia
DYT13 (607671)	1p36. 13–36. 32		AD	Mixed-type dystonia
DYT17 (612406)	20p11.2-q13.12		AR	Segmental or generalized dystonia with severe dysphonia
DTY21 (not assigned)	2q14.3-q21.3		AD	Mixed-type dystonia, late-onset multifocal with craniocervical involvement
Dystonia-plus				
DYT5/DYT14 (128230)	14q22	*GCH1*	AD	Dopa-responsive dystonia
	11p15.5	*TH*	AR	Dopa-responsive dystonia
	2p13.2	*SPR*	AR	Dopa-responsive dystonia
DYT11 (159900)	11q23. 1, 7q21	*SGCE*	AD	Myoclonus–dystonia
DYT12 (128235)	19q12-q13. 2	*ATP1A3*	AD	Rapid-onset dystonia–parkinsonism
DYT15 (607488)	18p11		AD	Myoclonus–dystonia
DYT16 (612067)	2q31. 3	*PRKRA*	AR	Dystonia–parkinsonism
Paroxysmal dystonia				
DYT8 (118800)	2q35	*MR1*	AD	Paroxysmal non-kinesigenic dyskinesia
DYT9/DYT18 (612126)	1p35-p31. 3	*SLC2A1*	AD	Paroxysmal exercise-induced dyskinesia
DYT10 (128200)	16p11. 2-q12. 1		AD	Episodic kinesigenic dyskinesia
DYT19 (611031)	16q13-q22. 1		AD	Episodic kinesigenic dyskinesia
DYT20 (611147)	2q31		AD	Paroxysmal exercise-induced dyskinesia
Heredodegenerative				
DYT3 (314250)	Xq13	*TAF1*	X-linked	Dystonia–parkinsonism

*The gene name is indicated when known; otherwise, the locus is reported.

AD, autosomal dominant; AR, autosomal recessive; ATP1A3, ATPase, Na^+/K^+ transporting; GCH1, guanosine triphosphate cyclohydrolase 1; *MR1*, myofibrillogenesis regulator 1; *PRKRA*, double-stranded RNA-activated protein kinase; *SGCE*, ε-sarcoglycan; *SLC2A1*, solute carrier family 2 (facilitated glucose transporter), member 1; *SPR*, sepiapterin reductase; *TAF1*, TATA boxing-binding protein associated factor; *TH*, tyrosine hydroxylase; *THAP1*, thanatos-associated protein; *TOR1A*, torsin A gene.

THAP1-associated DYT6 dystonia should be considered in patients with early-onset DYT1-negative generalized or segmental dystonia, particularly if cranial involvement is prominent. As a rule, age at onset is higher than in DYT1 dystonia, and the topographic distribution differs between the two forms. The exact prevalence of DYT6 dystonia is still undetermined.

Mapped loci

The DYT7 locus, mapping to the short arm of chromosome 18, was identified in a large German family with an autosomal dominant focal pure dystonia phenotype (50). The mean age of disease onset was 40 years with a prevalent phenotype characterized by focal cervical dystonia. In some patients a segmental distribution has been reported, where cervical dystonia is associated with Meige's syndrome or writer's cramp. No patient had generalized dystonia.

The DYT13 locus was mapped in a large Italian family with prominent craniocervical and upper limb involvement and a pure dystonia phenotype (51, 52). In the majority of cases onset was in infancy or adolescence. Of the eleven definitely affected individuals, two had generalized dystonia with early onset in the upper limb or the cervical region (53). Disability was mild even in generalized cases. A peculiar feature of the DYT13 phenotype is prominent cervical or upper limb involvement, similarly to the DYT6 phenotype, although the DYT13 family has tested negative for DYT6 mutations.

The DYT15 locus was mapped in a large Canadian kindred, whose thirteen affected members had alcohol-responsive myoclonic dystonia involving the upper limbs, hands, and axial muscles (54).

The DYT17 dystonia locus was mapped in a single consanguineous Lebanese family with three sisters suffering from recessively inherited primary pure dystonia and onset in adolescence (55). The site of onset was cervical, with progression to segmental distribution in two of the sisters and generalization in one. Prominent features were dystonia and dysarthria, unresponsive to levodopa.

The DYT21 locus was recently mapped on chromosome 2 in a family from northern Sweden with sixteen members affected by late-onset pure torsion dystonia. The disease is inherited in an autosomal dominant manner with a penetrance that may be as high as 90%. Age at onset ranges between 13 and 50 years, and the prevalent phenotype is a multifocal dystonia with prominent craniocervical involvement.

Classified phenotypes

DYT2 is a recessive pure dystonia phenotype originally described in three consanguineous pedigrees of Spanish gypsies. The disease was named 'autosomal recessive dystonia in gypsies' and listed as DYT2 (56, 57). In two of the families the presentation was similar to that of DYT1 dystonia, consisting of early limb onset and progression to generalization; in a third family dystonia presented with prominent oromandibular and cervical involvement (57). A Sephardic Jewish Iranian family with a similar phenotype and autosomal recessive inheritance was later described (58). Three siblings in this family had primary dystonia with limb onset in childhood, and slow progression to generalization with predominant craniocervical involvement. Two patients presented with foot dystonia and gait abnormalities as early features, and all had cervical involvement, facial grimacing, blepharospasm, and upper and lower limb dystonia. Two patients also had dystonic dysphagia. A third family with childhood-onset generalized dystonia and autosomal recessive inheritance also shared the broad DYT2 phenotype (59).

The DYT4 phenotype refers to a large Australian pedigree with twenty affected members and autosomal dominant inheritance (60). Penetrance was complete in all the obligate gene carriers examined; age at onset varied from 13 to 37 years. Many patients presented with 'whispering dysphonia', while others had cervical dystonia. Most patients eventually developed generalized dystonia. Wilson disease co-existed in the same pedigree, but was excluded as a cause of dystonia in the affected individuals (61).

Unclassified phenotypes

A number of scattered pedigrees not carrying the DYT1 mutation have been described. In some of these families, DYT6 dystonia has not been excluded. Linkage studies have not been performed or have not been informative, leaving these pedigrees unmapped.

A non-Jewish American family presented with adult-onset DYT1-negative primary dystonia (62). The disease started in the neck in six cases and in a leg in one. All patients developed cervical dystonia, and language impairment (dysarthria or dysphonia) occurred in five. Four patients developed generalization of symptoms. In a Swedish family transmission was autosomal dominant with a heterogeneous phenotype (63). There was involvement of the face and larynx, and generalization occurred in three of the ten patients. A family from South Tyrol had six affected individuals, four of whom developed generalization approximately 5 years after onset (64). The limbs were involved at onset in all cases except one, who started with cervical dystonia. Upper body involvement was observed in three of the four generalized cases. An Italian family had six affected individuals, one of whom had severe segmental dystonia (65). The prevalent phenotype was an adult-onset craniocervical dystonia with occasional axial involvement but no generalization.

A common phenotype was outlined in a series of forty-three Italian patients with non-DYT1 early-onset dystonia (24). This was characterized by cervical involvement, frequent non-limb onset, a relatively benign course, and uncommon generalization. This finding suggests that these non-DYT1 Italian families may share a common genetic defect. Their features are similar to the DYT6 genotype, although DYT6 gene mutations were excluded in these subjects.

Focal dystonia with onset in adulthood may be the only clinical sign in many patients, who usually have no or mild progression to a segmental pure dystonia. The most frequent forms of dystonia with typical sporadic occurrence that remain genetically unclassified are blepharospasm, spasmodic dysphonia, cervical dystonia, Meige's syndrome, and occupational upper limb dystonia.

Cervical dystonia is the most common of these forms. Different abnormal head positions can be observed, including horizontal head rotation (torticollis), head tilting (laterocollis), head flexion (antecollis), and head extension (retrocollis). These postures can be variably combined depending on the neck muscles involved. Repetitive head jerks can resemble head tremor, but can be differentiated when a directional preponderance and sustainment at peak of movement are observed. Pain occurs in 75% of patients with cervical dystonia (66). Cranial dystonias are less prevalent than cervical forms. Spasmodic dysphonia affects the vocal folds; abnormal adduction, which causes a strained strangled voice, is more common than abduction, in which the voice sounds whispering and breathy.

Patients with blepharospasm have abnormal contractions of the orbicularis oculi muscles. Mild cases are characterized by a simple increase in blink rate and occasional flurries of blinking; in more severe cases forceful eye closure can interfere with vision, leading to functional blindness. In oromandibular dystonia there is abnormal activity in lower facial, tongue, jaw, and pharyngeal muscles that can interfere with speaking or swallowing. Brachial dystonia is a form of focal dystonia that can be primarily, or exclusively, present with writing (writer's cramp).

Segmental dystonia can affect the upper and lower cranial muscles, as in the combination of blepharospasm with oromandibular dystonia, sometimes called Meige's syndrome. In craniocervical dystonia, another type of segmental dystonia, the cranial area is involved together with the neck muscles.

Pathophysiology

Dystonia is characterized by an abnormal co-contraction of agonist and antagonist muscles that is worsened by a selection of task-specific movements and is usually relieved by a selection of sensory tricks. The abnormal co-contraction is thought to be caused by a dysfunction at the spinal or cortical level or both (67). Reciprocal inhibition is the central nervous system process by which a muscle is inhibited when its antagonist is activated. A decreased reciprocal inhibition at different levels of the central nervous system might contribute to the excessive movement seen in dystonia. Dystonic patients may have faulty processing within the inhibitory interactions between antagonist muscles at the sensorimotor cortex level.

Neuroimaging studies have recently provided interesting insights to understanding the pathophysiological mechanisms of primary pure dystonia. Diffusion magnetic resonance studies found signal abnormalities in various brain areas (including corpus callosum, basal ganglia, pontine, and prefrontal cortical areas) in cervical dystonia, writer's cramp, and generalized dystonia, but not in blepharospasm (68–71). Functional MRI studies conducted in patients with blepharospasm (72), writer's cramp (73–75), or upper limb focal dystonia (76) demonstrated that several deep structures and cortical areas may be activated, depending on the different modalities of examination. Voxel-based morphometry showed an increase in grey matter density or volume in various areas, including the cerebellum, basal ganglia, and primary somatosensory cortex, which might represent plastic changes secondary to overuse (77–81). PET studies have provided information about areas of abnormal metabolism in different types of dystonia and in different conditions (e.g. during active involuntary movement or during sleep), providing insight into the role of cerebellar and subcortical structures compared with cortical areas (82, 83).

Several studies have analysed genetically classified dystonias to investigate functional and morphological changes. Non-DYT1 adult-onset dystonia patients and asymptomatic DYT1 carriers have significantly larger basal ganglia than symptomatic DYT1 mutation carriers, with a negative correlation between severity of dystonia and basal ganglia size in DYT1 patients (84). In DYT6 and DYT1 dystonia patients, D2 receptor availability is reduced in the caudate and putamen and [^{11}C]raclopride binding is also reduced in the ventrolateral thalamus (85). These changes were more pronounced in DYT6 than in DYT1 carriers, without any difference between manifesting and non-manifesting carriers. Several studies have failed to detect neuropathological changes in DYT1 dystonia. In particular, immunohistochemistry of the basal ganglia has not revealed morphological abnormalities (86). More recently, however, brainstem abnormalities were observed in four typical DYT1 patients who had perinuclear inclusion bodies in the midbrain reticular formation and periaqueductal grey matter. These inclusions stained positively for ubiquitin, torsinA, and the nuclear envelope protein lamin A/C. Similar findings were not reported in genetically unclassified adult-onset primary pure dystonia patients (87). These findings suggest that the underlying molecular pathological mechanisms might differ in different dystonia types. In another study, nigral dopaminergic neurons were found to be larger in the substantia nigra of dystonia patients compared with healthy controls, with no difference between DYT1 and non-DYT1 cases (88).

An emerging line of evidence indicates that dystonia could be a disorder of neuroplasticity. In some susceptible individuals, the mechanisms of neuroplasticity during the acquisition of new motor skills are subtly abnormal. In the presence of such a genetic predisposition, environmental factors, such as repetitive training or peripheral nervous system, injury may trigger an abnormal maladaptive plasticity, which can lead to overt dystonia.

Treatment

There is no aetiological or neuroprotective treatment for primary pure dystonia syndromes. Aetiological therapies are available for some dystonia-plus syndromes of metabolic origin, such as levodopa-responsive dystonia, or non-primary forms, such as Wilson disease. Symptomatic treatments aim to relieve involuntary movements, correct abnormal postures, prevent contractures, reduce pain and embarrassment, and improve function (89). Botulinum toxin is the first-line treatment for most types of focal dystonia. Neurosurgical treatments have an increasing role in the symptomatic treatment plan. Evidence-based treatment guidelines have recently been published by the European Federation of Neurological Sciences (11).

Botulinum toxins

Botulinum neurotoxins (BoNTs) inhibit the vesicular release of acetylcholine at the neuromuscular junction, resulting in a transient localized impairment of neurotransmission. Different forms of type A and one type B BoNT are available for clinical use (90) (Table 18.3).

In properly adjusted doses, BoNTs are an effective and safe treatment for cranial and cervical dystonia (91). According to one systematic review, no conclusions can be drawn on the efficacy of BoNT for different types of spasmodic dysphonia (92), although uncontrolled studies have found this treatment efficacious. BoNT/A is also efficacious for the treatment of writing dystonia (93).

BoNT injections can be performed directly or by EMG- or ultrasound-guided targeting, and there is no consensus on which is the most appropriate practice. In recent years, the results of long-term studies of the efficacy and safety of BoNT/A have become available, new formulations of BoNT/A have been marketed, and new studies of BoNT/B have been performed.

The efficacy and safety profile of BoNT treatments have been evaluated in long-term observational studies. BoNT/A is effective and safe in treating blepharospasm, with long-lasting efficacy for up to 15 years (94). In patients with different dystonia types followed for over 12 years there was no decline of efficacy and the main side effects were muscle weakness in or around the injected region (95). OnabotulinumtoxinA immunogenicity was found to be low after long-term use (96). A meta-analysis found that adverse events are more frequent among children with cerebral palsy than in individuals with other conditions (97). BoNTs are safe when repeated treatments are performed over many years, but doctors and patients should be aware that high cumulative doses may be dangerous, particularly in children.

Systemic treatments

Little evidence-based information is available for other medical treatments for primary dystonia.

Anticholinergic drugs at high dosage are reported to be effective in the treatment of childhood-onset primary or secondary generalized dystonias (98, 99). This therapy is generally well tolerated when the dose is started low and increased slowly. Trihexyphenidyl should be titrated up to a dosage of 30–40 mg/day, but some patients might require up to 60 100 mg/day, although dose-related side effects (e. g. drowsiness, memory difficulty, and urinary retention) might limit its usefulness, especially in adults.

Non-controlled trials are available for the effects of antidopaminergic drugs. Tetrabenazine was effective in one small double-blind randomized crossover study (100). The positive effect of this treatment was confirmed in a large series of patients with different types of movement disorders, including dystonia, followed up retrospectively for a mean duration of 6.6 years (101).

Deep brain stimulation (DBS)

Long-term electrical stimulation of the globus palliduus internus (GPi) is now established as an effective treatment for primary generalized or segmental dystonia (102, 103). A randomized 'sham stimulation-controlled' 6-month trial has shown that bilateral high-frequency stimulation of the GPi is efficacious in reducing

Table 18.3 Main muscles involved and typical BoNT doses in more common focal dystonias

	Ona-BoNT/A	Abo-BoNT/A	Inco-BoNT/A	Rima-BoNT/B
Blepharospasm	Orbicularis oculi: 1.25–2.5U for each site (4 sites)	Orbicularis oculi: 5–10U for each site (4 sites)	Orbicularis oculi 1.25–2.5U for each site (4 sites)	Orbicularis oculi: 50–100U for each site (4 sites)
Oromandibular dystonia	Perioral muscles: 2.5–5U for each site (4–5 sites) Masseter: 15–60U for each side (1–2 sites)	Perioral muscles: 10–20U for each site (2–3 sites) Masseter: 60–240U for each side (1–2 sites)	Perioral muscles: 2.5–5U for each site (4–5 sites) Masseter: 15–60U for each side (1–2 sites)	Perioral muscles: 100–200U for each site (4–5 sites) Masseter: 600–2400U for each side (1–2 sites)
Torticollis	Contralateral sternocleidomastoid: 25–50U for each site (2 sites) Omolateral nuchal muscles: 25–50U for each site (2 sites)	Contralateral sternocleidomastoid: 100–200U for each site (2 sites) Omolateral nuchal muscles: 100–200U for each site (2 sites)	Contralateral sternocleidomastoid: 25–50U for each site (2 sites) Omolateral nuchal muscles: 25–50U for each site (2 sites)	Contralateral sternocleidomastoid: 1000–2000U for each site (2 sites) Omolateral nuchal muscles: 1000–2000U for each site (2 sites)
Laterocollis	Omolateral splenius capitis: 12.5–37.5U for each site (2–3 sites) Omolateral sternocleidomastoid: 6.25–12.5U for each site (2 sites)	Omolateral splenius capitis: 50–150U for each site (2–3 sites) Omolateral sternocleidomastoid: 25–50U for each site (2 sites).	Omolateral splenius capitis: 12.5–37.5U for each site (2–3 sites) Omolateral sternocleidomastoid: 6.25–12.5U for each site (2 sites)	Omolateral splenius capitis: 500–1500U for each site (2–3 sites) Omolateral sternocleidomastoid: 250–500U for each site (2 sites)
Retrocollis	Bilateral splenius capitis: 18.75–50U for each side	Bilateral splenius capitis: 75–200U for each side	Bilateral splenius capitis: 18.75–50U for each side	Bilateral splenius capitis: 750–2000U for each side
Anterocollis	Bilateral scalenus anterior: 40–60U for each side	Bilateral scalenus anterior: 160–240U for each side	Bilateral scalenus anterior: 40–60U for each side	Bilateral scalenus anterior: 1600–2400U for each side
Laryngeal dystonia (adductor type)	Vocal cord (thyroarytenoid muscle): 1.25–2.5U for each side (5–10U if unilateral) Lateral cricoarytenoid: 2.5–5U for each side	Vocal cord (thyroarytenoid muscle): 5U for each side (20 if unilateral) Lateral cricoarytenoid: 10–20U for each side	Vocal cord (thyroarytenoid muscle): 1.25–2.5U for each side (5–10U if unilateral) Lateral cricoarytenoid: 2.5–5U for each side	Vocal cord (thyroarytenoid muscle): 50–100U for each side (200–500U if unilateral) Lateral cricoarytenoid: 100–200 for each side

motor impairment and disability in patients with primary generalized or cervical dystonia (103).

Surgery is indicated after medications or BoNT have failed to provide adequate improvement. There is limited experience for targets other than the GPi (104), such as the thalamus, the subthalamic nucleus (105), and the cerebral cortex (106). Chronic stimulation in dystonia uses higher pulse-widths and voltages than in Parkinson's disease, resulting in earlier battery depletion; replacement may sometimes be needed every 2 years or less. GPi DBS is generally less effective in secondary dystonia. This procedure requires a specialized expertise and a multidisciplinary team, and may be limited by the occurrence of side effects. Other indications are still being explored, such as status dystonicus, task-specific dystonias, camptocormia, secondary hemidystonia, pantothenate-kinase-associated neurodegeneration, Lesch–Nyhan disease, and cerebral-palsy-related dystonia–choreoathetosis.

According to a National Institute for Health and Clinical Excellence (NICE) guideline (107), GPi DBS provides marked benefit with improvement of dystonia motor scores (34–88%) and disability scores (40–50%). A meta-analysis using a regression analysis, published in 2006, revealed that longer duration of dystonia correlated negatively with surgical outcome (108). Improvement of dystonia after DBS commonly follows a specific pattern, with phasic (clonic or tremulous) elements improving earlier than tonic features, with improvement in the latter often developed by weeks or months (109–111). Overall, the most beneficial results with pallidal DBS were reported in children with primary generalized dystonia, particularly in DYT1 dystonia, which improves by 40–90% (112–114). Long-term efficacy was reported to be sustained after more than 5 years of follow-up (115). In patients with cervical dystonia, GPi DBS has so far been used mainly in those who were not thought to be ideal candidates for peripheral denervation, including patients with head tremor and myoclonus or marked phasic movements (116).

Safety aspects which have to be considered include surgery-related complications, stimulation-induced side effects, and hardware-related problems. Chronic high-voltage GPi DBS may induce a parkinsonian gait or bradykinesia in limbs unaffected by dystonia (117, 118). Bilateral pallidal stimulation does not impair cognitive performance (119).

Other neurosurgical procedures

According to the NICE guidelines (120), selective peripheral denervation in cervical dystonia requires specialized expertise, but is safe, with infrequent and minimal side effects, and is indicated exclusively in cervical dystonia. According to EFNS guidelines there is insufficient evidence to use this treatment in primary dystonia, although this procedure may be indicated in patients affected by secondary dystonia combined with spasticity (91). Intrathecal baclofen has been used in patients with severe generalized dystonia. Since this treatment is complicated by medication-related side effects, it is currently indicated only in patients where secondary dystonia is combined with spasticity (121).

References

1. Oppenheim H. Über eine eigenartige Krampfkrankheit des kindlichen und jugendlichen Alters (dysbasia lordotica progressiva, dystonia musculorum deformans). *Neurol Zentralbl* 1911; 30: 1090–107.
2. Fahn S, Eldridge R. Definition of dystonia and classification of the dystonic states. *Adv Neurol* 1976; 14: 1–5.
3. Marsden CD. Dystonia: the spectrum of the disease. *Res Publ Assoc Res Nerv Ment Dis* 1976; 55: 351–67.
4. Marsden CD. Blepharospasm-oromandibular dystonia syndrome (Brueghel's syndrome). A variant of adult-onset torsion dystonia? *J Neurol Neurosurg Psychiatry* 1976; 39: 1204–9.
5. Sheehy MP, Marsden CD. Writers' cramp: a focal dystonia. *Brain* 1982; 105: 461–80.
6. Fahn S, Marsden CD, Calne DB. Classification and investigation of dystonia. In: Marsden CD, Fahn S (eds) *Movement disorders 2*, pp. 332–58. London: Butterworths, 1987.
7. Albanese A. The clinical expression of primary dystonia. *J Neurol* 2003; 250: 1145–51.
8. Albanese A, Lalli S. Is this dystonia? *Mov Disord* 2009; 24: 1725–31.
9. Fahn S. Concept and classification of dystonia. *Adv Neurol* 1988; 50: 1–8.
10. Fahn S, Bressman SB, Marsden CD. Classification of dystonia. *Adv Neurol* 1998; 78: 1–10.
11. Albanese A, Asmus F, Bhatia KP, et al. EFNS guidelines on diagnosis and treatment of primary dystonias. *Eur J Neurol* 2011 Jan; 18: 5–18.
12. Marsden CD, Harrison MJ. Idiopathic torsion dystonia (dystonia musculorum deformans). A review of forty-two patients. *Brain* 1974; 97: 793–810.
13. Elia AE, Lalli S, Albanese A. Differential diagnosis of dystonia. *Eur J Neurol* 2010; 17 (Suppl 1): 1–8.
14. Lalli S, Albanese A. The diagnostic challenge of primary dystonia: evidence from misdiagnosis. *Mov Disord* 2010; 25: 1619–26.
15. Wissel J, Muller J, Ebersbach G, Poewe W. Trick maneuvers in cervical dystonia: investigation of movement- and touch-related changes in polymyographic activity. *Mov Disord* 1999; 14: 994–9.
16. Sitburana O, Jankovic J. Focal hand dystonia, mirror dystonia and motor overflow. *J Neurol Sci* 2008; 266: 31–3.
17. Jedynak PC, Tranchant C, de Beyl DZ. Prospective clinical study of writer's cramp. *Mov Disord* 2001; 16: 494–9.
18. Defazio G, Abbruzzese G, Livrea P, Berardelli A. Epidemiology of primary dystonia. *Lancet Neurol* 2004; 3: 673–8.
19. Zeman W, Kaelbling R, Pasamanick B. Idiopathic dystonia musculorum deformans. II. The formes frustes. *Neurology* 1960; 10: 1068–75.
20. Muller U. The monogenic primary dystonias. *Brain* 2009; 132: 2005–25.
21. Ozelius LJ, Hewett JW, Page CE, et al. The early-onset torsion dystonia gene (DYT1) encodes an ATP-binding protein. *Nat Genet* 1997; 17: 40–8.
22. Bressman SB, de Leon D, Brin MF, et al. Idiopathic dystonia among Ashkenazi Jews: evidence for autosomal dominant inheritance. *Ann Neurol* 1989; 26: 612–20.
23. Valente EM, Warner TT, Jarman PR, Mathen D, Fletcher NA, Marsden CD, et al. The role of DYT1 in primary torsion dystonia in Europe. *Brain* 1998; 121: 2335–9.
24. Fasano A, Nardocci N, Elia AE, Zorzi G, Bentivoglio AR, Albanese A. Non-DYT1 early-onset primary torsion dystonia: comparison with DYT1 phenotype and review of the literature. *Mov Disord* 2006; 21: 1411–18.
25. Opal P, Tintner R, Jankovic J, et al. Intrafamilial phenotypic variability of the DYT1 dystonia: from asymptomatic TOR1A gene carrier status to dystonic storm. *Mov Disord* 2002; 17: 339–45.
26. Bentivoglio AR, Loi M, Valente EM, Ialongo T, Tonali P, Albanese A. Phenotypic variability of DYT1-PTD: does the clinical spectrum include psychogenic dystonia? *Mov Disord* 2002; 17: 1058–63.
27. Gambarin M, Valente EM, Liberini P, et al. Atypical phenotypes and clinical variability in a large Italian family with DYT1-primary torsion dystonia. *Mov Disord* 2006; 21: 1782–4.
28. Kostic VS, Svetel M, Kabakci K, et al. Intrafamilial phenotypic and genetic heterogeneity of dystonia. *J Neurol Sci* 2006; 250: 92–6.
29. Fasano A, Elia A, Albanese A. Early onset primary torsion dystonia. In: Fernández-Alvarez E, Arzimanoglou A, Tolosa E (eds) *Paediatric movement disorders*, pp. 31–55. Esher: John Libbey, 2005.
30. Brassat D, Camuzat A, Vidailhet M, et al. Frequency of the DYT1 mutation in primary torsion dystonia without family history. *Arch Neurol* 2000; 57: 333–5.
31. Gatto EM, Pardal MM, Micheli FE. Unusual phenotypic expression of the DYT1 mutation. *Parkinsonism Relat Disord* 2003; 9: 277–9.
32. Chinnery PF, Reading PJ, McCarthy EL, Curtis A, Burn DJ. Late-onset axial jerky dystonia due to the DYT1 deletion. *Mov Disord* 2002; 17: 196–8.
33. Edwards M, Wood N, Bhatia K. Unusual phenotypes in DYT1 dystonia: a report of five cases and a review of the literature. *Mov Disord* 2003; 18: 706–11.
34. Bressman SB, Sabatti C, Raymond D, et al. The DYT1 phenotype and guidelines for diagnostic testing. *Neurology* 2000; 54: 1746–52.
35. Ikeuchi T, Shimohata T, Nakano R, Koide R, Takano H, Tsuji S. A case of primary torsion dystonia in Japan with the 3-bp (GAG) deletion in the DYT1 gene with a unique clinical presentation. *Neurogenetics* 1999; 2: 189–90.
36. Asanuma K, Ma Y, Okulski J, et al. Decreased striatal D2 receptor binding in non-manifesting carriers of the DYT1 dystonia mutation. *Neurology* 2005; 64: 347–9.
37. Fiorio M, Gambarin M, Valente EM, et al. Defective temporal processing of sensory stimuli in DYT1 mutation carriers: a new endophenotype of dystonia? *Brain* 2007; 130: 134–42.
38. Valente EM, Povey S, Warner TT, Wood NW, Davis MB. Detailed haplotype analysis in Ashkenazi Jewish and non-Jewish British dystonic patients carrying the GAG deletion in the DYT1 gene: evidence for a limited number of founder mutations. *Ann Hum Genet* 1999; 63: 1–8.
39. Doheny D, Danisi F, Smith C, et al. Clinical findings of a myoclonus-dystonia family with two distinct mutations. *Neurology* 2002; 59: 1244–6.
40. Hewett J, Gonzalez-Agosti C, Slater D, et al. Mutant torsinA, responsible for early-onset torsion dystonia, forms membrane inclusions in cultured neural cells. *Hum Mol Genet* 2000; 9: 1403–13.
41. Kustedjo K, Bracey MH, Cravatt BF. Torsin A and its torsion dystonia-associated mutant forms are lumenal glycoproteins that exhibit distinct subcellular localizations. *J Biol Chem* 2000; 275: 27 933–9.
42. Shashidharan P, Good PF, Hsu A, Perl DP, Brin MF, Olanow CW. TorsinA accumulation in Lewy bodies in sporadic Parkinson's disease. *Brain Res* 2000; 877: 379–81.
43. Almasy L, Bressman SB, Raymond D, et al. Idiopathic torsion dystonia linked to chromosome 8 in two Mennonite families. *Ann Neurol* 1997; 42: 670–3.
44. Fuchs T, Gavarini S, Saunders-Pullman R, et al. Mutations in the THAP1 gene are responsible for DYT6 primary torsion dystonia. *Nat Genet* 2009; 41: 286–8.
45. Bressman SB, Raymond D, Fuchs T, Heiman GA, Ozelius LJ, Saunders-Pullman R. Mutations in THAP1 (DYT6) in early-onset dystonia: a genetic screening study. *Lancet Neurol* 2009; 8: 441–6.
46. Bonetti M, Barzaghi C, Brancati F, et al. Mutation screening of the DYT6/THAP1 gene in Italy. *Mov Disord* 2009; 24: 2424–7.

47. Houlden H, Schneider SA, Paudel R, et al. THAP1 mutations (DYT6) are an additional cause of early-onset dystonia. *Neurology* 2010; 74: 846–50.
48. Gavarini S, Cayrol C, Fuchs T, et al. Direct interaction between causative genes of DYT1 and DYT6 primary dystonia. *Ann Neurol* 2010; 68: 549–53.
49. Kaiser FJ, Osmanoric A, Rakovic A, et al. The dystonia gene DYT1 is repressed by the transcription factor THAP1 (DYT6). *Ann Neurol* 2010; 68: 554–9.
50. Leube B, Rudnicki D, Ratzlaff T, Kessler KR, Benecke R, Auburger G. Idiopathic torsion dystonia: assignment of a gene to chromosome 18p in a German family with adult onset, autosomal dominant inheritance and purely focal distribution. *Hum Mol Genet* 1996; 5: 1673–7.
51. Bentivoglio AR, Del Grosso N, Albanese A, Cassetta E, Tonali P, Frontali M. Non-DYT1 dystonia in a large Italian family. *J Neurol Neurosurg Psychiatry* 1997; 62: 357–60.
52. Valente EM, Bentivoglio AR, Cassetta E, et al. DYT13, a novel primary torsion dystonia locus, maps to chromosome 1p36.13–36.32 in an Italian family with cranial-cervical or upper limb onset. *Ann Neurol* 2001; 49: 362–6.
53. Bentivoglio AR, Ialongo T, Contarino MF, Valente EM, Albanese A. Phenotypic characterization of DYT13 primary torsion dystonia. *Mov Disord* 2004; 19: 200–6.
54. Grimes DA, Han F, Lang AE, George-Hyssop P, Racacho L, Bulman DE. A novel locus for inherited myoclonus-dystonia on 18p11. *Neurology* 2002; 59: 1183–6.
55. Chouery E, Kfoury J, Delague V, et al. A novel locus for autosomal recessive primary torsion dystonia (DYT17) maps to 20p11.22-q13.12. *Neurogenetics* 2008; 9: 287–93.
56. Gimenez-Roldan S, Delgado G, Marin M, Villanueva JA, Mateo D. Hereditary torsion dystonia in gypsies. *Adv Neurol* 1988; 50: 73–81.
57. Gimenez-Roldan S, Lopez-Fraile IP, Esteban A. Dystonia in Spain: study of a gypsy family and general survey. *Adv Neurol* 1976; 14: 125–36.
58. Khan NL, Wood NW, Bhatia KP. Autosomal recessive, DYT2-like primary torsion dystonia: a new family. *Neurology* 2003; 61: 1801–3.
59. Moretti P, Hedera P, Wald J, Fink J. Autosomal recessive primary generalized dystonia in two siblings from a consanguineous family. *Mov Disord* 2005; 20: 245–7.
60. Parker N. Hereditary whispering dysphonia. *J Neurol Neurosurg Psychiatry* 1985; 48: 218–24.
61. Ahmad F, Davis MB, Waddy HM, Oley CA, Marsden CD, Harding AE. Evidence for locus heterogeneity in autosomal dominant torsion dystonia. *Genomics* 1993; 15: 9–12.
62. Bressman SB, Heiman GA, Nygaard TG, et al. A study of idiopathic torsion dystonia in a non-Jewish family: evidence for genetic heterogeneity. *Neurology* 1994; 44: 283–7.
63. Holmgren G, Ozelius L, Forsgren L, et al. Adult onset idiopathic torsion dystonia is excluded from the DYT 1 region (9q34) in a Swedish family. *J Neurol Neurosurg Psychiatry* 1995; 59: 178–81.
64. Klein C, Pramstaller PP, Castellan CC, Breakefield XO, Kramer PL, Ozelius LJ. Clinical and genetic evaluation of a family with a mixed dystonia phenotype from South Tyrol. *Ann Neurol* 1998; 44: 394–8.
65. Albanese A, Bentivoglio AR, Del Grosso N, et al. Phenotype variability of dystonia in monozygotic twins. *J Neurol* 2000; 247: 148–50.
66. Chan J, Brin MF, Fahn S. Idiopathic cervical dystonia: clinical characteristics. *Mov Disord* 1991; 6: 119–26.
67. Quartarone A, Rizzo V, Morgante F. Clinical features of dystonia: a pathophysiological revisitation. *Curr Opin Neurol* 2008; 21: 484–90.
68. Fabbrini G, Pantano P, Totaro P, et al. Diffusion tensor imaging in patients with primary cervical dystonia and in patients with blepharospasm. *Eur J Neurol* 2008; 15: 185–9.
69. Carbon M, Kingsley PB, Tang C, Bressman S, Eidelberg D. Microstructural white matter changes in primary torsion dystonia. *Mov Disord* 2008 Jan 30; 23: 234–9.
70. Delmaire C, Vidailhet M, Wassermann D, et al. Diffusion abnormalities in the primary sensorimotor pathways in writer's cramp. *Arch Neurol* 2009; 66: 502–8.
71. Bonilha L, de Vries PM, Vincent DJ, et al. Structural white matter abnormalities in patients with idiopathic dystonia. *Mov Disord* 2007; 22: 1110–16.
72. Schmidt KE, Linden DE, Goebel R, Zanella FE, Lanfermann H, Zubcov AA. Striatal activation during blepharospasm revealed by fMRI. *Neurology* 2003; 60: 1738–43.
73. Preibisch C, Berg D, Hofmann E, Solymosi L, Naumann M. Cerebral activation patterns in patients with writer's cramp: a functional magnetic resonance imaging study. *J Neurol* 2001; 248: 10–17.
74. Oga T, Honda M, Toma K, et al. Abnormal cortical mechanisms of voluntary muscle relaxation in patients with writer's cramp: an fMRI study. *Brain* 2002; 125: 895–903.
75. Peller M, Zeuner KE, Munchau A, et al. The basal ganglia are hyperactive during the discrimination of tactile stimuli in writer's cramp. *Brain* 2006; 129: 2697–708.
76. Butterworth S, Francis S, Kelly E, McGlone F, Bowtell R, Sawle GV. Abnormal cortical sensory activation in dystonia: an fMRI study. *Mov Disord* 2003; 18: 673–82.
77. Obermann M, Yaldizli O, de Greiff A, et al. Morphometric changes of sensorimotor structures in focal dystonia. *Mov Disord* 2007; 22: 1117–23.
78. Draganski B, Thun-Hohenstein C, Bogdahn U, Winkler J, May A. 'Motor circuit' gray matter changes in idiopathic cervical dystonia. *Neurology* 2003; 61: 1228–31.
79. Garraux G, Bauer A, Hanakawa T, Wu T, Kansaku K, Hallett M. Changes in brain anatomy in focal hand dystonia. *Ann Neurol* 2004; 55: 736–9.
80. Egger K, Mueller J, Schocke M, et al. Voxel based morphometry reveals specific gray matter changes in primary dystonia. *Mov Disord* 2007; 22: 1538–42.
81. Delmaire C, Vidailhet M, Elbaz A, et al. Structural abnormalities in the cerebellum and sensorimotor circuit in writer's cramp. *Neurology* 2007; 69: 376–80.
82. Hutchinson M, Nakamura T, Moeller JR, et al. The metabolic topography of essential blepharospasm: a focal dystonia with general implications. *Neurology* 2000; 55: 673–7.
83. Asanuma K, Ma Y, Huang C, et al. The metabolic pathology of dopa-responsive dystonia. *Ann Neurol* 2005; 57: 596–600.
84. Draganski B, Schneider SA, Fiorio M, et al. Genotype–phenotype interactions in primary dystonias revealed by differential changes in brain structure. *NeuroImage* 2009; 47: 1141–7.
85. Carbon M, Niethammer M, Peng S, et al. Abnormal striatal and thalamic dopamine neurotransmission: Genotype-related features of dystonia. *Neurology* 2009; 72: 2097–103.
86. Walker RH, Brin MF, Sandu D, Good PF, Shashidharan P. TorsinA immunoreactivity in brains of patients with DYT1 and non-DYT1 dystonia. *Neurology* 2002; 58: 120–4.
87. Holton JL, Schneider SA, Ganesharajah T, et al. Neuropathology of primary adult-onset dystonia. *Neurology* 2008; 70: 695–9.
88. Rostasy K, Augood SJ, Hewett JW, et al. TorsinA protein and neuropathology in early onset generalized dystonia with GAG deletion. *Neurobiol Dis* 2003; 12: 11–24.
89. Jankovic J. Treatment of hyperkinetic movement disorders. *Lancet Neurol* 2009; 8: 844–56.
90. Albanese A. Terminology for preparations of botulinum toxins. What a difference a name makes. *JAMA* 2011; 305: 89–90.
91. Albanese A, Barnes MP, Bhatia KP, et al. A systematic review on the diagnosis and treatment of primary (idiopathic) dystonia and dystonia plus syndromes: report of an EFNS/MDS-ES Task Force. *Eur J Neurol* 2006; 13: 433–44.
92. Watts CC, Whurr R, Nye C. Botulinum toxin injections for the treatment of spasmodic dysphonia. *Cochrane Database Syst Rev* 2004; CD004327.
93. Balash Y, Giladi N. Efficacy of pharmacological treatment of dystonia: evidence-based review including meta-analysis of the effect of botulinum toxin and other cure options. *Eur J Neurol* 2004; 11: 361–70.

94. Bentivoglio AR, Fasano A, Ialongo T, Soleti F, Lo Fermo S, Albanese A. Fifteen-year experience in treating blepharospasm with Botox or Dysport: same toxin, two drugs. *Neurotox Res* 2009; 15: 224–31.
95. Mejia NI, Vuong KD, Jankovic J. Long-term botulinum toxin efficacy, safety, and immunogenicity. *Mov Disord* 2005; 20: 592–7.
96. Brin MF, Comella CL, Jankovic J, Lai F, Naumann M. Long-term treatment with botulinum toxin type A in cervical dystonia has low immunogenicity by mouse protection assay. *Mov Disord* 2008; 23: 1353–60.
97. Albavera-Hernandez C, Rodriguez JM, Idrovo AJ. Safety of botulinum toxin type A among children with spasticity secondary to cerebral palsy: a systematic review of randomized clinical trials. *Clin Rehabil* 2009; 23: 394–407.
98. Burke RE, Fahn S. Double-blind evaluation of trihexyphenidyl in dystonia. *Adv Neurol* 1983; 37: 189–92.
99. Burke RE, Fahn S, Marsden CD. Torsion dystonia: a double blind, prospective trial of high-dosage trihexyphenidil. *Neurology* 1986; 36: 160–4.
100. Jankovic J. Treatment of hyperkinetic movement disorders with tetrabenazine: a double-blind crossover study. *Ann Neurol* 1982; 11: 41–7.
101. Jankovic J, Beach J. Long-term effects of tetrabenazine in hyperkinetic movement disorders. *Neurology* 1997; 48: 358–62.
102. Krauss JK, Yianni J, Loher TJ, Aziz TZ. Deep brain stimulation for dystonia. *J Clin Neurophysiol* 2004; 21: 18–30.
103. Kupsch A, Benecke R, Muller J, et al. Pallidal deep-brain stimulation in primary generalized or segmental dystonia. *N Engl J Med* 2006; 355: 1978–90.
104. Capelle HH, Krauss JK. Neuromodulation in dystonia: current aspects of deep brain stimulation. *Neuromodulation* 2009; 12: 8–21.
105. Lyons MK, Birch BD, Hillman RA, Boucher OK, Evidente VG. Long-term follow-up of deep brain stimulation for Meige syndrome. *Neurosurg Focus* 2010; 29: E5.
106. Romito LM, Franzini A, Perani D, et al. Fixed dystonia unresponsive to pallidal stimulation improved by motor cortex stimulation. *Neurology* 2007 13; 68: 875–6.
107. National Institute for Health and Clinical Excellence. Deep brain stimulation for tremor and dystonia (excluding Parkinson's disease). Available online at http: //www nice org uk/guidance/IPG188 (issued 2006).
108. Holloway KL, Baron MS, Brown R, Cifu DX, Carne W, Ramakrishnan V. Deep brain stimulation for dystonia: a meta-analysis. *Neuromodulation* 2006; 9: 253–61.
109. Coubes P, Cif L, El Fertit H, et al. Electrical stimulation of the globus pallidus internus in patients with primary generalized dystonia: long-term results. *J Neurosurg* 2004; 101: 189–94.
110. Krause M, Fogel W, Kloss M, Rasche D, Volkmann J, Tronnier V. Pallidal stimulation for dystonia. *Neurosurgery* 2004; 55: 1361–70.
111. Krauss JK, Pohle T, Weber S, Ozdoba C, Burgunder JM. Bilateral stimulation of globus pallidus internus for treatment of cervical dystonia. *Lancet* 1999; 354: 837–8.
112. Coubes P, Roubertie A, Vayssiere N, Hemm S, Echenne B. Treatment of DYT1-generalised dystonia by stimulation of the internal globus pallidus. *Lancet* 2000; 355: 2220–1.
113. Egidi M, Franzini A, Marras C, Cavallo M, Mondani M, Lavano A, et al. A survey of Italian cases of dystonia treated by deep brain stimulation. *J Neurosurg Sci* 2007; 51: 153–8.
114. Borggraefe I, Mehrkens JH, Telegravciska M, Berweck S, Botzel K, Heinen F. Bilateral pallidal stimulation in children and adolescents with primary generalized dystonia. Report of six patients and literature-based analysis of predictive outcomes variables. *Brain Dev* 2010; 32: 223–8.
115. Isaias IU, Alterman RL, Tagliati M. Deep brain stimulation for primary generalized dystonia: long-term outcomes. *Arch Neurol* 2009; 66: 465–70.
116. Krauss JK. Deep brain stimulation for cervical dystonia. *J Neurol Neurosurg Psychiatry* 2003; 74: 1598.
117. Ostrem JL, Marks WJ, Jr, Volz MM, Heath SL, Starr PA. Pallidal deep brain stimulation in patients with cranial-cervical dystonia (Meige syndrome). *Mov Disord* 2007; 22: 1885–91.
118. Berman BD, Starr PA, Marks WJ, Ostrem JL. Induction of bradykinesia with pallidal deep brain stimulation in patients with cranial–cervical dystonia. *Stereotact Funct Neurosurg* 2009; 87: 37–44.
119. Pillon B, Ardouin C, Dujardin K, et al. Preservation of cognitive function in dystonia treated by pallidal stimulation. *Neurology* 2006; 66: 1556–8.
120. National Institute for Health and Clinical Excellence. Selective peripheral denervation of cervical dystonia. Available online at http://guidance.nice.org.uk/IPG80 (issued 2004).
121. Albright AL, Barry MJ, Shafton DH, Ferson SS. Intrathecal baclofen for generalized dystonia. *Dev Med Child Neurol* 2001; 43: 652–7.

CHAPTER 19

Other Dystonias

Julie Phukan and Thomas Warner

Introduction

Primary forms of dystonia represent around 70% of all cases and are described in the preceding chapter. The remainder comprise those cases where dystonia is part of a more complex movement disorder or neurological syndrome. These can be divided into four broad categories: dystonia-plus syndromes, heredodegenerative disorders, secondary (or symptomatic dystonia), and dystonia that is a feature of another neurological condition. The key difference from primary dystonia is the presence of other neurological features in addition to dystonia. Many have underlying neurodegeneration, often genetic in origin.

Dystonia-plus syndromes

In these syndromes, torsion dystonia is associated with another movement disorder, typically myoclonus or parkinsonism. There is no evidence of neurodegeneration and they appear to be caused by neuronal dysfunction.

Dopa-responsive dystonia (DRD)

The classic phenotype of this rare disorder is of early-onset lower limb dystonia (4–8 years of age) causing gait disturbance, with diurnal fluctuation (worsening of symptoms toward the evening and improvement after sleep) and an excellent response to levodopa (1, 2). Parkinsonism can develop later and may be an early feature in adult-onset cases. Additional features include brisk reflexes, spasticity, ankle clonus, and extensor plantar responses (3).

Atypical cases include patients with craniocervical and oromandibular dystonia, early hypotonia with proximal weakness, spontaneously remitting dystonia, and spasticity mimicking cerebral palsy (4, 5). Associations with anxiety, depression, obsessive–compulsive disorder, and/or sleep disturbances have been reported (6).

Most cases are inherited as an autosomal dominant trait with reduced penetrance (30%). Females are two to four times more likely to be affected than males. Heterozygous mutations in the *GCH1* (*DYT5*) gene cause the majority of these cases (5, 7), although deletions have been described (8). The gene encodes GTP cyclohydrolase 1, an enzyme that catalyses the first step in the biosynthesis of tetrahydrobiopterin (BH4), an essential co-factor for tyrosine hydroxylase (TH), and the rate-limiting enzyme for dopamine synthesis. *In vitro* studies have shown that patients have reduced GTP cyclohydrolase 1 activity, leading to low levels of pterins and monoamines, which explains the dramatic beneficial treatment response to levodopa. Most of the missense mutations appear to lie within the core of the protein and impair its tertiary structure and/or stability (9).

Other rare forms of DRD caused by autosomal recessive mutations in genes for tyrosine hydroxylase and sepiapterin reductase have been reported (2, 10, 11). These forms usually have additional features such as parkinsonism, cognitive impairment, spastic paraplegia, hypotonia, myoclonus, seizures, and progressive neurological deterioration (12).

Diagnosis is by recognition of the clinical phenotype and response to levodopa. A phenylalanine loading test and cerebrospinal fluid (CSF) pterin studies can be useful. Dopamine transporter SPECT or fluorodopa PET scans are normal in DRD, differentiating it from young-onset Parkinson's disease presenting with foot dystonia (early use of levodopa is not usually recommended in these cases). Mutation analysis of *GCH1* (*DYT5*) gene is also available.

DRD demonstrates a dramatic and sustained response to small doses of levodopa (as low as 50–200 mg). Benefit is usually apparent within days to weeks, and the motor complications of levodopa treatment seen in Parkinson's disease rarely develop. Because of the benefit from levodopa treatment, every patient with early-onset dystonia without an alternative diagnosis should have a trial of levodopa.

Myoclonus–dystonia syndrome (MDS)

MDS is a rare autosomal dominant condition characterized by myoclonic jerks and dystonia, affecting mainly the neck, trunk, and arms. Prevalence is estimated at two per million in Europe (2). Onset is typically in the first or second decade (2, 13) and it usually follows a relatively benign course. Myoclonus tends to dominate the condition, but dystonia occurs in around two-thirds of patients, typically with cervical dystonia and writer's cramp. The jerks show dramatic improvement with alcohol and benzodiazepines (2, 14), although there is often a rebound effect. Myoclonus can be precipitated or aggravated by caffeine, active movement of the involved region, stress, sudden noise, and tactile stimuli. Depression, anxiety, obsessive–compulsive disorder, and panic attacks have been reported in MDS (15).

Inheritance is autosomal dominant with reduced penetrance. Numerous point mutations and small deletions have been identified in the epsilon-sarcoglycan gene (*SGCE, DYT11*) in many individuals (16–18). Maternal imprinting of the SGCE gene means that most cases are inherited from mutant paternal alleles (19). The sarcoglycans are a family of *trans*-membrane proteins that are part of the dystrophin-associated glycoprotein in cardiac and skeletal muscle. SGCE is expressed in a wide variety of tissues, but incorporation of exon 11b leads to a brain-specific SGCE splice variant, found mainly in midbrain monoaminergic neurons, cerebellar Purkinje cells, hippocampus, and cortex (20). Mutant SGCE appears to be abnormally trafficked and is retained intracellularly (instead of at its normal location at the neuronal plasma membrane) where it is degraded by the proteasome (21). The DYT1 gene product, torsinA, binds SGCE, promotes its degradation, and contributes to its quality control; mice carrying mutations in both TorsinA and SGCE show earlier onset of motor deficit (22).

Diagnosis is clinical, but can be confirmed by mutation analysis of the *SGCE* gene. Treatment is problematic. In patients with response to alcohol, GABAergic drugs such as clonazepam and gamma-hydroxybutyrate have marked, but transient, effects and addiction can be a problem. Cervical dystonia and writer's cramp may respond to botulinum toxin injections. Response to high-dose levodopa has been reported in two patients with SGCE deletions, with improvement even in myoclonus (23). In severe cases bilateral deep brain stimulation (DBS) of the globus pallidus internus (GPi) has conferred lasting improvement in both dystonia and myoclonus.

Rapid-onset dystonia–parkinsonism (RDP)

RDP is a rare, autosomal dominant movement disorder with reduced penetrance. Typically, there is abrupt onset of dystonia and parkinsonism, developing over a period of hours to weeks followed by little progression (2, 24, 25). Onset is associated with specific physical triggers such as fever, strenuous exercise, childbirth, excessive alcohol consumption, or psychological stress. RDP usually presents in adolescence or young adulthood. Common symptoms are postural instability, bradykinesia, and limb and cranial dystonia with a rostrocaudal gradient of involvement. The limited pathology studied to date has found no evidence of neurodegeneration, suggesting a functional mechanism. Some patients have reduced levels of CSF homovanillic acid, implying involvement of the dopaminergic system, but there is a poor response to dopaminergic medications.

The condition is caused by loss of function mutations in the alpha-3 subunit of the Na^+/K^+-ATPase pump (*ATP1A3* gene) (26), which is crucial for maintaining the electrochemical gradient across the cell membrane (27).

In a mouse model using striatal and cerebellar injections of ouabain (an inhibitor of the Na^+/K^+-ATPase pump) a phenotype similar to RDP was produced, with dystonia resulting from cerebellar injection and parkinsonism resulting from basal ganglia injection (28). These mild symptoms rapidly transformed into persistent dystonia and rigidity after stress, simulating the clinical features of this condition.

Treatment is generally supportive. Levodopa is not effective and response to GPi DBS has been poor.

Recently, two other dystonia–parkinsonism syndromes have been described: *DYT16* dystonia and dopamine transporter deficiency syndrome. *DYT16* dystonia–parkinsonism is an autosomal recessive condition reported in two consanguineous Brazilian families and one sporadic case (29). Progressive early-onset generalized dystonia occurs with axial, oromandibular, and laryngeal involvement in addition to parkinsonian features. Homozygous missense mutations within the stress response gene protein kinase interferon-inducible double-stranded RNA-dependent activator (*PRKRA*) were identified in affected individuals. A heterozygous frameshift mutation leading to protein truncation was also identified in a sporadic German case with early-onset dystonia (30). The *PRKRA* gene binds double-stranded RNA and is involved in the cellular stress response, although the mechanism that results in dystonia–parkinsonism is unknown.

The dopamine transporter deficiency syndrome is an autosomal recessive condition which manifests in infancy with severe dystonia–parkinsonism, an eye movement disorder, and pyramidal tract features (31). The ratio of homovanillic acid to 5-hydroxyindoleacetic acid in the CSF was raised. Loss of function mutations were identified in the gene encoding the dopamine transporter (SLC6A3).

Heredodegenerative disorders with dystonia

Dystonia can be part of a more widespread genetic neurological disorder where there is underlying neurodegeneration; these are referred to as heredodegenerative causes. Selected conditions are described below and others are summarized in Table 19.1.

X-linked dystonia–parkinsonism (XDP, DYT3)

This progressive X-linked neurodegenerative dystonia is predominantly found in Philippino males (32). Onset of symptoms is between 12 and 64 years, and either dystonia or parkinsonism may be the presenting clinical feature (32). Ninety per cent of cases present with focal dystonia affecting almost any body part which progresses over years, often becoming generalized. Parkinsonism develops in more than 50% of all cases often within 2 years of dystonia onset, and freezing may be a prominent feature (32, 33). Other features include myoclonus, chorea, focal tremor, myorhythmia, and chorea-ballism (33). Duration of illness is around 16 years, with death at a mean age of 55 years. Female heterozygotes can manifest mild dystonia or chorea.

PET scans have revealed decreased striatal glucose metabolism, but no evidence for loss of nigrostriatal dopaminergic projections (34). Neuropathological analysis demonstrates a multifocal mosaic pattern of astrocytosis in the caudate and lateral putamen, with relatively selective degeneration of the striosome compartment (35).

A founder mutation about 1000–2000 years ago is thought to explain the geographical clustering in the Philippines. The disease locus, DYT3, has been mapped to Xq13.1.

An SVA (short interspersed nuclear element, variable number of tandem repeats, and Alu composite) retro-transposon insertion has been identified in an intron of TAF1, a major transcription factor (36). This retro-transposon insertion appears to reduce neuron-specific expression of TAF1 in the caudate nucleus, possibly through DNA methylation changes. In turn, this impairs transcription of a number of neuronal genes related to cell division and proliferation, including the dopamine D2 receptor gene. The resulting imbalance in activity of striosomal and matrix-based pathways (the latter are relatively spared until the parkinsonian phase of the illness) is postulated to give rise to abnormal movement. The preferential

Table 19.1 Other neurodegenerative syndromes that can cause dystonia

Disorder	Inheritance/gene	Onset	Clinical features	Investigations/pathology
Ataxia telangiectasia	Autosomal recessive ATM gene	2–4 years	Cerebellar ataxia, oculomotor apraxia, choreoathetosis, grimacing, dysarthria, telangiectases Variable immunodeficiency Predisposition to malignancies Dystonia (late feature) Usually wheelchair bound by 10 years Death in the second decade	Increased serum alpha-fetoprotein Decreased serum levels IgA, IgE, IgG Pathology: cerebellar Purkinje cell loss; spinal cord degeneration; posterior and lateral columns and anterior horn cells
Hereditary chorea-acanthocytosis (neuroacanthocytosis)	Autosomal recessive Chorein gene	Third to fourth decade	Chorea (especially of mouth, tongue, lip- and tongue-biting), tics, dystonia, parkinsonism, behavioural disinhibition, cognitive decline Peripheral neuropathy	Acanthocytosis on EM Raised creatine kinase in blood EMG Pathology: basal ganglia neuronal loss
Rett syndrome	Sporadic or X-linked dominant Most commonly MECP gene	After 1 year in girls (fatal neonatal encephalopathy in boys)	'Acquired microcephaly' Severe regression of language and motor skills Autistic behaviour Stereotypies of the hands Prolonged QT interval Spasticity, dystonia, seizures, muscle wasting and scoliosis	Pathology: decreased brain size especially frontal lobe and later cerebellar atrophy
Infantile bilateral striatal necrosis and familial striatal necrosis	Sporadic, but some inherited in an autosomal recessive or maternal pattern		Chorea, dystonia, rigidity, ballism, stereotyped cry, grimace, hyperextension of the neck in response to stimuli	Spongy degeneration of caudate and putamen
Neuronal intranuclear inclusion disease	Typically occurs sporadically but inherited forms described	Childhood onset Adult onset less common	Ataxia, spasticity, parkinsonism, autonomic dysfunction and cognitive deficits, dystonia, chorea, motor neuropathy	Intranuclear inclusions composed of eosinophilic ubiquinated material in the central, peripheral, and autonomic nervous systems
Ataxia with vitamin E deficiency	Autosomal recessive Mutations in the gene encoding alpha-tocopherol transfer protein	Onset before 20 years	Similar to Friedreich's ataxia Ataxia, dystonia (more frequent than Friedreich's), dysarthria, loss of vibration sense and deep tendon reflexes Head titubation Xanthelasma, tendon xanthomas, retinitis pigmentosa, deafness, sphincter involvement	Laboratory findings: very low vitamin E levels; cholesterol and triglyceride levels may be high Vitamin E supplementation may retard progression of the disease

loss of striosomal medium spiny striatal projection neurons (MSNs) is consistent with the expression of the neuron-specific isoform of TAF1 that in the rat is enriched in striosomal MSNs (37).

Treatment of XDP with oral medication is disappointing, with variable benefit from levodopa. However, bilateral GPi DBS has been used successfully to treat the condition (38).

Metabolic disorders

Metal and mineral metabolism

A number of genetic disorders are characterized by deposition of metal in the brain, predominantly copper and iron. The basal ganglia appear particularly susceptible to metal deposition and hence these conditions have mixed movement disorders, with predominant dystonia and parkinsonism. The key conditions are Wilson disease for copper, and neurodegeneration with brain iron accumulation (NBIA) for iron, which can be subdivided into specific genetic conditions: pantothenate kinase-associated neurodegeneration, infantile neuroaxonal dystrophy, and neuroferritinopathy. Idiopathic basal ganglia calcification (Fahr's disease) is also discussed.

Wilson disease

Wilson disease is a rare autosomal recessive disorder of copper transport caused by mutation of the *ATP7B* gene which encodes a copper transporter. Clinical manifestations result from copper accumulation in the brain and liver and may present in childhood or adulthood, typically presenting with hepatic (40%), neurological (40%), or psychiatric (20%) symptoms. Prevalence is estimated at 1 in 30 000 in most populations, with higher prevalence in Japan and China. Wilson disease is covered in detail in Chapter 23, and this section will only consider the association with dystonia.

Three basic neurological presentations have been identified: parkinsonism, generalized dystonia, and a tremor-predominant form. Dystonia is common, and has been reported in up to

65% of patients. It often affects cranial structures, with prominent dysarthria, dysphagia, drooling, risus sardonicus (a fixed pseudo-smile), and abnormal posturing (39). With time the dystonia becomes more extensive, often becoming segmental or generalized.

Neurodegeneration with brain iron accumulation type 1 (NBIA-1)

This term encompasses a number of disorders of iron accumulation in the brain, including those previously labelled Hallervoden–Spatz disease. The most common form is pantothenate kinase-associated neurodegeneration (PKAN) which accounts for approximately 50% of cases. Other disorders of iron accumulation include neuroferritinopathy and infantile neuroaxonal dystrophy.

PKAN is a rare autosomal recessive disorder of co-enzyme A (CoA) metabolism. Estimated prevalence is 1–3 per million, suggesting a carrier frequency of 1 in 275–300. The majority have mutations in the pantothenate kinase 2 gene.

Onset is usually in the first decade, but adult-onset cases have been described (40). The course of the disease is progressive over 10–12 years, although survival can be longer. PKAN can be familial or sporadic. It is characterized clinically by prominent dystonia (in up to 87%), parkinsonism, cognitive impairment, pseudobulbar features, spasticity, and cerebellar ataxia (40, 41). Limb dystonia can lead to children being considered to be clumsy before other symptoms emerge (41). Cranial dystonia can lead to recurrent trauma of the tongue, even leading to dental extraction. Axial dystonia occurs later in the course of illness. Pigmentary retinopathy occurs in around two-thirds of cases, with night blindness and progressive peripheral visual field loss. Intellectual involvement is variable, as are seizures.

Neuropathological features include neuronal loss, gliosis, axonal spheroids, and iron deposition in the globus pallidus, red nucleus, and substantia nigra. The HARP syndrome (hypo-prebetalipoproteinaemia, acanthocytosis, retinitis pigmentosa) is part of the PKAN spectrum.

The diagnosis is suggested by MRI findings of bilateral hyperintense signal changes in the anteromedial globus pallidus with surrounding hypointensity in the globus pallidus and substantia nigra pars reticulata on T_2-weighted images. This 'eye-of-the-tiger' sign is highly specific to PKAN. Most patients have mutations in the *PANK2* gene (40, 41) and molecular analysis can confirm the diagnosis.

Treatment is symptomatic. Dystonia may occasionally benefit from baclofen, trihexyphenidyl, or botulinum toxin. Bilateral pallidal stimulation and thalamotomy have also been used for intractable generalized dystonia in PKAN with evidence of sustained benefit (42, 43). A recent phase II trial of the oral iron-chelating drug deferiprone in ten patients with PKAN, demonstrated reduced pallidal iron content at 6 months as assessed by MRI T2* relaxometry (44). However, there was no clinical change in dystonia or quality of life over the same period. It is possible that longer-term therapy, or earlier intervention, may affect neurological progress.

Neuroferritinopathy

Neuroferritinopathy is an adult-onset (mean age 40) autosomal dominant disorder which results in abnormal aggregates of iron and ferritin in the brain due to a mutation in the ferritin light chain gene (*FTL1*) (45). Fewer than 100 cases have been described.

Patients present with chorea or dystonia with asymmetric limb involvement and sometimes evidence of parkinsonism and ataxia (46). With time, orofacial dystonia develops, affecting speech, and dysphagia can be a significant problem. Eye movements are preserved. A progressive frontal and subcortical cognitive decline has been described.

Serum ferritin is low, typically ≤20 μg/dl (46), in the presence of normal serum iron, transferrin, and haemoglobin levels. MRI in all patients demonstrates excess brain iron accumulation on T2* MRI in the putamen and globus pallidus, often with cystic changes. Molecular genetic testing for FTL is available.

Neuropathology reveals iron and ferritin deposition both within neurons and extracellularly in the basal ganglia, forebrain, and cerebellum with accompanying neuronal loss. In mice expressing a mutant human form of the FTL gene, there was increased cytoplasmic FTL, ferritin heavy chain polypeptides, and iron (47). It was suggested that the pathogenesis in neuroferritinopathy resulted from a combination of reduction in iron-storage function and enhanced toxicity associated with iron-induced ferritin aggregates in the brain.

Treatment is symptomatic and supportive, and no drugs have been shown to alter the course of neuroferritinopathy. The role of iron chelation and venesection is under review.

Infantile and atypical neuroaxonal dystrophy (INAD)

INAD is an autosomal recessive condition that presents between the ages of 6 months and 3 years with truncal hypotonia, progressive psychomotor delay, cerebellar ataxia, pyramidal signs, strabismus, nystagmus, and optic atrophy. Tetraparesis and progressive cognitive decline and seizure follow, with death typically in the first decade (48). MRI demonstrates hypointensity of the globus pallidus (indicating iron accumulation) in addition to cerebellar atrophy. The signal abnormality differs from the 'eye of the tiger' sign of PKAN as there is no central hyperintensity (49).

Atypical forms present later (2–7 years) with a picture of static encephalopathy and later deterioration from 7 to 12 years, with progressive dystonia, ataxia, dysarthria, and neurobehavioural disturbance (41). Again, MRI demonstrates iron accumulation in the medial and lateral portions of the pallidum, and there may be EEG abnormalities.

Both infantile and later forms of neuroaxonal dystrophy are caused by mutations in the *PLA2G6* gene, which encodes $iPLA_2$-VIa, a calcium-independent phospholipase, which may disrupt membrane homeostasis (41, 48, 49).

Two cases of Pakistani and Indian descent with dystonia–parkinsonism have also been found to have mutations in *PLA2G6* (homozygous missense mutations) with an onset at 10–26 years of subacute dystonia–parkinsonism, pyramidal signs, eye movement abnormalities, and cognitive/psychiatric features (50). Cerebellar features which are present in typical INAD were absent in these cases. Also in contrast with INAD, iron was absent in the basal ganglia. Three individuals had good response to levodopa.

Idiopathic basal ganglia calcification

Idiopathic basal ganglia calcification (Fahr's disease) is an autosomal dominant neurodegenerative disease with basal ganglia calcification that typically presents between 30 and 50 years of age with chorea, dystonia, parkinsonism, ataxia, seizures, cognitive impairment, and neuropsychiatric disorder (51, 52). Pyramidal and cerebellar signs may also feature. It is slowly progressive. Over thirty affected families have been reported (53).

Calcification of the globus pallidus, putamen, caudate, thalamus, and dentate nucleus is evident on neuroimaging. Histopathology demonstrates perivascular iron deposits in the basal ganglia and dentate nucleus. A locus, IBGC1, has been identified on chromosome 14q (54) but the responsible gene has not been identified. Treatment is symptomatic.

Lysosomal storage disorders

This is a large group of disorders including the gangliosidoses, neuronal ceroid lipofuscinosis (Batten's disease), the fucosidoses, the leucodystrophies, Niemann–Pick disease type C, and Pelizaeus–Merzbacher disease. All have systemic features but can also present with movement disorders, including dystonia. In the sphingolipidoses the pathway of degradation of sphingolipids is disrupted, either by specific enzyme deficiency or by lack of activator protein. This results in sphingolipid accumulation in one or more organs, particularly the brain. The inheritance is autosomal recessive in all these conditions except Fabry's disease and Pelizaeus–Merzbacher disease, which are X-linked.

Niemann–Pick disease type C is described in detail below. The other lysosomal storage disorders are outlined in Table 19.2.

Niemann–Pick disease type C

Niemann–Pick disease type C is an autosomal recessive lipid storage disease. Two-thirds of affected infants are of Ashkenazi Jewish parentage. Prevalence in Europe is estimated as 1 in 150 000. Defective intracellular esterification leads to the accumulation of free cholesterol in lysosymes. This causes a cholesterol 'traffic jam', possibly leading to a deficiency in membrane cholesterol and resulting in membrane dysfunction in distal axons with subsequent apoptosis. There is progressive neurological and hepatic dysfunction.

Table 19.2 Other lysosomal storage disorders which can cause dystonia

	Enzyme defect/ genetics	Infantile and juvenile forms	Adult forms	Pathology, diagnosis, prognosis
GM1 gangliosidosis	β-galactosidase gene Autosomal recessive	Early infantile form: hypotonia, failure to thrive, spasticity, macular cherry red spot, hepatosplenomegaly, dysmorphic features, seizures, death during the second year Late infantile and juvenile forms show slower progression Systemic features are uncommon	Slowly progressive extrapyramidal features, dysarthria Dystonia is more common in adult onset disease (55, 56) Usually no organomegaly or cherry-red spots	Pathology: multilamellated neuronal inclusions primarily in the basal ganglia Macroscopic: widespread atrophy Diagnosis via vacuolated lymphocytes, foam cells in bone marrow and low β-galactosidase in white cells or cultured fibroblasts Prognosis: infantile has worst outcome; death between 2 and 5 years of age
GM2 gangliosidosis (a) Tay Sachs (b) Sandhoff disease	Autosomal recessive β-hexosaminidase A subunit absent in white cells; highest carrier rate in Ashkenazi Jews β-hexosaminidase A and B subunits absent in white cells. Also affects non-Jewish infants	Almost always evident by the fourth month Infantile form: hyperacusis/ abnormal startle, psychomotor regression, spasticity, seizures, macrocephaly, cherry-red spot, blindness Juvenile form: anterior horn cell disease, extrapyramidal signs ± intermittent psychosis As above but with hepatosplenomegaly	Dystonia prominent Slowly progressive MND-type picture, tremor, dysarthria, intermittent psychosis (57)	Pathology: megalencephaly, neuronal loss, reactive gliosis; nerve cells distended with glycolipid. Inclusions preferentially located in anterior horn cells and the cerebellum in adults Enzymatic defect in serum, white blood cells, and cultured fibroblasts from skin or amniotic fluid Prognosis: infantile has worst outcome: death between 2 and 5 years of age Untreatable but some states offer screening to individuals of Jewish origin for the recessive trait
Metachromatic leukodystrophy	Mutations in ASA/ARSA gene which encodes the lysosomal protein arylsulfatase A	Manifests between the first and fourth year; progressive loss of motor and intellectual functions; ataxia, optic atrophy, spasticity and seizures; death occurs by 5 years of age Juvenile cases: developmental regression, speech disturbance, ataxia, seizures, spastic quadraparesis	Adults: slow course of dementia, peripheral neuropathy, pyramidal signs, peripheral neuropathy, seizures, ataxia Dystonia may occur in any form, typically late in the course of the disease	Pathology: demonstrates demyelination, metachromatic granule deposition in oligodendrocytes, macrophages, and neurons Diagnosis: deficiency of arylsulfatase A activity in leucocytes or cultured fibroblasts; molecular genetic testing for ARSA gene; increased urinary excretion of sulfatides with absence of arylsulfatase Prognosis: late infantile form is fatal; otherwise in most cases there is progression to quadriplegic mute state over 1–3 years; slower progression in late-onset cases.

(Continued)

Table 19.2 (Continued)

	Enzyme defect/ genetics	Infantile and juvenile forms	Adult forms	Pathology, diagnosis, prognosis
Krabbe disease (globoid cell leucodystrophy)	Galactocerebroside β-galactosidase deficiency	Infantile onset >80% of cases Psychomotor regression, extreme irritability, recurrent pyrexia of unknown origins, vomiting, seizures, stiffness, opisthotonus, and spasms, peripheral neuropathy, optic atrophy, dystonia	Adult-onset cases very rare Clinical features more variable and rate of progression may be slower	Pathology: extensive demyelination and globoid cells throughout the white matter (globoid cells are large histiocytes containing galactocerebroside) Diagnosis: enzyme deficiency in leucocytes or cultured fibroblasts Prognosis: death usually within 2 years
Pelizaeus–Merzbacher disease	Mutations of proteolipid protein gene mutations X-linked	Manifests in first 3 months of life Dystonia, nystagmus titubation, hypotonia, stridor, tremor, choreoathetosis, psychomotor retardation, cognitive impairment, peripheral neuropathy, and later spastic quadriparesis and ataxia	Milder late-onset cases: possible visual loss, areflexia, spastic paraparesis	Neuropathology demonstrates central demyelination and axonal loss Diagnosis: direct mutation analysis Prognosis: most patients never walk or lose the ability in childhood or adolescence; may plateau in the second decade before subsequent psychomotor deterioration; some with later disease onset can survive to the sixth decade or longer
Fucosidosis	Alpha-L-fucosidase deficiency, leading to accumulation of fucose-containing glycolipids and oligosaccharides Numerous mutations of FUCA1 gene	Mild to moderate psychomotor regression begins at 12–15 months, growth retardation, dysmorphism, excessive sweating, dysostosis multiplex, organomegaly, and angiokeratoma corporis diffusum	Rare: less than 100 cases, 20 of them in South Italy	Diagnosis: abnormal enzyme activity in cultured fibroblasts or leucocytes; electron microscopy: vacuoles in multiple tissues including brain and liver Prognosis: death can occur within 4–6 years; rare variant with slower progression into late childhood and adulthood

Presentation may be antenatally with fetal hydrops. Fifty per cent of cases present in the neonatal period with hypotonia, prolonged cholestatic jaundice, ascites, hepatosplenomegaly, or severe infiltrative disease manifesting in liver and/or respiratory failure. Neurological features emerge in infancy, late adolescence, or occasionally adulthood. Supranuclear gaze palsy (a hallmark of the condition), psychomotor regression, progressive dystonia, progressive ataxia, spasticity, seizures, gelastic cataplexy, dysarthria and dysphonia, and dysphagia have been described. A macular cherry-red spot is evident in about a quarter of patients. Most infants die by the end of their second year due to an intercurrent infection. Adult cases are rare and are more likely to present with dementia or psychiatric symptoms (58). Later-onset cases die in the second to third decade and adult-onset cases progress more slowly.

Diagnosis is made by demonstration of abnormal cholesterol esterification and filipin staining in cultured fibroblasts (59). Foam cells and sea-blue histiocytes can be demonstrated in bone marrow, spleen, liver, lung, lymph nodes, and tonsils, and inclusions seen in skin biopsy. Diagnosis is confirmed by demonstrating lipid trafficking defects in cultured fibroblasts and should be followed by genotyping. Ninety-five per cent of cases are caused by mutations in the *NPC1* gene (18q11) which encodes a key protein in cholesterol trafficking (60). Mutations in *NPC2* (14q24.3) account for the remaining 5% of cases (61). Prenatal testing of cultured amniocytes or DNA is available.

MRI of the brain may be normal initially but later shows marked atrophy of the cerebellum, cerebellar vermis, and corpus callosum. Neuropathological examination demonstrates lipids, particularly in the large pyramidal neurons, ballooned neurons in the basal ganglia and thalamus, axonal spheroids in the thalamus, brainstem, and cerebellum, and neurofibrillary tangles in the hippocampus, entorhinal cortex, thalamus, and basal ganglia in adults with the disease.

Inborn errors of metabolism (Table 19.3)

Lesch–Nyhan syndrome

Lesch–Nyhan syndrome is an X-linked recessive disorder caused by deficiency of the purine salvage enzyme hypoxanthine-guanine phosphoribosyltransferase (HPRT) resulting in hyperuricaemia. Affected children appear normal at birth, but hypotonia and developmental delay are evident by 3–6 months. Self-injurious behaviour begins in the second year, followed by mental retardation, extrapyramidal involvement (action dystonia, choreoathetosis, opisthotonos), and pyramidal involvement (spasticity, hyperreflexia, extensor plantar reflexes) (62). The hallmark symptom is severe and involuntary self-mutilation (e.g. biting of lips and/or fingers, head banging, eye-poking). Speech is delayed and dysarthric. Limb dystonia is universal and severe (62). There may also be truncal dystonia with dystonic tremor and opisthotonus, oromandibular and lingual dystonia (causing cheek- and lip-biting), and laryngeal dystonia. Affected children may initially be diagnosed as having cerebral palsy and most never walk. Overproduction of uric acid and subsequent deposition of uric acid crystals leads to gouty arthritis and nephropathy.

Diagnosis is suggested by the finding of hyperuricaemia. HPRT enzyme activity less than 1.5% of normal in cells (e.g, blood,

Table 19.3 Other inborn errors of metabolism with motor phenotype including dystonia

	Mechanism	Clinical course	Diagnosis
Triosephosphate isomerase (TPI) deficiency	Mutations in TPI which converts glyceraldehyde phosphate and dihydro-oxyacetone phosphate	Age of onset, 2 years Chronic haemolytic anaemia, dystonia, tremor, muscular atrophy secondary to anterior horn cell disease, corticospinal signs Death usually occurs in early childhood	TPI levels in red blood cells
Aromatic amino acid decarboxylase (AADC) deficiency	Lack of AADC leading to reduced levels of biogenic amines dopamine, serotonin, noradrenaline, and adrenaline	Onset in first year Developmental delay, oculogyric crises, opisthotonic posturing, autonomic dysfunction Bradykinesia, athetosis, myoclonic jerks, tongue-thrusting, flexor spasms Cognitive deficits are variable Variable response to dopamine agonist or non-selective MAOIs	High plasma levels of levodopa and low levels of plasma dopamine and noradrenaline metabolites CSF: low levels of homovanillic acid and 5-hydroxyindoleacetic acid and elevated 3-*O*-methyldopa Direct genetic analysis is available on a research basis
Glucose transport defects	Guanidinoacetate methyltransferase deficiency, molybdenum co-factor deficiency, and glucose transporter protein type 1 deficiency may also exhibit dystonia as part of their clinical phenotypes		

cultured fibroblasts, lymphoblasts) is diagnostic. Sequence analysis of HPRT1 is also available.

Management is symptomatic and includes the use of allopurinol (a xanthine oxidase inhibitor) to reduce uric acid and thus the risk of nephrolithiasis, gouty arthritis, and tophi. However, this does not affect the development or severity of the neurobehavioural manifestations.

Amino and organic aciduria (Table 19.4)

Disruption of the normal catabolism of amino acid or organic acid pathways should be considered in any child presenting with an encephalopathy and metabolic acidosis, or in the child with more general developmental delay. All are individually rare. Almost all these disorders are autosomal recessive.

Dystonia has been described in various other disorders of amino acid and organic acid metabolism, including methylmalonic aciduria, 4-hydroxybutyric aciduria, 3-methylglutaconic acidaemia, 2-oxoglutaric aciduria, and Hartnup disease. Measurement of serum and urinary amino and organic acids is indicated in children with no other identifiable cause of dystonia.

Mitochondrial disorders

Leigh syndrome, or subacute necrotizing encephalomyelopathy, typically occurs as the result of mutations in the gene encoding

Table 19.4 Amino and organic aciduria

Disorder	Clinical features	Investigations	Management
Glutaric aciduria type 1: mutations in the mitochondrial enzyme glutaryl-co-enzyme A dehydrogenase disrupt the metabolism of lysine, hydroxylysine, and tryptophan	Macrocephaly Subsequent encephalopathic crises (triggered by an intercurrent febrile illness) Severe generalized dystonia is common ± choreoatheotosis, progressive extrapyramidal symptoms, spasticity and seizures, and a variable degree of intellectual impairment	Neuroimaging: frontotemporal atrophy; 'batwing' or 'box-like' sylvian fissures; often subdural effusions or haematomas and retinal haemorrhages Diagnosis: increased glutaric and 3-hydroxyglutaric acid in the urine; plasma-free carnitine is reduced and glutaryl carnitine is elevated; reduced enzyme activity in fibroblasts Pathology: neuronal loss and decreased GABA levels have been demonstrated in the putamen, caudate, and pallidum with striatal degeneration and spongiform white matter	Newborn screening is used in some high-risk populations Identification is crucial before development of neurological signs Dietary restriction of lysine and tryptophan, supplemented with L-carnitine and riboflavin, prevents progression Supportive therapy (fluid, glucose, insulin repletion) during intercurrent infections Prognosis varies: death in first decade during intercurrent illness or survival into adulthood
Homocystinuria: cystathionine β-synthase deficiency	Neurodevelopmental delay, often with behavioural problems, seizures in 20%, and extrapyramidal features Marfanoid habitus Osteoporosis and scoliosis Ectopia lentis Mild mental retardation Later thromboembolic vaso-occlusive disease	Raised urinary homocysteine levels and abnormal plasma amino acid levels with elevated methionine and homocysteine and low cystine; confirmation is via assay of cystathionine β-synthase activity in fibroblast culture	Treatment with pyridoxine reduces/normalizes amino acid levels in up to 50%, may improve cognition and delay onset of thromboembolic events, ± low methionine diet with cystine and betaine supplementation Prognosis: increased risk of thromboembolic events

(Continued)

Table 19.4 (Continued)

Disorder	Clinical features	Investigations	Management
Propionic acidaemia: propionyl CoA carboxylase deficiency	Infants develop episodic severe metabolic acidosis and ketosis and encephalopathy Surviving children subsequently have severe extrapyramidal movement disorders, seizures, and developmental delay, thrombocytopenia, and neutropenia	Diagnosis: measurement of organic acids and demonstration of a decrease in propionyl-CoA carboxylase in leucocytes or fibroblasts	Supportive care Frequent feeding Low-protein diet Acidotic crises treated with protein restriction, sodium bicarbonate, carnitine, and glucose Peritoneal dialysis may be required; carnitine and biotin supplementation Prognosis varies: neurological sequelae common despite treatment
Methylmalonic aciduria: defective methylmalonyl CoA mutase	Neonatal encephalopathy Erythematous rash Hepatomegaly Later developmental delay Nephritis with renal failure 'Metabolic stroke' (acute and chronic basal ganglia involvement) Choreoathetosis, dystonia, quadriparesis, pancreatitis, growth failure, functional immune impairment, optic nerve atrophy	Analysis of organic acids in plasma and/or urine Molecular genetic testing for definitive diagnosis	Intravenous administration of alkali and L-carnitine supplements in addition to high-dose vitamin B_{12} during crises During periods of stability, diet should be low in the amino acids leucine, isoleucine, and valine

SURF-1, which is important for cytochrome-*c* oxidase assembly. Other mitochondrial enzymatic abnormalities include defects in pyruvate dehydrogenase and respiratory complexes I, II, IV, and V (63). It may be inherited in a maternal, X-linked, or autosomal recessive fashion. Onset is typically acute or subacute in infancy or childhood, often following a viral infection, with developmental regression, seizures, brainstem dysfunction, dystonia, ataxia, optic atrophy, and peripheral neuropathy. Abnormalities of ocular movement and respiration (e.g. episodic hyperventilation, apnoea) also feature. Death typically occurs by the age of 3 years. The diagnosis is supported by finding elevated levels of lactate and pyruvate in serum and CSF, an abnormal pattern of cytochrome-*c* oxidase expression on muscle biopsy, and an abnormal MRI signal and necrosis in the basal ganglia, thalamus, and brainstem. It is confirmed by molecular genetic testing. Treatment is supportive.

Leber's hereditary optic neuropathy

Mutations in mitochondrial respiratory chain complexes I, III, or IV lead to this disorder, characterized by rapid bilateral painless vision loss beginning between ages 18 and 23 (63). Males are four times more frequently affected than females. Transmission is maternal. Dystonia, ataxia, or spastic paraplegia may also occur (64, 65). The diagnosis is supported by an elevated serum lactate and microangiopathic changes in the optic fundus. Direct DNA mutation analysis is available.

Mohr–Tranebjaerg syndrome (dystonia/deafness)

This unusual disorder results from mutations in the genes encoding DDP1 or DDP2, proteins involved in mitochondrial transport. It is inherited in a recessive X-linked fashion and is characterized by sensorineural hearing loss in early childhood, progressive dystonia (which usually develops in the teens), cortical blindness, dysphagia, and paranoia (66).

Trinucleotide repeat disorders

Dystonia can also feature as part of the movement disorder phenomenology encountered in Huntington's disease, spinocerebellar ataxias (3 and 17), and dentatorubral-pallidoluysian atrophy.

Dystonia as a feature of other neurological conditions

Parkinsonian disorders

Dystonia is not uncommon in parkinsonism, including idiopathic Parkinson's disease (IPD), progressive supranuclear palsy, multiple system atrophy, and corticobasal degeneration, in addition to X-linked dystonia–parkinsonism and rapid-onset dystonia–parkinsonism described above.

In IPD it features frequently during OFF periods in patients with Parkinson's disease with motor fluctuations, and it is also seen in patients with multiple system atrophy. Corticobasal degeneration classically features a dystonic hand or foot in addition to apraxia and myoclonus; retrocollis of the neck is common in progressive supranuclear palsy (67). Dystonia is also common in autosomal recessive juvenile Parkinson disease.

Secondary dystonia

The secondary forms of dystonia (Table 19.5) are typically caused by injury to the basal ganglia and thalamus and include infarcts, tumours, vascular malformations, and trauma. Injury to cortical and brainstem structures and the cerebellum, spinal cord, and even peripheral nerves has also been associated with development of dystonia. Exposure to drugs and toxins can also cause either acute or chronic dystonia.

Table 19.5 Secondary causes of dystonia

CNS tumour	
Vascular lesion	Stroke Arteriovenous malformation
Demyelination and inflammatory	Multiple sclerosis Central pontine myelinolysis Sjügren's syndrome
Perinatal cerebral injury	Cerebral palsy Kernicterus
Infections	Encephalitis (including viral and paraneoplastic) Abscess Subacute sclerosing panencephalitis Creutzfeldt–Jakob disease
Trauma	Head or cervical cord trauma
Other	Syringomyelia Arnold–Chiari malformation Spinal stenosis Pachygyria
Drugs and toxins	See text

Hemidystonia is one of the most common manifestations of secondary dystonia associated with structural lesions (68), typically involving the caudate and the putamen (69–71). In many of these cases, dystonia is accompanied by other movement disorders such as parkinsonism, chorea, and tics.

The traditional view that dystonia arises only from basal ganglia injury has expanded to involve other brain structures. Pathoanatomical correlates of hemidystonia have been identified in the thalamus, the internal capsule, and the cortex, often in association with lesions of the basal ganglia (72). Thalamic lesions can cause limb dystonia, and the responsible lesions occur most frequently in subnuclei linked to the cerebellum, not the basal ganglia (73). Further evidence points to cerebellar circuitry involvement (74). Structural lesions associated with cervical dystonia have most commonly localized to the brainstem and cerebellum, with fewer cases localizing to the cervical spinal cord and basal ganglia. In addition, structural and functional imaging studies link damage to the cerebellum or its connections to the emergence of dystonia (75). Prominent dystonia occurs in the spinocerebellar ataxias, including some where the known neuropathology is limited to the cerebellum. Recently, abnormalities in cerebellothalamocortical pathways have been identified in torsinA DYT1 knock-in mice (76).

Drug-induced dystonia

Drug-induced dystonia may be of acute or delayed (tardive) onset and most commonly occurs with dopamine receptor blocking agents, such as neuroleptics (phenothiazines, butyrophenones, haloperidol, olanzapine, quetiapine) and antiemetics (metoclopramide, prochlorperazine, promethazine). Agents which deplete dopamine, such as tetrabenazine, may also cause dystonia, and there are also reports of dystonia occurring with use of antidepressants (SSRIs, MAOIs), calcium antagonists, general anaesthetic agents, anticonvulsants (carbamazepine, phenytoin), antimalarials, levodopa, ranitidine, ecstasy, and cocaine.

Acute dystonic reactions occur within hours or days of starting or rapidly increasing the dose of antipsychotic medications (77). Most reactions are idiosyncratic. Although less common than tardive dyskinesia, acute dystonic reactions affect approximately 6% of patients exposed to 'typical' neuroleptics and 1–2% of those exposed to 'atypical' neuroleptics (78). Risk factors for the development of acute dystonia include younger age, male sex, previous occurrence of acute dystonia, recent cocaine use, race (white vs Asian), and presence of affective disorder. Craniocervical involvement is most common; oculogyria and jaw and neck dystonias are frequently painful. Symptoms spontaneously subside over hours.

Tardive dystonia is defined as chronic dystonia present for at least a month occurring either during or within 3 months of discontinuation of neuroleptic use. Other causes of secondary dystonia must be excluded, and there should be no family history of dystonia (79). The severity of dystonia does not correlate with the duration of exposure to the medication, and young males are particularly susceptible (80). The most frequently observed clinical picture is of retrocollis (but also torticollis) or opisthotonic trunk movements. However, spread is common with segmental or generalized dystonia in most patients.

Acute dystonic reactions usually respond quickly (within 20 minutes) to intravenous anticholinergic drugs (e.g. diphenhydramine or benztropine). A subsequent short oral course of either drug is usually recommended to prevent recurrence. Tardive dystonia is often refractory, although discontinuation of neuroleptics increases the chance of remission fourfold. More promisingly, pallidal DBS has been reported to improve symptoms of patients with tardive dystonia (81).

Conclusions

The clinical assessment and diagnosis of non-primary dystonias can be difficult, and are not helped by a rather cumbersome classification system. The key point is to determine whether dystonia is a major clinical feature, or just a more minor component of the phenotype. The nature of the dystonia is also important; hemidystonia strongly suggests a contralateral basal ganglia lesion, whilst dystonia which worsens as the day progresses points to dopa-responsive dystonia, which should never be missed as it is eminently treatable. Indeed, all cases where there is predominant dystonia of young onset merit a therapeutic trial of levodopa. Where dystonia is associated with other neurological features, a broader differential diagnosis is needed, which may be guided by family history or the presence of other features. Table 19.6 attempts to guide this process by summarizing syndromic associations.

Table 19.6 Clinical clues for diagnosing dystonia syndromes

Features accompanying dystonia	Condition
Ataxia ± peripheral neuropathy	Friedreich's ataxia Ataxia telangiectasia Niemann–Pick type C Spinocerebellar ataxia (e.g. SCA3) Metachromatic leucodystrophy Wilson disease Neuroacanthocytosis

(Continued)

Table 19.6 (Continued)

Features accompanying dystonia	Condition
Dementia	Huntington's disease Spinocerebellar atrophy type 17 (SCA17) Creutzfeldt–Jakob disease PKAN Niemann–Pick type C Neuroacanthocytosis
Parkinsonism	Drugs (e.g. neuroleptics) Dopa-responsive dystonia Progressive supranuclear palsy Multiple system atrophy Corticobasal degeneration Wilson disease Rapid onset dystonia–parkinsonism Young-onset Parkinson's disease (e.g. Parkin mutations) Neuroferritinopathy Idiopathic basal ganglia calcification (Fahr's disease) Kufor–Rakeb disease PLA2G6-associated neurodegeneration (PARK14) X-linked dystonia-parkinsonism
Supranuclear gaze palsy	Progressive supranuclear palsy Niemann–Pick type C PKAN Kufor–Rakeb disease
Oculomotor apraxia	Ataxia telangiectasia Huntington's disease
Retinitis pigmentosa	PKAN (HARP) Metachromatic leucodystrophy GM2 gangliosidosis
Deafness	Mohr–Tranebjaerg syndrome Woodhouse–Sakati syndrome
Oro-bulbar involvement	Drugs (e.g. neuroleptics) PKAN Neuroferritinopathy Lesch–Nyhan syndrome Neuroacanthocytosis

References

1. Segawa M, Hosaka A, Miyagawa F, Nomura Y, Imai H. Hereditary progressive dystonia with marked diurnal fluctuation. *Adv Neurol* 1976; 14: 215–33.
2. Asmus F, Gasser T. Dystonia-plus syndromes. *Eur J Neurol* 2010; 17 (Suppl 1): 37–45.
3. Trender-Gerhard I, Sweeney MG, Schwingenschuh P, et al. Autosomal-dominant GTPCH1-deficient DRD: clinical characteristics and long-term outcome of 34 patients. *J Neurol Neurosurg Psychiatry* 2009; 80: 839–45.
4. Kong CK, Ko CH, Tong SF, Lam CW. Atypical presentation of dopa-responsive dystonia: generalized hypotonia and proximal weakness. *Neurology* 2001; 57: 1121–4.
5. Bandmann O, Valente EM, Holmans P, et al. Dopa-responsive dystonia: a clinical and molecular genetic study. *Ann Neurol* 1998; 44: 649–56.
6. Van Hove JL, Steyaert J, Matthijs G, et al. Expanded motor and psychiatric phenotype in autosomal dominant Segawa syndrome due to GTP cyclohydrolase deficiency. *J Neurol Neurosurg Psychiatry* 2006; 77: 18–23.
7. Ichinose H, Ohye T, Takahiashi E, et al. Hereditary progressive dystonia with marked diurnal fluctuation caused by mutations in the GTP cyclohydrolase I gene. *Nat Genet* 1994; 8: 236–42.
8. Furukawa Y, Guttman M, Sparagana SP, et al. Dopa-responsive dystonia due to a large deletion in the GTP cyclohydrolase I gene. *Ann Neurol* 2000; 47: 517–20.
9. Maita N, Hatakeyama K, Okada K, Hakoshima T. Structural basis of biopterin induced inhibition of GTP cyclohydrolase 1 by GFRP, its feedback regulatory protein. *J Biol Chem* 2004; 279: 51 524–40.
10. Ludecke B, Knappskog PM, Clayton PT, et al. Recessively inherited L-DOPA-responsive parkinsonism in infancy caused by a point mutation (L205P) in the tyrosine hydroxylase gene. *Hum Mol Genet* 1996; 5: 1023–8.
11. Bonafé L, Thöny B, Penzien JM, et al. Mutations in the sepiapterinreductase gene cause a novel tetrahydrobiopterin-dependent monoamine-neurotransmitter deficiency without hyperphenylalaninemia. *Am J Hum Genet* 2001; 69: 269–77.
12. Blau N, Bonafe L, Thöny B. Tetrahydrobiopterin deficiencies without hyperphenylalaninemia: diagnosis and genetics of dopa-responsive dystonia and sepiapterin reductase deficiency. *Mol Genet Metab* 2001; 74: 172–85.
13. Vidailhet M, Tassin J, Durif F, et al. A major locus for several phenotypes of myoclonus–dystonia on chromosome 7q. *Neurology* 2001; 56: 1213–16.
14. Kyllerman M, Forsgren L, Sanner G, Holmgren G, Wahlstrom J, Drugge U. Alcohol responsive myoclonic dystonia in a large family: dominant inheritance and phenotypic variation. *Mov Disord* 1990; 5: 270–9.
15. Saunders-Pullman R, Shriberg J, Heiman G, et al. Myoclonus dystonia: possible association with obsessive–compulsive disorder and alcohol dependence. *Neurology* 2002; 58: 242–5.
16. Zimprich A, Grabowski M, Asmus F, et al. Mutations in the gene encoding epsilon-sarcoglycan cause myoclonus-dystonia syndrome. *Nat Genet* 2001; 29: 66–9.
17. Marechal L, Raux G, Dumanchin C, et al. Severe myoclonus–dystonia syndrome associated with a novel epsilon-sarcoglycan gene truncating mutation. *Am J Med Genet* 2003; 119B: 114–17.
18. Kinugawa K, Vidailhet M, Clot F, et al. Myoclonus dystonia: an update. *Mov Disord* 2008; 24: 479–89.
19. Grabowski M, Zimprich A, Lorenz D, et al. The SGCE gene mutated in myoclonus dystonia is maternally imprinted. *Eur J Hum Genet* 2003; 11: 138–44.
20. Chan P, Gonzalez-Maeso J, Ruff F, Bishop DM, Hof P, Sealfon S. Epsilon-sarcoglycan immunoreactivity and mRNA expression in mouse brain. *J Comp Neurol* 2005; 482: 50–73.
21. Esapa CT, Waite A, Locke M, et al. SGCE missense mutations that cause myoclonus-dystonia syndrome impair epsilon-sarcoglycan trafficking to the plasma membrane: modulation by ubiquitination and torsinA. *Hum Mol Genet* 2007; 16: 327–42.
22. Yokoi F, Yang G, Li J, et al. Earlier onset of motor deficits in mice with double mutations in DYT1 and SGCE. *J Biochem* 2010; 148: 459–66.
23. Luciano MS, Ozelius L, Sims K, Raymond D, Liu L, Saunders-Pullman R. Responsiveness to l-dopa in epsilon sarcoglycan deletion. *Mov Disord* 2009; 24: 425–8.
24. Dobyns WB, Ozelius LJ, Kramer PL, et al. Rapid-onset dystonia–parkinsonism. *Neurology* 1993; 43: 2596–602.
25. Brashear A, de Leon D, Bressman SB, Thyagarajan D, Farlow MR, Dobyns WB. Rapid-onset dystonia parkinsonism in a second family. *Neurology* 1997; 48: 1066–9.
26. de Carvalho Aguiar P, Sweadner KJ, et al. Mutations in the Na^+/K^+-ATPase alpha3 gene ATP1A3 are associated with rapid-onset dystonia parkinsonism. *Neuron* 2004; 43: 169–75.
27. Rodacker V, Toustrup-Jensen M, Vilsen B. Mutations Phe785Leu and Thr618Met in the Na^+, K^+ ATPase, associated with familial rapid onset

dystonia-parkinsonism, interfere with Na^+ interaction by distinct mechanisms. *J Biol Chem* 2006; 281: 18 539–48.
28. Calderon DP, Fremont R, Kraenzlin F, Khodakhah K. The neural substrate of rapid onset dystonia parkinsonism. *Nat Neurosci* 2011; 14: 357–65.
29. Camargos S, Scholz S, Simon-Sanchez J, et al. DYT16, a novel young onset dystonia–parkinsonism disorder: identification of a segregating mutation in the stress response protein. *Lancet Neurol* 2008; 7: 215–22.
30. Seibler P, Djarmati A, Langpap B, et al. A heterozygous frame- shift mutation in PRKRA (DYT16) associated with generalised dystonia in a German patient. *Lancet Neurol* 2008; 7: 380–1.
31. Kurian MA, Li Y, Zhen J, et al. Clinical and molecular characterisation of hereditary dopamine transporter deficiency syndrome: an observational cohort and experimental study. *Lancet Neurol* 2011; 10: 54–62.
32. Lee LV, Munoz EL, Tan KT, Reyes MT. Sex linked recessive dystonia parkinsonism of Panay, Philippines (XDP). *Mol Pathol* 2001; 54: 362–8.
33. Evidente VGH, Advincula J,Esteban R,et al. The phenomenology of "Lubag" or x-linked dystonia-parkinsonism. *Mov Disord.* 2002; 17: 1271–7.
34. Eidelberg D, Takikawa S, Wilhelmsen K, Dhawan V, Chaly T, Robeson W, et al. Positron emission tomographic findings in Filipino X-linked dystonia-parkinsonism. *Ann Neurol* 1993; 34(2): 185–91.
35. Goto S, Lee LV, Minoz FL, et al. Functional anatomy of the basal ganglia in X-linked recessive dystonia parkinsonism. *Ann Neurol* 2005; 58: 7–17.
36. Makino S, Kaji R, Ando S, et al. Reduced neuron-specific expression of the TAF1 gene is associated with X-linked dystonia-parkinsonism. *Am J Hum Genet* 2007; 80: 393–406.
37. Sako W, Morigaki R, Kaji R, et al. Identification and localization of neuron-specific isoform of TAF1 in rat brain: implications for neuropathology of DYT3 dystonia. *Neuroscience* 2011; 189: 100–7.
38. Martinez-Torres I, Limousin P, Tisch S, et al. Early and marked benefit with GPi deep brain stimulation for Lubag syndrome presenting with rapidly progressive life threatening dystonia. *Mov Disord* 2009; 24: 1710–12.
39. Svetel M, Kozić D, Stefanova E, Semnic R, Dragasevic N, Kostic VS. Dystonia in Wilson's disease. *Mov Disord* 2001; 16: 719–23.
40. Schneider S, Hardy J, Bhatia KP. Syndromes of neurodegeneration with brain iron accumulation (NBIA): an update on clinical presentation, histological and genetic underpinnings and treatment considerations. *Mov Disord* 2012; 27: 42–53.
41. Gregory A, Polster BJ, Hayflick SJ. Clinical and genetic delineation of neurodegeneration with brain iron accumulation. *J Med Genet* 2009; 46: 73–80.
42. Castelnau P, Cif L, Valente EM, Vayssiere N, Hemm S, Gannau A, Digiorgio A, Coubes P. Pallidal stimulation improves pantothenate kinase-associated neurodegeneration. *Ann Neurol* 2005; 57: 738–41.
43. Krause M, Fogel W, Tronnier V, Pohle S, Hörtnagel K, Thyen U, Volkmann J. Long-term benefit to pallidal deep brain stimulation in a case of dystonia secondary to pantothenate kinase-associated neurodegeneration. *Mov Disord* 2006; 21: 2255–7.
44. Zorzi G, Zibordi F, Chiapparini L, et al. Iron-related MRI images in patients with pantothenate kinase–associated neurodegeneration (PKAN) treated with deferiprone: Results of a phase II pilot trial. *Movement Disorders* 2011; 26: 1755–9.
45. Curtis AR, Fey C, Morris CM, et al. Mutation in the gene encoding ferritin light polypeptide causes dominant adult-onset basal ganglia disease. *Nat Genet* 2001; 28: 350–4.
46. Chinnery PF, Crompton DE, Birchall D, et al. Clinical features and natural history of neuroferritinopathy caused by the FTL1 460InsA mutation. *Brain* 2007; 130: 110–19.
47. Barbeito AG, Levade T, Delisle M, Ghetti B, Vidal R. Abnormal iron metabolism in fibroblasts from a patient with the neurodegenerative disease hereditary ferritinopathy. *Mol Neurodegener* 2010; 5: 50.
48. Gregory A, Westaway SK, Holm IE, et al. Neurodegeneration associated with genetic defects in phospholipase A(2). *Neurology* 2008; 71: 1402–9.
49. Schneider, SA, Bhatia KP, Hardy J. Complicated recessive dystonia parkinsonism syndromes. *Mov Disord* 2009; 24: 490–9.
50. Paisan-Ruiz C, Bhatia KP, Li A, et al. Characterization of PLA2G6 as a locus for dystonia-parkinsonism. *Ann Neurol* 2009; 65: 19–23.
51. Flint J, Goldstein LH. Familial calcification of the basal ganglia: a case report and review of the literature. *Psychol Med* 1992; 22: 581–95.
52. Larsen TA, Dunn HG, Jan JE, Calne DB. Dystonia and calcification of the basal ganglia. *Neurology* 1985; 35: 533–7.
53. Manyam BV, Walters AS, Keller IA, Ghobrial M. Parkinsonism associated with autosomal dominant bilateral striopallidodentate calcinosis. *Parkinsonism Relat Disord* 2001a; 7: 289.
54. Geschwind DH, Loginov M, Stern JM. Identification of a locus on chromosome 14q for idiopathic basal ganglia calcification (Fahr disease). *Am J Hum Genet* 1999; 65: 764–72.
55. Goldman JE, Katz D, Rapin I, Purpura DP, Suzuki K. Chronic GM1-gangliosidosis presenting as dystonia: I. clinical and pathological features. *Ann Neurol* 1981; 9: 465–75.
56. Nakano T, Ikeda S, Kondo K, Yanagisawa N, Tsuji S. Adult GM1-gangliosidosis: clinical patterns and rectal biopsy. *Neurology* 1985; 35: 875–80.
57. Oates CE, Bosch EP, Hart MN. Movement disorders associated with chronic GM2 gangliosidosis. *Eur Neurol* 1986; 25: 154–9.
58. Imrie J, Vijayaraghaven S, Whitehouse C, et al. Niemann–Pick disease type C in adults. *J Inherit Metab Dis* 2002; 25: 491–500.
59. Roff CF, Goldin E, Comly ME, et al. Niemann–Pick type C disease: Deficient intracellular transport of exogenously derived cholesterol. *Am J Med Genet* 1992; 42: 593–8.
60. Carstea ED, Morris JA, Coleman KG, et al. Niemann–Pick C1 disease gene: homology to mediators of cholesterol homeostasis. *Science* 1997; 277: 228–31.
61. Naureckiene S, Sleat DE, Lackland H, et al. Identification of HE1 as the second gene of Niemann–Pick C disease. *Science* 2000; 290: 2298–301.
62. Jinnah HA, Visser JE, Harris JC, et al. Delineation of the motor disorders of Lesch–Nyhan syndrome. *Brain* 2006; 129: 1201–17.
63. Schmiedel J, Jackson S, Schafer J, Reichmann H. Mitochondrial cytopathies. *J Neurol* 2003; 250: 267–77.
64. Novotny EJ, Jr, Singh G, Wallace DC, et al. Leber's disease and dystonia: a mitochondrial disease. *Neurology* 1986; 36: 1053–60.
65. Watanabe M, Mita S, Takita T, Goto Y, Uchino M, Imamura S. Leber's hereditary optic neuropathy with dystonia in a Japanese family. *J Neurol Sci* 2006; 243: 31–4.
66. Jin H, May M, Tranebjaerg L, et al. A novel X-linked gene, DDP, shows mutations in families with deafness (DFN-1), dystonia, mental deficiency and blindness. *Nat Genet* 1996; 14: 177–80.
67. Jankovic J, Tintner R. Dystonia and parkinsonism. *Parkinsonism Relat Disord* 2001; 8: 109–21.
68. Svetel M, Ivanovic N, Marinkovic J, Jovic J, Dragasevic N, Kostic VS. Characteristics of dystonic movements in primary and symptomatic dystonias. *J Neurol Neurosurg Psychiatry* 2004; 75: 329–30.
69. Krauss JK, Mohadjer M, Braus DF, Wakhloo AK, Nobbe F, Mundinger F. Dystonia following head trauma: a report of nine patients and review of the literature. *Mov Disord* 1992; 7: 263–72.
70. Bhatia KP, Marsden CD. The behavioral and motor consequences of focal lesions of the basal ganglia in man. *Brain* 1994; 117: 859–76.
71. Munchau A, Mathen D, Cox T, Quinn NP, Marsden CD, Bhatia KP. Unilateral lesions of the globus pallidus: report of four patients presenting with focal or segmental dystonia. *J Neurol Neurosurg Psychiatry* 2000; 69: 494–8.
72. Chuang C, Fahn S, Frucht SJ. The natural history and treatment of acquired hemidystonia: report of 33 cases and review of the literature. *J Neurol Neurosurg Psychiatry* 2002; 72: 59–67.

73. Lehericy S, Grand S, Pollak P, et al. Clinical characteristics and topography of lesion in movement disorders due to thalamic lesions. *Neurology* 2001; 57: 1055–66.
74. Jinnah HA, Hess EJ. A new twist on the anatomy of dystonia: the basal ganglia and the cerebellum. *Neurology* 2006; 67: 1740–1.
75. Hallett M. Pathophysiology of dystonia. *J Neural Transm Suppl* 2006; 70: 485–8.
76. Ulug AM, Vo A, Argyelan M, et al. Cerebellar thalamocortical pathways are abnormal in torsinA DYT1 knock-in mice. *Proc Natl Acad Sci USA* 2011; 108: 6638–43.
77. Diederich NJ, Goetz CG. Drug-induced movement disorders. *Neurol Clin* 1998; 16: 125–39.
78. Pierre JM. Extrapyramidal symptoms with atypical antipsychotics: incidence,prevention and management. *Drug Saf* 2005; 28: 191–208.
79. Burke RE, Fahn S, Jankovic J, et al. Tardive dystonia: late-onset and persistent dystonia caused by antipsychotic drugs. *Neurology* 1982; 32: 1335–46.
80. Kiriakakis V, Bhatia KP, Quinn NP, Marsden CD. The natural history of tardive dystonia. A long-term follow-up study of 107 cases. *Brain* 1998; 121: 2053–66.
81. Capelle H, Blahak C, Schrader C, et al. Chronic deep brain stimulation in patients with tardive dystonia without a history of major psychosis. *Mov Disord* 2010; 25: 1477–81.

CHAPTER 20

Huntington's Disease

Roger A. Barker and Josef Priller

Summary

Huntington's disease (HD) is a rare autosomal dominant neurodegenerative condition that commonly presents in mid life with a combination of a movement disorder, psychiatric, and cognitive problems. The identification of the gene underlying HD in 1993 has led to many major breakthroughs in our understanding of this disease, but it remains incurable and fatal to the present time. Our better understanding of the range of clinical features seen in this complex neuropsychiatric disorder and our ability to detect those earliest changes is leading to a new era of drugs trials for HD with the prospect of identifying disease-modifying agents. There is also a new impetus to look at drugs to better treat the symptoms and signs of HD as well as better support the patients and their families in the community. In this chapter we outline some of these therapies as well as providing clinical tips on how best to assess the HD patient.

Essential background

Epidemiology

HD is a rare genetic disorder which affects men and women equally (1). The prevalence rates are between 4 and 10 per 100 000 in Europe and the USA (2, 3), while HD is less frequent in Finland and Asian countries (around 0.5 per 100 000). In contrast, it is highly prevalent in some isolated populations, e.g. Lake Maracaibo in Venezuela (>5000 per 100 000) and in secluded parts of Europe (4–6). Recent data from the UK Huntington's Disease Association suggests that the true prevalence of HD may be >12 per 100 000 (7). HD prevalence rates are beginning to rise with improved care and life expectancy (8), although the numbers are confounded by the low rates of predictive testing in the HD at-risk population. Moreover, the frequency of HD is likely to have been underestimated in the black American and African populations, where considerable genetic heterogeneity exists and the variant Huntington's disease-like 2 is more frequent (9, 10).

Aetiology and genetics

HD is caused by a CAG (cytosine–adenine–guanine) trinucleotide repeat expansion in the first exon of the *huntingtin* gene on chromosome 4p (11). Inheritance is autosomal dominant with full penetrance when the number of CAG repeats is >39 and with incomplete penetrance for 36–39 CAG repeats (12, 13). The normal alleles range from 9 to 11 CAG repeats at the low end to 34–35 at the high end (14), and so every human being carries CAG repeats in the *huntingtin* gene. HD shows complete dominance, as no difference of phenotype is observed between homozygotes and heterozygotes apart from the fact that the homozygotes may progress more quickly (15, 16). There is, however, a strong correlation between the age of onset in HD and the number of CAG repeats (13, 17). Furthermore, the trinucleotide repeat is unstable on replication and shows a propensity to expand, particularly during spermatogenesis (18, 19). This accounts for the phenomenon of *genetic anticipation*, in which the age of onset of HD tends to diminish in successive generations, with juvenile-onset cases (i.e. HD before the age of 21 years) commonly arising from paternal transmission. A *cis*-acting haplogroup A comprising 22 single-nucleotide polymorphisms was identified, which may predispose Europeans to CAG instability (20). New-onset cases of HD with a negative family history can arise from a parent with an intermediate-size CAG repeat (27–35), which has expanded into the pathological range in gametes (21). On the other hand, there is also evidence for contraction of CAG repeats during transmission (21).

Recently, normal and mutant *huntingtin* were found to interact to affect disease severity in HD, which weakens the association between mutant CAG repeat length and age of onset. Normal alleles at the high end are associated with an earlier age of onset when mutant CAG repeat length is low (36–44) and with a later age of onset when mutant CAG repeat length is >44 (17). In general, the CAG repeat number only explains 60–70% of the variance in age of onset, with the remainder being influenced by modifier genes and the environment (22). Therefore we strongly recommend against making prognostic statements based on the number of CAG repeats in the *huntingtin* gene. Indeed, to reinforce this point, it has been reported that there is a remarkable phenotypic discordance for HD in monozygotic twins (23, 24), and CAG repeat length mosaicism may account for some of this (24). In terms of genetic modifiers, polymorphisms in the glutamate receptor GluR6, the *N*-methyl-D-aspartate (NMDA) receptor subunits 2A/B (GRIN2A/B), and the huntingtin-associated protein 1 (HAP-1) genes have all been described (25, 26).

Pathophysiology

It was hoped that the identification of the gene causing HD in 1993 would quickly lead to an understanding of the pathophysiology of the condition and with this a cure. However, nearly 20 years later it is still unclear exactly how the mutant huntingtin causes disease, and indeed what the function of normal huntingtin is (see Fig. 20.1).

Huntingtin is a ubiquitously expressed protein of high molecular weight (348 kDa). The CAG repeat in the huntingtin gene translates into a polyglutamine (polyQ) strand in the N-terminal part of this protein, which may have emerged more recently in evolution compared with the ancient rest of the molecule, along with more complex brain development (27). Huntingtin is a vital protein; mice deficient in the huntingtin gene show early embryonic death prior to the formation of the nervous system (28). Reductions of huntingtin levels below 50% result in structural abnormalities of the cortex and striatum (29), suggesting that huntingtin is implicated in normal brain development and that loss of normal huntingtin function may be at least in part involved in HD pathogenesis. In fact, huntingtin is an anti-apoptotic protein, which protects neurons from excitotoxic cell death (30). Normal huntingtin also stimulates the transcription of brain-derived neurotrophic factor (BDNF) and secures the vital delivery of BDNF to striatal neurons via corticostriatal afferents, which may explain the particular vulnerability of these brain regions in HD (31). Importantly, normal huntingtin is

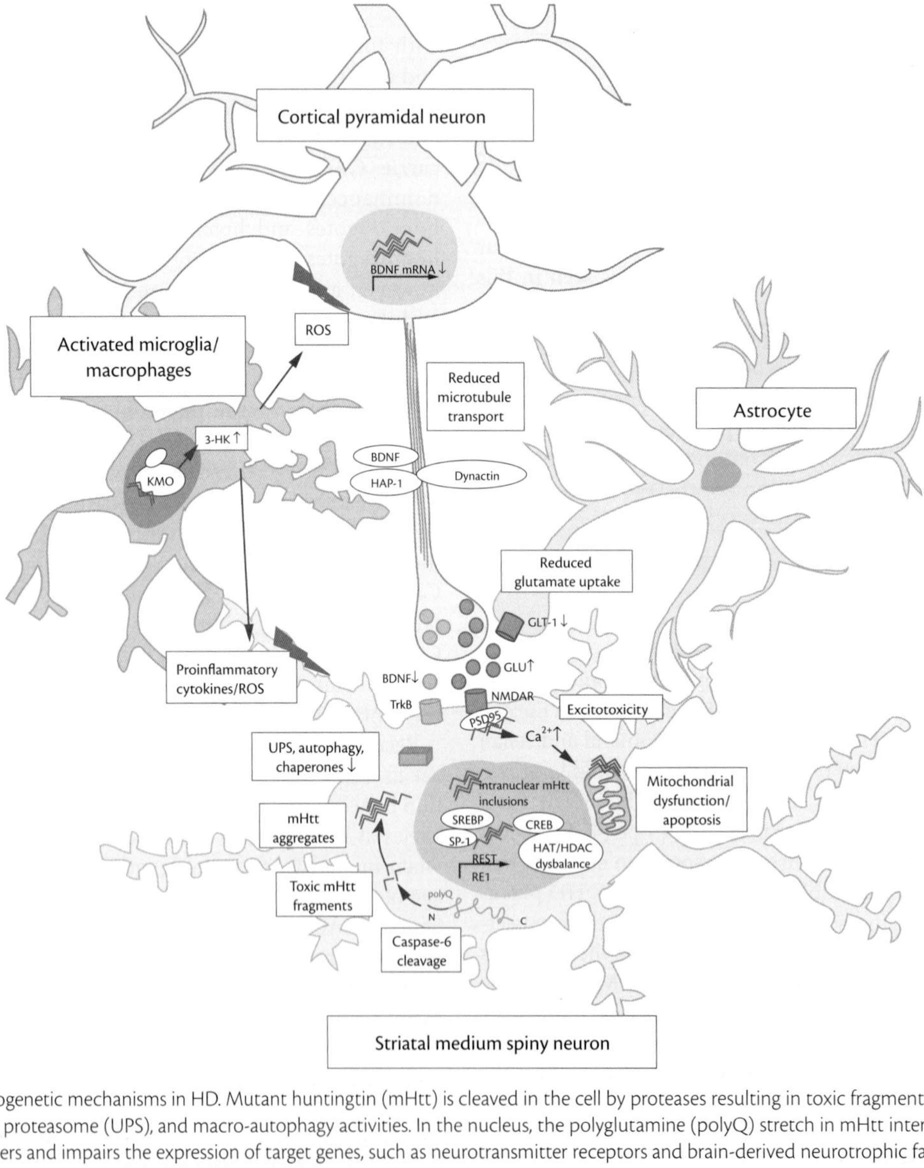

Fig. 20.1 Potential pathogenetic mechanisms in HD. Mutant huntingtin (mHtt) is cleaved in the cell by proteases resulting in toxic fragments, which aggregate and interfere with chaperone, proteasome (UPS), and macro-autophagy activities. In the nucleus, the polyglutamine (polyQ) stretch in mHtt interacts with transcription factors/epigenetic modifiers and impairs the expression of target genes, such as neurotransmitter receptors and brain-derived neurotrophic factor (BDNF). Medium spiny neurons in the striatum are particularly vulnerable in HD. They depend on BDNF which is delivered by cortical neurons, but less so in HD since vesicular transport along microtubules is disturbed by mHtt. Medium spiny neurons also depend on glutamate release from cortical afferents. In HD, excitotoxic damage results from enhanced NMDA glutamate receptor sensitivity on striatal neurons, reduced clearance of extracellular glutamate by the astroglial glutamate transporter (GLT)-1, and mHtt-mediated impairment of mitochondrial calcium buffering capacity, which promotes apoptosis. Microglia and macrophages are activated in HD and secrete proinflammatory cytokines. Kynurenine 3-monooxygenase (KMO) also produces 3-hydroxykynurenine (3-HK), a free radical generator (ROS) that mediates neuronal cell death.

involved in intraneuronal vesicular transport and axonal trafficking (32), as well as synaptic transmission.

An overwhelming body of evidence suggests that HD results from a toxic gain of function of the mutant huntingtin protein. Huntingtin has numerous sites for post-translational modifications (e.g. phosphorylation, palmitoylation, acetylation, ubiquitination, and sumoylation) which control protein stability, localization, and function. These processes can be impaired by mutant huntingtin, resulting in enhanced neurotoxicity due to reduced clearance by the proteasome, the lysosome, or autophagy (33, 34). Post-translational modifications also play a role in the proteolytic cleavage of huntingtin by caspases, calpain, and other proteases. Cleavage of huntingtin by caspase-6 appears to be a critical event in HD pathogenesis (35). Proteolysis of huntingtin liberates toxic fragments with expanded polyQ, which are prone to aggregate. In fact, ubiquitinated mutant huntingtin aggregates are a neuropathological hallmark of HD, and are present as nuclear and cytoplasmic inclusions in cortical neurons and in the medium-sized spiny neurons in the striatum, which are particularly vulnerable to degeneration (36). Nuclear aggregates are mainly composed of N-terminal huntingtin fragments comprising the polyQ strand, whereas cytoplasmic inclusions contain full-length and truncated mutant huntingtin (37). Aggregate formation occurs via soluble and non-soluble intermediates, including oligomers, globular intermediates, protofibrils, and amyloid-like fibres. The propensity of mutant huntingtin fragments to form amyloid-like aggregates depends on the polyQ repeat length, the protein concentration, and time (38), which may help to explain why disease manifestation requires a certain CAG repeat length. Failure of the ubiquitin–proteasome system (UPS) to degrade mutant huntingtin is implicated in aggregate formation and may explain the preferential vulnerability of neurons in HD, which have lower UPS activity compared with glia (39). However, controversy still exists over whether mutant huntingtin aggregates are neurotoxic or neuroprotective. Toxicity could arise from the sequestration of transcription factors in the nucleus or from interference with the axonal transport machinery. On the other hand, aggregation of mutant huntingtin could also represent an attempt by neurons to sequester toxic soluble oligomers and globular and protofibril intermediates. Along these lines, pharmacological promotion of inclusion formation was found to reduce the toxicity of mutant huntingtin (40). Aggregate formation could also be protective by stimulating the clearance of mutant huntingtin via autophagy, i.e. the process of sequestration of intracellular proteins and organelles by autophagosomes and their subsequent degradation upon fusion with lysosomes (41). There is ample evidence to suggest that mutant huntingtin directly interferes with the cellular transcription machinery. Expanded polyQ repeat huntingtin can bind to DNA to repress transcription (42), or it can inhibit the activity of transcription factors and co-activators on gene promoters—for example, SP1 and TFIID/TFIIF (43), CBP and CREB (44), and SREBP and SRE (45). The latter also implicate impaired brain cholesterol biosynthesis in the pathogenesis of HD (46). Target genes of REST/NRSF, including BDNF (promoter II), are downregulated in HD as a result of loss of normal huntingtin function, increased REST/NRSF release, and activation of the nuclear RE1/NRSE silencer (46). Epigenetic modifications, such as acetylation and deacetylation of histones, also play a role in HD. The expanded polyQ binds to the acetyltransferase domain of the CREB-binding protein (CBP) and blocks its activity, resulting in reduced gene transcription (47). This can be overcome by the administration of histone deacetylase (HDAC) inhibitors. Besides transcriptional dysregulation, loss of BDNF in corticostriatal afferents also results from impaired vesicular transport of BDNF in HD, possibly as a result of reduced association of the huntingtin–HAP-1–p150 dynactin complex with microtubules (48).

Mutant huntingtin may promote problems within the local neuronal microenvironment and the dialogue between neurons and glia, causing excitotoxicity in glutamate-rich areas, such as the striatum. In fact, astrocytes, which express mutant huntingtin, fail to remove extracellular glutamate because of the downregulation of the glial glutamate transporter GLT-1 (49). Moreover, striatal neurons show increased sensitivity of NMDA receptors as a result of reduced gene expression and increased calpain cleavage of the NR2B subunit (50). The polyQ in mutant huntingtin also impairs the ability of normal huntingtin to bind to the postsynaptic density (PSD) 95 molecule, resulting in the sensitization of NMDA receptors (51). Loss of striatal cannabinoid CB1 receptors (52) and downregulation of dopamine D1 and D2 receptors (53) also render striatal neurons more sensitive to excitotoxicity. The overactivation of glutamate receptors results in increased intracellular calcium concentrations in neurons, worsened by the fact that mutant huntingtin also enhances calcium release via intracellular inositol (1,4,5)-triphosphate receptors (54). In addition, mitochondria from patients with HD exhibit defects in calcium homeostasis, and they depolarize at lower calcium loads (55). The alterations in mitochondrial function may be due to direct deleterious effects of mutant huntingtin on mitochondria, changes in energy metabolism and/or interaction of mutant huntingtin with transcription factors that regulate the expression of genes responsible for mitochondrial function, e.g. PGC-1 alpha (56). Mutant huntingtin also increases p53 levels and promotes apoptosis (57).

In addition, there is now great interest in the role of inflammation in neurodegenerative processes within the brain. PET studies revealed that microglia are activated in HD, and the degree of microglial activation correlates with disease severity and striatal atrophy (58). Involvement of the innate immune system in HD is also emphasized by findings of elevated cytokine levels, such as interleukin 6, in the peripheral blood of pre-manifest HD gene carriers (59). Recently, a link between the kynurenine pathway generated by tryptophan degradation and neurodegeneration was established (60). Kynurenine 3-mono-oxygenase (KMO) is expressed at high levels in macrophages and functions as a branching point of the kynurenine pathway. KMO metabolizes kynurenine to 3-hydroxykynurenine (3-HK), a free-radical generator (ROS) that mediates neuronal cell death. Peripheral inhibition of KMO confers neuroprotection through the accumulation of kynurenic acid (60).

Whatever the exact pathophysiological mechanisms in HD, the net result is neuronal dysfunction, shrinkage, and ultimately loss in a wide range of structures, which have traditionally been classified using striatal atrophy and Vonsattel staging (61). This approach, whilst being a useful way to stage tissue for analysis, can be misleading as it relegates the atrophy and cell loss at other sites to being of secondary importance, when this might well not be the case given much of the recent imaging and clinical work in pre-manifest and established disease (62, 63). Whatever the exact sequence of pathological events and cell loss, the advanced HD brain is characterized by extensive neuronal loss, atrophy, and the formation of intracellular inclusions with a marked astrogliosis (64).

Clinical features (see videos and Table 20.1)

The clinical features of HD are well described and classically consist of a triad of problems involving disorders of movement, cognition, and mood (65). However, which of these is predominant varies from patient to patient, and indeed there are a host of other features that are now increasingly recognized as being a part of HD, and which may even occur before the overt motor features of the illness.

The earliest features of HD vary depending on the extent to which one searches for deficits (63), but in clinic they are often the choreiform movements (see Videos 20.1 and 20.2) which typically are brought out by walking or other motor actions, such as repetitive hand-tapping. These movements often consist of slight flicks of chorea around the head, shoulder, or fingers, and are often not noticed by the patient themselves. Indeed it is worth asking the patient's partner whether they have noticed abnormal fidgety movements at night in bed or in the evening when the patient is resting. With time, these movements become more prominent and involve all body parts symmetrically; it is very unusual to see any major asymmetry. The resultant picture is of patients with involuntary facial grimaces and smiles, a tongue that they cannot keep protruded (see Video 20.3), and slightly slurred speech. Their gait becomes abnormal in a way that is hard to characterize, as it has elements of chorea, dystonia, and some ataxia (see Video 20.4). As the patients advance, they often move into a phase of the illness where the chorea becomes less prominent and is replaced by a more bradykinetic dystonic movement disorder (see Fig. 20.2), with signs of spasticity in the legs and, in some instances, a degree of hemiballismus which is very hard to treat (see below). In younger-onset cases, especially the juvenile Westphal variant of HD, the patient typically develops a parkinsonian syndrome with relatively little if any chorea (66).

Whilst these are the typical movement disorders seen in HD, some patients, especially younger-onset cases, can develop myoclonus, but tremor is very rare and any focal motor deficits should

Table 20.1 Clinical features of HD

Motor	Chorea; ballismus; dystonia; parkinsonism
Cognitive	Frontal executive dysfunction with problems of set-shifting and attention; dementia in advanced cases
Psychiatric	Depression; mood swings; impulsiveness and irritability; suicidality; paranoia and psychotic episodes; obsessive behaviour; apathy
Non classical features: • epilepsy • circadian rhythm abnormalities with insomnia and daytime somnolence • weight loss • vomiting • constipation	

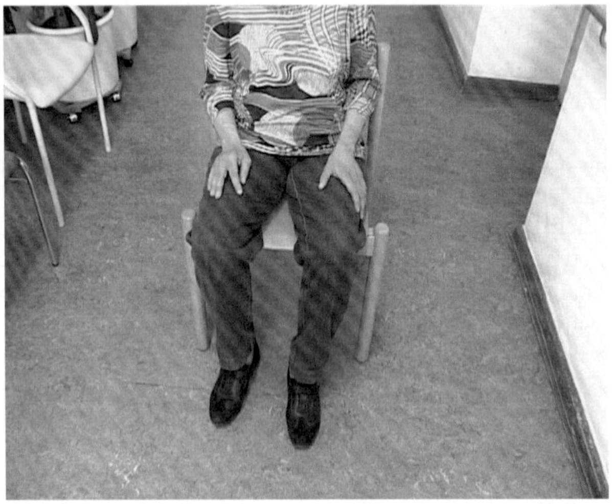

Video 20.2 Common choreiform movements of the extremities and trunk.

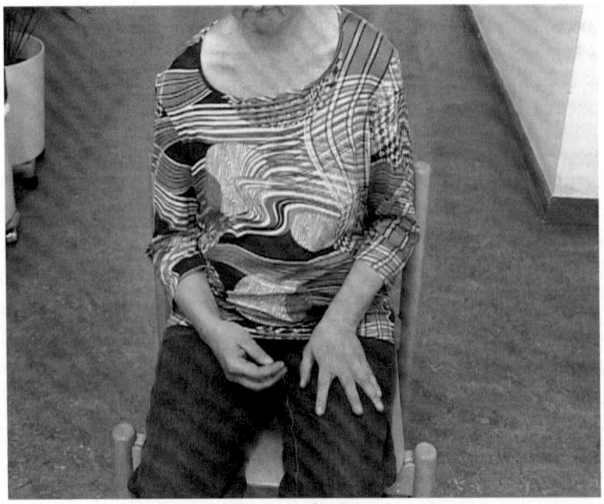

Video 20.1 Intermittent choreiform movements of the extremities and trunk.

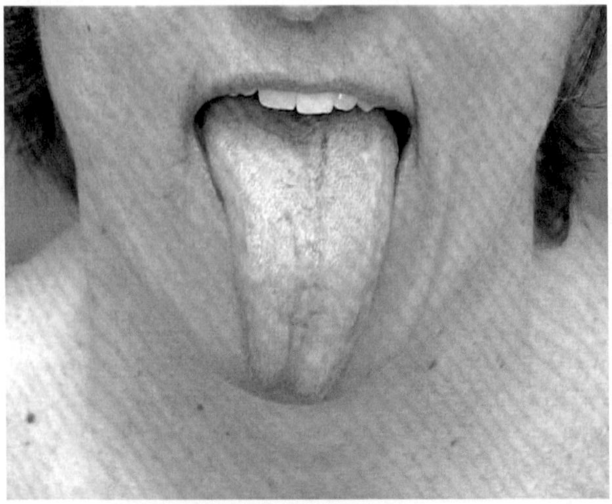

Video 20.3 Impersistence of tongue protrusion.

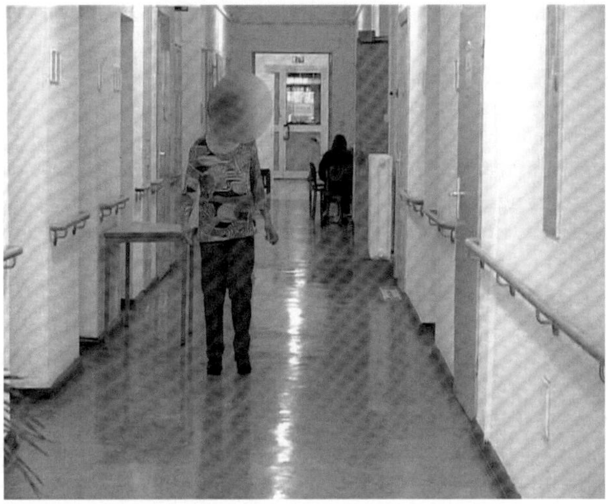

Video 20.4 Choreiform and dystonic gait.

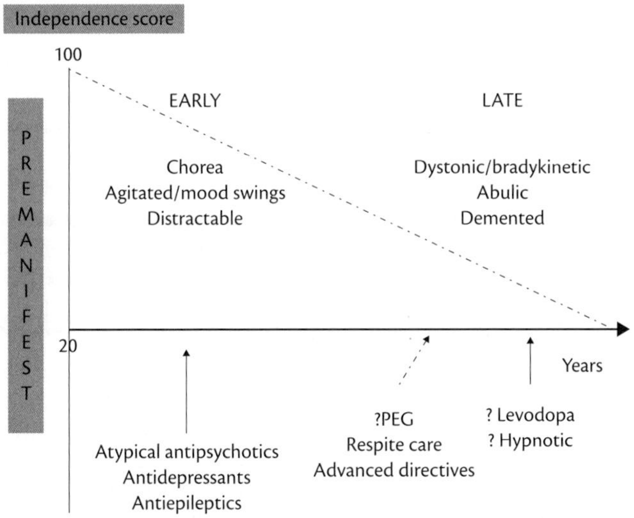

Fig. 20.2 Schematic diagram of the progress of HD over time.

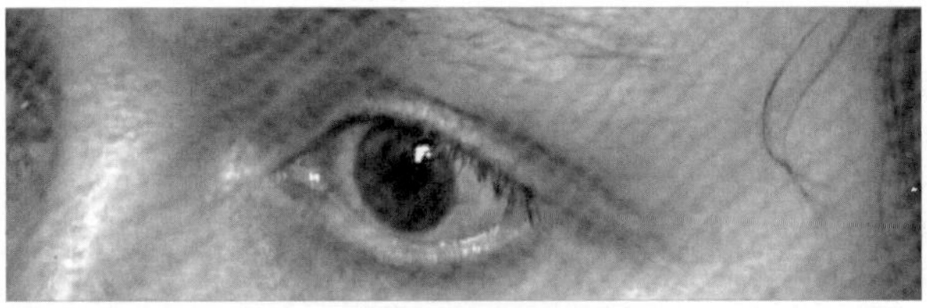

Video 20.5 Impaired ocular pursuit and saccades.

be investigated as they are not a feature of HD. Eye-movement abnormalities in terms of problems of saccadic movements are common—initially slowed, leading on to problems of initiation with head movements to compensate (see Video 20.5). The same is also true of smooth pursuit eye movements: in the early stages they can be jerky and/or interrupted (see Video 20.5) before becoming more impaired and almost absent in advanced disease. These eye-movement abnormalities are often more obvious in younger-onset cases and should always be specifically assessed in any patient with suspected HD.

Cognitively, the earliest deficits in HD are an inability to make decisions about issues that are often not that important, such as choosing outfits to wear or food items to buy. Some patients can articulate these types of deficit, but more typically patients and their families complain that the patient has lost the ability to make decisions over complex issues or that they are fine as long as they follow routines. Thus a change in circumstance (job change etc.) can sometimes precipitate and expose the cognitive problems which become more apparent as the disease progresses, with all patients developing dementia in the advanced stages of the disease. These cognitive abnormalities can be seen by using formal neuropsychological tests such as the STROOP or trail-making tasks and highlight that the early cognitive deficits have a mainly frontostriatal basis (67, 68). It is very rare for patients with HD to present with major memory or language deficits, and it is worth remembering that a patient who has become almost mute could be depressed. This may also be important in some patients who, for some reason, seem to have suddenly become much more cognitively impaired.

Psychiatric features can be very varied (69, 70). Some patients remain well throughout their illness, with no florid psychiatric features. However, some patients can develop depression, which may be exacerbated by some of the medications used to treat the motor features of HD (e.g. tetrabenazine). In other cases the depression seems to run independently of the disease (i.e. precedes the development of overt motor features of the illness by years). The most common problems in the early stages of HD are much more likely to be irritability and impulsiveness as well as major mood swings, with patients getting very worked up over often trivial issues. This can lead to violent outbursts and problems with the law. Moreover, one in four HD patients attempts suicide (71, 72). With time these problems resolve and are often replaced by a more abulic apathetic stage of disease which can be very frustrating for the carers and family, as it can be perceived as the patient being lazy.

Psychotic problems can be seen in HD but are less common than perseverations. When present, these can cause profound problems, as can the more frontal presentation of HD when patients have no insight into their problems so that they do not seek help or take the required medication for their condition (73). Finally, in juvenile HD, behavioural problems can be the dominant problem with development of obsessive behaviours associated with violent outbursts when confronted about them.

Other features which can also be seen in HD include the following.

- Circadian rhythm disturbances may begin early in the course of the illness and become more obvious once an imposed sleep–wake regime is lost (e.g. end of employment) (74, 75). This can create major management problems as the partner of the patient may have to adopt a similar sleep–wake cycle whilst still trying to work normally.
- Weight loss is very common and can be due to problems of dysphagia, mood, and motivation as well as depression. However, there may also be a more fundamental problem with metabolism in this condition which predisposes patients to lose weight (76).
- Epilepsy is rarely seen, and when present tends to occur in young-onset cases.
- Vomiting and constipation are common in advanced patients, but whether this reflects a degree of autonomic or enteric nervous system involvement is unclear.

Diagnosis

The diagnosis of HD is straightforward in the right clinical context, given the ease with which one can test for the mutant gene. There are two main situations in which a genetic test is needed or requested: the first is in the manifest patient when a diagnostic test is needed to confirm the diagnosis; the second situation is when an individual at risk of developing HD wishes to have a genetic test to ascertain if they carry the mutant gene (77). In both cases genetic counselling is needed, given the implications of a positive test to the patients and their family.

In the case of a manifest patient, the need to ascertain the family history is important—check that when there is no apparent family history, the age at which the parents died is known as their early death may hide the family history. However, given that HD is the most common cause of chorea (apart from levodopa-induced dyskinesias in Parkinson's disease), undertaking the genetic test is logical and it is only worth looking for the other rarer causes of chorea if it is negative (see Chapters 21 and 22).

There are clear guidelines as to how predictive testing can best be done, given the implications of a positive test to future employment, life assurance, etc (78). If a patient tests positive for the abnormal gene, it is our practice to follow them up so that they can be assessed for early features and often reassured that many symptoms that they have are normal with ageing. There are currently two major studies looking at pre-manifest patients, TRACK-HD (79) and PREDICT-HD (80), with the aim of identifying cognitive, motor, imaging, and biomarker tests. Such a result would not only help in informing patients as to whether the disease has actually begun, but would also open up a window for introducing disease-modifying therapies earlier.

Management

The management of HD patients (70, 81, 82) is best done in a multidisciplinary clinic which should include a number of different medical specialities (see Table 20.2). The involvement of such a team enables all aspects of patient care to be addressed, and not just from a pharmacological perspective. Having the team available outside the clinic appointment is also helpful, given that most family doctors understandably have limited knowledge and lack confidence in managing this condition.

In the early stages of the disease, management is mainly supportive and provision of reassurance; treating the movement disorder is not necessary unless the patient has a disability secondary to it. When the chorea becomes severe enough to merit therapy, a number of possible agents can be considered, but those used most commonly are the antipsychotic drugs, olanzapine and tiapride, or the catecholamine-depleting agent, tetrabenazine (TBZ). Olanzapine can be given once a day starting at 2.5 mg and increasing to a maximum dose of 20 mg. Tiapride is often given at 50–100 mg tds with a maximum daily dose of 1200 mg. TBZ is given two or three times a day, starting at around 12.5 mg bd/tds with a maximum dose of 200 mg/day. In addition to the antichorea effects, olanzapine has a number of other desirable properties in that it helps patients sleep if it is given at night and it calms down the mood swings that are common in HD. The drug effectively suppresses chorea in most people, but it causes increased appetite and therefore weight gain, which may be of value given the problems of weight loss in many cases. The main side effects of olanzapine are unacceptable weight gain and daytime sedation. In contrast, TBZ is the only proven drug to treat the chorea of HD, but can cause daytime sedation and, in some cases, depression. Tiapride is also efficacious in controlling the hyperkinesias and gait disturbance associated with HD. Other drugs that can be used to help treat the chorea are sulpiride, amisulpiride, risperidone, and other antipsychotics. Some patients do not respond to these drugs, and anecdotally other agents have been tried with some success including baclofen, amantadine, and nabilone in refractory cases. The role for pallidal deep brain stimulation is contentious, with the first clinical studies underway to test its use in treating the chorea of HD.

Table 20.2 Members of the multidisciplinary HD clinic

◆ Neurologist
◆ Neuropsychologist
◆ Neuropsychiatrist
◆ Clinical geneticist/Genetics counsellor
◆ HDA worker
◆ Physiotherapist
◆ Speech and language therapist
◆ Dietician
◆ Occupational therapist

The dystonic aspects of HD occasionally respond to TBZ. Although levodopa is often tried for parkinsonian features, especially in juvenile HD, the effects are not convincing. Other agents are occasionally tried, including baclofen and benzodiazepines, but generally speaking they have a marginal subjective benefit without much evidence of a major clinical effect.

The psychiatric features of HD generally respond to standard therapies. Thus depressive features can be treated with standard antidepressants, of which our preferred choice is citalopram because of its anxiolytic properties. However, sertraline, paroxetine, venlafaxine, and mirtazapine can be used to good effect. When mood swings are an issue, olanzapine can often help; if not, then standard mood-stabilizing antiepileptic medications such as lamotrigine, sodium valproate, and carbamazepine can be used. Carbamazepine can cause problems of somnolence as well as skin rashes. Lithium is rarely used for mood stabilization because of problems of compliance and anxieties about side effects if it is not taken properly.

Treatment of the cognitive aspects of HD is much more problematic, unless there is an affective element to the problem. Cholinesterase inhibitors have been tried without much in the way of documented benefits.

Other drugs which can be of use in HD include modafinil for daytime somnolence, zopiclone or even sodium oxybate for insomnia (which can be a major problem in HD), oxybutynin for bladder instability, and standard laxatives for constipation.

In addition, patients can often benefit from speech and language therapists, mainly to check on swallowing, dieticians to help advise on the best diet from a calorific perspective (as well as which supplements to use) and to avoid choking and aspiration, and occupational therapists to ensure that appropriate measures are put in place to deal with the home situation to maximize independence and safety. Physiotherapy can be helpful in assessing and helping gait problems, and social workers and regional Huntington's

Disease Association advisers are also invaluable in supporting the patient and their family in the community.

Finally, two other issues are always worth bringing up sooner rather than later: advanced directives and percutaneous endoscopic gastrostomy (PEG) feeding. The former deals with the issue of what the patient and their family would like to be done as the disease enters the final phases, and this also helps shape discussions about power of attorney, nursing home placement/respite, and PEG placement. This last issue is something that will arise in all patients as their illness progresses, and some will decide early on that they would not want a PEG when the situation merits this. However, in other cases, this is sought and our own advice is to go for PEG placement sooner rather than later, with the main indications being weight loss, recurrent chest infections, or mounting anxieties about the time needed to maintain sufficient feeding to ensure that the calorific input is adequate (83).

Key advances

The major advances in HD in the last 20 years have been substantial and are listed below.

- Identification of the genetic basis of HD in 1993. This seminal international collaborative piece of research identified the mutant gene in HD as a CAG expansion in exon 1 of the *huntingtin* gene. This discovery has had a number of major implications: (a) patients can now be diagnosed with certainty; (b) patients at risk of the disease can now be tested to see if they are gene carriers, which has implications for their own future as well as family planning; (c) where relevant, *in vitro* fertilization can be performed with selection of non-affected embryos; (d) transgenic models of HD have been developed which have revealed unique pathological and pathogenic insights into the disease (see above) as well as providing a model by which to test for novel disease-modifying agents. This has shown that the route to cell death in HD follows many different pathways and involves cells other than neurons.
- The establishment of specialist clinics and integrated networks of HD research (Huntington Study Group in North America (http://www.huntington-study-group.org) and EURO-HD in Europe (http://www.euro-hd.net). This has ensured that patients are properly supported and treated, and that research into this rare condition is more integrated at an international level in terms of both a better understanding of the natural history of the disease and the development of drug trials.
- The adoption and successful completion of a number of drug therapies in large numbers of patients, including ethyl-eicosapentaenoic acid (negative outcome) (84), pridopidine (possibly some benefits) (85), and latrepirdine (negative outcome after initial positive small trial) (86). This work has laid the foundation for conducting more trials with possible disease-modifying therapies, which are emerging from a number of laboratories using transgenic models of HD.
- The recognition that HD has problems outside the classical area of disorders of movement, cognition, and affect. It is now clear that HD patients have problems with sleep and metabolism. Attention to these features of the illness may be important, as many of these problems significantly affect quality of life for the patients and their carers/families.
- The detailed study of pre-manifest HD individuals with the aim of trying to identify the earliest problems that mark the onset of the disease process, with the hope that these markers of disease onset could be used to help monitor the efficacy of disease-modifying drugs.

Future developments

The main developments that are likely to occur in HD over the next few years will be the emergence of disease-modifying therapies that will involve cocktails of drugs designed to target different aspects of the pathogenic cascade. This will include standard drug therapies designed, for example, to upregulate autophagy (rapamycin) or inhibit excitotoxicity (memantine), as well as more innovative therapies such as gene-silencing approaches (87). The latter approach will involve delivering some form of interfering RNA against the mutant gene mRNA with the aim of silencing its effects, whilst ensuring that the expression of normal *huntingtin* (which is vital for normal cellular function) remains unaffected. The main problem with this approach will be (a) ensuring that the iRNA silences only the mutant form, (b) that it can do this in all the relevant cell types in the CNS, (c) that it can do this for the lifetime of the patient, and (d) that it causes no side effects by interfering with other RNAs. This is a tall order, but is becoming more feasible with evolving and improving gene delivery technologies.

Other novel therapeutic approaches include the use of growth factors to help rescue dysfunctional cells, of which the most obvious candidate is BDNF, as this has been shown to be down-regulated in HD (88). This is likely to be delivered using a gene delivery system, although interestingly this growth factor is upregulated in the brain after exercise/environmental enrichment. Thus another approach could be through using programmes of intense physiotherapy/enrichment in patients with HD (89).

The development of cell-based therapies for treating HD is less clear cut, given some of the recent data showing that transplants of fetal striatal tissue survive poorly in the long term in the HD brain (90, 91). Nevertheless cells may have some role to play, possibly through improved disease modelling *in vitro* using neurons derived from induced pluripotent stem (iPS) cells from patients with HD. This is important as it will help to dissect the pathogenic process and pathways that take place in cells carrying the mutant gene, so that logical cocktails of agents can be used to target these relevant pathways, akin to what has been achieved in HIV therapeutics.

The use of these new therapeutics will require the development of better biomarkers with which one can follow disease progression at a pathogenic level. This may necessitate a combination of measures including imaging (MRI and PET), wet biomarkers (blood and possibly CSF samples subject to -omics analysis (like transcriptomics, proteomics, etc.), and more objective clinical measures (92). These are likely to become more evident as longitudinal data emerge from ongoing studies.

Finally, the identification of genetic and environmental modifiers of disease will be important in establishing how we can better alter the disease course as well as informing us about how individual patients are likely to progress over time.

Conclusion

Since the gene for HD was identified in 1993, great progress has been made in better modelling this disorder and understanding its pathogenic basis. This has generated a large number of candidate therapies that are now starting to enter the clinic. Moreover, the necessary international infrastructure is now being developed to allow clinical trials to be performed more easily. However, these trials are hampered by problems of disease heterogeneity and the absence of robust and easy to use biomarkers that accurately mirror disease pathogenesis and progression.

Nevertheless the management of HD has been transformed over the last 10 years by the widespread adoption of specialist clinics that are now being linked up into large international networks. This ensures that all patients are assessed equally using similar tools, which enables good natural history data to be collected whilst also facilitating drug trials. The latter include those designed to address best symptomatic therapies as well as those more concerned with disease modification.

All of this sets the stage for the next phase of HD therapeutics which, it is hoped, will start to make inroads into disease modification by slowing down the progression of this disorder. Indeed, simply slowing the disease down by 50% would make a huge difference, given the average age at which it presents and that it typically progresses over a 20-year period. This knowledge may also encourage more at-risk patients to come to clinic, because the landscape of HD is changing every year. What we will be doing in 10 years' time may be very different from what we do now, with most patients in trials of combinations of drugs designed to slow the disease down.

Top clinical tips

- HD is best managed in specialist clinics.
- Diagnosing HD is straightforward but requires clinical genetics input early in the diagnostic process.
- The early features of HD are hard to define but the partner reporting abnormal movements at night is helpful.
- The best way to pick up early chorea is to watch the fingers when the patient is walking, or to listen whilst the patient does repetitive hand tapping and to watch the legs/feet for chorea when they are performing this test.
- The best first-line therapy for HD is often olanzapine, tiapride, or tetrabenazine.
- Planning for the future is useful, and it should be ensured that all patients have equal access to research/clinical trials.

References

1. Ramos-Arroyo MA, Moreno S, Valiente A. Incidence and mutation rates of Huntington's disease in Spain: experience of 9 years of direct genetic testing. *J Neurol Neurosurg Psychiatry* 2005; 76 :337–42.
2. Kokmen E, Ozekmekçi FS, Beard CM, O'Brien PC, Kurland LT. Incidence and prevalence of Huntington's disease in Olmsted County, Minnesota (1950 through 1989). *Arch Neurol* 1994; 51: 696–8.
3. Morrison PJ, Johnston WP, Nevin NC. The epidemiology of Huntington's disease in Northern Ireland. *J Med Genet* 1995; 32: 524–30.
4. Palo J, Somer H, Ikonen E, Karila L, Peltonen L. Low prevalence of Huntington's disease in Finland. *Lancet* 1987; 330: 805–6.
5. Masuda N, Goto J, Murayama N, Watanabe M, Kondo I, Kanazawa I. Analysis of triplet repeats in the huntingtin gene in Japanese families affected with Huntington's disease. *J Med Genet* 1995; 32: 701–5.
6. Wexler NS, Lorimer J, Porter J, et al. Venezuelan kindreds reveal that genetic and environmental factors modulate Huntington's disease age of onset. *Proc Natl Acad Sci USA* 2004; 101: 3498–503.
7. Spinney L. Uncovering the true prevalence of Huntington's disease. *Lancet Neurol* 2010; 9: 760–1.
8. Morrison PJ. Accurate prevalence and uptake of testing for Huntington's disease. *Lancet Neurol* 2010; 9: 1147.
9. Magazi DS, Krause A, Bonev V, et al. Huntington's disease: genetic heterogeneity in black African patients. *S Afr Med J* 2008; 98: 200–3.
10. Margolis RL, Holmes SE, Rosenblatt A, et al. Huntington's Disease-like 2 (HDL2) in North America and Japan. *Ann Neurol* 2004; 56: 670–4.
11. Huntington's Disease Collaborative Research Group. A novel gene containing a trinucleotide repeat that is expanded and unstable on Huntington's disease chromosomes. *Cell* 1993; 72: 971–83.
12. Rubinsztein DC, Leggo J, Coles R, et al. Phenotypic characterization of individuals with 30–40 CAG repeats in the Huntington disease (HD) gene reveals HD cases with 36 repeats and apparently normal elderly individuals with 36–39 repeats. *Am J Hum Genet* 59: 16–22.
13. Brinkman RR, Mezei MM, Theilmann J, Almqvist E, Hayden MR. The likelihood of being affected with Huntington disease by a particular age, for a specific CAG size. *Am J Hum Genet* 1997; 60: 1202–10.
14. Read AP. Huntington's disease: testing the test. *Nat Genet* 1993; 4: 329–30.
15. Wexler NS, Young AB, Tanzi RE, et al. Homozygotes for Huntington's disease. *Nature* 1987; 326: 194–7.
16. Squitieri F, Gellera C, Cannella M, et al. Homozygosity for CAG mutation in Huntington disease is associated with a more severe clinical course. *Brain* 2003; 126: 946–55.
17. Aziz NA, Jurgens CK, Landwehrmeyer GB, et al. Normal and mutant HTT interact to affect clinical severity and progression in Huntington disease. *Neurology* 2009; 73: 1280–5.
18. Ranen NG, Stine OC, Abbott MH, et al. Anticipation and instability of IT-15 (CAG)N repeats in parent–offspring pairs with Huntington disease. *Am J Hum Genet* 1995; 57: 593–602.
19. Trottier Y, Biancalana V, Mandel J-L. Instability of CAG repeats in Huntington's disease: relation to parental transmission and age of onset. *J Med Genet* 1994; 31: 377–82.
20. Warby SC, Montpetit A, Hayden AR, et al. CAG expansion in the Huntington disease gene is associated with a specific and targetable predisposing haplogroup. *Am J Hum Genet* 2009; 84: 351–66.
21. Semaka A, Collins JA, Hayden MR. Unstable familial transmissions of Huntington disease alleles with 27–35 CAG repeats (intermediate alleles). *Am J Med Genet* 2010; 153B: 314–20.
22. Rosenblatt A, Brinkman RR, Liang KY, et al. Familial influence on age of onset among siblings with Huntington disease. *Am J Med Genet* 2001; 105: 399–403.
23. Norremolle A, Hasholt L, Petersen CB, et al. Mosaicism of the CAG repeat sequence in the Huntington disease gene in a pair of monozygotic twins. *Am J Med Genet* 2004; 130A: 154–9.
24. Panas M, Karadima G, Markianos M, Kalfakis N, Vassilopoulos D. Phenotypic discordance in a pair of monozygotic twins with Huntington's disease. *Clin Genet* 2008; 74: 291–2.
25. Andresen JM, Gayan J, Cherny SS, et al. Replication of twelve association studies for Huntington's disease residual age of onset in large Venezuelan kindreds. *J Med Genet* 2007; 44: 44–50.
26. Metzger S, et al. Huntingtin-associated protein-1 is a modifier of the age-at-onset of Huntington's disease. *Hum Mol Genet* 2008; 17: 1137–46.
27. Tartari M, Gissi C, Lo Sardo V, et al. Phylogenetic comparison of huntingtin homologues reveals the appearance of a primitive polyQ in sea urchin. *Mol Biol Evol* 2008; 25: 330–8.

28. Duyao MP, Auerbach AB, Ryan A, et al. Inactivation of the mouse Huntington's disease gene homolog HdH. *Science* 1995; 269: 407–10.
29. Auerbach W, Hurlbert MS, Hilditch-Maguire P, et al. The HD mutation causes progressive lethal neurological disease in mice expressing reduced levels of huntingtin. *Hum Mol Genet* 2001; 10: 2515–23.
30. Leavitt BR, van Raamsdonk JM, Shehadeh J, et al. Wild-type huntingtin protects neurons from excitotoxicity. *J Neurochem* 2006; 96: 1121–9.
31. Zuccato C, Ciammola A, Rigamonti D, et al. Loss of huntingtin-mediated BDNF gene transcription in Huntington's disease. *Science* 2001; 293: 493–8.
32. Trushina E, Dyer RB, Badger JD, et al. Mutant huntingtin impairs axonal trafficking in mammalian neurons *in vivo* and *in vitro*. *Mol Cell Biol* 2004; 24: 8195–209.
33. Thompson LM, Aiken CT, Kaltenbach LS, et al. IKK phosphorylates huntingtin and targets it for degradation by the proteasome and lysosome. *J Cell Biol* 2009; 187: 1083–99.
34. Jeong H, Then F, Melia TJ, Jr, et al. Acetylation targets mutant huntingtin to autophagosomes for degradation. *Cell* 2009; 137: 60–72.
35. Graham RK, Deng Y, Slow EJ, et al. Cleavage at the caspase-6 site is required for neuronal dysfunction and degeneration due to mutant huntingtin. *Cell* 2006; 125: 1179–91.
36. DiFiglia M, Sapp E, Chase KO, et al. Aggregation of huntingtin in neuronal intranuclear inclusions and dystrophic neurites in the brain. *Science* 1997; 277: 1990–3.
37. Martindale D, Hackam A, et al. Length of huntingtin and its polyglutamine tract influences localization and frequency of intracellular aggregates. *Nat Genet* 1998; 18:150–4.
38. Scherzinger E, Sittler A, Schweiger K, et al. Self-assembly of polyglutamine-containing huntingtin fragments into amyloid-like fibrils: implications for Huntington's disease pathology. *Proc Natl Acad Sci USA* 1999; 96: 4604–9.
39. Tydlacka S, Wang CE, Wang X, Li S, Li XJ. Differential activities of the ubiquitin-proteasome system in neurons versus glia may account for the preferential accumulation of misfolded proteins in neurons. 2008; 28: 13 285–95.
40. Bodner RA, Outeiro TF, Altmann S, et al. Pharmacological promotion of inclusion formation: a therapeutic approach for Huntington's and Parkinson's diseases. *Proc Natl Acad Sci USA* 2006; 103: 4246–51.
41. Ravikumar B, Vacher C, Berger Z, et al. Inhibition of mTOR induces autophagy and reduces toxicity of polyglutamine expansions in fly and mouse models of Huntington disease. *Nat Genet* 2004; 36: 585–95.
42. Benn CL, Sun T, Sadri-Vakili G, et al. Huntingtin modulates transcription, occupies gene promoters in vivo, and binds directly to DNA in a polyglutamine-dependent manner. *J Neurosci* 2008; 28: 10 720–33.
43. Zhai W, Jeong H, Cui L, Krainc D, Tjian R. *In vitro* analysis of huntingtin-mediated transcriptional repression reveals multiple transcription factor targets. *Cell* 2005; 123: 1241–53.
44. Nucifora FC, Jr, Sasaki M, Peters MF, et al. Interference by huntingtin and atrophin-1 with cbp-mediated transcription leading to cellular toxicity. *Science* 2001; 291: 2423–8.
45. Valenza M, Rigamonti D, Goffredo D, et al. Dysfunction of the cholesterol biosynthetic pathway in Huntington's disease. *J Neurosci* 2005; 25: 9932–9.
46. Zuccato C, Tartari M, Crotti A, et al. Huntingtin interacts with REST/NRSF to modulate the transcription of NRSE-controlled neuronal genes. *Nat Genet* 2003; 35: 76–83.
47. Steffan JS, Bodai L, Palos J, et al. Histone deacetylase inhibitors arrest polyglutamine-dependent neurodegeneration in Drosophila. *Nature* 2001; 413: 739–43.
48. Gauthier LR, Charrin BC, Borrell-Pagès M, et al. Huntingtin controls neurotrophic support and survival of neurons by enhancing BDNF vesicular transport along microtubules. Cell 2004; 118: 127–38.
49. Shin JY, Fang ZH, Yu ZX, Wang CE, Li SH, Li XJ. Expression of mutant huntingtin in glial cells contributes to neuronal excitotoxicity. *J Cell Biol* 2005; 171: 1001–12.
50. Cowan CM, Fan MM, Fan J, et al. Polyglutamine-modulated striatal calpain activity in YAC transgenic huntington disease mouse model: impact on NMDA receptor function and toxicity. *J Neurosci* 2008; 28: 12 725–35.
51. Sun Y, Savanenin A, Reddy PH, Liu YF. Polyglutamine-expanded huntingtin promotes sensitization of *N*-methyl-D-aspartate receptors via post-synaptic density 95. *J Biol Chem* 2001; 276: 24 713–18.
52. Blázquez C, Chiarlone A,Sagredo O, et al. Loss of striatal type 1 cannabinoid receptors is a key pathogenic factor in Huntington's disease. *Brain* 2011; 134: 119–36.
53. Cummings DM, Milnerwood AJ, Dallérac GM, et al. Aberrant cortical synaptic plasticity and dopaminergic dysfunction in a mouse model of Huntington's disease. *Hum Mol Genet* 2006; 15: 2856–68.
54. Tang TS, Tu H, Chan EY, et al. Huntingtin and huntingtin-associated protein 1 influence neuronal calcium signaling mediated by inositol-(1,4,5) triphosphate receptor type 1. *Neuron* 2003; 39: 227–39.
55. Panov AV, Gutekunst CA, Leavitt BR, et al. Early mitochondrial calcium defects in Huntington's disease are a direct effect of polyglutamines. *Nat Neurosci* 2002; 5: 731–6.
56. Cui L, Jeong H, Borovecki F, Parkhurst CN, Tanese N, Krainc D. Transcriptional repression of PGC-1alpha by mutant huntingtin leads to mitochondrial dysfunction and neurodegeneration. *Cell* 2006; 127: 59–69.
57. Bae BI, Xu H, Igarashi S, et al. p53 mediates cellular dysfunction and behavioral abnormalities in Huntington's disease. *Neuron* 2005; 47: 29–41.
58. Pavese N, Gerhard A, Tai YF, et al. Microglial activation correlates with severity in Huntington disease: a clinical and PET study. *Neurology* 2006; 66: 1638–43.
59. Björkqvist M, Wild EJ, Thiele J, et al. A novel pathogenic pathway of immune activation detectable before clinical onset in Huntington's disease. *J Exp Med* 2008; 205: 1869–77.
60. Zwilling D, Huang SY, Sathyasaikumar KV, et al. Kynurenine 3-monooxygenase inhibition in blood ameliorates neurodegeneration. *Cell* 2011; 145: 863–74.
61. Vonsattel JP, Myers RH, Stevens TJ, et al. Neuropathological classification of Huntington's disease. *J Neuropathol Exp Neurol* 1985; 44: 559–77.
62. Rosas HD, Salat DH, Lee SY, et al. Cerebral cortex and the clinical expression of Huntington's disease: complexity and heterogeneity. *Brain* 2008; 131: 1057–68.
63. Tabrizi SJ, Scahill RI, Durr A, et al. Biological and clinical changes in premanifest and early stage Huntington's disease in the TRACK-HD study: the 12-month longitudinal analysis. *Lancet Neurol* 2011; 10: 31–42.
64. Vonsattel JP, DiFiglia M. Huntington disease. *J Neuropathol Exp Neurol* 1998; 57: 369–84.
65. Bates G, Harper P, Jones L. *Huntington's disease* (3rd edn). Oxford: Oxford University Press, 2002.
66. Quarrell OWJ, Brewer HM, Squitieri F, Barker RA, Nance MA, Landwehrmeyer GB (eds). *Juvenile Huntington's disease and other trinucleotide repeat disorders*. Oxford: Oxford University Press, 2009.
67. Ho AK, Sahakian BJ, Brown RG, et al. Profile of cognitive progression in early Huntington's disease. *Neurology* 2003; 61: 1702–6.
68. Mason SL, Wijeyekoon R, Swain R, et al. Cognitive follow up of a small cohort of Huntington's disease patients over a 5 year period. *PLoS Curr* 2010; 2: RRN1174.
69. van Duijn E, Kingma EM, van der Mast RC. Psychopathology in verified Huntington's disease gene carriers. *J Neuropsychiatry Clin Neurosci* 2007; 19: 441–8.
70. Ross CA, Tabrizi SJ. Huntington's disease: from molecular pathogenesis to clinical treatment. *Lancet Neurol* 2011; 10: 83–98.
71. Fiedorowicz JG, Mills JA, Ruggle A, et al. Suicidal behavior in prodromal Huntington disease. *Neurodegener Dis* 2011; 8: 483–90.
72. Bindler L, Travers D, Millet B. Suicide in Huntington's disease: a review. *Rev Med Suisse* 2009; 5: 646–8.
73. Ho AK, Robbins AO, Barker RA. Huntington's disease patients have selective problems with insight. *Mov Disord* 2006; 21: 385–9.

74. Goodman AO, Rogers L, Pilsworth S, et al. Asymptomatic sleep abnormalities are a common early feature in patients with Huntington's disease. *Curr Neurol Neurosci Rep* 2011; 11: 211–17.
75. Morton AJ, Wood NI, Hastings MH, Hurelbrink C, Barker RA, Maywood ES. Disintegration of the sleep–wake cycle and circadian timing in Huntington's disease. *J Neurosci* 2005; 25: 157–63.
76. Goodman AO, Murgatroyd PR, Medina-Gomez G, et al. The metabolic profile of early Huntington's disease—a combined human and transgenic mouse study. *Exp Neurol* 2008; 210: 691–8.
77. Tibben A. Predictive testing for Huntington's disease. *Brain Res Bull* 2007; 72: 165–71.
78. International Huntington Association (IHA) and the World Federation of Neurology (WFN) Research Group on Huntington's Chorea. Guidelines for the molecular genetics predictive test in Huntington's disease. *Neurology* 1994; 44: 1533–6.
79. Tabrizi SJ, Langbehn DR, Leavitt BR, et al. Biological and clinical manifestations of Huntington's disease in the longitudinal TRACK-HD study: cross-sectional analysis of baseline data. *Lancet Neurol* 2009; 8: 791–801.
80. Paulsen JS, Hayden M, Stout JC, et al. Preparing for preventive clinical trials: the Predict-HD study. *Arch Neurol* 2006; 63: 883–90.
81. Phillips W, Shannon KM, Barker RA. The current clinical management of Huntington's disease. *Mov Disord* 2008; 23: 1491–504.
82. Mason SL, Barker RA. Emerging drug therapies in Huntington's disease. *Expert Opin Emerg Drugs* 2009; 14: 273–97.
83. Klager J, Duckett A, Sandler S, Moskowitz C. Huntington's disease: a caring approach to the end of life. *Care Manag J* 2008; 9: 75–81.
84. Huntington Study Group TREND-HD Investigators. Randomized controlled trial of ethyl-eicosapentaenoic acid in Huntington disease: the TREND-HD study. *Arch Neurol* 2008; 65: 1582–9.
85. Lundin A, Dietrichs E, Haghighi S, et al. Efficacy and safety of the dopaminergic stabilizer pridopidine (ACR16) in patients with Huntington's disease. *Clin Neuropharmacol* 2010; 33: 260–4.
86. Kieburtz K, McDermott MP, Voss TS, et al. A randomized, placebo-controlled trial of latrepirdine in Huntington disease. *Arch Neurol* 2010; 67: 154–60.
87. Sah DW, Aronin N. Oligonucleotide therapeutic approaches for Huntington disease. *J Clin Invest* 2011; 121: 500–7.
88. Xie Y, Hayden MR, Xu B. BDNF overexpression in the forebrain rescues Huntington's disease phenotypes in YAC128 mice. *J Neurosci* 2010; 30: 14 708–18.
89. Nithianantharajah J, Hannan AJ. Enriched environments, experience-dependent plasticity and disorders of the nervous system. *Nat Rev Neurosci* 2006; 7: 697–709.
90. Clelland CD, Barker RA, Watts C. Cell therapy in Huntington disease. *Neurosurg Focus* 2008; 24: E9.
91. Cicchetti F, Soulet D, Freeman TB. Neuronal degeneration in striatal transplants and Huntington's disease: potential mechanisms and clinical implications. *Brain* 2011; 134: 641–52.
92. Weir DW, Sturrock A, Leavitt BR. Development of biomarkers for Huntington's disease. *Lancet Neurol* 2011; 10: 573–90.

CHAPTER 21

Huntington's Disease Look-alikes

Edward J. Wild and Sarah J. Tabrizi

Summary

Around 1% of patients in whom Huntington's disease (HD) is suspected clinically, lack the genetic mutation that causes HD. Such patients, referred to as having HD look-alike syndromes, HD phenocopies or HD-like disorders, present a diagnostic challenge. This chapter offers a definition of HD look-alikes and reviews the causes and features of HD look-alike syndromes, including HD-like syndromes 1, 2, and 3, familial prion disease, spinocerebellar ataxias 17, 1, 2, and 3, dentatorubral-pallidoluysian atrophy (DRPLA), brain iron accumulation disorders including pantothenate kinase associated neurodegeneration (PKAN) and neuroferritinopathy, choreoacanthocytosis, MacLeod syndrome, Wilson disease, Friedreich's ataxia, mitochondrial disease, and benign hereditary chorea, and considers possible acquired causes. The evidence for the relative frequencies of each genetic cause is reviewed. The yield from exhaustive genetic investigation of such patients is only 2%, which is important when it comes to genetic counselling. We propose a rational framework for the investigation of HD look-alike patients, based on genetic frequencies and associated clinical features. The exclusion of treatable causes is a top priority. Expert genetic counselling and multidisciplinary care via a neurogenetics clinic remain the mainstay of care for such patients.

Introduction

Soon after the discovery of the genetic mutation responsible for Huntington's disease (HD) in 1993, enabling the definitive genetic testing of all patients with a clinical diagnosis of HD, it became apparent that a minority of patients presenting with symptoms and signs suggestive of the condition lacked its causative genetic abnormality—an expanded CAG repeat in the *HTT* gene. Such cases, resembling HD but lacking the HD mutation—are referred to, variously, as HD-like (HDL) syndromes, HD phenocopies, or Huntington's look-alikes. The term 'phenocopy' was coined to mean a phenotype characteristic of a particular genetic syndrome, but produced environmentally; used more broadly, it can be used to refer to syndromes suggestive with any cause—genetic or environmental—other than the expected genotype. This chapter describes the conditions that can produce HD-like presentations, reviews the evidence for their relative frequency, and proposes a rational framework for their investigation and management.

Prevalence and definition

Overall, Huntington look-alike syndromes are thought to represent about 1% of patients where HD is suspected clinically (see Fig. 21.1), and they can be extremely challenging in terms of diagnosis, management, and counselling for patients and family members (1). Specific prevalence figures for HD look-alike syndromes are not available, but the prevalence of manifest HD is estimated at 10 per 100 000 in most Western populations, and so the prevalence of look-alikes ought to be about one per million (2). However, recent figures have suggested that the prevalence of HD is likely to be substantially greater than previously estimated (3). Moreover, exactly what constitutes a Huntington look-alike syndrome is poorly defined. No formal definition exists, but the figure of 1% comes from early studies where patients subsequently redefined as look-alikes had previously had a firm clinical diagnosis of Huntington's disease.

However, beyond the classical triad of chorea, subcortical dementia, and psychiatric disturbance, Huntington's disease is now recognized as producing a wide range of phenotypes, including purely psychiatric, akinetic–rigid, dystonic, and ataxic variants. Therefore we have proposed a more flexible working definition of HD look-alike syndromes as shown in Box 21.1 (4, 5).

The extent to which the combination of the likely increased prevalence of HD and this broader definition alters the prevalence of HD look-alike syndromes remains to be seen, but our experience suggests that such patients are far more common than the one per million suggested by traditional approaches.

Note that autosomal dominant inheritance, or indeed a family history, is not an absolute requirement for a patient to be considered an HD look-alike. As many as 25% of new HD patients presenting to specialist clinics have no such family history (6)—a figure brought about by HD's historically entrenched stigma, the emergence of new cases through intergenerational CAG repeat expansion, and complications such as non-paternity and adoption.

Of course, there are no treatments that have been proved to slow down the progression of Huntington's disease in humans, and

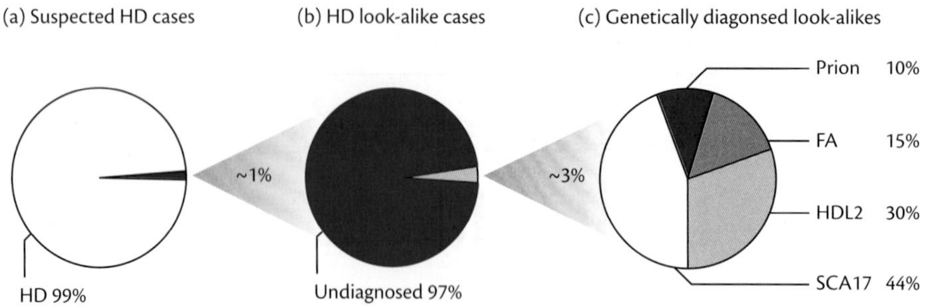

Fig. 21.1 Relative frequencies of (a) Huntington's disease and look-alike cases, (b) undiagnosed and genetically diagnosed look-alikes, and (c) individual look-alike syndromes. FA, Friedreich's ataxia; HD, Huntington's disease; Prion, familial prion disease. (Modified from Wild E, Tabrizi S. Huntington's disease phenocopy syndromes. *Curr Opin Neurol* 2007; 20: 681–7, by permission of Wolters Kluwer Health/Lippincott–Williams & Wilkins)

Box 21.1 Working definition of Huntington's disease look-alike syndromes

1. A movement disorder consistent with HD as determined by an experienced neurologist AND
2. A negative test for the pathogenic CAG repeat expansion in the *HTT* gene AND
3. At least one of the following:
   - family history suggestive of autosomal dominant inheritance;
   - cognitive impairment;
   - behavioural or psychiatric symptoms.

unfortunately the same is true of many of its described look-alike syndromes. This is not universally the case, and disease-modifying treatments *are* available for some conditions, such as Wilson disease, provided that a diagnosis is made in a timely manner.

However, even in the absence of a specific treatment, there is still benefit in seeking a diagnosis for these rare conditions. It is useful for patients and relatives to have a specific name for their condition, both psychologically and in order to obtain access to appropriate symptomatic, supportive, and social assistance. Obtaining a genetic diagnosis enables family members to be counselled with accuracy on their genetic risk, offered predictive or diagnostic genetic testing, and given access to assisted fertility techniques that may prevent them passing on an incurable genetic condition to their children. Finally, an accurate diagnosis gives patients and those at risk the option of taking part in specific clinical and genetic research programmes that may benefit them or future generations.

Individual Huntington look-alikes

In addition to the three conditions named HDL1–3, various other genetic disorders can produce phenotypes resembling HD. These are summarized in Table 21.1 and discussed individually below.

HDL1 and familial prion disease

HDL1 was the first HD look-alike syndrome for which a genetic cause was identified. It is a form of familial prion disease, caused by a mutation in the *PRNP* gene resulting in an eight-octapeptide insertion in the prion protein. The disease has autosomal dominant inheritance with early-adult onset and causes chorea, ataxia, cognitive decline, personality change, and basal ganglia atrophy. The name HDL1 refers specifically to this genotype–phenotype combination, which is restricted to just a handful of reported pedigrees (7). However, it is now known that an HD-like syndrome with prominent rigidity and ataxia can be caused by other *PRNP* mutations, such as the more common six-octapeptide repeat insertion. Such mutations are known to produce a variety of phenotypes, even within a single pedigree, including behavioural change, dementia, myoclonus, seizures, chorea, and pyramidal, cerebellar, and extrapyramidal signs, so it is perhaps unsurprising that Huntington look-alikes are within their gamut (8). Therefore screening of the entire *PRNP* gene (15 kb), rather than focused testing for the specific mutation causing HDL1, is recommended in the evaluation of Huntington look-alike patients.

HDL2

HDL2 is one of the more common genetic causes of a Huntington look-alike syndrome. It is caused by GTC/CAG triplet expansions in the *JPH3* gene encoding junctophilin-3, a component of junctional complexes that mediates crosstalk between cell surface and intracellular ion channels. Its inheritance is autosomal dominant; *JPH3* alleles with over 41 repeats are pathogenic, while normal alleles have 6–28 repeats.

HDL2 was first described in the USA in 2001 in an African American family and subsequent pedigrees have revealed it to be almost exclusively confined to populations of African descent. It is now known to be more common than HD itself in some black African populations (9). However, more recent cases have been reported in Middle Eastern and European patients (4, 10).

Clinically, HDL2 is a very close phenocopy of HD, especially the Westphal rigid variant of HD typically seen in juvenile patients and adults with younger onset. Onset of HDL2 is typically in the fourth decade. Most patients experience cognitive and psychiatric dysfunction, dystonia, extrapyramidal rigidity, and weight loss; many also display chorea. There is said to be a lower frequency of eye-movement abnormalities of the kind seen in HD, and seizures are less frequent than in juvenile HD (11).

Neuroimaging in HDL2 is somewhat similar to HD, showing atrophy of the caudate, putamen, and cerebral hemispheres. Microscopically there are also similarities with ubiquitin-positive neuronal intranuclear inclusions and a loss of medium-sized neurons in the striatum in a dorsal–ventral gradient. Some patients with HDL2 develop acanthocytosis in peripheral blood.

Table 21.1 Principal causes of Huntington's disease look-alike syndromes

Condition	Gene	Protein	Inheritance	Notes
Familial prion disease	*PRNP*	Prion	AD	Includes HDL1
HDL2	*JPH3*	Junctophilin 3	AD	African ancestry
HDL3	Unknown	Unknown	AR	Two pedigrees only
SCA17	*TBP*	TATA-binding protein	AD	Cerebellar atrophy and ataxia
SCA1	*ATXN1*	Ataxin 1	AD	
SCA2	*ATXN2*	Ataxin 2	AD	
SCA3	*ATXN3*	Ataxin 3	AD	
DRPLA	*ATN1*	Atrophin 1	AD	Myoclonic epilepsy
PKAN (NBIA1)	*PANK2*	Pantothenate kinase	AR	MRI 'eye of the tiger sign', pigmentary retinopathy
Neuroferritinopathy	*FTL*	Ferritin light chain	AD	Early dysarthria and persistent asymmetry
Choreoacanthocytosis	*CHAC*	Chorein	AR	Mutilating orofacial dystonia
MacLeod syndrome	*XK*	Kell antigen	XR	Systemic features
Wilson disease	*ATP7B*	Copper-transporting ATPase	AR	Kayser–Fleischer rings etc.
Friedreich's ataxia	*FRDA*	Frataxin	AR	Rarely resembles HD
Mitochondrial disease	mtDNA or nuclear mitochondrial genes			
Benign hereditary chorea	*TITF1*	Thyroid transcription factor 1	AD	Non-choreic features, rare
Acquired causes	e.g. Sydenham's chorea, antibasal ganglia antibodies, neuro-SLE, thyrotoxicosis, vascular disease, medications			

AD, autosomal dominant; AR, autosomal recessive; XR, X-linked recessive. For other abbreviations, see text.

However, the pathogenesis of HDL2 is curious. As in myotonic dystrophy type 1 (DM1), and quite unlike in HD, there is no evidence that the mutant protein is harmful; rather, foci containing *JPH3* RNA are seen neuronal nuclei, and it appears that the triplet-expanded RNA itself may be the toxic species in HDL2 (12). A recently developed mouse model of HDL2, expressing a bacterial artificial chromosome (BAC), promises to shed light on the pathogenesis of the condition and may reveal shared mechanisms for HD-like disorders including HD itself (13).

HDL3

HDL3 is an autosomal recessive HD-like disorder linked to chromosome 4p15.3. The causative gene is unknown and the disorder has been reported in only two pedigrees (14).

SCA17 and other spinocerebellar ataxias

The spinocerebellar ataxias are a heterogeneous group of hereditary degenerative disorders causing cerebellar ataxia and a spectrum of associated features. Although cerebellar ataxia is seldom the sole feature of Huntington's disease, it is commonly seen as a component of the compound movement disorder. SCA17 is caused by CAG or CAA repeat expansions in the *TBP* gene, resulting in lengthened polyglutamine tracts in the TATA binding protein, a key transcription factor (15). Overall, SCA17 is rare, with a prevalence of around 0.2 per 100 000.

Unaffected individuals have 42 or fewer repeats, with most affected patients having over 50; milder symptoms have been reported with as few as 43 repeats. The interrupted configuration of the triplet-repeat alleles appears to be responsible for a relatively low incidence of genetic anticipation, which is common in HD with its contiguous CAG repeats.

SCA17 causes a wide variety of phenotypes. The most common features are intellectual decline (in 100% of patients), ataxia (90%), and epilepsy (50%), so the majority of cases of SCA17 are not particularly HD-like and calls for the disease to be renamed HDL4 may not, overall, be well-founded (15). However, in the 20% of SCA17 patients who develop chorea, it can be an extremely close HD look-alike. Moreover, SCA17 tends to be phenotypically homogeneous within individual families, so affected offspring of an HD-like SCA17 patient are likely to resemble HD themselves (16).

Unlike HD, SCA17 almost invariably causes cerebellar atrophy which can be visualized on MR scanning. Selective enhancement of the putamen has also been reported, which is not seen in HD or the other SCAs (17).

Pathologically, SCA17 causes neuronal loss in the cortex, striatum, and cerebellum. Protein aggregates containing polyglutamine and TBP accumulate widely in neuronal nuclei (18). The fact that SCA17 is caused by a mutated transcription factor makes it an exciting target for providing insights into the role of gene transcription dysregulation in neurodegenerative disease as a whole, and HD in particular. Recent work in a mouse model expressing polyglutamine-expanded TBP has shown that SCA17 is associated with downregulation of the high-affinity nerve growth factor receptor TrkA (19), which has been implicated in the pathogenesis of both Alzheimer's and Huntington's diseases (20, 21).

Because of the clinical heterogeneity of both Huntington's disease and the spinocerebellar ataxias, many of the other SCAs can mimic HD to different extents. In particular, SCAs 1, 2, and 3 (caused by abnormal CAG repeat expansions in the genes encoding ataxin 1, 2, and 3) can cause a combination of hypokinetic and hyperkinetic movement disorders, including chorea, that may resemble HD (22).

Dentatorubral-pallidoluysian atrophy

Although DRPLA was probably first described in 1958 by Smith and colleagues (23), it bears the eponym Naito–Oyanagi disease and is most commonly seen in families of Japanese descent. It has autosomal dominant inheritance. In 1994, shortly after the HD gene was cloned, the genetic cause of DRPLA was found—another CAG triplet repeat expansion, in the atrophin 1 gene (*ATN1*) on chromosome 12 (24). Like HD, the length of the CAG repeat expansion correlates inversely with age at onset; in fact, among the CAG triplet repeat disorders, DRPLA most prominently exhibits genetic anticipation because of the tendency of its CAG repeat tract to lengthen when inherited paternally (25).

In common with many of the diseases mentioned in this chapter, DRPLA may present with a diversity of phenotypes. The core features are myoclonic epilepsy, dementia, ataxia, and choreoathetosis. Onset is typically earlier than in Huntington's disease (in the twenties), although the course of the disease is usually about the same (15–20 years). The frequent presence of myoclonic epilepsy is a distinguishing feature of DRPLA; epilepsy is only rarely a prominent feature of HD, although seizures are quite common in juvenile HD patients. Intractable myoclonic epilepsy should prompt suspicion of a diagnosis other than HD.

As the name suggests, DRPLA produces degenerative brain atrophy, predominantly affecting the dentatorubral system, which connects the cerebellar dentate to the midbrain red nucleus, and the pallidoluysian system, which unites the globus pallidus and the subthalamic nucleus (nucleus of Luys).

Like HD, DRPLA is a disease of protein accumulation. Polyglutamine-expanded atrophin 1 aggregates in DRPLA brain as intracytoplasmic ubiquitinated neuronal inclusions (25). Atrophin-1 interacts with many other proteins, but appears to function as a transcriptional repressor, an activity which becomes attenuated in the presence of an expanded CAG repeat tract (26).

As well as atrophy of the affected brain regions, especially the brainstem and cerebellum, MRI scanning in DRPLA may show hyperintense cerebral white matter T_2 lesions (25).

Interestingly, the same CAG repeat expansion in the *ATN1* gene can also cause a pathologically distinct illness called 'Haw River syndrome' after the North Carolina town where its large inaugural pedigree was described. Patients display clinical features similar to 'classical' DRPLA but without myoclonic seizures. Pathologically, there is calcification of the basal ganglia, subcortical demyelination, and neuroaxonal dystrophy—features not typically seen in DRPLA (27).

Iron accumulation disorders

Neurodegeneration with brain iron accumulation (NBIA) is the term for a family of conditions in which a progressive neurological syndrome with neurodegeneration is accompanied by the abnormal deposition of iron in brain tissues, especially the basal ganglia. NBIA disorders are clinically and genetically heterogeneous and can arise in early childhood or adult life, but share a tendency to produce extrapyramidal syndromes with cognitive and behavioural features (see also Chapter 12).

The iron accumulation disorders are generally, though not invariably, distinguishable from HD and the other look-alike syndromes through the ability of MRI to detect deposited iron in brain tissue. In the absence of a known family history, targeted genetic testing is most useful after MRI to elucidate the specific cause of the iron accumulation (28).

The majority of NBIA cases are accounted for by NBIA1, an autosomal recessive disorder caused by mutations in the *PANK2* gene encoding pantothenate kinase. The condition is now called PKAN (pantothenate kinase-associated neurodegeneration) rather than its previous eponym, Hallervorden–Spatz disease, which is now considered ethically inappropriate.

Rather confusingly, *PANK2* mutations also cause HARP syndrome, which constitutes hypoprebetalipoproteinaemia, acanthocytosis, retinitis pigmentosa, and pallidal degeneration. Increasingly it is recognized that HARP syndrome, which resembles PKAN but also produces lipoprotein abnormalities, is part of the PKAN disease spectrum (29).

Most cases of PKAN do not closely resemble HD. Classically, PKAN presents in early childhood with gait difficulty and progresses rapidly to a picture of prominent dystonia and corticospinal tract involvement producing upper motor neuron signs. In contrast, corticospinal signs are not a feature of juvenile HD (jHD) and, conversely, PANK2 does not cause the eye-movement disorder and propensity to seizures of jHD. Moreover, jHD seldom presents *de novo* within a family with no prior history (except in cases of non-paternity) because it is most unusual for an *HTT* triplet repeat expansion to increase, in a single transmission, from a range consistent with a symptom-free parent to an expansion large enough to cause jHD in their child.

However, the spectrum of PKAN presentations certainly overlaps with that of HD. Atypical PKAN can present in early adult life, progress slowly, and produce dysarthria, psychiatric symptoms including depression, emotional lability, and impulsivity, in addition to extrapyramidal dysfunction (28). Clues to a diagnosis of PKAN over HD include a paucity of chorea and the presence of pigmentary retinopathy.

MRI of such patients generally reveals iron deposition in a typical pattern: symmetric regions of hypointensity in the medial globus pallidus containing central areas of hyperintensity. This 'eye of the tiger' sign (Fig. 21.2) is said to be pathognomonic of PKAN (30). Dedicated MR sequences can confirm the presence of abnormal iron deposits with more specificity, and may also be more sensitive than basic T_2 imaging. These are T_2*, also known as gradient echo (GRE), and susceptibility-weighted imaging (SWI) sequences (Fig. 21.2).

Neuroferritinopathy, caused by mutations in the ferritin light chain gene *FTL*, is a relatively recent addition to the canon of HD look-alikes. Aside from being the only autosomal dominant brain iron accumulation disorder, it is a close clinical mimic, often producing an adult-onset syndrome with chorea, dystonia, cognitive decline, and behavioural features. Limb chorea in neuroferritinopathy may be strikingly asymmetric and, unlike in HD, such asymmetry persists throughout the disease course. Another distinguishing feature is the early development of dysarthria due to action-specific orofacial dystonia triggered by speech. In males, neuroferritinopathy may be disclosed by low serum ferritin, but this may be obscured by menstrual-related changes in females. Abnormalities on MRI are invariable, however, and can also distinguish neuroferritinopathy cases from other causes of NBIA. Iron accumulation is seen on T_2* or SWI sequences even in asymptomatic mutation-positive individuals (Fig. 21.2), and later progresses to cause cystic change in the caudate and putamen (31).

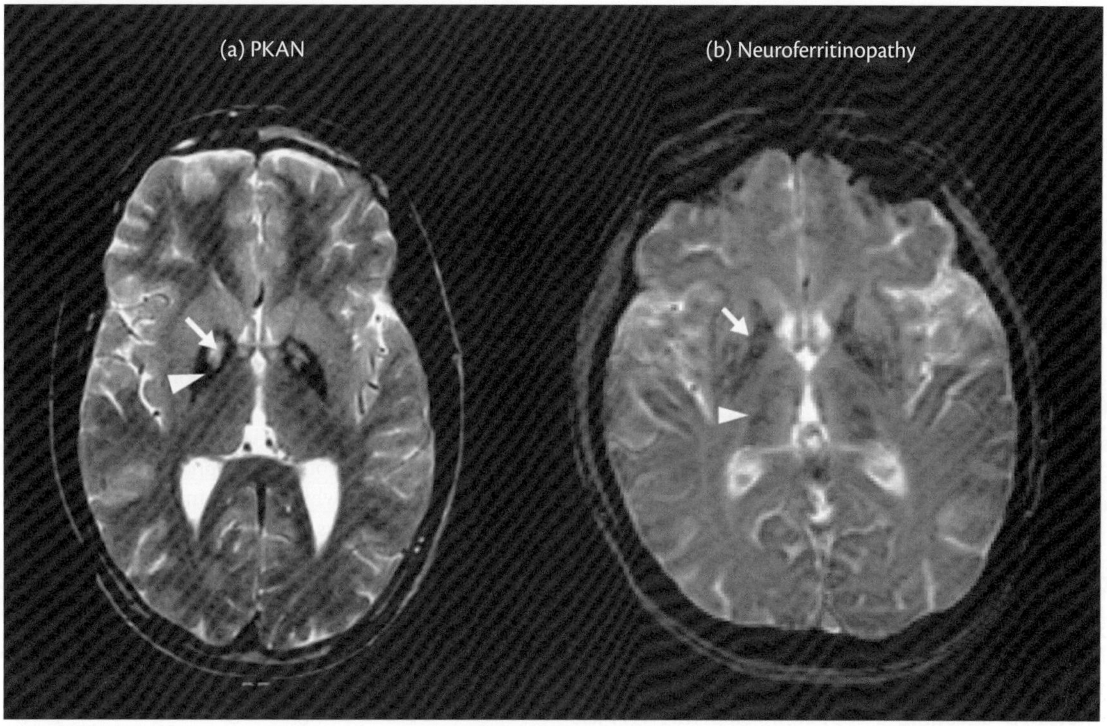

Fig. 21.2 MRI in brain iron accumulation disorders: (a) axial T_2-weighted brain MRI in PKAN demonstrating the 'eye of the tiger' sign due to globus pallidus hypointensity (arrow head) containing a high intensity focus (arrow). (Image reproduced from Hartig MB et al. Genotypic and phenotypic spectrum of PANK2 mutations in patients with neurodegeneration with brain iron accumulation. *Ann Neurol* 2007; 59: 248–56, by permission of Wiley Interscience) (b) T_2* MRI scan in neuroferritinopathy, showing reduced signal in the basal ganglia (arrow) and thalamus (arrow head). (Image reproduced from Chinnery PF et al. Clinical features and natural history of neuroferritinopathy caused by the FTL1 460InsA mutation, *Brain* 2007; 130: 110–19, by permission of Oxford University Press)

The other brain iron accumulation diseases, although heterogeneous, are sufficiently different from Huntington's disease that they need not be considered look-alikes. Aceruloplasminaemia, caused by *CP* mutations resulting in systemic absence of ceruloplasmin, has adult onset and can produce chorea, but is dominated by retinal degeneration and diabetes mellitus in addition to blepharospasm, facial and neck dystonia, tremor, and ataxia. *PLA2G6*-associated neurodegeneration (PLAN), of which the most common presentation is infantile neuroaxonal dystrophy (INAD), generally causes rapidly progressive psychomotor, corticospinal, cerebellar, and dystonic features in the presence of high brain iron. Likewise, fatty acid hydroxylase-associated neurodegeneration (FAHN), Woodhouse–Sakati syndrome, and Kufor–Rakeb syndrome are dominated by dystonia and neurological and systemic features not seen in HD (28).

Neuroacanthocytosis

Conditions in which neurological symptoms are seen in the presence of acanthocytes (erythrocytes with thorn-like protrusions) in peripheral blood are collectively referred to as neuroacanthocytosis syndromes. This classification is awkward, as several conditions meeting these criteria belong primarily to other disease families because acanthocytosis was not part of the initial description, or because acanthocytes are seen only rarely. Hyperkinetic movement disorders appear to be a feature of the 'core' neuroacanthocytosis syndromes; in addition to choreoacanthocytosis and MacLeod syndrome, acanthocytes may be seen in both NBIA and HDL2, described above.

Choreoacanthocytosis is an autosomal recessive condition caused by mutations in the *CHAC* gene, encoding the chorein protein, which may resemble HD clinically. It causes a range of movement disorders including chorea, tics, and dystonia. Later, patients develop dementia and psychiatric features similar to those seen in HD. Age at onset is younger than HD, on average, but there is substantial overlap. The defining characteristic of choreoacanthocytosis is dominant orofacial dystonia, commonly with tongue protrusion, with biting of the tongue and lips, resulting in permanent damage in some cases. In addition, seizures are seen in around half of cases, and other features such as neuropathy, distal amyotrophy, and elevation of serum creatine kinase are not shared with HD (32).

MacLeod syndrome is another neuroacanthocytosis that may mimic HD. Caused by mutations in the *XK* gene encoding the Kell erythrocyte antigen, its inheritance is X-linked recessive; symptoms are restricted to hemizygous males, while females with a single mutant allele are asymptomatic carriers. However, in small pedigrees, the inheritance may be ambiguous. MacLeod syndrome patients experience limb chorea, facial tics, subcortical dementia, and neuropsychiatric problems, with less dystonia than is seen in choreoacanthocytosis. However, it also produces non-HD-like features including axonal neuropathy, hepatosplenomegaly, cardiomyopathy, and haemolytic anaemia (32).

Demonstrating the presence of acanthocytes in peripheral blood may be instructive in the clinical assessment of an HD-like patient, but is not necessarily straightforward. Acanthocytes are seen in many common systemic conditions, including hypothyroidism and chronic renal failure, and therefore may be an incidental finding, statistically speaking, as often they are of no neurological significance. In addition, even in cases of neuroacanthocytosis, several blood films may be required and sample handling has a bearing on yield. 'True' acanthocytosis may be missed in a significant proportion of cases because of the use of dry blood smears or EDTA blood tubes. Instead, it is recommended that whole blood is mixed in a one-to-one ratio with a solution containing 10 units of heparin per millilitre of normal saline; after 30 minutes of agitation, phase-contrast microscopy of a wet preparation should be used to examine for spiculated cells (the normal value is less than 6.3%) (33). This approach offers diagnostic sensitivity approaching 100% but is not universally available; thus biochemical techniques such as Western blotting for chorein protein, and of course genetic testing, may be needed in suspected neuroacanthocytosis cases whether or not acanthocytes have been found.

Wilson disease

Wilson disease (hepatolenticular degeneration), which is described in detail in Chapter 23, is a genetic disorder of copper metabolism with autosomal recessive inheritance caused by mutations in *ATP7B* encoding a copper-transporting ATPase protein. It produces a wide range of clinical phenotypes consisting of hepatic dysfunction, neurological symptoms, and psychiatric disorder. The presence of all three is rare, and pure neurological or neuropsychiatric presentations are common. The neurological spectrum of Wilson disease includes chorea, choreoathetosis, and dystonia, while the psychiatric features include depression, anxiety, and psychosis; frontal and subcortical cognitive decline is also seen. Thus, with the right combination of features, Wilson's disease may mimic Huntington's disease, closely or otherwise.

It is particularly crucial to seek a diagnosis of Wilson disease in any HD-like patient lacking an autosomal dominant family history because the condition can be effectively treated by copper chelating treatments and other approaches. The majority of patients with neurological manifestations—though not all, as is sometimes claimed—have pathognomonic Kayser–Fleischer rings caused by copper deposition in the cornea; these are best seen on slit-lamp examination by an experienced ophthalmologist. Biochemical testing may reveal typical abnormalities of copper metabolism: low serum caeruloplasmin, high urinary copper, and high hepatic copper are the most reliable tests, but are best used in combination. Molecular genetic testing may be targeted to specific mutations depending on ethnicity; sequence analysis of the entire *ATP7B* is also available (34).

Friedreich's ataxia

Friedreich's ataxia has autosomal recessive inheritance and is the most prevalent cause of inherited ataxia. The vast majority of cases do not resemble Huntington's disease at all, but it is now accepted that chorea may be a feature alongside ataxia (35), while, conversely, Huntington's disease may produce cerebellar ataxia and atrophy (36). We reported a patient homozygous for abnormal GAA tract expansions in the *FRDA* gene, who developed generalized chorea, eye-movement restriction, and cognitive impairment, alongside the more typical features of ataxia and sensory neuropathy, and in whom negative genetic testing for Huntington's disease preceded a positive test for Friedreich's ataxia (4). The situation is not common but should be borne in mind.

Other causes

We recently reinvestigated our cohort in the light of the discovery of an expanded hexapeptide repeat in the first intron of the *C9orf72* gene in familial frontotemporal dementia and motor neuron disease (39, 40). Of 514 subjects, ten (2%) had the expansion. In our cohort, this is therefore the commonest genetic cause of HD-like clinical presentations (unpublished data). We therefore tentatively propose screening for this expansion in the diagnostic workup of HD-like patients.

Mutations in mitochondrial DNA, and in nuclear genes encoding mitochondrial proteins, can produce a notoriously broad spectrum of symptoms, which is ever increasing as more mutations are described. Myoclonus and dystonia are the most common movement disorders seen in *mitochondrial disease*, but chorea can occur and may be accompanied by cognitive decline or psychiatric features (37).

Benign hereditary chorea, an autosomal dominant disorder caused by mutations in *TITF1* encoding thyroid transcription factor 1, is, as the name suggests, generally a slowly progressive condition of isolated chorea, albeit with relatively young onset. However, atypical cases have been described with dystonia and gait disturbance. Intellectual impairment (as distinct from cognitive decline) may also be seen (38). Certain cases may resemble HD, at least transiently, and the condition should be borne in mind.

Acquired causes of HD look-alike syndromes are seldom seen because of the chronic degenerative nature of HD and its mimics. Chorea and neuropsychiatric symptoms are seen in Sydenham's chorea and other syndromes associated with anti-basal ganglia antibodies, although these are usually subacute and self-limiting, or at least non-progressive. Systemic lupus erythematosus (SLE) with CNS involvement and thyrotoxicosis can both produce chorea and psychiatric manifestations, but are likewise distinguishable from HD on the basis of tempo and associated systemic features. Rarely, chronic small vessel disease may produce a hyperkinetic movement disorder with cognitive involvement, but not without pyramidal signs and typical MRI changes (39).

Diagnostic yield

A number of studies have sought to identify large cohorts of patients with HD look-alike syndromes by applying different panels of genetic tests to each subject in order to screen for previously described and novel genetic causes of such syndromes. These cohorts generally consist of patients where there was a suspicion of HD sufficient to justify genetic testing for that disorder, but the test was negative.

Such studies cannot be taken as being representative of HD look-alikes as a whole because they usually exclude very rare disorders, like DRPLA, and conditions where clinical features or non-genetic approaches, such as metabolic testing and slit-lamp examination in Wilson disease or blood film examination in choreoacanthocytosis, may reveal a diagnosis before HD genetic testing is contemplated. Nonetheless, such studies offer insights into the relative frequencies of those conditions where genetic testing is useful. However, the overwhelming impression they give is pessimistic. Combining the results of five HD look-alike cohorts, tested for a variable number of conditions, with 285 patients of our own, tested for nine genetic conditions, produced a diagnostic yield of only 2% for genetic testing (see Fig. 21.1). This contrasts dramatically with the 99% probability that a suspicion of Huntington's disease will be confirmed by genetic testing, and suggests two conclusions: first, the majority of HD look-alike cases are caused by as yet unknown genetic (or non-genetic) factors; secondly, the patient in whom HD genetic testing is unexpectedly negative should be counselled to prepare for a long diagnostic process with a very low probability of success.

Nonetheless, the 2% of patients in whom a diagnosis is ultimately found do give an idea of the relative frequencies of each genetic cause. In that handful of patients, the most common diagnosis was SCA17, accounting for 44% of diagnoses; HDL2 accounted for 32%; the single Friedreich's ataxia case represented 15% of diagnoses; and familial prion disease (including HDL1) was found in 10% (see Fig. 21.1) (5).

Diagnostic approach

Although the yield from genetic testing is starkly low, combining these relative frequencies with the clinical features and available diagnostic techniques does suggest a rational strategy for the assessment of HD look-alike patients, combining clinical assessment with non-genetic and genetic tests. This approach is summarized in Fig. 21.3. Above all, it should be borne in mind that positive and negative genetic test results may have widespread ramifications for patients and family members, so expert neurogenetic counselling is essential throughout the process of investigation. Such counselling is just as important in the symptomatic patient as when performed for predictive testing, and when performed for an HD-like condition rather than for Huntington's disease itself.

The presence of associated clinical features may be sufficient to prompt directed genetic testing—for instance, Kayser–Fleischer rings in Wilson disease, myoclonic epilepsy in DRPLA, or prominent orofacial dystonia in choreoacanthocytosis. Directed non-genetic testing is often cheaper and quicker than genetic testing, and may also be more sensitive; thus, peripheral blood films, repeated several times or prepared as suggested earlier in this chapter, should be considered in all HD look-alike patients, and MRI scanning with T_2* or SWI sequences may disclose a wide variety of abnormalities such as focal atrophy, signal change, or brain iron accumulation.

Where genetic testing is carried out, it should be approached rationally according to the patient's clinical presentation and the likelihood of a positive result. In turn, this depends on the relative frequencies presented above and in Fig. 21.1, and factors such as

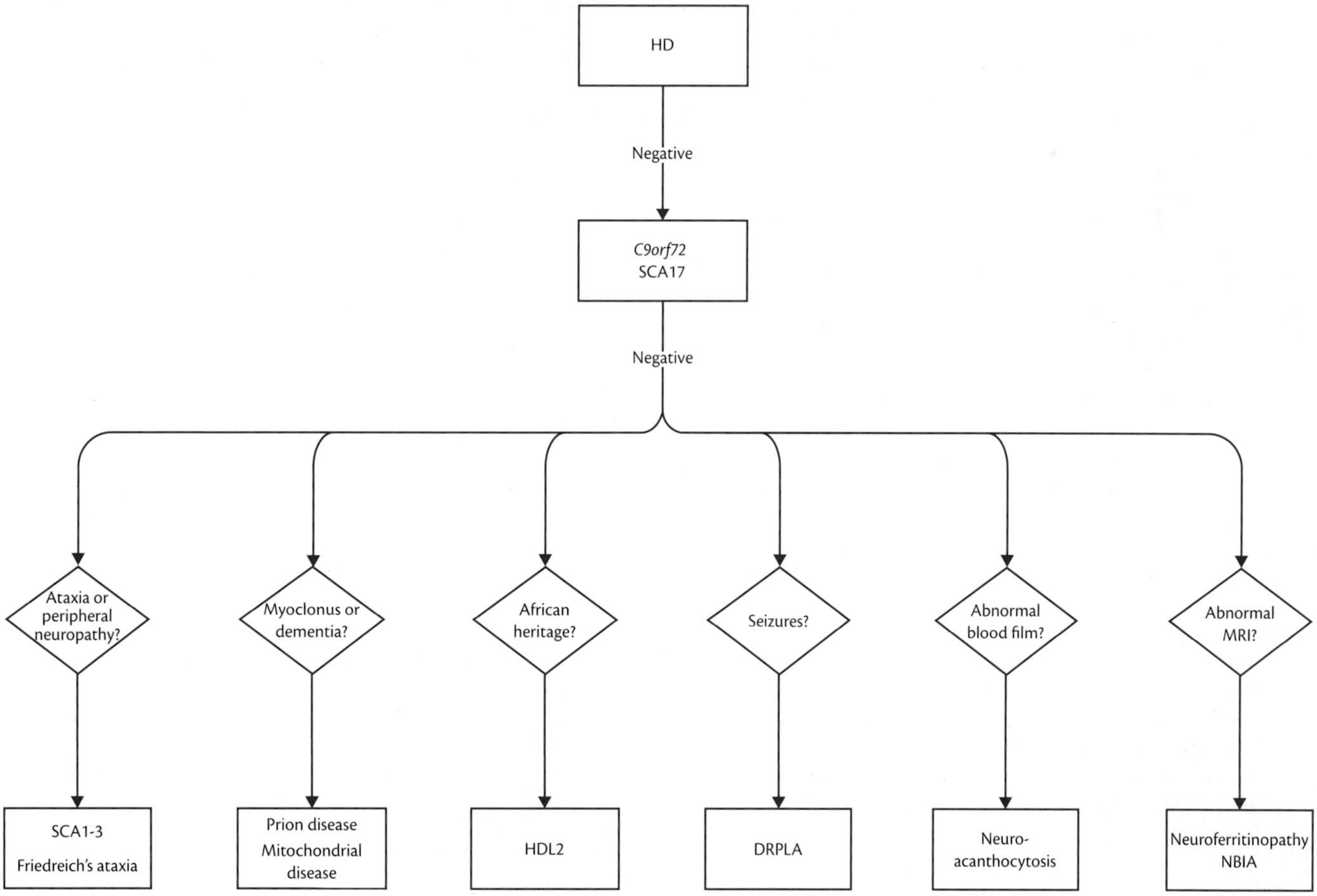

Fig. 21.3 Suggested approach to directed genetic testing in Huntington's disease look-alike syndromes. (Modified from Wild E, Tabrizi S. Huntington's disease phenocopy syndromes. *Curr Opin Neurol* 2007; 20: 681–7, by permission of Wolters Kluwer Health/Lippincott–Williams & Wilkins)

family history and ethnicity. SCA17 is the most frequent cause of HD look-alike syndromes and should form the first line of genetic testing, especially in patients with ataxia. HDL2, although relatively common, is essentially confined to people with African ancestry. The presence of myoclonus or early dementia should prompt genetic testing for familial prion disease, through *PRNP* sequencing rather than targeted mutation analysis. Genetic testing for other disorders should be considered on the basis of the clinical features described earlier and in Fig. 21.3 (5).

Management

The management of HD look-alike patients depends on whether a specific diagnosis is found (in which case the patient ceases to be an HD look-alike) and, if so, whether (as in the case of Wilson disease) the diagnosis suggests particular treatments. In practice, for the vast majority of patients, management consists of supportive multidisciplinary care, combined with an ongoing series of directed investigations and, where possible, storage of DNA for research use and future clinical testing as it becomes available. As noted above, such care is best delivered through the specialist neurogenetics clinic.

References

1. Kremer B, Goldberg P, Andrew SE, et al. A worldwide study of the Huntington's disease mutation: the sensitivity and specificity of measuring CAG repeats. *N Engl J Med* 1994; 330: 1401–6.
2. Bates G, Harper PS, Jones L (eds) *Huntington's disease* (3rd edn). Oxford: Oxford University Press, 2002.
3. Douglas I, Evans S, Rawlins MD, et al. Prevalence of adult Huntington's disease in the UK based on diagnoses recorded in general practice records. *J Neurol Neurosurg Psychiatry* 2013: doi:10.1136/jnnp-2012-304636
4. Wild EJ, Mudanohwo EE, Sweeney MG, et al. Huntington's disease phenocopies are clinically and genetically heterogeneous. *Mov Disord* 2008; 23: 716–20.
5. Wild EJ, Tabrizi SJ. Huntington's disease phenocopy syndromes. *Curr Opin Neurol* 2007; 20: 681–7.
6. Almqvist EW, Elterman DS, MacLeod PM, Hayden MR. High incidence rate and absent family histories in one quarter of patients newly diagnosed with Huntington disease in British Columbia. *Clin Genet* 2001; 60: 198–205.
7. Moore RC, Xiang F, Monaghan J, et al. Huntington disease phenocopy is a familial prion disease. *Am J Hum Genet* 2001; 69: 1385–8.
8. Mead S, Poulter M, Beck J, et al. Inherited prion disease with six octapeptide repeat insertional mutation—molecular analysis of phenotypic heterogeneity. *Brain* 2006; 129: 2297–317.
9. Krause A, Hetem C, Holmes SE, Margolis RL. HDL2 mutations are an important cause of Huntington's disease in patients with African ancestry. *J Neurol Neurosurg Psychiatry* 2005; 76 (Suppl 4): A16–26.
10. Santos C, Wanderley H, Vedolin L, Pena SD, Jardim L, Sequeiros J. Huntington disease-like 2: the first patient with apparent European ancestry. *Clin Genet* 2008; 73: 480–5.
11. Walker RH, Jankovic J, O'Hearn E, Margolis RL. Phenotypic features of Huntington's disease-like 2. *Mov Disord* 2003; 18: 1527–30.
12. Rudnicki DD, Holmes SE, Lin MW, Thornton CA, Ross CA, Margolis RL. Huntington's disease-like 2 is associated with CUG repeat-containing RNA foci. *Ann Neurol* 2007; 61: 272–82.
13. Wilburn B, Rudnicki DD, Zhao J, et al. An antisense CAG repeat transcript at JPH3 locus mediates expanded polyglutamine protein toxicity in Huntington's disease-like 2 mice. *Neuron* 2011; 70: 427–40.
14. Kambouris M, Bohlega S, Al-Tahan A, Meyer BF. Localization of the gene for a novel autosomal recessive neurodegenerative Huntington-like disorder to 4p15.3. *Am J Hum Genet* 2000; 66: 445–52.
15. Stevanin G, Fujigasaki H, Lebre A-S, et al. Huntington's disease-like phenotype due to trinucleotide repeat expansions in the TBP and JPH3 genes. *Brain* 2003; 126: 1599–603.
16. Schneider SA, van de Warrenburg BPC, Hughes TD, et al. Phenotypic homogeneity of the Huntington disease-like presentation in a SCA17 family. *Neurology* 2006; 67: 1701–3.
17. Loy CT, Sweeney MG, Davis MB, et al. Spinocerebellar ataxia type 17: extension of phenotype with putaminal rim hyperintensity on magnetic resonance imaging. *Mov Disord* 2005; 20: 1521–3.
18. Rolfs A, Koeppen AH, Bauer I, et al. Clinical features and neuropathology of autosomal dominant spinocerebellar ataxia (SCA17). *Ann Neurol* 2003; 54: 367–75.
19. Shah AG, Friedman MJ, Huang S, Roberts M, Li XJ, Li S. Transcriptional dysregulation of TrkA associates with neurodegeneration in spinocerebellar ataxia type 17. *Hum Mol Genet* 2009; 18: 4141–52.
20. Counts SE, Mufson EJ. The role of nerve growth factor receptors in cholinergic basal forebrain degeneration in prodromal Alzheimer disease. *J Neuropathol Exp Neurol* 2005; 64: 263–72.
21. Rong J, McGuire JR, Fang ZH, et al. Regulation of intracellular trafficking of huntingtin-associated protein-1 is critical for TrkA protein levels and neurite outgrowth. *J Neurosci* 2006; 26: 6019–30.
22. Schols L, Bauer P, Schmidt T, Schulte T, Riess O. Autosomal dominant cerebellar ataxias: clinical features, genetics, and pathogenesis. *Lancet Neurol* 2004; 3: 291–304.
23. Smith JK, Gonda VE, Malamud N. Unusual form of cerebellar ataxia; combined dentato-rubral and pallido-luysian degeneration. *Neurology* 1958; 8: 205–9.
24. Koide R, Ikeuchi T, Onodera O, et al. Unstable expansion of CAG repeat in hereditary dentatorubral-pallidoluysian atrophy (DRPLA). *Nat Genet* 1994; 6: 9–13.
25. Yamada M. Dentatorubral-pallidoluysian atrophy (DRPLA). *Neuropathology* 2010; 30: 453–7.
26. Zhang S, Xu L, Lee J, Xu T. Drosophila atrophin homolog functions as a transcriptional corepressor in multiple developmental processes. *Cell* 2002; 108: 45–56.
27. Burke JR, Wingfield MS, Lewis KE, et al. The Haw River syndrome: dentatorubropallidoluysian atrophy (DRPLA) in an African–American family. *Nat Genet* 1994; 7: 521–4.
28. Gregory A, Hayflick SJ. Genetics of neurodegeneration with brain iron accumulation. *Curr Neurol Neurosci Rep* 2011; 11: 254–61.
29. Ching KH, Westaway SK, Gitschier J, Higgins JJ, Hayflick SJ. HARP syndrome is allelic with pantothenate kinase-associated neurodegeneration. *Neurology* 2002; 58: 1673–4.
30. Hartig MB, Hörtnagel K, Garavaglia B, et al. Genotypic and phenotypic spectrum of PANK2 mutations in patients with neurodegeneration with brain iron accumulation. *Ann Neurol* 2006; 59: 248–56.
31. Chinnery PF, Crompton DE, Birchall D, et al. Clinical features and natural history of neuroferritinopathy caused by the FTL1 460InsA mutation. *Brain* 2007; 130: 110–19.
32. Danek A, Walker RH. Neuroacanthocytosis. *Curr Opin Neurol* 2005; 18: 386–92.
33. Storch A, Kornhass M, Schwarz J. Testing for acanthocytosis. A prospective reader-blinded study in movement disorder patients. *J Neurol* 2005; 252: 84–90.
34. Ferenci P. Pathophysiology and clinical features of Wilson disease. *Metab Brain Dis* 2004; 19: 229–39.
35. Hanna MG, Davis MB, Sweeney MG, et al. Generalized chorea in two patients harboring the Friedreich's ataxia gene trinucleotide repeat expansion. *Mov Disord* 1998; 13: 339–40.
36. Rodda RA. Cerebellar atrophy in Huntington's disease. *J Neurol Sci* 1981; 50: 147–57.
37. Caer M, Viala K, Levy R, et al. Adult-onset chorea and mitochondrial cytopathy. *Mov Disord* 2005; 20: 490–2.
38. Kleiner-Fisman G, Rogaeva E, Halliday W, et al. Benign hereditary chorea: Clinical, genetic, and pathological findings. *Ann Neurol* 2003; 54: 244–7.
39. DeJesus-Hernandez, M, et al. Expanded GGGGCC hexanucleotide repeat in noncoding region of C9ORF72 causes chromosome 9p-linked FTD and ALS. *Neuron* 2011. 72(2): p. 245–56.
40. Renton, AE, et al. A hexanucleotide repeat expansion in *C9ORF72* is the cause of chromosome 9p21-linked ALS-FTD. *Neuron* 2011. 72(2): p. 257–68.

CHAPTER 22

Non-degenerative Choreas

Francisco Cardoso

Summary

Non-genetic choreas can have myriad causes which fit into the following categories: autoimmune, vascular, drug-induced, infectious, metabolic and toxic encephalopathy, and miscellaneous. Sydenham's chorea, an autoimmune condition related to streptococcal infection, is the most common cause of chorea in children worldwide. In contrast, vascular disease, particularly in association with diabetes mellitus type 2, accounts for the majority of non-genetic choreas in adults. HIV infection, systemic lupus erythematosus, drugs, paraneoplastic syndromes, hyperthyroidism, brain neoplasms, etc. are also causes of chorea. The aim of this chapter is to discuss the epidemiology, clinical features, diagnosis, pathogenesis, and management of acquired causes of chorea.

Essential background

Chorea is a hyperkinetic syndrome characterized by brief, abrupt involuntary movements resulting from a continuous flow of random muscle contractions. The pattern of movement may sometimes appear playful, conveying a feeling of restlessness to the observer. When choreic movements are more severe, assuming a flinging, sometimes violent, character, they are called ballism. Regardless of its aetiology, overall chorea has the same motor features, although the muscle tone varies depending on the underlying aetiology (1). As several basal ganglia circuits are often involved in conditions associated with chorea, non-motor features such as subcortical cognitive decline, obsessions, compulsions, attention deficit, etc. are often present in choreic syndromes. Chorea has both genetic causes, described in other chapters of this book, and non-genetic causes (Table 22.1). The latter include vascular choreas, autoimmune choreas, metabolic and toxic choreas, and drug-induced choreas. The aim of this chapter is to provide an overview of the main causes of non-hereditary choreas, discussing their clinical features, aetiology, and pathogenesis, and management. As they represent separate entities, each category will be discussed separately, although always following the same outline: aetiology, pathophysiology, clinical features, diagnosis, and management.

Epidemiology

Although there are very few community-based studies available regarding the prevalence and incidence of choreas as a whole, there is information regarding the situation in tertiary care centres. According to a recent study from Pennsylvania, Sydenham's chorea (SC) accounts for almost 100% of acute cases of chorea seen in children (2). Recent studies from Australia confirm that it is a relatively common cause of acute chorea in children (3, 4). In contrast, the situation is quite distinct in adult patients. Although no published data are available, it is likely that levodopa-induced chorea in Parkinson's disease (PD) patients is the most common cause of chorea seen by neurologists. One study of consecutive patients seen at a tertiary hospital found that stroke accounted for 50% of all cases, drug abuse was identified in a third of patients, and the remaining patients had chorea related to AIDS and other infections as well as metabolic problems (5).

Autoimmune choreas

Sydenham's chorea

SC, the most common form of autoimmune chorea worldwide, is a major feature of acute rheumatic fever (ARF), a non-suppurative complication of group A beta-haemolytic streptococcus infection. Despite the decline of ARF, it remains as the most common cause of acute chorea in children in the USA and a major public health problem in developing areas of the world. Clinically, it is characterized by a combination of chorea, other movement disorders, behavioural abnormalities, and cognitive changes (1, 2, 6).

Aetiology and pathogenesis

Taranta and Stollerman (7) established the casual relationship between infection with group A beta-haemolytic streptococci and the occurrence of SC (7). Based on the assumption of molecular mimicry between streptococcal and central nervous system antigens, it has been proposed that the bacterial infection in genetically predisposed subjects leads to formation of cross-reactive antibodies that disrupt basal ganglia function. Several studies have demonstrated the presence of such circulating antibodies in 50–90% of patients with SC (8, 9). A specific epitope of streptococcal M proteins that cross-reacts with basal ganglia has been identified (10). In one study it was demonstrated that all patients with active SC have antibasal ganglia antibodies demonstrated by ELISA and Western blot. In subjects with persistent SC (duration of disease greater than 2 years despite best medical treatment) the positivity was about 60% (11). Recently it was determined that neuronal tubulin is the target of antineuronal antibodies (12). It must be

Table 22.1 Non-genetic causes of chorea

Immunological ◆ Sydenham's chorea and variants (chorea gravidarum and contraceptive-induced chorea) ◆ Systemic lupus erythematosus ◆ Antiphospholipid antibody syndrome ◆ Paraneoplastic syndromes ◆ Acute disseminated encephalomyelopathy ◆ Coeliac disease
Drug-related ◆ Amantadine ◆ Amphetamine ◆ Anticonvulsants (carbamazepine, phenytoin, lamotrigine, valproic acid) ◆ Carbon monoxide ◆ Calcium-channel blockers (cinnarizine, flunarizine) ◆ CNS stimulants (methylphenidate, pemoline, cyproheptadine) ◆ Cocaine ◆ Dopamine agonists ◆ Dopamine receptor blockers ◆ Ethanol ◆ Levodopa ◆ Levofloxacin ◆ Lithium ◆ Sympathomimetics ◆ Theophylline ◆ Tricyclic antidepressants
Infections ◆ AIDS related (toxoplasmosis, progressive multifocal leucoencephalopathy, HIV encephalitis) ◆ Bacteria • Diphtheria • Scarlet fever • Whooping cough ◆ Encephalitis • B19 parvovirus • Japanese encephalitis • Measles • Mumps • West Nile River encephalitis • Others ◆ Parasites • Neurocysticercosis ◆ Protozoan • Malaria • Syphilis
Endocrine-metabolic dysfunction ◆ Adrenal insufficiency ◆ Hyper/hypocalcaemia ◆ Hyper/hypoglycaemia ◆ Hypomagnesaemia ◆ Hypernatraemia ◆ Liver failure
Vascular ◆ Post-pump chorea (cardiac surgery) ◆ Stroke ◆ Subdural haematoma
Miscellaneous ◆ Anoxic encephalopathy ◆ Cerebral palsy ◆ Kernicterus ◆ Multiple sclerosis ◆ Normal maturation (<12 months old) ◆ Nutritional (e.g. B_{12} deficiency) ◆ Posttraumatic (brain injury)

emphasized that the biological value of the antibasal ganglia antibodies remains to be determined. However, one study suggests that they may interfere with neuronal function. Kirvan and colleagues demonstrated that the IgM of one patient with SC induced expression of calcium-dependent calmodulin in a culture of neuroblastoma cells (13). Our finding that there is a linear correlation between the increase of intracellular calcium levels in PC12 cells and antibasal ganglia antibody titre in the serum from SC patients further strengthens the hypothesis that these antibodies have a pathogenic role (14).

Although some investigations suggest that susceptibility to rheumatic chorea is linked to human leucocyte antigen-linked antigen expression (15), others fail to identify any relationship between SC and human leucocyte antigen class I and II alleles (16). However, an investigation has shown that there is an association between HLA-DRB1*07 and recurrent streptococcal pharyngitis and rheumatic heart disease (17). The genetic marker for ARF and related conditions was the B-cell alloantigen D8/17 (18). Despite reports claiming high specificity and sensitivity from the group which developed the assay (19, 20), the findings of other authors suggest that the D8/17 marker lacks both specificity and sensitivity (1). Another suggested genetic risk factor for the development of ARF, but not SC, is polymorphisms within the promoter region of the tumour necrosis factor-alpha gene (21).

Because of difficulties in accounting for the pathogenesis of SC with the molecular mimicry hypothesis, studies have addressed the role of immune cellular mechanisms in this condition. In an investigation of sera and cerebrospinal fluid (CSF) samples from patients of the Movement Disorders Clinic, Federal University of Minas Gerais, Brazil, Church and colleagues (22) found elevation of cytokines that take part in the Th2 (antibody-mediated) response, interleukins 4 (IL-4) and 10 (IL-10), in the serum of acute SC compared with persistent SC (22). They also described raised IL-4 and Il-10 in 31% of the CSF of patients with acute SC, whereas only IL-4 was raised in the CSF of patients with persistent SC. The authors concluded that SC is characterized by a Th2 response. However, as they found an elevation of IL-12 in acute SC and, more recently, an increased concentration of chemokines CXCL9 and CXCL10 in the serum of patients with acute SC (23), it can be concluded that Th1 (cell-mediated) mechanisms may also be involved in the pathogenesis of this disorder. A recent investigation confirmed that cellular immune mechanisms might be relevant to the pathogenesis of SC because there is a monocyte dysfunction (24).

Currently, the weight of evidence suggests that the pathogenesis of SC is related to circulating cross-reactive antibodies. Streptococcus-induced antibodies can be associated with a form of acute disseminated encephalomyelitis characterized by a high frequency of dystonia and other movement disorders as well as basal ganglia lesions on neuroimaging (25). Antineural and antinuclear antibodies have also been found in patients with Tourette's syndrome, but their relationship with prior streptococcus infection remains equivocal (26).

It remains unclear why up to 50% of patients with SC develop a persistent course of the illness. In this subset of individuals, the titres of antibasal ganglia antibodies are low. Taking into account this finding as well as our observation that serum brain-derived neurotrophic factor (BDNF) levels are high in this group of patients, it can be hypothesized that the acute immune process causes structural brain lesions, resulting in permanent dysfunction of the basal ganglia (27).

Clinical features

The usual age of onset of SC is 8–9 years, but there are reports of patients who developed chorea during the third decade of life. In most series, there is a female preponderance (28). Typically, patients develop this disease 4–8 weeks after an episode of group A beta-haemolytic streptococcal pharyngitis. It does not occur after streptococcal infection of the skin. The chorea spreads rapidly and becomes generalized, but 20% of patients remain hemichoreic (28, 29). Patients display motor impersistence, particularly noticeable during tongue protrusion and ocular fixation. The muscle tone is usually decreased; in severe and rare cases (8% of all patients seen at the Movement Disorders Clinic of the Federal University of Minas Gerais, Brazil), this is so pronounced that the patient may become bedridden (chorea paralytica).

Patients often display other neurological and non-neurological symptoms and signs. There are reports of common occurrence of tics in SC. However, it is virtually impossible to distinguish simple tics from fragments of chorea. Even vocal tics, found in 70% or more of patients with SC in one study, are not a simple diagnosis in patients with hyperkinesias (30). In a cohort of 108 SC patients carefully followed up at our unit, we have identified vocalizations in just 8% of subjects. We have avoided the term 'tic' because there was no premonitory sign or complex sound and, conversely, the vocalizations were associated with severe cranial chorea. Taken together, these findings suggest that the involuntary sounds present in a few patients with SC result from choreic contractions of the upper respiratory tract muscles rather than true tics (31, 32). There is evidence that many patients with active chorea have hypometric saccades, and a few of them also show oculogyric crisis. Dysarthria is common and there is also impairment of verbal fluency. In fact, a case-control study of patients described a pattern of decreased verbal fluency which reflected reduced phonetic, but not semantic, output (33). This result is consistent with dysfunction of the dorsolateral prefrontal–basal ganglia circuit. In a recent study of adults with SC, we have extended this finding, showing that many functions that depend on the prefrontal area are impaired in these patients. The conclusion of this study is that SC should be included among the causes of dysexecutive syndrome (34, 35). Prosody is also affected in SC. One investigation of 20 patients with SC has shown decreased vocal tessitura and increased duration of the speech (36–38). Interestingly, these findings are similar to those observed in PD (39). In a survey of 100 patients with rheumatic fever, half of whom had chorea, we found that migraine is more frequent in SC (21.8%) than in normal controls (8.1%, $p = 0.02$) (40). This is similar to what has been described in Tourette's syndrome (41). In the older literature, there are also references to papilloedema, central retinal artery occlusion, and seizures in a few patients with SC.

Attention has also been drawn to behavioural abnormalities. Swedo and colleagues (42) found obsessive–compulsive behaviour in five of thirteen SC patients, three of whom met the criteria for obsessive–compulsive disorder, whereas no patient in the rheumatic fever group presented with obsessive–compulsive behaviour (42). In another study of 30 patients with SC, Asbahr and colleagues (43) demonstrated that 70% of subjects presented with obsessions and compulsions, whereas 16.7% met the criteria for obsessive–compulsive disorder. None of 20 patients with ARF without chorea had obsessions or compulsions (43). These results were generally replicated by a more recent study which found that patients with ARF without chorea had more obsessions and compulsions than healthy controls (44). This study also tackled the issue of hyperactivity and attention deficit disorder in SC and found that 45% of 22 patients met criteria for this condition. Maia and colleagues (45) investigated behavioural abnormalities in 50 healthy subjects, 50 patients with rheumatic fever without chorea, and 56 patients with SC (45). The authors found that obsessive–compulsive behaviour, obsessive–compulsive disorder, and attention deficit and hyperactivity disorder were more frequent in the SC group (19%, 23.2%, and 30.4%, respectively) than in the healthy controls (11%, 4%, and 8%, respectively) and in the patients with ARF without chorea (14%, 6%, and 8%, respectively). In this study, the authors demonstrated that obsessive–compulsive behaviour displays little degree of interference in the performance of the activities of daily living. Another study compared the phenomenology of obsessions and compulsions of patients with SC with subjects diagnosed with tic disorders. The authors showed that the symptoms observed among the SC patients were different from those reported by patients with tic disorders, but were similar to those previously noted among samples of paediatric patients with primary obsessive–compulsive disorder (46). Another investigation comparing healthy controls with patients with rheumatic fever showed that obsessive–compulsive behaviour is more commonly seen in patients with SC with relatives who also have obsessions and compulsions (47). This study makes clear that there is interplay between genetic factors and environment in the development of behavioural problems in SC. We recently reported that SC may rarely induce psychosis or trichotillomania during the acute phase of the illness (48, 49).

The peripheral nervous system is not targeted in SC (50). Finally, it must be kept in mind that SC is a major manifestation of rheumatic fever. Between 60 and 80% of patients display cardiac involvement, particularly mitral valve dysfunction, in SC, whereas the association with arthritis is less common (seen in 30% of patients). However, in approximately 20% of patients, chorea is the sole finding (28, 51). A prospective follow-up of patients with SC with and without cardiac involvement in the first episode of chorea suggests that the heart remains spared in those without lesion at the onset of rheumatic fever (52).

Diagnosis

The current diagnostic criteria for SC are a modification of the Jones criteria: chorea with acute or subacute onset and lack of clinical and laboratory evidence of an alternative cause. The diagnosis is further supported by the presence of additional major or minor manifestations of rheumatic fever (33, 53, 54). Of note, according to the current criteria, the diagnosis of SC is still possible in the absence of any other feature of rheumatic fever.

The UFMG Sydenham's Chorea Rating Scale (USCRS), the first validated scale to rate SC, provides a detailed quantitative description of the performance of activities of daily living, behavioural abnormalities, and motor function. It comprises 27 items; each is scored from 0 (no symptom or sign) to 4 (severe disability or finding) (55). Of note, the USCRS is not intended to be used as a diagnostic tool but rather to assess patients who already have an established diagnosis of SC.

Several conditions may present with clinical manifestations similar to SC (1). The most important differential diagnosis is systemic lupus erythematosus (SLE), which will be discussed later in this chapter. From a clinical point of view, a majority of subjects with SLE will have other non-neurological manifestations such as arthritis, pericarditis, and other serosites as well as skin abnormalities. Moreover, the neurological picture of SLE tends to be more complex and may include psychosis, seizures, other movement disorders, and even mental status and consciousness level changes. Only in rare instances will chorea, with a tendency for spontaneous remissions and recurrences, be an isolated manifestation of SLE. The difficulty in distinguishing these two conditions is increased since at least 20% of patients with SC display recurrence of the movement disorder. Eventually, patients with SLE will develop other features, meeting diagnostic criteria for this condition (1). Primary antiphospholipid antibody syndrome (PAPS) is differentiated from SC by the absence of other clinical and laboratory features of rheumatic fever as well as the usual association with repeated abortions, venous thrombosis, and other vascular events, and the presence of typical laboratory abnormalities. Encephalitides, either as a result of direct viral invasion or by means of an immune-mediated post-infectious process, can cause chorea. However, this usually happens in younger children; the clinical picture is more diverse and includes seizures, pyramidal signs, and impaired psychomotor development. There are also laboratory abnormalities suggestive of the underlying condition. Drug-induced choreas are readily distinguished by a careful history demonstrating a temporal relationship between onset of the movement disorder and exposure to the agent.

Children and young adults with chorea should undergo complete neurological examination and diagnostic testing to determine the aetiology of various causes of chorea. As there is no specific biological marker of SC, the aim of the diagnostic work-up in patients suspected to have rheumatic chorea is threefold: (1) to identify evidence of recent streptococcal infection or acute phase reaction, (2) to search for cardiac injury associated with RF, and (3) to rule out alternative causes. Tests of acute phase reactants such as erythrocyte sedimentation rate, C-reactive protein, leucocytosis, other blood tests like rheumatoid factor, mucoproteins, protein electrophoresis, and supporting evidence of preceding streptococcal infection (increased antistreptolysin-O, antiDNAse-B, or other antistreptococcal antibodies; positive throat culture for group A streptococcus; recent scarlet fever) are much less helpful in diagnosing SC than in other forms of rheumatic fever because of the usual long latency between the infection and onset of the movement disorder. Elevated antistreptolysin-O titre may be found commonly in populations with a high prevalence of streptococcal infection. Furthermore, the antistreptolysin-O titre declines if the interval between infection and rheumatic fever is more than 2 months. However, anti-DNase-B titres may remain elevated for up to a year after streptococcal pharyngitis. Heart evaluation (i.e. Doppler echocardiography) is mandatory because the association of SC with carditis is found in up to 80% of patients. Cardiac lesions are the main source of serious morbidity in SC. Serological studies for SLE and PAPS must be ordered to rule out these conditions. EEG has little importance in the evaluation of these patients, showing non-specific generalized slowing acutely or after clinical recovery. Spinal fluid analysis is usually normal, but it may show a slightly increased lymphocyte count. In general, neuroimaging will help rule out vascular and other structural causes such as moyamoya disease. CT scan of the brain invariably fails to display abnormalities. Similarly, head MRI is often normal, although there are case reports of reversible hyperintensity in the basal ganglia area. In one study, Giedd and colleagues (56) showed increased signal in just two of twenty-four patients, although morphometric techniques revealed mean values for the size of the striatum and pallidum that were larger than controls. Unfortunately, these findings are of little help on an individual basis because there was an extensive overlap between controls and patients. PET and SPECT imaging may prove to be useful tools in the evaluation, revealing transient increases in striatal metabolism during the acute phase of the illness, a finding confirmed by a recent study (57–62). This contrasts with other choreic disorders (such as Huntington's disease) that are associated with hypometabolism. Of note, however, a recent investigation showed hyperperfusion in two patients with SC whereas the remaining five had hypometabolism (63). It is possible that the inconsistencies in these studies reflect heterogeneity of the population of patients. In our own unit, we have observed a correlation between hypermetabolism of the basal ganglia on SPECT during acute SC, whereas patients with persistent chorea often display hypometabolism in the basal ganglia. Increasing interest is now directed to autoimmune markers which may eventually be useful for diagnosis. However, the test of antineuronal antibodies is not commercially available, and is performed only for research purposes. Moreover, preliminary evidence suggests that these antibodies are not specific for SC. Similarly, the low sensitivity and specificity of the alloantigen D8/17 renders it unsuitable as a diagnostic test.

Management

In the past, physicians emphasized the need for bed rest for the treatment of SC. Currently there is no place for this measure. Quarantine to prevent contamination of others is usually unnecessary because SC is an autoimmune condition, and does not result from direct bacterial attack against the central nervous system (CNS) (64).

The first aim of the treatment of SC is to provide control of chorea and behavioral problems often associated with this condition. Regardless of the choice of agent for symptomatic control, the physician should attempt a gradual decrease of the dosage of the medication (25% reduction every 2 weeks) after the patient has remained free from the symptoms for at least a month. Another important point is that in some patients the symptoms are so mild that they do not cause meaningful disability. In these cases, it is possible not to introduce any pharmacological intervention, since spontaneous remission of SC is the rule (54, 65). The second aim is prophylaxis against new bouts of ARF. Although it remains unproven whether prophylaxis of streptococcal infection prevents recurrences of SC (66), clearly it decreases the development of new cardiac lesions which are the source of the most important disability in rheumatic fever.

There are no controlled studies of symptomatic treatment of SC, and the reader must be aware that all recommendations are off-label use of the cited drugs (64). The first choice of the authors is valproic acid with an initial dosage of 250 mg/day that is increased during a 2-week period to 250 mg three times a day. If the response is not satisfactory, dosage can be increased gradually up to 1500 mg/day. As this drug has a rather slow onset of action, we usually wait for 2 weeks before concluding that the regimen is ineffective. This is usually well tolerated, although some patients may develop dyspepsia and diarrhoea initially. Chronic exposure may be associated with action tremor of the hands and, more rarely, liver toxicity. An open-label study demonstrated that carbamazepine (15 mg/kg/day) is as effective as valproic acid (20–25 mg/kg/day) to induce remission of chorea (1, 67, 68). If the patient fails to respond to valproic acid or as first-line treatment in patients who present with chorea paralytica, the next option is to prescribe neuroleptics. Risperidone, a relatively potent dopamine D2 receptor blocker, is usually effective. The usual initial regimen is 1 mg twice a day. If the chorea is still troublesome 2 weeks later, the dosage can be increased to 2 mg twice a day. Haloperidol and pimozide are also occasionally used in the management of chorea in SC. However, they are less well tolerated than risperidone. Dopamine D2 receptor blockers must be used with great caution in patients with SC. After observation of the development of parkinsonism, dystonia, or both in patients treated with neuroleptics, we performed a case–control study comparing the response to these drugs in patients with SC and Tourette's syndrome. We demonstrated that 5% of 100 patients with chorea developed extrapyramidal complications, whereas these findings were not seen among patients with tics matched for age and dosage of neuroleptics (67). Other potential side effects of these agents are sedation, depression, and tardive dyskinesia.

There are no published guidelines concerning the discontinuation of antichoreic agents. Our policy is to attempt a gradual decrease of the dosage (25% reduction every 2 weeks) after the patient has been free from chorea for at least a month. Finally, the most important measure in the treatment of patients with SC is secondary prophylaxis.

Because of the presumably autoimmune origin of SC, there have been attempts to treat patients with rheumatic chorea with corticosteroids. However, this is a controversial area. Despite mention of effectiveness of prednisone in suppressing chorea, this drug is only used when there is associated severe carditis. We recently reported that methylprednisolone at a dose of 25 mg/kg/day in children and 1 g/day in adults for 5 days followed by 1 mg/kg/day of prednisone is an effective and well-tolerated treatment for patients with SC refractory to conventional treatment with antichoreic drugs and penicillin (68). At least one other group has replicated our findings of good response to steroids in selected patients with SC (69). In one of the few randomized controlled trials in SC, the authors compared oral prednisone (2mg/kg/day) with placebo in a double-blind fashion. Simultaneous use of haloperidol was allowed. They concluded that steroids accelerate recovery but the rate of remission and recurrence is similar in both groups (70). However, this study had some limitations. Haloperidol use was not controlled in the two groups, and it is uncertain whether the development of side effects such as weight gain and moon face in the steroid group could have potentially compromised the blinding of the study (this is of particular concern considering the high dosage of prednisone). In addition, the authors used a non-validated scale to rate the severity of chorea. The current recommendation is to reserve steroids for patients with persistent disabling chorea refractory to antichoreic agents or those who develop unacceptable side effects with other agents. Finally, there is one open controlled study of a small number of patients which reports that plasma exchange or intravenous immunoglobulin are as effective as oral prednisone in controlling the severity of chorea in SC (71). Surprisingly, the authors report a lack of side effects in all groups. Because of the lack of additional studies to confirm the safety and effectiveness of these treatments, their high cost, and the existence of alternative efficacious therapeutic options, plasmapheresis and immunoglobulin are presently considered as investigational and do not have a place in routine medical practice.

Other autoimmune choreas

Other immunological causes of chorea are SLE, PAPS, vasculitis, and paraneoplastic syndromes. SLE and PAPS are classically described as the prototypes of autoimmune choreas (72). However, several reports show that chorea is seen in no more than 1–2% of large series of patients with these conditions (73, 74). A PET study showed that there is hypometabolism of the basal ganglia in chorea associated with SLE (75). Rarely, autoimmune chorea has been reported in the context of paraneoplastic syndromes associated with CV2/CRMP5 antibodies in patients with small cell lung carcinoma, malignant thymoma, and, less frequently, breast cancer (76–79). Chorea associated with SLE or PAPS has been treated with immunosuppressive measures, especially intravenous methylprednisolone following a dosage regimen as described for SC, as well as intravenous immunoglobulin (80). As it is accepted that neurological complications, including chorea, in PAPS are related to ischaemic events, antiplatelet agents and even anticoagulants are often prescribed to treat chorea in this condition (81). However, these recommendations are based on reports of open-label studies involving small numbers of patients as well as the clinical experience of physicians (1). There is a report of the association of generalized chorea with bilateral basal ganglia lesions in Sjögren's syndrome (82).

Vascular choreas

A study in a tertiary referral center showed that cerebrovascular disease was the most common cause of non-genetic chorea, accounting for 21 out of 42 cases (5). Conversely, chorea is an unusual complication of acute vascular lesion, seen in less than 1% of patients with acute stroke.

Aetiology and pathogenesis

Vascular hemichorea, or hemiballism, is usually related to ischaemic or haemorrhagic lesion of the basal ganglia and adjacent white matter in the territory of the middle or the posterior cerebral artery (83). In contrast with classical textbook descriptions of hemiballism, the majority of patients with vascular chorea have lesions outside the subthalamus (84). An uncommon cause of chorea is moyamoya disease, an intracranial vasculopathy which presents with ischaemic lesion or, less commonly, haemorrhagic stroke of the basal ganglia (85). Another rare form of vascular chorea is 'post-pump chorea', a complication of extracorporeal circulation. The pathogenesis of this movement disorder is believed to be related to vascular insult of the basal ganglia during the surgical procedure. Finally, it is possible that polycythaemia vera, a rare cause of chorea, induces hyperkinesia via a vascular mechanism (86).

Clinical features and diagnosis

Vascular chorea usually has an abrupt onset with the majority of patients displaying severe choreic movements, which are labelled ballism, on one hemibody. Careful examination often reveals that patients have an underlying mild hemiparesis. Typically, hemiballism hemichorea affects elderly diabetic patients. Despite the dramatic onset, spontaneous remission is the rule. In contrast, post-pump chorea is almost exclusively a complication of cardiac surgery in infants who commonly develop cognitive deficits. The long-term prognosis of post-pump chorea is rather poor. For example, in one series of eight patients, five subjects had persistent chorea and one of them died. In another study there was a clear distinction between those eight patients with onset at earlier age (median, 4.3 months), all of whom recovered fully, and eleven others with older onset (median, 16.8 months). Four of the latter died and only one of the survivors made a complete neurological recovery (87). Rarely, paroxysmal chorea triggered by emotional stress and hyperventilation may also be caused by moyamoya syndrome, a condition of unknown cause characterized by vascular malformation in the base of the brain (88, 89).

The diagnosis of vascular chorea relies on the clinical features and typical imaging findings, i.e. ischaemic or haemorrhagic lesions of the basal ganglia, particularly the subthalamic area. Of note, particularly among patients of Asian background with diabetes, MRI scans show a bilateral hypersignal in the lentiform nucleus, presumed to represent microhaemorrhage.

Management

Despite the usual favourable long-term prognosis of vascular chorea, treatment with antichoreic drugs such as neuroleptics or dopamine depletors may be necessary in the acute phase. Persistent movement disorder may remain in a few patients with vascular chorea. In this circumstance, they can be effectively treated with stereotactic surgery such as thalamotomy or posteroventral pallidotomy (90, 91).

Drug-induced choreas

Chorea can result from exposure to a variety of drugs, and drug-induced chorea is probably the most commonly encountered type of chorea in neurological practice and in the community (92).

Aetiology and pathogenesis

A list of drugs which may cause chorea is included in Table 22.1 (1, 92). Certain drugs seem to require pre-existing basal ganglia dysfunction to induce chorea, whereas others appear to be more universally choreogenic. Examples of the former are oral contraceptives, which are particularly likely to induce chorea in patients with previous choreic episodes such as SC, chorea with SLE, or chorea gravidarum (93, 94), and levodopa, which only induces chorea in patients with idiopathic PD or other parkinsonian disorders (95). Dopamine antagonists (DA), on the other hand, are capable of inducing dyskinesias without pre-existing basal ganglia abnormality. In one study of 100 consecutive patients with tardive dyskinesia, we demonstrated that, in contrast with the traditional assumption, chorea is rarely seen in association with use of DA antagonists (96). The most prevalent types of drug-induced chorea result from treatment of PD patients with levodopa. Levodopa-induced chorea develops in more than 40% of PD patients, depending on age and duration and dose of levodopa treatment. Furthermore, a variety of other agents has been associated with chorea in retrospective studies or anecdotal case reports. These include tricyclic antidepressants and the SSRIs (97–99). Phenytoin may also induce involuntary movements, including orofacial chorea, particularly when other antiepileptic drugs are administered (100). There are occasional reports of choreic dyskinesias induced by other antiepileptic drugs, such as carbamazepine (101) and lamotrigine (102). There is a recent report relating valproate use to the onset of chorea which is surprising, considering the established antichoreic action of this agent in SC (103). Chronic exposure to amphetamines and other stimulants may induce orofacial dyskinesias and choreic movements of the trunk and extremities (105). There is also a report of the onset of chorea in association with intrathecal infusion of methotrexate (106).

Clinical features and diagnosis

Chorea induced by drugs does not usually have distinctive features. The exception to this statement is chorea in tardive dyskinesia, where the majority of patients have a combination of chorea and other phenomena, particularly stereotypies and dystonia. Another exception is levodopa-induced dyskinesia because patients also display parkinsonian features as well as other hyperkinesias, mainly dystonia. Obviously, the diagnosis depends on the history of onset of the movement disorder after exposure to the offending agent. Improvement or remission with withdrawal of the drug further supports the diagnosis. However, one should be aware that in tardive dyskinesia there may be initial worsening of the movement disorder after the discontinuation of the antidopaminergic agent.

Management

The mainstay of the treatment of drug-induced choreas is the withdrawal of the offending agent. Chorea in the context of tardive dyskinesia is usually responsive to treatment with tetrabenazine, a presynaptic dopamine depletor. The management of levodopa-related chorea and other movement disorders is beyond the scope of the chapter.

Infectious choreas

SC could be considered a form of infectious chorea as it is induced by group A beta-haemolytic streptococcus. However, in a strict sense the term is limited to instances where chorea results from injury to the brain directly produced by a micro-organism. Human immunodeficiency virus (HIV) and its complications is the most frequently reported infectious cause of chorea. For example, in one series of 42 consecutive patients with non-genetic chorea, AIDS was found to be the cause in 12% of the subjects (5). In HIV-positive patients, chorea is the result of either the direct action of the virus or other mechanisms such as opportunistic infections (toxoplasmosis, syphilis, etc.) or drugs (107). However, with the advent of highly active antiretroviral therapy, there has been a decline in HIV-related neurological complications, including movement disorders. Other infections related to chorea are new variant Creutzfeldt–Jakob disease, tuberculosis, syphilis, and herpes simplex encephalitis (108–111).

Chorea in metabolic and toxic encephalopathy

Chronic acquired hepatolenticular degeneration was the first well-characterized metabolic cause of chorea. Originally described in the context of alcoholic encephalopathy, it can occur in any form of acquired liver disease. The clinical picture is heterogeneous, since patients may present with a variable combination of neurological and hepatic manifestations. In most instances, there is a combination of different movement disorders, but a few subjects may present with isolated chorea. MRI of the brain shows not only images compatible with cavitations in the basal ganglia (hyperintense signal on T_2 and hypointense on T_1) but also a hyperintense T_1 signal in the pallidum, putamen, and upper brainstem. The latter has been interpreted as being caused by deposition of manganese (112).

More recently, there is growing interest in the association of chorea and non-ketotic hyperglycaemia in type 2 diabetes mellitus, a condition particularly common among patients with an Asian ethnic background. Unlike the usual neurological manifestations of non-ketotic hyperglycaemia, patients do not have change in the level of consciousness but develop unilateral or generalized chorea–ballism. The MRI findings are characteristic, with a hyperintense signal in the pallidum on T_1 possibly reflecting microhaemorrhages, although it has been suggested that inflammation may also play a role in the pathogenesis (113, 114). Once glycaemic control is achieved, there is gradual remission of chorea (115, 116).

A few patients with hyperthyroidism may develop generalized chorea, or even ballism, related to this endocrine dysfunction. The lack of structural changes in the brain, the appearance with onset of thyrotoxicosis, and remission with endocrine control suggest that the basal ganglia dysfunction is induced by hormonal influences (117, 118). Other possible metabolic causes of chorea are even rarer and include hypoglycaemia, renal failure, and ketogenic diet (1).

Miscellaneous

Focal choreic limb movements or hemichorea can be a rare presenting symptom of primary or secondary brain neoplasms involving the basal ganglia, subthalamic nucleus, or adjacent areas. This type of presentation has been described most often for primary CNS lymphoma, but may occur with any type of subcortical tumor or even nonneoplastic structural disease disrupting striato-pallido-thalamo-cortical motor circuitry (119, 120). Therefore brain imaging is mandatory in any new-onset focal or hemichoreic syndrome. Uncommon causes of chorea recently reported include giant tumefactive perivascular spaces (121), intracranial sewing needles (122), and psychiatric diseases (123). Finally, although there is a decline in the frequency of cerebral palsy, a multicentre study demonstrated that pallidal deep brain stimulation is an effective treatment for chorea and dystonia related to this condition (124). Despite the fact that the results of this study are preliminary, it is an important investigation considering the current limited treatment options for chorea and dystonia associated with cerebral palsy.

Key advances

SC has been considered to be an autoimmune form of chorea related to rheumatic fever since the 1970s. In the last few years growing evidence supporting such a theory has been reported. The use of contemporary immunological methods has demonstrated that the majority of patients with the acute form of SC have high titres of circulating antibodies, which recognize antigens of streptococcus as well as the basal ganglia (11). There is also some evidence indicating that these anti-basal ganglia antibodies are capable of inducing functional changes in neural cells (13, 14). Recent studies indicate that parkinsonism and myoclonus, rather than chorea, are the most common movement disorders associated with SLE (125).

Diabetes mellitus is the most common risk factor for vascular chorea–hemiballism, a condition almost invariably seen among the elderly (83). Diabetes mellitus type 2 induces unilateral or bilateral chorea in association with hypersignal in the basal ganglia mostly, for unknown reasons, in patients of Asian background. Although the issue remains contentious, most studies suggest that these neuroimaging findings are related to microhaemorrhages (113–116).

At the onset of the AIDS epidemic, neurological complications were often diagnosed in HIV-positive patients. Physicians diagnosed chorea–ballism related to toxoplasmosis in around 3% of patients (107). With the introduction of highly active antiretroviral therapy, there has been a decline in the incidence of neurological complications among HIV-positive subjects (126). There are no recent data specifically related to the epidemiology of movement disorders, including chorea, in this particular population. Nevertheless, judging from clinical experience as well as the limited number of new publications related to the issue, one can assume that chorea and other extrapyramidal syndromes have become much rarer among HIV-positive patients.

Future developments

Despite the accumulating evidence pointing to the autoimmune nature of SC, it still remains to be proved beyond any reasonable doubt that circulating anti-basal ganglia antibodies are relevant to the pathogenesis of this condition. This is not a question with interest limited to the academic world. It is beyond the scope of this chapter to tackle the concept of PANDAS (paediatric autoimmune neuropsychiatric disorders related to streptococcus). However, it is worth mentioning that some have suggested that streptococcus-induced antibodies are responsible for triggering conditions such as tics, obsessive–compulsive disorders, etc. (127). If such a hypothesis is proved to be true, the epidemiological relevance of streptococcus-related neurological complications will increase substantially. Currently, the majority of studies fail to support such a causal relationship between streptococcus and clinical phenomena other than chorea (128). However, there is a need to address whether anti-basal ganglia antibodies are capable of inducing functional changes *in vivo*. Controlled studies to investigate treatments for movement disorders associated with SLE as well as PAPS are limited because of their rarity. As they are ubiquitous conditions, it is quite likely that collaborative multicentre studies may lead to new developments in their management. In the field of AIDS-related chorea, there has been a decline in its occurrence with the use of highly active antiretroviral agents. However, it is rather disappointing that these drugs have not succeeded in completely preventing the development of CNS complications of HIV infection. This suggests that there is a need for more active agents, or perhaps drugs that act via mechanisms distinct from those that are tackled by currently available medications.

Conclusions

SC remains as the most common cause of chorea in children worldwide. In addition to chorea, patients with SC often have behavioural disorders, such as obsessions and hyperactivity. In most patients there is spontaneous remission after a few months.

However, in 25% of subjects the condition remains persistent. Treatment is based on use of antichoreic drugs as well as prophylaxis of new streptococcus infections with penicillin. SLE and related conditions cause chorea and other movement disorders in less than 5% of patients. Despite the lack of controlled studies, these patients are treated with immunosuppressive agents combined with anticoagulants when there are circulating antiphospholipid antibodies. Vascular disease is the most common cause of acute non-hereditary chorea among adults. Most patients are elderly with diabetes mellitus type 2 who present with sudden-onset hemichorea–hemiballism. Although spontaneous recovery is the rule, severe hyperkinesia requires treatment with antidopaminergic agents. Levodopa and dopamine agonists are the most common agents leading to chorea in clinical practice, although the list of agents implicated in the causation of this phenomenon is quite long. HIV remains as the most frequent infectious cause of chorea, despite the decline of neurological complications in AIDS with the introduction of highly active antiretroviral therapy. Finally, there are other less common causes of acquired chorea such as paraneoplastic syndromes, moyamoya disease, hyperthyroidism, liver failure, subdural haematoma, and brain neoplasms.

Top clinical tips

- Sydenham's chorea is the most common cause of non-genetic chorea in children.
- Treatment of Sydenham's chorea involves antichoreic agents and prophylaxis against streptococcal infection.
- Chorea is a rare complication of systemic lupus erythematosus.
- Vascular disease is the most common cause of non-genetic chorea in adults.
- Diabetes mellitus is the most common risk factor for vascular chorea.
- Drug-induced chorea is usually a complication of dopaminergic agents.

References

1. Cardoso F, Seppi K, Mair KJ, Wenning GK, Poewe W. Seminar on choreas. *Lancet Neurol* 2006; 5: 589–602.
2. Zomorrodi A, Wald ER. Sydenham's chorea in western Pennsylvania. *Pediatrics* 2006; 117: e675–9.
3. Dale RC, Singh H, Troedson C, Pillai S, Gaikiwari S, Kozlowska K. A prospective study of acute movement disorders in children. *Dev Med Child Neurol* 2010; 52: 739–48.
4. Smith MT, Lester-Smith D, Zurynski Y, Noonan S, Carapetis JR, Elliott EJ. Persistence of acute rheumatic fever in a tertiary children's hospital. *J Paediatr Child Health* 2011; 47: 198–203.
5. Piccolo I, Defanti CA, Soliveri P, et al. Cause and course in a series of patients with sporadic chorea. *J Neurol* 2003; 250: 429–35.
6. Cardoso F. Chorea. In: Hallett M, Poewe W (eds) *Therapeutics of Parkinson's disease and other movement disorders*, pp. 212–27. Philadelphia, PA: John Wiley, 2008.
7. Taranta A, Stollerman GH. The relationship of Sydenham's chorea to infection with group A streptococci. *Am J Med* 1956; 20: 1970.
8. Husby G, Van De Rijn U, Zabriskie JB, Abdin ZH, Williams RC, Jr. Antibodies reacting with cytoplasm of subthalamic and caudate nuclei neurons in chorea and acute rheumatic fever. *J Exp Med* 1976; 144: 1094–110.
9. Cardoso F. Chorea gravidarum. *Arch Neurol* 2002; 59: 868–70.
10. Bronze MS, Dale JB. Epitopes of streptococcal M proteins that evoke antibodies that cross-react with human brain. *J Immunol* 1993; 151: 2820–8.
11. Church AJ, Cardoso F, Dale RC, et al. Anti-basal ganglia antibodies in acute and persistent Sydenham's chorea. *Neurology* 2002; 59: 227–31.
12. Kirvan CA, Cox CJ, Swedo SE, Cunningham MW. Tubulin is a neuronal target of autoantibodies in Sydenham's chorea. *J Immunol* 2007; 178: 7412–21.
13. Kirvan CA, Swedo SE, Heuser JS, Cunningham MW. Mimicry and autoantibody-mediated neuronal cell signaling in Sydenham chorea. *Nat Med* 2003; 9: 914–20.
14. Teixeira AL, Jr, Guimaraes MM, Romano-Silva MA, Cardoso F. Serum from Sydenham's chorea patients modifies intracellular calcium levels in PC12 cells by a complement-independent mechanism. *Mov Disord* 2005; 20: 843–5.
15. Ayoub EM, Barrett DJ, Maclaren NK, Krischer JP. Association of class II human histocompatibility leukocyte antigens with rheumatic fever. *J Clin Invest* 1986; 77: 2019–26.
16. Donadi EA, Smith AG, Louzada-Junior P, Voltarelli JC, Nepom GT. HLA class I and class II profiles of patients presenting with Sydenham's chorea. *J Neurol* 2000; 247: 122–8.
17. Haydardedeoglu FE, Tutkak H, Kose K, Duzgun N. Genetic susceptibility to rheumatic heart disease and streptococcal pharyngitis: association with HLA-DR alleles. *Tissue Antigens* 2006; 68: 293–6.
18. Feldman BM, Zabriskie JB, Silverman ED, Laxer RM. Diagnostic use of B-cell alloantigen D8/17 in rheumatic chorea. *J Pediatr* 1993; 123: 84–6.
19. Eisen JL, Leonard HL, Swedo SE, et al. The use of antibody D8/17 to identify B cells in adults with obsessive–compulsive disorder. *Psychiatry Res* 2001; 104: 221–5.
20. Harel L, Zeharia A, Kodman Y, et al. Presence of the d8/17 B-cell marker in children with rheumatic fever in Israel. *Clin Genet* 2002; 61: 293–8.
21. Ramasawmy R, Fae KC, Spina G, et al. Association of polymorphisms within the promoter region of the tumor necrosis factor-alpha with clinical outcomes of rheumatic fever. *Mol Immunol* 2007; 44: 1873–8.
22. Church AJ, Dale RC, Cardoso F, et al. CSF and serum immune parameters in Sydenham's chorea: evidence of an autoimmune syndrome? *J Neuroimmunol* 2003; 136: 149–53.
23. Teixeira AL, Jr, Cardoso F, Souza AL, Teixeira MM. Increased serum concentrations of monokine induced by interferon-gamma/CXCL9 and interferon-gamma-inducible protein 10/CXCL-10 in Sydenham's chorea patients. *J Neuroimmunol* 2004; 150: 157–62.
24. Torres KC, Dutra WO, de Rezende VB, Cardoso F, Gollob KJ, Teixeira AL. Monocyte dysfunction in Sydenham's chorea patients. *Hum Immunol* 2010; 71: 351–4.
25. Dale RC, Church AJ, Cardoso F, et al. Poststreptococcal acute disseminated encephalomyelitis with basal ganglia involvement and auto-reactive antibasal ganglia antibodies. *Ann Neurol* 2001; 50: 588–95.
26. Morshed SA, Parveen S, Leckman JF, et al. Antibodies against neural, nuclear, cytoskeletal, and streptococcal epitopes in children and adults with Tourette's syndrome, Sydenham's chorea, and autoimmune disorders. *Biol Psychiatry* 2001; 50: 566–77.
27. Teixeira AL, Bretas TL, Kummer A, et al. Serum levels of brain-derived neurotrophic factor in Sydenham's chorea. *Neurol Sci* 2010; 31: 399–401.
28. Cardoso F, Silva CE, Mota CC. Sydenham's chorea in 50 consecutive patients with rheumatic fever. *Mov Disord* 1997; 12: 701–3.
29. Nausieda PA, Grossman BJ, Koller WC, Weiner WJ, Klawans HL. Sydenham's chorea: an update. *Neurology* 1980; 30: 331–4.
30. Mercadante MT, Campos MC, Marques-Dias MJ, et al. Vocal tics in Sydenham's chorea. *J Am Acad Child Adolesc Psychiatry* 1997; 36: 305–6.
31. Jankovic J. Differential diagnosis and etiology of tics. *Adv Neurol* 2001; 85: 15–29.
32. Teixeira AL, Jr, Cardoso F, Maia DP, et al. Frequency and significance of vocalizations in Sydenham's chorea. *Parkinsonism Relat Disord* 2009; 15: 62–3.

33. Cunningham MC, Maia DP, Teixeira AL, Jr, Cardoso F. Sydenham's chorea is associated with decreased verbal fluency. *Parkinsonism Relat Disord* 2006; 12: 165–7.
34. Beato R, Maia D, Teixeira A, Cardoso F. Executive functioning in adult patients with Sydenham's chorea. *Mov Disord* 2010; 25: 853–7.
35. Cavalcanti A, Hilário MO, dos Santos FH, Bolognani SA, Bueno OF, Len CA. Subtle cognitive deficits in adults with a previous history of Sydenham's chorea during childhood. *Arthritis Care Res* 2010; 62: 1065–71.
36. Cardoso F, Oliveira PM, Reis CC, et al. Prosody in Sydenham chorea—I: Tessitura. *Mov Disord* 2006; 21: S359–60.
37. Cardoso F, Oliveira PM, Reis CC, et al. Prosody in Sydenham chorea—II: Duration. f statements. *Mov Disord* 2006; 21: S360.
38. Oliveira PM, Cardoso F, Maia DP, Cunningham MC, Teixeira AL, Jr, Reis C. Acoustic analysis of prosody in Sydenham's chorea. *Arq Neuropsiquiatr* 2010; 68: 744–8.
39. Azevedo LL, Cardoso F, Reis C. Acoustic analysis of prosody in females with Parkinson's disease: comparison with normal controls. *Arq Neuropsiquiatr* 2003; 61: 999–1003.
40. Teixeira AL, Jr, Meira FC, Maia DP, Cunningham MC, Cardoso F. Migraine headache in patients with Sydenham's chorea. *Cephalalgia* 2005; 25: 542–4.
41. Kwack C, Vuong KD, Jankovic J. Migraine headache in patients with Tourette syndrome. *Arch Neurol* 2003; 60: 1595–8.
42. Swedo SE, Leonard HL, Garvey M, et al. Pediatric autoimmune neuropsychiatric disorders associated with streptococcal infections: clinical description of the first 50 cases. *Am J Psychiatry* 1988; 155: 264–71.
43. Asbahr FR, Negrao AB, Gentil V, et al. Obsessive–compulsive and related symptoms in children and adolescents with rheumatic fever with and without chorea: a prospective 6-month study. *Am J Psychiatry* 1998; 155: 1122–4.
44. Mercadante MT, Busatto GF, Lombroso PJ, et al. The psychiatric symptoms of rheumatic fever. *Am J Psychiatry* 2000; 157: 2036–8.
45. Maia DP, Teixeira AL, Jr, Quintao Cunningham MC, Cardoso F. Obsessive–compulsive behavior, hyperactivity, and attention deficit disorder in Sydenham chorea. *Neurology* 2005; 64: 1799–801.
46. Asbahr FR, Garvey MA, Snider LA, et al. Obsessive–compulsive symptoms among patients with Sydenham chorea. *Biol Psychiatry* 2005; 57: 1073–6.
47. Hounie AG, Pauls DL, do Rosario-Campos MC, et al. Obsessive-compulsive spectrum disorders and rheumatic fever: a family study. *Biol Psychiatry* 2007; 61: 266–72.
48. Kummer A, Maia DP, Cardoso F, Teixeira, AL. Trichotillomania in acute Sydenham's chorea. *Aust NZ J Psychiatry* 2007; 41: 1013–14.
49. Teixeira, AL Jr, Maia DP, Cardoso F. Psychosis following acute Sydenham's chorea. *Eur Child Adolesc Psychiatry* 2007; 16: 67–9.
50. Cardoso F, Dornas L, Cunningham M, Oliveira JT. Nerve conduction study in Sydenham's chorea. *Mov Disord* 205; 20: 360–3.
51. Vijayalakshmi IB, Mithravinda J, Deva AN. The role of echocardiography in diagnosing carditis in the setting of acute rheumatic fever. *Cardiol Young* 2005; 15: 583–8.
52. Panamonta M, Chaikitpinyo A, Auvichayapat N, et al. Evolution of valve damage in Sydenham's chorea during recurrence of rheumatic fever. *Int J Cardiol* 2007; 119: 73–9.
53. Guidelines for diagnosis of rheumatic fever, Jones criteria, 1992 update. Special Writing Group of the Committee of Rheumatic Fever, Endocarditis, and Kawasaki Disease of the Council on Cardio-Vascular Disease of the Young of the American Heart Association. Guidelines for the diagnosis of rheumatic fever. *JAMA* 1992; 268: 2069–73.
54. Cardoso F, Vargas AP, Oliveira LD, Guerra AA, Amaral SV. Persistent Sydenham's chorea. *Mov Disord* 1999; 14: 805–7.
55. Teixeira AL, Jr, Maia DP, Cardoso F. UFMG Sydenham's chorea rating scale (USCRS): reliability and consistency. *Mov Disord* 2005; 20: 585–91.
56. Giedd JN, Rapoport JL, Kruesi MJ, et al. Sydenham's chorea: magnetic resonance imaging of the basal ganglia. *Neurology* 1995; 45: 2199–202.
57. Giedd JN, Rapoport JL, Kruesi MJ, et al. Sydenham's chorea: magnetic resonance imaging of the basal ganglia. *Neurology* 1995; 45: 2199–202.
58. Goldman S, Amrom D, Szliwowski HB, et al. Reversible striatal hypermetabolism in a case of Sydenham's chorea. *Mov Disord* 1993; 8: 355–8.
59. Weindl A, Kuwert T, Leenders KL, et al. Increased striatal glucose consumption in Sydenham's chorea. *Mov Disord* 1993; 8: 437–44.
60. Lee PH, Nam HS, Lee KY, Lee BI, Lee JD. Serial brain SPECT images in a case of Sydenham chorea. *Arch Neurol* 1999; 56: 237–40.
61. Barsottini OG, Ferraz HB, Seviliano MM, Barbieri A. Brain SPECT imaging in Sydenham's chorea. *Braz J Med Biol Res* 2002; 35: 431–6.
62. Paghera B, Caobelli F, Giubbini R, Premi E, Padovani A. Reversible striatal hypermetabolism in a case of rare adult-onset Sydenham chorea on two sequential 18F-FDG PET studies. *J Neuroradiol* 2011; 38: 325–6.
63. Ho L. Hypermetabolism in bilateral basal ganglia in Sydenham chorea on F-18 FDG PET-CT. *Clin Nucl Med* 2009; 34: 114–16.
64. Cardoso F. Sydenham's chorea. *Curr Treat Options Neurol* 2008; 10: 230–5.
65. Tumas V, Caldas CT, Santos AC, Nobre A, Fernandes RM. Sydenham's chorea: clinical observations from a Brazilian movement disorder clinic. *Parkinsonism Relat Disord* 2007; 13: 276–83.
66. Korn-Lubetzki I, Brand A, Steiner I. Recurrence of Sydenham chorea: implications for pathogenesis. *Arch Neurol* 2004; 61: 1261–4.
67. Teixeira AL, Cardoso F, Maia DP, Cunningham MC. Sydenham's chorea may be a risk factor for drug induced parkinsonism. *J Neurol Neurosurg Psychiatry* 2003; 74: 1350–1.
68. Cardoso F, Maia D, Cunningham MC, Valenca G. Treatment of Sydenham chorea with corticosteroids. *Mov Disord* 2003; 18: 1374–7.
69. Barash J, Margalith D, Matitiau A. Corticosteroid treatment in patients with Sydenham's chorea. *Pediatr Neurol* 2005; 32: 205–7.
70. Paz JA, Silva CA, Marques-Dias MJ. Randomized double-blind study with prednisone in Sydenham's chorea. *Pediatr Neurol* 2006; 34: 264–9.
71. Garvey MA, Snider LA, Leitman SF, Werden R, Swedo SE. Treatment of Sydenham's chorea with intravenous immunoglobulin, plasma exchange, or prednisone. *J Child Neurol* 2005; 20: 424–9.
72. Quinn N, Schrag A. Huntington's disease and other choreas. *J Neurol* 1998; 245: 709–16.
73. Asherson RA, Cervera R. The antiphospholipid syndrome: multiple faces beyond the classical presentation. *Autoimmun Rev* 2003; 2: 140–51.
74. Avcin T, Benseler SM, Tyrrell PN, Cucnik S, Silverman ED. A follow up study of antiphospholipid antibodies and associated neuropsychiatric manifestations in 137 children with systemic lupus erythematosus. *Arthritis Rheum* 2008; 59: 206–13.
75. Krakauer M, Law I. FDG PET brain imaging in neuropsychiatric systemic lupus erythematosus with choreic symptoms. *Clin Nucl Med* 2009; 34: 122–3.
76. Grant R, Graus F. Paraneoplastic movement disorders. *Mov Disord* 2009; 24: 1715–24.
77. Martinková J, Valkovic P, Benetin J. Paraneoplastic chorea associated with breast cancer. *Mov Disord* 2009; 24: 2296–7.
78. Honnorat J, Cartalat-Carel S, Ricard D, et al. Onco-neural antibodies and tumor type determine survival and neurological symptoms in paraneoplastic neurological syndromes with Hu or CV2/CRMP5 antibodies. *J Neurol Neurosurg Psychiatry* 2009; 80: 412–16.
79. Giometto B, Grisold W, Vitaliani R, et al. Paraneoplastic neurologic syndrome in the PNS Euronetwork database: a European study from 20 centers. *Arch Neurol* 2010; 67: 330–5.
80. Lazurova I, Macejova Z, Benhatchi K, et al. Efficacy of intravenous immunoglobulin treatment in lupus erythematosus chorea. *Clin Rheumatol* 2007; 26: 2145–7.
81. Levine SR, Brey RL. Neurological aspects of antiphospholipid antibody syndrome. *Lupus* 1996; 5: 347–53.
82. Min JH, Youn YC. Bilateral basal ganglia lesions of primary Sjogren syndrome presenting with generalized chorea. *Parkinsonism Relat Disord* 2009; 15: 398–9.

83. Park SY, Kim HJ, Cho YJ, Cho JY, Hong KS. Recurrent hemichorea following a single infarction in the contralateral subthalamic nucleus. *Mov Disord* 2009; 24: 617–18.
84. Ghika-Schmid F, Ghika J, Regli F, Bogousslavsky J. Hyperkinetic movement disorders during and after acute stroke: the Lausanne Stroke Registry. *J Neurol Sci* 1997; 146: 109–16.
85. Gonzalez-Alegre P, Ammache Z, Davis PH, Rodnitzky RL. Moyamoya-induced paroxysmal dyskinesia. *Mov Disord* 2003; 18: 1051–6.
86. Kumar H, Masiowski P, Jog M. Chorea in the elderly with mutation positive polycythemia vera: a case report. *Can J Neurol Sci* 2009; 36: 370–2.
87. Medlock MD, Cruse RS, Winek SJ, et al. A 10-year experience with post-pump chorea. *Ann Neurol* 1993; 34: 820–6.
88. Baik JS, Lee MS. Movement disorders associated with moyamoya disease: a report of 4 new cases and a review of literatures. *Mov Disord* 2010; 25: 1482–6.
89. Pandey P, Bell-Stephens T, Steinberg GK. Patients with moyamoya disease presenting with movement disorder. *J Neurosurg Pediatr* 2010; 6: 559–66.
90. Cardoso F, Jankovic J, Grossman RG, Hamilton WJ. Outcome after stereotactic thalamotomy for dystonia and hemiballismus. *Neurosurgery* 1995; 36: 501–7.
91. Choi SJ, Lee SW, Kim MC, et al. Posteroventral pallidotomy in medically intractable postapoplectic monochorea: case report. *Surg Neurol* 2003; 59: 486–90.
92. Wenning GK, Kiechl S, Seppi K, et al. Prevalence of movement disorders in men and women aged 50–89 years (Bruneck Study cohort): a population-based study. *Lancet Neurol* 2005; 4: 815–20.
93. Miranda M, Cardoso F, Giovannoni G, Church A. Oral contraceptive induced chorea: another condition associated with anti-basal ganglia antibodies. *J Neurol Neurosurg Psychiatry* 2004; 75: 327–8.
94. Karageyim AY, Kars B, Dansuk R, et al. Chorea gravidarum: a case report. *J Matern Fetal Neonatal Med* 2002; 12: 353–4.
95. Fahn S. The spectrum of levodopa-induced dyskinesias. *Ann Neurol* 2000; 47: S2–9.
96. Stacy M, Cardoso F, Jankovic J. Tardive stereotypy and other movement disorders in tardive dyskinesias. *Neurology* 1993; 43: 937–41.
97. Miller LG, Jankovic J. Neurologic approach to drug-induced movement disorders: a study of 125 patients. *South Med J* 1990; 83: 525–32.
98. Fox GC, Ebeid S, Vincenti G. Paroxetine-induced chorea. *Br J Psychiatry* 1997; 170: 193–4.
99. Bharucha KJ, Sethi KD. Complex movement disorders induced by fluoxetine. *Mov Disord* 1996; 11: 324–6.
100. Harrison MB, Lyons GR, Landow ER. Phenytoin and dyskinesias: a report of two cases and review of the literature. *Mov Disord* 1993; 8: 19–27.
101. Bimpong-Buta K, Froescher W. Carbamazepine-induced choreoathetoid dyskinesias. *J Neurol Neurosurg Psychiatry* 1982; 45: 560.
102. Zaatreh M, Tennison M, D'Cruz O, Beach RL. Anticonvulsants-induced chorea: a role for pharmacodynamic drug interaction? *Seizure* 2001; 10: 596–9.
103. Srinivasan S, Lok AW. Valproate-induced reversible hemichorea. *Mov Disord* 2010; 25: 1511–12.
104. Stork CM, Cantor R. Pemoline induced acute choreoathetosis: case report and review of the literature. *J Toxicol Clin Toxicol* 1997; 35: 105–8.
105. Morgan JC, Winter WC, Wooten GF. Amphetamine-induced chorea in attention deficit-hyperactivity disorder. *Mov Disord* 2004; 19: 840–2.
106. Necioğlu Orken D, Yldrmak Y, Kenangil G, et al. Intrathecal methotrexate-induced acute chorea. *J Pediatr Hematol Oncol* 2009; 31: 57–8.
107. Cardoso F. HIV-related movement disorders: epidemiology, pathogenesis and management. *CNS Drugs* 2002; 16: 663–8.
108. Kalita J, Ranjan P, Misra UK, Das BK. Hemichorea: a rare presentation of tuberculoma. *J Neurol Sci* 2003; 208: 109–11.
109. McKee D, Talbot P. Chorea as a presenting feature of variant Creutzfeldt–Jakob disease. *Mov Disord* 2003; 18: 837–8.
110. Ozben S, Erol C, Ozer F, Tiras R. Chorea as the presenting feature of neurosyphilis. *Neurol India* 2009; 57: 347–9.
111. Fernández Cooke E, Simón de Las Heras R, Muñoz González A, Allende Martinez L, Camacho Salas A. Choreoathetosis after herpes simplex encephalitis. *An Pediatr (Barc)* 2009; 71: 153–6.
112. Jog MS, Lang AE. Chronic acquired hepatocerebral degeneration: case reports and new insights. *Mov Disord* 1995; 10: 714–22.
113. Cherian A, Thomas B, Baheti NN, Chemmanam T, Kesavadas C. Concepts and controversies in nonketotic hyperglycemia-induced hemichorea: further evidence from susceptibility-weighted MR imaging. *J Magn Reson Imaging* 2009; 29: 699–703.
114. Wang JH, Wu T, Deng BQ, et al. Hemichorea-hemiballismus associated with nonketotic hyperglycemia: a possible role of inflammation. *J Neurol Sci* 2009; 284: 198–202.
115. Chu K, Kang DW, Kim DE, Park SH, Roh JK. Diffusion-weighted and gradient echo magnetic resonance findings of hemichorea–hemiballismus associated with diabetic hyperglycemia: a hyperviscosity syndrome? *Arch Neurol* 2002; 59: 448–52.
116. Lin JJ, Chang MK. Hemiballism-hemichorea and non-ketotic hyperglycaemia. *J Neurol Neurosurg Psychiatry* 1994; 57: 748–50.
117. Ristic AJ, Svetel M, Dragasevic N, Zarkovic M, Koprivsek K, Kostic VS. Bilateral chorea–ballism associated with hyperthyroidism. *Mov Disord* 2004; 19: 982–3.
118. Yu JH, Weng YM. Acute chorea as a presentation of Graves disease: case report and review. *Am J Emerg Med* 2009; 27: 369.e1–369.e3.
119. Poewe WH, Kleedorfer B, Willeit J, Gerstenbrand F. Primary CNS lymphoma presenting as a choreic movement disorder followed by segmental dystonia. *Mov Disord* 1988; 3: 320–5.
120. Moore FG. Bilateral hemichorea–hemiballism caused by metastatic lung cancer. *Mov Disord* 2009; 24: 1405–6.
121. Zacharia TT. Giant tumefactive perivascular spaces manifesting as chorea bilaterally. *J Neuroimaging* 2011; 21: 205–7.
122. Alp R, Ilhan Alp S, Ure H. Two intracranial sewing needles in a young woman with hemi-chorea. *Parkinsonism Relat Disord* 2009; 15: 795–6.
123. Ertan S, Uluduz D, Ozekmekçi S, et al. Clinical characteristics of 49 patients with psychogenic movement disorders in a tertiary clinic in Turkey. *Mov Disord* 2009; 24: 759–62.
124. Vidailhet M, Yelnik J, Lagrange C, et al. Bilateral pallidal deep brain stimulation for the treatment of patients with dystonia-choreoathetosis cerebral palsy: a prospective pilot study. *Lancet Neurol* 2009; 8: 709–17.
125. Joseph FG, Lammie GA, Scolding NJ. CNS lupus: a study of 41 patients. *Neurology* 2007; 69: 644–54.
126. McArthur JC, Brew BJ, Nath A. Neurological complications of HIV infection. *Lancet Neurol* 2005; 4: 543–5.
127. Gilbert DL, Kurlan R. PANDAS: horse or zebra? *Neurology* 2009; 73: 1252–3.
128. Brilot F, Merheb V, Ding A, Murphy T, Dale RC. Antibody binding to neuronal surface in Sydenham chorea, but not in PANDAS or Tourette syndrome. *Neurology* 2011; 76: 1508–13.

CHAPTER 23

Wilson Disease

Oliver Bandmann

Summary

Wilson disease (WD) is an autosomal recessively inherited monogenic copper storage disease. At least 50% of all patients with WD first present with neurological or psychiatric problems. If treated early, patients can make a full recovery and then lead a near-normal life, but failure to make the diagnosis can result in severe irreversible brain damage and untimely death.

The illness is named after S.A. Kinnier Wilson (1878–1937) who was born in the USA, but studied Medicine in Edinburgh and trained under Joseph Babinski in Paris. In 1905, whilst working at the National Hospital for Nervous Diseases, London, he saw a female patient who had developed severe dysarthria, a fixed smile, and a coarse tremor of her hands and feet. She died at the age of 29 years. Wilson performed the autopsy himself and described a cirrhotic liver and bilateral symmetrical destruction of the lenticular nucleus. He subsequently extended his study to other patients with similar presentations (1).

A role for copper as a possible pathogenic agent was first suggested by Rumpel in 1913 who described increased copper content in the liver. Cummings then demonstrated that excess copper is present in both liver and brain of WD patients (2).

Essential background

Epidemiology

The prevalence of WD is estimated to be 1:30 000 with a (heterozygote) *ATP7B* mutation carrier frequency in the general population of 1:90 (3). Our own genetic studies confirm that the genetic prevalence of *ATP7B* mutations in newborns is at least as high as this (unpublished data). One can then extrapolate these data to predict approximately 2000 cases of WD in the UK, or 10 000 cases in the USA. However, the number of clinically diagnosed cases of WD is substantially lower. Why? Reduced penetrance is well recognized in other autosomal recessively inherited metabolic disorders, and case reports suggest that it may also occur in individuals with two *ATP7B* mutations (4, 5). Alternatively, unusual presentations of WD, perhaps mimicking late-onset neurodegenerative or psychiatric disorders, may be more common than previously thought. The most worrying, but purely speculative, explanation would be that a substantial proportion of WD patients die undiagnosed in infancy or childhood. In our view, reduced penetrance is the most likely explanation. Of note, the prevalence can be substantially higher in isolated populations (6).

Genetics

WD is a monogenic autosomal recessively inherited disorder. The causative gene encodes a copper-transporting P-type ATPase named *ATP7B* on chromosome 13q14.3 (7–9). In non-isolated populations, disease-causing *ATP7B* mutations are scattered across the entire coding region and the adjacent splice sites, but there may be particular 'mutation hot spots'. The distribution and frequency of the individual mutations varies between populations, with H1069Q being the most common mutation in European patients of Caucasian origin (10). Mutations in the promoter region and large-scale *ATP7B* rearrangements have been reported, but are extremely rare (11, 12).

In the past, the use of inaccurate genetic screening techniques, which are now outdated, and occasional over-generous inclusion of patients with clinically unconfirmed WD suggested that a substantial proportion of WD patients only had one or indeed no detectable *ATP7B* mutation. However, a recently undertaken service evaluation of the UK WD/*ATP7B* diagnostic genetic service confirmed the detection of two mutations in >95% of all patients, but only if the entire coding region is sequenced (Ann Dalton, personal communication). In our view, it is much more likely that the very few remaining patients with clinically confirmed WD but only one (currently) detectable *ATP7B* mutation have an additional unusual mutation within *ATP7B*, such as sequence changes in as yet unidentified regulatory regions within its introns, rather than suggesting genetic heterogeneity (i.e. the presence of a second WD gene).

Pathophysiology

Copper is required for a wide range of crucial biochemical mechanisms such as cellular respiration, iron oxidation, neurotransmitter synthesis, antioxidant defence and connective tissue formation (13). The average diet provides about 2–5 mg of copper per day, but only about 1 mg/day is needed (14). Copper is mostly absorbed in the duodenum and proximal small intestine. Bound to albumin and the amino acid histidine, it is then transported to the liver in the portal circulation. Excess copper is excreted into the bile, and it is this excretion which is impaired in WD. The protein encoded by the WD gene, the ATP7B protein, is a copper-transporting P-type ATPase. ATP7B protein is mainly expressed in hepatocytes and functions in the transmembrane transport of copper within hepatocytes. The copper translocation cycle occurs in several stages, during which ATP hydrolysis drives the translocation of the copper: (1) binding of target ion; (2) binding of ATP to the nucleotide-binding (N) domain; (3) ATP hydrolysis and phosphorylation of the phosphorylation (P) domain; (4) translocation of the target ion; (5) dephosphorylation of the P-domain by the actuator (A) domain (15).

ATP7B mutations lead to impaired function of the ATP7B protein with reduced excretion of copper into the bile, leading to increased copper levels in the liver and other organs, in particular the brain. Excess copper leads to increased oxidative stress, mitochondrial dysfunction, and cell death.

Clinical presentation

WD typically presents in the second or third decade of life. Patients with hepatic problems tend to present earlier than those with neuropsychiatric symptoms, the mean age of onset being 11 years for patients with hepatic problems compared with a mean age of 17 years for those with neurological symptoms in a large case series (16). A recent multinational study comprising 1223 patients confirmed that about 90% of all patients become symptomatic below the age of 30 years (17). However, statistics and mean ages of onset help little if you are confronted with a patient in your own clinic who may or may not have WD. WD can start very early, the youngest case probably being a two-year-old child who presented with impaired liver function (18). More worryingly for adult neurologists, a first presentation of WD has also been reported in septuagenarians (19). Presentation as late as this is likely to be very rare indeed but 'late-onset' WD, arbitrarily defined as patients only becoming symptomatic at age >40 years, is now well recognized and, with 46/1223 (3.8%) of all WD patients included in the multinational study mentioned above, more common than perhaps previously thought (17).

The grand master of WD in the UK, John Walshe, once stated: 'There appears to be only one thing which all (WD) patients have in common ... namely that they are all different' (20). It has been proposed that the neurological manifestations of WD can be divided into three distinct syndromes: (1) a dystonic syndrome characterized by choreoathetosis and dystonic postures, (2) an ataxic syndrome with postural and intention tremor as well as ataxia of the limbs, and (3) a parkinsonian syndrome with hypokinesia, rigidity, and resting tremor (21). In our view, this classification is unhelpful—the considerable majority of WD patients who present with neurological problems will manifest with a combination of these features. The frequency of the respective neurological features varies widely from one case series to the next and is summarized in Table 23.1.

Terms such as 'flapping tremor' or 'wing-beating tremor' are frequently described as pathognomonic features for WD in the literature, but any other, more common, type of tremor such as rest, action, and intention tremor can occur as well. The most common form of tremor may be an irregular, jerky, and somewhat asymmetrical dystonic tremor combined with dystonic posturing and (action-induced) dystonia in the hands such as writer's cramp with abnormal fine finger movements on formal testing. Indeed, WD can result in any form or distribution of dystonia, including generalized, segmental, and multifocal dystonia (22). Common subtypes of focal dystonia, such as blepharospasm or torticollis, can be part of the dystonic presentation but isolated cervical dystonia is unlikely to be due to WD (23).

Dysarthria is a further very common symptom and can have ataxic, hypokinetic, and dysphonic features. It can be the first neurological symptom and is present in the vast majority of all WD patients who have a neurological presentation (24, 25). The speech may not only be difficult, or indeed impossible, to understand because the words are not formed properly, but also because the patient may speak rather fast with reduced volume and a strained hoarse voice. WD patients with dysarthria typically have slow tongue movements and may also display particular orofacial dyskinesias, namely involuntary grimacing with the mouth open and the upper lip contracted, resulting in the so-called risus sardonicus. Dysphagia can also be part of the clinical presentation. It may not only be due to slow and poorly coordinated lip, tongue, pharynx, and jaw movements, but also caused by impaired oesophageal motility (26). Parkinsonian features such as slowness of movement, including hypomimia, reduction in amplitude and rhythm of fine finger movements or foot tapping and shuffling, and small stepped gait are further typical features. Textbooks frequently include WD in the differential diagnostic list of causes for chorea. However, classical choreiform movements are rare compared with choreoathetotic movements with slow writhing movements (with a strong dystonic component).

Cerebellar dysfunction with ataxia, intention tremor, and dysdiadochokinesia may be under-recognized in WD and can be masked by the presence of additional dystonia or parkinsonism. However, it is not clear whether all WD patients reported to have ataxia in the literature really did have a cerebellar syndrome or simply could

Table 23.1 Comparison of the frequency of common neurological abnormalities in different case series

Ref.	*n*	Dystonia	Dysarthria	Parkinsonism	Ataxia	Chorea/Athetosis	Pyramidal signs
(20)*	136	15%	Juvenile: 52% Adult: 27%	45%	NA	11%	NA
(48)	31	65%	97%	52%	(42%)**	Rare	29%
(49)	22	36%	?	82%	50%	?	32%
(16)	282	35%	?	62%	28%	11%	16%
(25)	119	69%	91%	66%	(75%)**	Chorea 16% Athetosis 14%	Rare

*This case series concentrated on the neurological abnormalities at presentation.

**These figures refer to 'gait abnormalities'; the authors did not differentiate between ataxia and other gait abnormalities such as parkinsonian gait.

Modified from ref. 25.

not walk heel to toe because of prominent (lower limb) dystonia in isolation or combined with other extrapyramidal features.

Seizures have been reported to be the presenting symptom of WD, but can occur at any stage of the disease in about 5% of all patients and are more common after initiation of treatment (27). Pyramidal features such as pathologically brisk tendon reflexes can occur (see Table 23.1), but paralysis is not a feature of WD and the presence of sensory impairment practically excludes the diagnosis of WD (in the absence of dual pathology). Impaired ocular motility is a probably under-recognized, feature of WD, impaired vertical pursuit being the most common abnormality (28). In contrast, deterioration of vision as such is not part of WD and the pupils are normal.

Wilson described prominent psychiatric symptoms in eight of the twelve cases he reported in his thesis. A retrospective analysis of 195 cases came to the conclusion that 51% of these patients displayed psychopathological features (29). A wide range of different psychiatric problems including anxiety, depression, psychosis, and personality disorders can occur. Of note, anxiety and depression, but also irritability and apathy, continue to be common even in treated and otherwise clinically stable patients (30, 31).

A neurologist may not only encounter a WD patient in his own clinic, but also as a ward referral of the patient who initially comes to medical attention because of a general medical problem. Whilst the hepatic presentation is more common in children, it can still be the first presentation of 'late-onset' WD when patients are in their forties or fifties (17). Thus, the diagnosis of WD needs to be considered in any patient seen as a ward referral on a general medical ward with the working diagnosis of 'hepatic encephalopathy of unexplained cause'. Other, non-hepatic, general medical presentations include haemolytic crisis and a variety of joint and bone diseases including spontaneous fractures and premature osteoarthrosis (32). Rarely, WD can result in cardiomyopathy and arrhythmias. Endocrine abnormalities and renal manifestations have also been reported, but are rare as well (33).

Investigations

The Kayser–Fleischer ring (KFR) is caused by copper deposition in Descemet's membrane of the cornea and usually starts at the upper pole (33). KFRs are present in 100% of some, but not all, case series of WD patients with neurological presentation (14). It is not always clear whether a slit lamp was routinely used in all patients who did not have a KFR on bedside testing. It is easier to detect KFRs if the light of the ophthalmoscope is shone tangentially at the eyes, but the threshold should be low to refer a patient with possible WD to ophthalmology for slit-lamp examination. Rarely, KFRs can also occur in other liver diseases such as primary biliary cirrhosis (34).

Ceruloplasmin is the major copper-transporting protein in the blood with >90% of circulating copper bound to it in healthy individuals. Very low (<5 mg/dl) serum ceruloplasmin levels are strong evidence for WD. A mild to moderate reduction (<20 mg/dl) is consistent with the diagnosis of WD and diagnostic in the presence of KFRs (14). Ceruloplasmin may be low in other general medical conditions with marked renal or enteric protein loss, and also in endstage liver failure and in patients with Menkes disease, an X-linked disorder of copper uptake. An additional important cause of low ceruloplasmin is aceruloplasminaemia due to mutations in the *ceruloplasmin* gene. Patients with this condition can present to the neurologist with cognitive impairment (42%), craniofacial dyskinesias (28%), cerebellar ataxia (46%), and retinal degeneration (75%) (35). Patients with homozygote mutations tend to have more severe disease, but heterozygote mutation carriers can develop neurological symptoms as well. Serum ceruloplasmin is undetectable in homozygous cases, ferritin is elevated, and copper as well as iron levels in serum are very low. Microcytic anaemia is frequently present. Of note, heterozygote *ATP7B* mutation carriers can also exhibit a mild decrease in ceruloplasmin levels (36).

Copper levels in the blood of WD patients are typically low, despite the fact that WD is a copper-overload disease, because of the marked lowering of the (copper-transporting) ceruloplasmin protein. In contrast, serum non-ceruloplasmin-bound copper concentrations are usually elevated above 25 μg/dl (normal <15 μg/dl) (14).

Copper levels in a 24 hour urine collection reflect the amount of non-ceruloplasmin bound copper in circulation and are very useful both as a diagnostic procedure and to monitor treatment. Typically, >100 μg (1.6 μmol) is excreted during a 24-hour period in symptomatic patients, but >40 μg (0.6 μmol) in 24 hours may already indicate WD and requires further investigation (14).

The penicillamine challenge (urine copper excretion after penicillamine administration) has only been standardized in children.

MRI is a further very powerful investigation in patients with the neurological presentation of WD. The largest case series to date reported MRI abnormalities in 100%, but the characteristic 'face of the giant panda' sign was only present in 14%. Tectal plate hyperintensity (75%), central pontine myelinolysis-like abnormalities (62%), and concurrent signal changes in basal ganglia, thalamus, and brainstem (55%) were considerably more common (37). We would strongly advise against relying on the results of CT imaging in cases of suspected WD.

We do not see any justification for a liver biopsy in WD patients with neurological presentation in whom the clinical assessment and investigations listed above have already provided substantial evidence for the diagnosis of WD. We would advise caution against undertaking a liver biopsy only because a patient has a neurological condition of undetermined aetiology with a mild decrease of his ceruloplasmin levels, but normal MRI and normal 24 hour urine copper excretion. Of note, increased hepatic copper is not diagnostic for WD since a mild increase can also be observed in heterozygote *ATP7B* mutation carriers. Furthermore, other diseases such as primary biliary cirrhosis may also lead to increased hepatic copper levels.

Treatment

British anti-lewisite (BAL), or dimercaptopropanol, was introduced as the first chelating agent for WD by Denny Brown in 1951 (38). John Walshe's introduction of penicillamine as the first oral chelating agent then revolutionized the treatment of WD. Trientine, also a chelating agent, was subsequently introduced as an alternative to penicillamine, especially for those patients who cannot tolerate penicillamine (2). Treatment with copper chelators to facilitate copper excretion from the body continues to be the key principle of pharmacological treatment of WD, but has been complemented by use of zinc which reduces the copper levels in the body by inducing intestinal metallothionein in the duodenal enterocytes. Metallothionein preferentially binds copper, and so dietary copper is subsequently lost due to the frequent shedding of the enterocytes during normal cell turnover. The advantages and disadvantages of penicillamine, trientine, and zinc are now described in some more detail. A third chelating agent, ammonium tetrathiomolybdate, has only been used in clinical trials and is neither licensed nor commercially available for the treatment of WD in the UK or the USA. Therefore it will not be discussed any further.

Penicillamine is the most widely used drug for WD. Decades of experience have shown that it is not only a powerful de-coppering agent in the initial stage of the therapy but is also an excellent therapeutic agent for maintenance therapy in many patients, provided that they are monitored carefully for possible side effects of this compound. At the beginning of the therapy a hypersensitivity reaction can develop with fever, rash, lymphadenopathy, neutropenia, and proteinuria. Non-specific nausea can also occur. However, the most serious early side effect is a deterioration in neurological status, which may be severe (39). This has been reported in 20–50% of patients with a neurological presentation and is not always reversible (33). It is thought to be due to mobilization of copper in the tissue by the chelating therapy with resulting increase in oxidative stress. However, an acute deterioration can also be observed after initiation of treatment with trientine (40). Long-term side effects of penicillamine treatment include bone marrow suppression with thrombocytopenia and aplasia, nephrotoxicity, and skin complications such as elastosis perforans serpiginosa and aphthous stomatitis. Risk of neurological deterioration after initiation of therapy may be lower if penicillamine is increased gradually (e.g. start the patient on 250 mg/day for the first week and then increase by 250 mg per week until he/she reaches the initial final dose of the de-coppering stage, 1000–1500 mg in adults). This should ideally be divided into three doses, but some patients find it easier to take the drug twice daily. The drug is better absorbed if not taken with food, but many patients find it easier to take the medication with food. We start patients on vitamin E (400 IE per day) for the first 3–6 months, hoping that the antioxidant effect of this vitamin might abolish or at least reduce some of the immediate penicillamine side effects. The typical maintenance dose is 750–1000 mg in adults. Pencillamine treatment carries at least the theoretical risk of affecting pyridoxine metabolism. Therefore we also recommend 50 μg of vitamin B_6 twice weekly.

Trientine is perceived to be a less potent chelating agent than penicillamine but also appears to have a better side-effect profile. Current evidence suggests that it is at least a valid alternative to penicillamine as first-line drug treatment and certainly a very useful alternative for those patients who cannot tolerate penicillamine. It is important to stress that the transient neurological deterioration seen after initiation with penicillamine treatment can also occur after a patient has been started on trientine (40). Therefore, similarly to our approach for the initiation of penicillamine treatment, we advise starting the patient on a low dose of trientine, such as 300 mg/day for the first week, and then increasing the dose by 300 mg each week until the patient has reached the final initial dose of 1200–1800 mg/day. The maintenance dose is usually 600 mg twice daily. Other complications of trientine are iron deficiency with sideroblastic anaemia. Lupus-like reactions have also been reported in some WD patients on trientine, but most of them had been on penicillamine before (14).

Zinc is increasingly used as first-line therapy for asymptomatic or presymptomatic patients. It is generally very well tolerated and typically only has a few side effects such as abdominal discomfort (41, 42). The usual dose for adults is 150 mg/day in three doses (14).

Which drug should you then choose for the WD patient in your clinic? It is important to realize that the 'top three' drugs, penicillamine, trientine, and zinc, have never been compared in modern head-to-head trials. At least some of the manuscripts and books published on this issue are rather dogmatic and unilaterally favour one drug above all others. Fortunately, the American Association for the Study of Liver Diseases (AASLD) has published (in our view) eminently sensible treatment recommendations (14):

> Initial treatment for symptomatic patients should include a chelating agent (penicillamine or trientine). Trientine may be better tolerated (Class I, Level B) ... Treatment of pre-symptomatic patients or those on maintenance therapy can be accomplished with a chelating agent or with zinc ... (Class I, Level B)

We appreciate that these guidelines may lack precision (no clear preference for penicillamine vs trientine for the treatment of symptomatic patients, no clear preference for zinc vs chelating agent for maintenance therapy) but they accurately reflect the current uncertainty.

At the beginning of therapy, it is important to not only warn patients about possible side effects of the medication, but also to make them aware of the fact that it might take months until the first improvement is noticed. With all the therapeutic enthusiasm for one of the few near-curable movement disorders, it is crucial to be patient. It is then absolutely crucial to monitor all WD patients for the rest of their lives. The minimum requirement in stable patients should include an annual neurological and general medical examination. In addition, we would strongly recommend annual assessment of copper excretion via a 24 hour urine collection. Treatment with any chelating agent should be stopped 48 hours prior to the start of the urine collection and then only be started again after the urine collection has finished. We use the target values of <0.6 μmol/24 hour copper excretion in patients on penicillamine and <2.0 μmol/24 hour in patients on trientine. Significantly higher copper excretion may reflect either poor compliance or simply the fact that the dose of the respective therapeutic agent is too low. Our annual reviews include a large number of additional blood tests including ceruloplasmin, copper, liver function tests, full blood count, iron and ferritin, renal function tests, and urinalysis.

Official guidelines state that food with very high concentrations of copper (shellfish, nuts, chocolate, mushrooms, and offal) should be avoided, at least in the first year of treatment. However, common sense needs to be used when dietary advice is given. Doctors should show empathy for patients who already face the prospect of having to take medication for the rest of their lives. A gentle increase in the dose of the respective drug may be more appropriate than over-zealous dietary advice and criticism of the patient's lifestyle.

Liver transplantation is the only effective option for those WD patients who present with acute liver failure (14). Both clinical and radiological improvement has been reported in patients with the neurological presentation of WD, but outcome has not always been beneficial (14, 43, 44). It is hard to justify liver transplantation in a WD patient with pure neurological presentation unless he/she has developed severe side effects on all the different WD drugs.

Key advances

Unfortunately, there have not really been any major breakthroughs in the diagnosis and treatment of WD over the past 5–10 years. The most important step forward would be a well-designed drug study comparing the efficacy of penicillamine and trientine in the acute stage of the illness and a comparison of chelating agents versus zinc for maintenance therapy. A unified WD rating scale has now been developed and evaluated which may prove useful in future drug studies (45).

Future developments

Liver cirrhosis and anaemia in WD are at least partially due to copper-mediated activation of acid sphingomyelinase and release of ceramide. Treatment with the acid sphingomyelinase inhibitor amitriptyline prevented liver failure and prolonged survival in *atp7b*-deficient rats, but it is currently unclear whether amitriptyline treatment may also be of benefit in human WD patients (46). Rescue of ATP7B protein function in hepatocyte-like cells from WD-induced pluripotent stem cells using viral gene therapy has been reported, but it is uncertain whether gene therapy will ever be a useful tool for the treatment of WD (47). Any new experimental therapeutic approach would need to be tested against best current medical practice. The single most desirable improvement for WD patients with a neurological presentation would be a form of therapy which would result in a more complete recovery of brain function, compared with those people who only partially recover despite optimal conventional drug therapy. However, it may be futile to target this goal since this residual neurological dysfunction may reflect irreversible brain damage.

Top clinical tips

- Always investigate patients with tremor and dysarthria for WD (in the absence of classical cerebellar features).
- Do not disregard the diagnosis of WD only because liver function tests are normal and you could not see a KFR yourself in clinic. In case of doubt, refer the patient to Ophthalmology for slit-lamp examination.
- Do not disregard the possible diagnosis of WD only because the ceruloplasmin levels are normal. Ceruloplasmin is an acute-phase protein. and any acute general medical illness such as liver failure may result in elevation and thus false normal levels of ceruloplasmin.
- Do not assume that it cannot be WD because the patient is 'too old'.
- WD is complicated. Try to see these patients in a multidisciplinary clinic together with hepatologists or metabolic physicians.
- Life-long close monitoring of WD patients may be more important than the initial decision as to which drug the patient should be started on.

References

1. Hoogenraad TU. S.A. Kinnier Wilson (1878–937). *J Neurol* 2001; 248: 71–2.
2. Walshe JM. The conquest of Wilson's disease. *Brain* 2009; 132: 2289–95.
3. Behari M, Pardasani V. Genetics of Wilson's disease. *Parkinsonism Relat Disord* 2010; 16: 639–44.
4. Czlonkowska A, Gromadzka G, Chabik G. Monozygotic female twins discordant for phenotype of Wilson's disease. *Mov Disord* 2009; 24: 1066–9.
5. Czlonkowska A, Rodo M, Gromadzka G. Late onset Wilson's disease: therapeutic implications. *Mov Disord* 2008; 23: 896–8.
6. Dedoussis GV, Genschel J, Sialvera, et al. Wilson disease: high prevalence in a mountainous area of Crete. *Ann Hum Genet* 2005; 69: 268–74.
7. Bull PC, Thomas GR, Rommens JM, Forbes JR, Cox DW. The Wilson disease gene is a putative copper transporting P-type ATPase similar to the Menkes gene. *Nat Genet* 1993; 5: 327–37.
8. Petrukhin K, Fischer SG, Pirastu M, et al. Mapping, cloning and genetic characterization of the region containing the Wilson disease gene. *Nat Genet* 1993; 5: 338–43.
9. Tanzi RE, Petrukhin K, Chernov I, et al. The Wilson disease gene is a copper transporting ATPase with homology to the Menkes disease gene. *Nat Genet* 1993; 5: 344–50.
10. Ferenci P. Regional distribution of mutations of the ATP7B gene in patients with Wilson disease: impact on genetic testing. *Hum Genet* 2006; 120: 151–9.
11. Cullen LM, Prat L, Cox DW. Genetic variation in the promoter and 5′ UTR of the copper transporter, ATP7B, in patients with Wilson disease. *Clin Genet* 2003; 64: 429–32.
12. Møller LB, Ott P, Lund C, Horn N. Homozygosity for a gross partial gene deletion of the C-terminal end of ATP7B in a Wilson patient with hepatic and no neurological manifestations. *Am J Med Genet A* 2005; 138: 340–3.
13. Madsen E, Gitlin JD. Copper and iron disorders of the brain. *Annu Rev Neurosci* 2007; 30: 317–37.
14. Roberts EA, Schilsky ML. Diagnosis and treatment of Wilson disease: an update. *Hepatology* 2008; 47: 2089–111.
15. de Bie P, Muller P, Wijmenga C, Klomp LW. Molecular pathogenesis of Wilson and Menkes disease: correlation of mutations with molecular defects and disease phenotypes. *J Med Genet* 2007; 44: 673–88.
16. Taly AB, Meenakshi-Sundaram S, Sinha S, Swamy HS, Arunodaya GR. Wilson disease: description of 282 patients evaluated over 3 decades. *Medicine (Baltimore)* 2007; 86: 112–21.
17. Ferenci P, Członkowska A, Merle U, et al. Late-onset Wilson's disease. *Gastroenterology* 2007; 132: 1294–8.
18. Beyersdorff A, Findeisen A. Morbus Wilson: Case report of a two-year-old child as first manifestation. *Scand J Gastroenterol* 2006; 41: 496–7.
19. Ala A, Borjigin J, Rochwarger A, Schilsky M. Wilson disease in septuagenarian siblings: raising the bar for diagnosis. *Hepatology* 2005; 41: 668–70.
20. Walshe JM, Yealland M. Wilson's disease: the problem of delayed diagnosis. *J Neurol Neurosurg Psychiatry* 1992; 55: 692–6.
21. Marsden CD. Wilson's disease. *QJM* 1987; 65: 959–66.
22. Svetel M, Kozić D, Stefanova E, Semnic R, Dragasevic N, Kostic VS. Dystonia in Wilson's disease. *Mov Disord* 2001; 16: 719–23.
23. Risvoll H, Kerty E. To test or not? The value of diagnostic tests in cervical dystonia. *Mov Disord* 2001; 16: 286–9.
24. Oder W, Grimm G, Kollegger H, Ferenci P, Schneider B, Deecke L. Neurological and neuropsychiatric spectrum of Wilson's disease: a prospective study of 45 cases. *J Neurol* 1991; 238: 281–7.
25. Machado A, Chien HF, Deguti MM et al. Neurological manifestations in Wilson's disease: report of 119 cases. *Mov Disord* 2006; 21: 2192–6.
26. Haggstrom G, Hirschowitz BI. Disordered esophageal motility in Wilson's disease. *J Clin Gastroenterol* 1980; 2: 273–5.
27. Dening TR, Berrios GE, Walshe JM. Wilson's disease and epilepsy. *Brain* 1988; 111: 1139–55.
28. Ingster-Moati I, Bui Quoc E, Pless M, et al. Ocular motility and Wilson's disease: a study on 34 patients. *J Neurol Neurosurg Psychiatry* 2007; 78: 1199–201.

29. Dening TR, Berrios GE. Wilson's disease: psychiatric symptoms in 195 cases. *Arch Gen Psychiatry* 1989; 46: 1126–34.
30. Portala K, Westermark K, von Knorring L, Ekselius L. Psychopathology in treated Wilson's disease determined by means of CPRS expert and self-ratings. *Acta Psychiatr Scand* 2000; 101: 104–9.
31. Svetel M, Potrebić A, Pekmezović T, et al. Neuropsychiatric aspects of treated Wilson's disease. *Parkinsonism Relat Disord* 2009; 15: 772–5.
32. Golding DN, Walshe JM. Arthropathy of Wilson's disease: study of clinical and radiological features in 32 patients. *Ann Rheum Dis* 1977; 36: 99–111.
33. Ala A, Walker AP, Ashkan K, Dooley JS, Schilsky ML. Wilson's disease. *Lancet* 2007; 369: 397–408.
34. Tauber J, Steinert RF. Pseudo-Kayser–Fleischer ring of the cornea associated with non-Wilsonian liver disease: a case report and literature review. *Cornea* 1993; 12: 74–7.
35. McNeill A, Pandolfo M, Kuhn J, Shang H, Miyajima H. The neurological presentation of ceruloplasmin gene mutations. *Eur Neurol* 2008; 60: 200–5.
36. Gromadzka G, Chabik G, Mendel T, et al. Middle-aged heterozygous carriers of Wilson's disease do not present with significant phenotypic deviations related to copper metabolism. *J Genet* 2010; 89: 463–7.
37. Prashanth LK, Sinha S, Taly AB, Vasudev MK. Do MRI features distinguish Wilson's disease from other early onset extrapyramidal disorders? An analysis of 100 cases. *Mov Disord* 2010; 25: 672–8.
38. Vilensky JA, Robertson WM, Gilman S. Denny-Brown, Wilson's disease, and BAL (British antilewisite (2,3-dimercaptopropanol)). *Neurology* 2002; 59: 914–16.
39. Brewer GJ, Terry CA, Aisen AM, Hill GM. Worsening of neurologic syndrome in patients with Wilson's disease with initial penicillamine therapy. *Arch Neurol* 1987; 44: 490–3.
40. Dahlman T, Hartvig P, Löfholm M, Nordlinder H, Lööf L, Westermark K. Long-term treatment of Wilson's disease with triethylene tetramine dihydrochloride (trientine). *QJM* 1995; 88: 609–16.
41. Brewer GJ, Dick RD, Johnson VD, Brunberg JA, Kluin KJ, Fink JK. Treatment of Wilson's disease with zinc. XV: Long-term follow-up studies. *J Lab Clin Med* 1998; 132: 264–78.
42. Czlonkowska A, Gajda J, Rodo M. Effects of long-term treatment in Wilson's disease with D-penicillamine and zinc sulphate. *J Neurol* 1996; 243: 269–73.
43. Schumacher G, Platz KP, Mueller AR, et al. Liver transplantation in neurologic Wilson's disease. *Transplant Proc* 2001; 33: 1518–19.
44. Wu JC, Huang CC, Jeng LB, Chu NS. Correlation of neurological manifestations and MR images in a patient with Wilson's disease after liver transplantation. *Acta Neurol Scand* 2000; 102: 135–9.
45. Leinweber B, Möller JC, Scherag A, et al. Evaluation of the Unified Wilson's Disease Rating Scale (UWDRS) in German patients with treated Wilson's disease. *Mov Disord* 2008; 23: 54–62.
46. Lang PA, Schenck M, Nicolay JP, et al. Liver cell death and anemia in Wilson disease involve acid sphingomyelinase and ceramide. *Nat Med* 2007; 13: 164–70.
47. Zhang S, Chen S, Li W, et al. Rescue of ATP7B function in hepatocyte-like cells from Wilson's disease induced pluripotent stem cells using gene therapy or the chaperone drug curcumin. *Hum Mol Genet* 2011; 20: 3176–87.
48. Starosta-Rubinstein S, Young AB, Kluin K, et al. Clinical assessment of 31 patients with Wilson's disease: correlations with structural changes on magnetic resonance imaging. *Arch Neurol* 1987; 44: 365–70.
49. Jha SK, Behari M, Ahuja GK. Wilson's disease: clinical and radiological features. *J Assoc Physicians India* 1998; 46: 602–5.

CHAPTER 24

Tic Disorders and Stereotypies

Erika F. Augustine and Jonathan W. Mink

Tics and stereotypies are among the most common movement disorders in childhood. These early-onset involuntary movements are stereotyped in nature, but differ in phenomenology, age at onset, and co-morbid conditions. This chapter will outline the key identifying features, natural history, and treatment of each.

Stereotypies

Stereotypies are involuntary, patterned, co-ordinated, repetitive, and non-reflexive movements that occur in the same fashion with each repetition (1). Although these non-functional movements are typically simple, fleeting, and rhythmic in appearance, more complex, sustained, and non-rhythmic movements can be seen. Stereotypies occur multiple times daily, particularly in settings of excitement, nervousness, fatigue, or engrossment. These predictable and sometimes suppressible movements are brief, lasting seconds to minutes, and most commonly involve the head, torso, and upper extremities in a symmetric manner.

The Diagnostic and Statistical Manual of Mental Disorders-IV TR (DSM-IV TR) criteria for stereotyped movement disorder include interference with normal activities or self-injury (2). These features are unusual for most typically developing children. Although stereotypies may briefly interrupt activity, they do not generally interfere with intended motor movements or impose functional limitations. Examples of common stereotypies include hand flapping, clapping, finger wiggling, body rocking, head nodding, and walking in circles, sometimes in conjunction with facial grimacing or vocalizations (3–5).

Differential diagnosis

It may be difficult to differentiate stereotypies from other involuntary movements, particularly complex motor tics. Although both types of movement are distractible and suppressible, the absence of premonitory urge in stereotypies is a helpful distinguishing feature. However, much like very young children with tics, young children with stereotypies may not be able to describe the feelings present during the movements, or may be unaware of the movements altogether. In these circumstances, close review of other involuntary movements, family history, and thorough examination may provide clues to the diagnosis. An individual child may have multiple stereotypies; however, the overall repertoire of movements is relatively constant over time, in contrast with chronic tic disorders where the catalogue of tics evolves (see Table 24.1 for other features differentiating stereotypies from tics). Stereotypies may demonstrate rhythmicity similar to tremor. Whereas tremor involves oscillation around a single joint, stereotypies involve multiple limb parts. Also, the duration of expression of stereotypies is often shorter than that of tremor. As it relates to prominent head stereotypies without other common motor stereotypies, especially in the setting of motor delay or clumsiness, cerebellar pathology or alternate diagnoses (spasmus nutans, bobble-head doll, head tremor, or hydrocephalus) should be considered (6, 7).

Neurobiology

The neurobiology of complex motor stereotypy is not well understood. Conventional imaging and electrophysiological studies are unrevealing in healthy children with stereotypy. Psychological factors, including self-stimulation and response to social deprivation, have been proposed. Dopamine and both direct and indirect dopamine receptor agonists can induce stereotypy, suggesting disruption of the striatal dopaminergic system as a factor. The efficacy of selective serotonin reuptake inhibitors (SSRIs) in the treatment of stereotypy raises a possible role for serotonin in the production of stereotypy, although it remains unclear whether this is through indirect effects on the dopaminergic system. Reductions in frontal white matter and caudate volume in healthy boys with stereotypies may implicate abnormalities of the cortico-striatal-thalamo-cortical (CSTC) circuitry, as seen in other movement disorders (8, 9).

Epidemiology

Stereotypies almost always begin before the age of 3 years and occur with higher frequency in boys (male-to-female ratios range from 1.6 to 3:1). Familial tendencies suggest a genetic component, with a positive family history in 25–30% (4, 10).

Table 24.1 Stereotypies versus tics

	Stereotypies	Tics
Age at onset	<3 years	5–7 years
Premonitory urge	No	Yes
Suppressible	Sometimes	Yes
Duration	Seconds to minutes	Second(s)
Rhythmicity	Yes	No
Typical anatomical distribution	Hands, arms, whole body	Eyes, face, neck, shoulders
Evolution over time	Little	Considerable
Persistence in sleep	No	Possible
Time course of improvement	Early childhood	Adolescence
Response to medication	Poor	Good

Clinical features and course

Motor stereotypies occurred in 2–3% of a cohort of 3- to 6-year-old children without developmental delay. Nail biting and thumb sucking, which are often considered to be stereotypies, were categorized separately, occurring in 23% and 25%, respectively (11). In a cohort of 100 typically developing children with motor stereotypies, involuntary movements began before age 2 years in over 80% of the sample. Distractibility was reported by 99% of parents. After a mean 6.8 years of follow-up, only 6% of subjects reported cessation of stereotypies which were present for 11–12 years in two subjects prior to resolution. Those with head nodding were more likely to report resolution than those with other types of stereotypy. Symptoms were stable for the majority of children, with worsening in only a small subset (10).

Prognosis has traditionally been thought to be very good for stereotypies in typically developing children, with improvement in involuntary movements beginning by the age of 4 years. However, some studies show that stereotypies often persist, and that neuropsychiatric co-morbidity is common, occurring in up to 46–70% (4, 10, 12). In the cohort mentioned above, 9% demonstrated early motor delay, and 6% demonstrated early language delay. Forty-six% of children over age 7 years in the same cohort carried a co-morbid diagnosis, including attention deficit–hyperactivity disorder (ADHD), tics, and/or obsessive–compulsive behaviours (10). Thus stereotypies may not be quite as benign as once thought.

Long standing stereotypies such as foot tapping, hair twirling, and nail biting have been reported in adults with normal cognition.

Stereotypies in neurodevelopmental and neurodegenerative disorders

Many types of repetitive behaviour are seen in autism, including restricted interests, compulsions, routines, and stereotypies. In a study of 60 children with autism spectrum disorders aged 2–5 years, some of whom were later diagnosed with autism, stereotypies were present with increasing frequency in pervasive developmental delay (PDD) (9%), high-functioning autism (31%), and low-functioning autism (56%) ($p < 0.05$). The presence and severity of stereotypies may correlate with the severity of the underlying disorder (13). Goldman et al. (14) reported similar findings from a study of videotaped sessions of the play of 129 autistic and 148 non-autistic developmentally delayed (NADD) children aged 2–8 years. Stereotypy was associated with the diagnosis of autism (odds ratio (OR) 7.20, $p < 0.001$). Children with autism demonstrated a mean 13.42 stereotypies compared with 8.24 in the non-autism group ($p = 0.03$). Analogous patterns were observed with respect to number of stereotypies and non-verbal IQ. Children with autism demonstrate a wider range of stereotypic behaviours with respect to type and diversity of movement (14–17).

Stereotypies are a cardinal feature of Rett syndrome and one of the diagnostic criteria, present in virtually all patients (18). Midline hand-wringing movements are most common followed by bruxism; both can be frequent to constant in occurrence (19). Almost unique to Rett syndrome, stereotypies often involve the hand and mouth and can be quite complex, with independent stereotypies performed simultaneously with each hand. Prominent stereotypies precede or arise along with loss of purposeful hand movement between 6 months and 3 years of age. Mutation-positive girls with Rett syndrome tend to display a greater number of stereotypies than mutation-negative patients with a Rett phenotype (20). There are conflicting reports regarding persistence of stereotypies over time in Rett syndrome. Some centres have observed a decrease in expression of stereotypies after age 10 years or approximately 5 years of disease evolution in mutation-positive patients (19, 21), particularly stereotypies that do not involve the hands (20). Another centre has observed persistence of stereotypies into adolescence and adulthood, although they were simpler because of the development of rigidity (22).

Stereotyped behaviours occur frequently in blind children. Although the same range of motor stereotypies seen in typically developing and developmentally impaired children does occur, blind children also have certain fairly specific oculodigital stereotypies including eye rubbing, pressing, and poking. These occur with greatest frequency in those with peripheral causes of blindness. In a sample of 26 children with congenital blindness, 73.1% demonstrated stereotypies, including eye pressing or poking in 30% (23).

Stereotypies have also been described in association with genetic, metabolic, neurodegenerative, paraneoplastic, and infectious conditions, including Down's syndrome, cri du chat (24), Prader–Willi syndrome (25), CDKL5 mutations (26), Primrose syndrome (27), Smith–Magenis syndrome (28, 29), Rubinstein–Taybi syndrome (30), fragile X syndrome (31), FOXG1 mutations (32), phenylketonuria (33), Wilson disease (34), herpes encephalitis (35), encephalitis lethargica (36), and congenital cerebellar malformations (7). Complex motor stereotypies are found in a majority (84%) of patients presenting with anti-NMDA receptor encephalitis (37).

Evaluation

Evaluation is largely based on observation of the movement in question, understanding the settings in which it occurs, and response to redirection. When the movement does not occur during the course of the office visit, home video can be an invaluable tool to aid in diagnosis. The opportunity to observe the movement and recognize it as stereotypy may avoid unnecessary work-up with EEG, MRI, and/or lumbar puncture. Diagnostic evaluation should be guided by the history and findings, if any, on neurological examination. Given the potential prominence of stereotypies in children with developmental disabilities or visual impairment, it is not uncommon for parents to express concern. A greater frequency and repertoire of stereotypies in a developmentally delayed child may raise concern for an underlying disorder such as autism or genetic syndromes.

Treatment

Most children with stereotypies do not require treatment, particularly if the movements do not interfere with daily activities and are not causing self-harm or discomfort. However, when movements are severe and cause injury or social impairment, treatment may be considered. In terms of behavioural strategies, habit reversal, as used in tic disorders, has been a successful strategy for stereotypies. Habit reversal combined with differential reinforcement of other behaviours in a cohort of 10 non-autistic children aged 6–12 years with stereotypies resulted in improvements in stereotypy severity. Improvement correlated with the number of treatment sessions completed and motivation (38). Additional behavioural strategies include response interruption and redirection (39–41).

Pharmacological benefit from benzodiazepines, SSRIs (42, 43), neuroleptics (44), opiate antagonists, alpha-adrenergic agents, beta-blockers, and antiepileptic medications have been reported (12, 45). Three randomized controlled trials demonstrated benefit of risperidone over placebo for treatment of autistic children with stereotypy; one randomized trial showed no difference from placebo (46).

Tics

Tics are sudden, repetitive, stereotyped, and non-rhythmic movements that can be a manifestation of childhood-onset neurobehavioural disorders. Tics are categorized as motor or phonic if laryngeal, pharyngeal, nasal, or respiratory muscles are involved. In 74–92% of children, these involuntary movements are preceded by a premonitory urge, described as a general tightening, discomfort, sensation of internal build-up, or localizable pain, itching, burning, or pressure (47). The premonitory urge is relieved at least temporarily by the tic in the majority of patients. There is often a lag between tic onset and the onset of recognized premonitory urges (up to 3 years in one series). Tics can persist in all stages of sleep and are suppressible which, in addition to the premonitory urge, are features that help to differentiate tics from other movement disorders. Tics are suggestible, may demonstrate rebound phenomena after suppression, and may be exacerbated by positive or negative stress or relaxation after stress, such as return to home after school. Work by Conelea and colleagues (48) suggests that, when examined objectively, tic frequency does not actually increase in the setting of stress; rather, successful tic suppression is disrupted. Tics fluctuate in frequency and severity, and evolve in type and anatomical distribution over time such that the constellation of tics present in a child in early childhood may be quite different from those demonstrated years later.

Simple motor tics are brief, purposeless, and typically involve only one muscle group. Examples include blinking, eye rolling, head nodding, and shoulder shrugging. Tics may be clonic (sudden jerks), tonic (sustained muscle contractions), or dystonic (sustained abnormal postures). Abdominal tightening is a common tonic tic, while sustained mouth opening, oculogyric movements, blepharospasm, and torticollis are examples of dystonic tics. In contrast with stereotypies that mainly occur in the upper limbs or entire body, simple motor tics predominate in the head and neck.

Simple phonic tics are meaningless utterances or sounds such as sniffing, coughing, throat clearing, clicks, humming, animal sounds, or whistling. Children with sniffing, coughing, or throat-clearing tics may first present to the allergist or otolaryngologist with concerns about seasonal allergies or asthma. Following failure of initial treatments or appearance of other classic tics, the focus is then redirected towards neurological evaluation.

Complex motor tics represent more intricate co-ordinated patterns of movement involving more than one muscle group. Bending, jumping, kicking, spitting, smelling, obscene gestures (copropraxia), and elaborate repertoires of movement are examples. Some patients manifest blocking—sudden cessation of all motor activity. The separation of complex tics from compulsions or habit disorders can be quite challenging.

Complex phonic tics are more involved utterances, including words, phrases, profanity, or racial slurs (coprolalia), repetition of others' words (echolalia), or repetition of one's own words (palilalia). The latter two symptoms may also be a manifestation of compulsive behaviour.

Tics wax and wane and vary in anatomical distribution. Children with mild tics are typically free of functional impairment. Very young children may even be unaware of the movements. However, more frequent and intricate tics can result in social embarrassment, speech interruption, and difficulty with everyday tasks. Less commonly, tics result in pain or frank injury (49).

Neurobiology

There has been significant focus on the role of the basal ganglia in tic disorders, given its involvement in other movement disorders as well as the development or exacerbation of tics in the setting of acquired basal ganglia lesions (50–52). Anatomical studies have demonstrated decreased caudate nucleus volumes in children and adults with Tourette's syndrome (TS) compared with controls, and inverse correlation between childhood caudate volume and tic severity in early adulthood (53–55). Thinning of the sensorimotor cortex compared with controls was positively correlated with tic severity in a cohort of 25 children with TS (56). A study of tic suppression using functional MRI found changes in signal intensity in the basal ganglia, thalamus, and related cortical regions (57). Decreased parvalbumin positive GABAergic and choline acetyltransferase positive cholinergic interneurons in the caudate and putamen suggest impaired regulation of striatal neuronal firing (58). Tics may be a consequence of abnormal corticothalamic activation of specific groups of striatal neurons, resulting in increased focal inhibition of globus pallidus internus (GPi) or substantia nigra pars reticulata (SNr) output neurons.

Clinically, response to dopamine-receptor antagonists and potential exacerbation of tics by dopamine and dopamine receptor agonists suggest involvement of the dopaminergic neurotransmitter system. PET and SPECT studies demonstrate conflicting results, but there is evidence for increased dopamine activity in the striatum (59). Post-mortem pathology supports functional imaging findings, with evidence of increased dopamine uptake sites in the caudate and putamen (60).

An enhanced immune response and post-streptococcal autoimmunity are among numerous proposed aetiological factors. Tics are described as part of paediatric autoimmune neuropsychiatric disorders associated with streptococcal infections (PANDAS) in which there is abrupt onset of multiple neuropsychiatric symptoms following pharyngeal streptococcal infection. Symptoms may subsequently flare in association with repeated streptococcal infection. Although recent studies show elevations in anti-streptolysin (ASO) titres and frequency of streptococcal infections in children with TS compared with controls, these same studies fail to show a clear relationship between streptococcal infection and neuropsychiatric symptom exacerbations (61). Thus, PANDAS remains a controversial entity.

Tic disorders

Primary tic disorders are categorized based on type of tic (motor, phonic, or both) and duration of symptoms (less or greater than 1 year). TS is a clinical diagnosis based on the presence of at least one phonic and multiple motor tics that have been present on a near daily basis for at least a year based on history and/or observation. See Table 24.2 for distinctions between transient tic disorder, chronic motor and chronic phonic tic disorders, Tourette's syndrome, and tic disorder not otherwise specified (NOS).

Epidemiology of tics and Tourette's syndrome

Estimates of the prevalence of tic disorders in childhood vary widely, from 0.9 to 28%. In contrast, estimated adult prevalence is approximately 1%, emphasizing that tics are predominantly, although not completely, an issue of childhood. Challenges in establishing accurate estimates include changing criteria and definitions of tics, assessment using existing diagnoses versus observation, and identification of mild cases. Although tic phenomenology is similar across different cultures, there is a question of lower tic prevalence in African Americans and sub-Saharan black Africans (62, 63).

Tics occur with higher frequency in special education populations, at a frequency of 27% compared with 19.7% in a general education sample (63); TS similarly occurs at higher frequency in this population.

For TS, prevalence estimates similarly vary based on population and methodology, 0.4–3.8% in general paediatric populations. An overall estimate of 1% was generated by Robertson et al. in a meta-analysis of 14 studies including 420,312 subjects (62). Males are affected more than females, 3–4:1 (64).

Tourette's syndrome

Clinical course

Tic onset is in early childhood, on average at age 5–7 years, with significant improvement in symptoms, if not resolution, by age 18 years. The mean age at onset of phonic tics is later than that of motor tics, 10–11 years versus 7 years, respectively (64, 65). The age of greatest tic severity is typically 10 years, and tics tend to improve in adolescence. In a cohort of 42 children with TS, almost 50% were tic free by age 18 years. Early tic severity may not be a predictor of later tic severity (66). Although tics generally demonstrate a favourable course over time, the same may not be true for co-morbid disorders, which can exhibit lifelong manifestations. Despite common association with psychopathology, TS was not common in assessment of adults in an adult inpatient psychiatry setting with major psychiatric disorders (67). When tics do persist into adulthood, facial and truncal tics tend to predominate over other tics, and there may be an increased risk of mood disorders and substance abuse (68).

Despite portrayal in the media of coprolalia and copropraxia as common in TS, relatively few patients exhibit this symptom. In an evaluation of lifetime occurrence of coprophenomena in 597 individuals with TS, coprolalia occurred in 19.3% of males and 14.6% of females, consistent with other reports (65, 69). Copropraxia occurred at a lower frequency, in 5.9% of males and 4.9% of females. It is an unusual presenting symptom; the mean age at onset is 10.5–11 years (64, 69). Coprophenomena may be associated with more severe TS, as manifested by a broader array of co-morbidities including associations with aggression, earlier onset of tics, greater number of tics, spitting, inappropriate sexual behaviour, and self-injury (65, 69).

Co-morbid disorders

There is a high co-occurrence of neuropsychological disorders with tics, including problems of attention, mood, anxiety, socialization, learning, impulse control, oppositionality, and obsessions and compulsions (70).

ADHD is a common comorbidity which may present 2–3 years prior to the onset of tics. In the Tourette Syndrome International Database Consortium (TIC) database of over 6000 subjects, the frequency of ADHD was 61% in children and 39%

Table 24.2 DSM-IV TR criteria for tic disorders (2)

	Transient tic disorder	Chronic motor tic disorder	Chronic vocal tic disorder	Tourette's syndrome	Tic disorder not otherwise specified
Tic types	Motor *or* phonic	Motor	Phonic	Motor (≥2) *and* phonic (≥1)	Motor *or* phonic
Frequency	Many times daily or near daily	Many times daily or near daily	Many times daily or near daily	Many times daily or near daily	No frequency criterion
Duration	4 weeks–12 months	≥12 months	≥12 months	≥12 months	<4 weeks or ongoing but <12 months
Tic-free intervals	<3 months	<3 months	<3 months	<3 months	No criterion
Age of onset	<18 years	<18 years	<18 years	<18 years	No age criterion
Other factors	Not due to effects of a substance or general medical condition	Not due to effects of a substance or general medical condition	Not due to effects of a substance or general medical condition	Not due to effects of a substance or general medical condition	Tics that do not meet criteria for a specific disorder

in adults, with males having a slightly higher occurrence of ADHD than females. Earlier onset of tics (64) and greater burden of co-morbid disorders, including anger, mood disorder, obsessive–compulsive disorder (OCD), oppositional–defiant disorder (ODD), anxiety, specific learning disability, and sleep disturbance have all been associated with the presence of ADHD. Although ADHD correlates with greater overall functional impairment, there is no evidence that it has a direct impact on tic severity. In TS subjects with ADHD, 82% had one or more additional co-morbid disorders (71). ADHD is one of many factors associated with coprophenomena and social skills deficits. Other studies have found a similar frequency of ADHD occurrence (64).

Approximately 30% of children with TS suffer from OCD, although a much higher frequency of low-impairment non-specific obsessive–compulsive (OC) symptoms may exist (sub-syndromal OC behaviours). Common compulsive symptoms include smelling, checking, counting, and touching. Obsessions in TS are less likely to be related to cleanliness, contamination, illness, or washing. Some compulsions, such as symmetry, evening up, and repeating activities may be related to 'just-right' phenomena, where patients with TS repeat, rearrange, or adjust items, speech, or actions until things feel 'just right'. OCD peaks in severity approximately 2 years after tic peak severity (64).

Patients with TS are at increased risk for non-OCD generalized anxiety disorder, panic disorder, specific phobias, and mood disorders, including depression (72). Separation anxiety is common among children with TS and may be exacerbated by use of neuroleptic agents which can cause a specific school phobia (73).

Episodic rage is often provoked by unmet expectation or a change in plan, is out of proportion to the inciting incident, is directed, is brief in duration (<30 min), and is followed by remorse and regret. Parents or siblings are the most common targets, and rage attacks occur almost exclusively at home (74). Many children feel out of control during attacks, but some are able to sense when a rage attack is impending, which may be a tool for behavioural therapies. Parents often describe the spells as being incongruent with the child's personality and temperament between attacks. Stephens and Sandor (73) evaluated 33 consecutive medication-free children with TS and found that children with TS plus ADHD or OCD were at increased risk for aggressive behaviours compared with children with TS only. Children with TS alone were similar to controls in aggressive behaviour profile. ADHD and OCD, but not tic severity, best correlate with aggression in TS. Similarly, children with TS only are comparable to controls in the occurrence of disruptive behaviours, which are more frequent in children with TS plus ADHD or ADHD alone (75).

Tics are often non-impairing, and certainly life-threatening tics are rare. When tics or associated disorders and behaviours result in emergency room visits or hospitalizations, the syndrome may be categorized as malignant TS. In a review of 333 individuals with TS, 5.1% were considered to have malignant TS. Emergency visits typically relate to anger, violence, self-injurious behaviour, or suicidality. Malignant TS, often refractory to standard treatments, has been associated with more complex tic symptomatology, suicidal ideation, and a greater burden of co-morbid disorders, especially OCD (76). Self-abusive tics were reported to be present in 13% of one sample of 250 children with TS (64). Serious TS-related sequelae reported in the literature include third-degree burns, pica, eye injuries, self-biting, cervical myelopathy, fractures, and subdural haematoma (76). Individuals with malignant TS may benefit from a higher level of therapeutic intervention such as botulinum toxin for cervical tics or deep brain stimulation (DBS).

Tourettism and secondary tic disorders

Although primary tic disorders, including TS, are the most common cause of tics, insults to the basal ganglia from tumour (77), stroke, encephalitis, and head trauma may result in secondary tic disorders or 'tourettism'. Less often, tics occur in association with neurodegenerative disorders, and genetic syndromes such as Down's syndrome. Finally, medications (levodopa, SSRIs, neuroleptics, anticonvulsants), drugs of abuse (amphetamines, opiates), and toxins (carbon monoxide) may induce or exacerbate tics. Taken as a group, individuals with secondary tics demonstrate a lesser burden of neuropsychiatric co-morbidities of ADHD, behavioural problems, and sleep disorders when compared with individuals with TS (78). Primary tic disorders uniformly begin in childhood. The new onset of tics in late adolescence or adulthood should prompt evaluation for secondary causes of tics.

Evaluation

In a typically developing child with tics and an otherwise normal neurological examination, ancillary studies such as EEG, nerve conduction studies (NCS) and EMG, and brain MRI are usually normal, and thus are not recommended unless there is some doubt about the diagnosis, there are atypical features, or the onset is later in childhood than would be expected for primary tic disorders. However, given the high burden of co-morbid psychopathology, particularly in TS, identification of the presence of tics is an opportunity to explore and address other diagnoses. Careful evaluation of academic performance, socialization, and mood is warranted.

Treatment

For many children with tics, identification of the problem and education regarding tics, low likelihood of impairment, and natural history are sufficient. If tics are not functionally impairing, do not cause significant social embarrassment or school dysfunction, and are not bothersome to the patient, treatment may not be warranted. Treatment is symptomatic only; it is not clear that treatment of tics alters the natural history of the disorder. When symptomatic treatment is required, the most troublesome symptom should be established and targeted first, which may be a symptom other than tics.

Given the waxing and waning nature of tics, it may be challenging to decide when to initiate treatment. If a patient presents with worsening tics at a time consistent with prior flares, such as at the beginning of the school year, a period of waiting and supportive management may be appropriate. It is unlikely that tics will be completely eliminated by a particular treatment regimen, but significant improvement can occur, with return to premorbid functioning.

For children with problematic tics, alpha-2-adrenergic agonists, which are typically well tolerated, are reasonable first-line agents, even though they demonstrate only moderate efficacy. Guanfacine may be preferred to clonidine because of its longer half-life, and thus fewer daily doses and lesser sedative effects. Both tics and ADHD may respond to intervention with alpha-2-adrenergic agents. Guanfacine and clonidine should be tapered after prolonged use to avoid rebound hypertension.

Dopamine receptor antagonists demonstrate greater efficacy, but use may be limited by side-effect profile. If first-line therapy is insufficient, addition or substitution of a dopamine receptor blocker is an appropriate next step. Haloperidol and pimozide are the only two neuroleptics approved by the FDA for treatment of TS. Three trials have demonstrated superiority of pimozide to placebo in the treatment of tics. Two studies found no significant difference between haloperidol and pimozide, while one study showed inferiority of pimozide. Pimozide may demonstrate better overall tolerability and fewer extrapyramidal side effects than haloperidol (79). Risperidone has also shown efficacy in the management of tics (80). Tic suppression correlates with D2 receptor binding affinity, and thus some atypical antipsychotics such as quetiapine show limited benefit. No significant difference was observed between risperidone and pimozide in a randomized clinical trial (81).

There are reports of efficacy with use of tetrabenazine (82–84), baclofen (85), and topiramate (86, 87), and in open-label trials of levetiracetam (88, 89). Of note, in blinded randomized trials versus placebo or clonidine, levetiracetam did not demonstrate benefit (90, 91). Tetrabenazine, in contrast with dopamine receptor antagonists, does not carry the risk of development of tardive dyskinesia. However, its use may be limited by the side effect of depression.

Specific agents, doses, and common side effects are listed in Table 24.3. In a recent randomized observer-blind trial of behavioural intervention versus supportive therapy and education, over 50% of those randomized to behavioural intervention demonstrated benefit described as 'very much improved' or 'much improved'. Most continued to demonstrate benefit 6 months after the initial intervention. Comprehensive behavioural intervention for tics (CBIT) consists of habit reversal training with tic awareness and competing response components, relaxation training, and functional interventions to target environments and situations where tics worsen (92). Although beneficial for targeting specific problematic tics, barriers to implementation of CBIT include lack of access to trained providers and commitment to practice on the part of the patient. Very young and/or highly inattentive children may not be appropriate candidates for this behavioural intervention.

Treatment with botulinum toxin can be a very effective therapy for specific tics that are confined to a focal anatomical region, such as cervical tics or very loud vocalizations. Botulinum toxin may reduce the frequency and severity of tic as well as diminishing the premonitory urge (49, 93, 94).

Consideration of an invasive or surgical approach for paediatric TS is a complex decision, given the natural history of improvement in tics in late adolescence or adulthood. However, some patients with severe TS fail to demonstrate such a trajectory of improvement and have life-threatening tics that are refractory to treatment. Another consideration is that quality of life may be determined to a greater degree by other factors than tics, even when they are severe.

In a series of 18 patients with long-standing refractory TS, all responded to bilateral thalamic DBS with decreased tic severity and decreased medication requirement. However, 12 experienced tic recurrence, with significant waning of initial benefit after 3–6 months in three subjects. Most required frequent reprogramming after 6 months to address symptom fluctuation. Serious adverse events included poor wound healing related to compulsive touching of the incision ($n = 1$) and abdominal haematoma at the pulse generator site ($n = 1$) (95). Three of five patients who underwent

Table 24.3 Tic pharmacotherapy

Medication: generic name	Class	Starting dose	Maintenance daily dose	Common side effects
Clonidine	α_2-adrenergic agonist	0.025–0.05 mg bid–tid	0.05–0.5 mg/day	Sedation, dizziness
Guanfacine	α_2-adrenergic agonist	0.5 mg qd	0.5–4 mg/day	Sedation, headache, irritability, dry mouth, syncope
Clonazepam	Benzodiazepine	0.125–0.5 mg qd–bid	0.5–10 mg/day	Sedation
Haloperidol*	Dopamine receptor antagonist, typical antipsychotic	0.25–0.5 mg bid–tid	0.5–20 mg/day	Sedation, weight gain, metabolic syndrome, cardiac arrhythmias, school phobia, hepatotoxicity
Pimozide*	Dopamine receptor antagonist, typical antipsychotic	0.5–1 mg bid	0.5–10 mg/day	Sedation, weight gain, metabolic syndrome, cardiac arrhythmias**, school phobia, hepatotoxicity
Risperidone	Dopamine receptor antagonist, atypical antipsychotic	0.25–0.5 mg qd	0.5–16 mg/day	Sedation, weight gain, metabolic syndrome, cardiac arrhythmias**
Aripiprazole	Dopamine receptor antagonist, atypical antipsychotic	2–5 mg qd	5–30 mg/day	Sedation, weight gain, metabolic syndrome
Tetrabenazine	Dopamine depletor, dopamine receptor antagonist	12.5–25 mg qd	25–200 mg/day	Depression, sedation
Baclofen	$GABA_B$ agonist	5–10 mg bid–tid	10–120 mg/day	Sedation
Topiramate	Carbonic anhydrase inhibitor, antiepileptic	15–25 mg qd–bid	25–400 mg/day	Sedation, cognitive slowing, nephrolithiasis, dizziness

qd, once daily; bid, twice daily; tid, three times daily.

*FDA approved for treatment of tics.

**Consider baseline and serial ECGs to monitor for prolongation of the QT interval.

bilateral thalamic DBS achieved marked improvement in tics, as measured by tic count and quality of life. There were non-significant trends towards improvement in anxiety, depression, and OC behaviours. Unilateral stimulation did not produce an effect on tic frequency or severity (96). Others have achieved similar results with bilateral thalamic stimulation (97). Until further data are available, surgical interventions are currently reserved for medically refractory cases, ideally in adults.

References

1. Singer HS, Mink JW, Gilbert DL. *Movement disorders in childhood*. St Louis,MO: Saunders (Elsevier), 2010.
2. *Diagnostic and statistical manual of mental disorders* (4th edn) (DSM-IV-TR). Washington, DC: American Psychiatric Association, 2000.
3. Singer HS. Motor stereotypies. *Semin Pediatr Neurol* 2009; 16:77–81.
4. Freeman RD, Soltanifar A, Baer S. Stereotypic movement disorder: easily missed. *Dev Med Child Neurol* 2010; 52: 733–8.
5. Mahone EM, Bridges D, Prahme C, Singer HS. Repetitive arm and hand movements (complex motor stereotypies) in children. *J Pediatr* 2004; 145: 391–5.
6. Hottinger-Blanc PM, Ziegler AL, Deonna T. A special type of head stereotypies in children with developmental (?cerebellar) disorder: description of 8 cases and literature review. *Eur J Paediatr Neurol* 2002; 6: 143–52.
7. Poretti A, Alber FD, Burki S, Toelle SP, Boltshauser E. Cognitive outcome in children with rhombencephalosynapsis. *Eur J Paediatr Neurol* 2009; 13: 28–33.
8. Kates WR, Lanham DC, Singer HS. Frontal white matter reductions in healthy males with complex stereotypies. *Pediatr Neurol* 2005; 32(2): 109–12.
9. Lanovaz MJ. Towards a comprehensive model of stereotypy: integrating operant and neurobiological interpretations. *Res Dev Disabil.* 2011; 32(2): 447–55.
10. Harris KM, Mahone EM, Singer HS. Nonautistic motor stereotypies: clinical features and longitudinal follow-up. *Pediatr Neurol* 2008; 38: 267–72.
11. Foster LG. Nervous habits and stereotyped behaviors in preschool children. *J Am Acad Child Adolesc Psychiatry* 1998; 37: 711–17.
12. Tan A, Salgado M, Fahn S. The characterization and outcome of stereotypical movements in nonautistic children. *Mov Disord* 1997; 12: 47–52.
13. Akshoomoff N, Farid N, Courchesne E, Haas R. Abnormalities on the neurological examination and EEG in young children with pervasive developmental disorders. *J Autism Dev Disord* 2007; 37(5): 887–93. Epub 2006/10/19.
14. Goldman S, Wang C, Salgado MW, Greene PE, Kim M, Rapin I. Motor stereotypies in children with autism and other developmental disorders. *Dev Med Child Neurol* 2009; 51: 30–8.
15. Morgan L, Wetherby AM, Barber A. Repetitive and stereotyped movements in children with autism spectrum disorders late in the second year of life. *J Child Psychol Psychiatry* 2008; 49: 826–37.
16. Loh A, Soman T, Brian J, et al. Stereotyped motor behaviors associated with autism in high-risk infants: a pilot videotape analysis of a sibling sample. *J Autism Dev Disord* 2007; 37: 25–36.
17. MacDonald R, Green G, Mansfield R, Geckeler A, Gardenier N, Anderson J, et al. Stereotypy in young children with autism and typically developing children. *Res Dev Disabil* 2007; 28(3): 266–77.
18. Carter P, Downs J, Bebbington A, et al. Stereotypical hand movements in 144 subjects with Rett syndrome from the population-based Australian database. *Mov Disord* 2010; 25: 282–8.
19. Temudo T, Ramos E, Dias K, et al. Movement disorders in Rett syndrome: an analysis of 60 patients with detected MECP2 mutation and correlation with mutation type. *Mov Disord* 2008; 23: 1384–90.
20. Temudo T, Santos M, Ramos E, et al. Rett syndrome with and without detected MECP2 mutations: an attempt to redefine phenotypes. *Brain Dev* 2011; 33: 69–76.
21. Temudo T, Oliveira P, Santos M, et al. Stereotypies in Rett syndrome: analysis of 83 patients with and without detected MECP2 mutations. *Neurology* 2007; 68: 1183–7.
22. Vignoli A, La Briola F, Canevini MP. Evolution of stereotypies in adolescents and women with Rett syndrome. *Mov Disord* 2009; 24: 1379–83.
23. Fazzi E, Lanners J, Danova S, et al. Stereotyped behaviours in blind children. *Brain Dev* 1999; 21: 522–8.
24. Collins MS, Cornish K. A survey of the prevalence of stereotypy, self-injury and aggression in children and young adults with Cri du Chat syndrome. *J Intellect Disabil Res* 2002; 46(Pt 2): 133–40.
25. Ogura K, Shinohara M, Ohno K, Mori E. Frontal behavioral syndromes in Prader–Willi syndrome. *Brain Dev* 2008; 30: 469–76.
26. Bahi-Buisson N, Nectoux J, Rosas-Vargas H, et al. Key clinical features to identify girls with CDKL5 mutations. *Brain* 2008; 131: 2647–61.
27. Dalal P, Leslie ND, Lindor NM, Gilbert DL, Espay AJ. Motor tics, stereotypies, and self-flagellation in primrose syndrome. *Neurology* 2010; 75: 284–6.
28. Gropman AL, Duncan WC, Smith AC. Neurologic and developmental features of the Smith-Magenis syndrome (del 17p11.2). *Pediatr Neurol* 2006; 34: 337–50.
29. Laje G, Bernert R, Morse R, Pao M, Smith AC. Pharmacological treatment of disruptive behavior in Smith–Magenis syndrome. *Am J Med Genet C Semin Med Genet* 2010; 154C: 463–8.
30. Galera C, Taupiac E, Fraisse S, et al. Socio-behavioral characteristics of children with Rubinstein–Taybi syndrome. *J Autism Dev Disord* 2009; 39: 1252–60.
31. Boyle L, Kaufmann WE. The behavioral phenotype of FMR1 mutations. *Am J Med Genet C Semin Med Genet* 2010; 154C: 469–76.
32. Bahi-Buisson N, Nectoux J, Girard B, et al. Revisiting the phenotype associated with FOXG1 mutations: two novel cases of congenital Rett variant. *Neurogenetics* 2010; 11: 241–9.
33. Gouider-Khouja N, Kraoua I, Benrhouma H, Fraj N, Rouissi A. Movement disorders in neuro-metabolic diseases. *Eur J Paediatr Neurol* 2010; 14: 304–7.
34. Yorio AA, Mesri JC, Pagano MA, Lera G. Stereotypies in Wilson's disease. *Mov Disord* 1997; 12: 614–16.
35. Twardowschy CA, De Paola L, Teive HA, Silvado C. Stereotypies after herpetic encephalitis with bitemporal lesions. *Mov Disord* 2010; 25: 2888–9.
36. Dale RC, Webster R, Gill D. Contemporary encephalitis lethargica presenting with agitated catatonia, stereotypy, and dystonia–parkinsonism. *Mov Disord* 2007; 22: 2281–4.
37. Florance NR, Davis RL, Lam C, Szperka C, Zhou L, Ahmad S, et al. Anti-*N*-methyl-d-aspartate receptor (NMDAR) encephalitis in children and adolescents. *Ann Neurol* 2009; 66: 11–18.
38. Miller JM, Singer HS, Bridges DD, Waranch HR. Behavioral therapy for treatment of stereotypic movements in nonautistic children. *J Child Neurol* 2006; 21: 119–25.
39. Ahrens EN, Lerman DC, Kodak T, Worsdell AS, Keegan C. Further evaluation of response interruption and redirection as treatment for stereotypy. *J Appl Behav Anal* 2011; 44: 95–108.
40. Cassella MD, Sidener TM, Sidener DW, Progar PR. Response interruption and redirection for vocal stereotypy in children with autism: a systematic replication. *J Appl Behav Anal* 2011; 44: 169–73.
41. Ahearn WH, Clark KM, MacDonald RP, Chung BI. Assessing and treating vocal stereotypy in children with autism. *J Appl Behav Anal* 2007; 40: 263–75.
42. Vogel W, Stein DJ. Citalopram for head-banging. *J Am Acad Child Adolesc Psychiatry* 2000; 39: 544–5.
43. Kalapatapu RK. Escitalopram treatment of stereotypic movement disorder in an adolescent with mitochondrial disorder and mental retardation. *J Child Adolesc Psychopharmacol* 2009; 19: 313–16.

44. Capone GT, Goyal P, Grados M, Smith B, Kammann H. Risperidone use in children with Down syndrome, severe intellectual disability, and comorbid autistic spectrum disorders: a naturalistic study. *J Dev Behav Pediatr* 2008; 29: 106–16.
45. Hashizume Y, Yoshijima H, Uchimura N, Maeda H. Case of head banging that continued to adolescence. *Psychiatry Clin Neurosci* 2002; 56: 255–6.
46. Rajapakse T, Pringsheim T. Pharmacotherapeutics of Tourette syndrome and stereotypies in autism. *Semin Pediatr Neurol* 2010; 17: 254–60.
47. Leckman JF, Walker DE, Cohen DJ. Premonitory urges in Tourette's syndrome. *Am J Psychiatry* 1993; 150: 98–102.
48. Conelea CA, Woods DW, Brandt BC. The impact of a stress induction task on tic frequencies in youth with Tourette Syndrome. *Behav Res Therapy* 2011; 49: 492–7.
49. Krauss JK, Jankovic J. Severe motor tics causing cervical myelopathy in Tourette's syndrome. *Mov Disord* 1996; 11: 563–6.
50. Dale RC, Church AJ, Heyman I. Striatal encephalitis after varicella zoster infection complicated by Tourettism. *Mov Disord* 2003; 18: 1554–6.
51. Peterson BS, Bronen RA, Duncan CC. Three cases of symptom change in Tourette's syndrome and obsessive-compulsive disorder associated with paediatric cerebral malignancies. *J Neurol Neurosurg Psychiatry* 1996; 61: 497–505.
52. Gomis M, Puente V, Pont-Sunyer C, Oliveras C, Roquer J. Adult onset simple phonic tic after caudate stroke. *Mov Disord* 2008; 23: 765–6.
53. Hyde TM, Stacey ME, Coppola R, Handel SF, Rickler KC, Weinberger DR. Cerebral morphometric abnormalities in Tourette's syndrome: a quantitative MRI study of monozygotic twins. *Neurology* 1995; 45: 1176–82.
54. Peterson BS, Thomas P, Kane MJ, et al. Basal ganglia volumes in patients with Gilles de la Tourette syndrome. *Arch Gen Psychiatry* 2003; 60: 415–24.
55. Bloch MH, Leckman JF, Zhu H, Peterson BS. Caudate volumes in childhood predict symptom severity in adults with Tourette syndrome. *Neurology* 2005; 65: 1253–8.
56. Sowell ER, Kan E, Yoshii J, et al. Thinning of sensorimotor cortices in children with Tourette syndrome. *Nat Neurosci* 2008; 11: 637–9.
57. Peterson BS, Skudlarski P, Anderson AW, et al. A functional magnetic resonance imaging study of tic suppression in Tourette syndrome. *Arch Gen Psychiatry* 1998; 55: 326–33.
58. Kataoka Y, Kalanithi PS, Grantz H, et al. Decreased number of parvalbumin and cholinergic interneurons in the striatum of individuals with Tourette syndrome. *J Comp Neurol* 2010; 518: 277–91.
59. Rickards H. Functional neuroimaging in Tourette syndrome. *J Psychosom Res* 2009; 67: 575–84.
60. Singer HS, Hahn IH, Moran TH. Abnormal dopamine uptake sites in postmortem striatum from patients with Tourette's syndrome. *Ann Neurol* 1991; 30: 558–62.
61. Martino D, Chiarotti F, Buttiglione M, et al. The relationship between group A streptococcal infections and Tourette syndrome: a study on a large service-based cohort. *Dev Med Child Neurol* 2011; 53: 951–7.
62. Robertson MM. The prevalence and epidemiology of Gilles de la Tourette syndrome. Part 1: the epidemiological and prevalence studies. *J Psychosom Res* 2008; 65: 461–72.
63. Kurlan R, McDermott MP, Deeley C, et al. Prevalence of tics in schoolchildren and association with placement in special education. *Neurology* 2001; 57: 1383–8.
64. Comings DE, Comings BG. Tourette syndrome: clinical and psychological aspects of 250 cases. *Am J Hum Genet* 1985; 37: 435–50.
65. Robertson MM, Trimble MR, Lees AJ. The psychopathology of the Gilles de la Tourette syndrome: a phenomenological analysis. *Br J Psychiatry* 1988; 152: 383–90.
66. Leckman JF, Zhang H, Vitale A, et al. Course of tic severity in Tourette syndrome: the first two decades. *Pediatrics* 1998; 102: 14–19.
67. Eapen V, Laker M, Anfield A, Dobbs J, Robertson MM. Prevalence of tics and Tourette syndrome in an inpatient adult psychiatry setting. *J Psychiatry Neurosci* 2001; 26: 417–20.
68. Jankovic J, Gelineau-Kattner R, Davidson A. Tourette's syndrome in adults. *Mov Disord* 2010; 25: 2171–5.
69. Freeman RD, Zinner SH, Muller-Vahl KR, et al. Coprophenomena in Tourette syndrome. *Dev Med Child Neurol* 2009; 51: 218–27.
70. Kurlan R, Como PG, Miller B, et al. The behavioral spectrum of tic disorders: a community-based study. *Neurology* 2002; 59: 414–20.
71. Freeman RD. Tic disorders and ADHD: answers from a world-wide clinical dataset on Tourette syndrome. *Eur Child Adolesc Psychiatry* 2007; 16 (Suppl 1): 15–23.
72. Robertson MM, Banerjee S, Eapen V, Fox-Hiley P. Obsessive compulsive behaviour and depressive symptoms in young people with Tourette syndrome. *Eur Child Adolesc Psychiatry* 2002; 11: 261–5.
73. Stephens RJ, Sandor P. Aggressive behaviour in children with Tourette syndrome and comorbid attention-deficit hyperactivity disorder and obsessive-compulsive disorder. *Can J Psychiatry* 1999; 44: 1036–42.
74. Budman CL, Rockmore L, Stokes J, Sossin M. Clinical phenomenology of episodic rage in children with Tourette syndrome. *J Psychosom Res* 2003; 55: 59–65.
75. Sukhodolsky DG, Scahill L, Zhang H, et al. Disruptive behavior in children with Tourette's syndrome: association with ADHD comorbidity, tic severity, and functional impairment. *J Am Acad Child Adolesc Psychiatry* 2003; 42: 98–105.
76. Cheung MY, Shahed J, Jankovic J. Malignant Tourette syndrome. *Mov Disord* 2007; 22: 1743–50.
77. Luat AF, Behen ME, Juhasz C, Sood S, Chugani HT. Secondary tics or tourettism associated with a brain tumor. *Pediatr Neurol* 2009; 41: 457–60.
78. Mejia NI, Jankovic J. Secondary tics and tourettism. *Rev Bras Psiquiatr* 2005; 27: 11–17.
79. Sallee FR, Nesbitt L, Jackson C, Sine L, Sethuraman G. Relative efficacy of haloperidol and pimozide in children and adolescents with Tourette's disorder. *Am J Psychiatry* 1997; 154: 1057–62.
80. Dion Y, Annable L, Sandor P, Chouinard G. Risperidone in the treatment of Tourette syndrome: a double-blind, placebo-controlled trial. *J Clin Psychopharmacol* 2002; 22: 31–9.
81. Pringsheim T, Marras C. Pimozide for tics in Tourette's syndrome. *Cochrane Database Syst Rev* 2009: CD006996.
82. Jankovic J, Glaze DG, Frost JD, Jr. Effect of tetrabenazine on tics and sleep of Gilles de la Tourette's syndrome. *Neurology* 1984; 34: 688–92.
83. Jankovic J, Orman J. Tetrabenazine therapy of dystonia, chorea, tics, and other dyskinesias. *Neurology* 1988; 38: 391–4.
84. Porta M, Sassi M, Cavallazzi M, Fornari M, Brambilla A, Servello D. Tourette's syndrome and role of tetrabenazine: review and personal experience. *Clin Drug Investig* 2008; 28: 443–59.
85. Singer HS, Wendlandt J, Krieger M, Giuliano J. Baclofen treatment in Tourette syndrome: a double-blind, placebo-controlled, crossover trial. *Neurology* 2001; 56: 599–604.
86. Kuo SH, Jimenez-Shahed J. Topiramate in treatment of tourette syndrome. *Clin Neuropharmacol* 2010; 33: 32–4.
87. Jankovic J, Jimenez-Shahed J, Brown LW. A randomised, double-blind, placebo-controlled study of topiramate in the treatment of Tourette syndrome. *J Neurol Neurosurg Psychiatry* 2010; 81: 70–3.
88. Awaad Y, Michon AM, Minarik S. Use of levetiracetam to treat tics in children and adolescents with Tourette syndrome. *Mov Disord* 2005; 20: 714–18.
89. Fernandez-Jaen A, Fernandez-Mayoralas DM, Munoz-Jareno N, Calleja-Perez B. An open-label, prospective study of levetiracetam in children and adolescents with Tourette syndrome. *Eur J Paediatr Neurol* 2009; 13: 541–5.
90. Smith-Hicks CL, Bridges DD, Paynter NP, Singer HS. A double blind randomized placebo control trial of levetiracetam in Tourette syndrome. *Mov Disord* 2007; 22: 1764–70.
91. Hedderick EF, Morris CM, Singer HS. Double-blind, crossover study of clonidine and levetiracetam in Tourette syndrome. *Pediatr Neurol* 2009; 40: 420–5.

92. Piacentini J, Woods DW, Scahill L, et al. Behavior therapy for children with Tourette disorder. *JAMA* 2010; 303: 1929–37.
93. Jankovic J. Botulinum toxin in the treatment of dystonic tics. *Mov Disord* 1994; 9: 347–9.
94. Simpson DM, Blitzer A, Brashear A, et al. Assessment: botulinum neurotoxin for the treatment of movement disorders (an evidence-based review): report of the Therapeutics and Technology Assessment Subcommittee of the American Academy of Neurology. *Neurology* 2008; 70: 1699–706.
95. Servello D, Porta M, Sassi M, Brambilla A, Robertson MM. Deep brain stimulation in 18 patients with severe Gilles de la Tourette syndrome refractory to treatment: the surgery and stimulation. *J Neurol Neurosurg Psychiatry* 2008; 79: 136–42.
96. Maciunas RJ, Maddux BN, Riley DE, et al. Prospective randomized double-blind trial of bilateral thalamic deep brain stimulation in adults with Tourette syndrome. *J Neurosurg* 2007; 107: 1004–14.
97. Lee MWY, Au-Yeung MM, Hung KN, Wong CK. Deep brain stimulation in a Chinese Tourette's syndrome patient. *Hong Kong Med J* 2011; 17: 147–50.

CHAPTER 25

Myoclonus

Marina A. J. Tijssen

Summary

Myoclonus is characterized by quick and involuntary jerks and classified as one of the hyperkinetic movement disorders. Myoclonus can be caused by muscle contractions (positive myoclonus) or by interruptions of tonic muscle (negative myoclonus). The main classification of myoclonus is based on the anatomical origin of the myoclonic jerks: cortical, subcortical, spinal, and peripheral myoclonus, each with distinctive physiological mechanisms. Clinical characteristics, aetiology, and treatment options are related to the anatomical classification of myoclonus.

The epidemiology of myoclonus is poorly documented, as myoclonus has many different causes and a spectrum of clinical presentations. A single study showed a lifetime prevalence of 8.6 cases per 100 000. The aetiology of myoclonus is diverse and in 70% of cases is symptomatic. Over the last 10 years new genes have been discovered for several myoclonic disorders. Recent pathophysiological studies illustrate an important role for the cerebellum in generating both cortical and subcortical myoclonus, but further studies addressing the precise mechanism of myoclonus are required. Therapy is usually symptomatic, as treatment of an underlying cause is often impossible or ineffective. Therapeutic options are mainly based on a low level of evidence, as randomized controlled trials are not available.

Essential background

Myoclonus literally means 'a quick movement of muscle' and is clinically defined by sudden, brief, and shock-like involuntary movements caused by muscle contractions (positive myoclonus) or muscle inhibition (negative myoclonus) (1, 2). The term paramyoclonus multiplex for the sudden jerks was introduced in 1881 by Friedreich in a patient with essential myoclonus (3). In 1963, Lance and Adams first described negative myoclonus in patients with post-hypoxic myoclonus (4).

Clinically, myoclonus is quite distinct. In most cases the diagnosis can be established on clinical grounds with a relatively high degree of diagnostic certainty. Alternative diagnoses include tics, tremor, dystonia, chorea, simple partial seizures, and psychogenic jerks. Clinical clues help to differentiate it from other movement disorders (5–8). For example, stimulus sensitivity can be present in patients with myoclonus, but is rare in other movement disorders. Myoclonus often interferes with voluntary movements and increases with muscle activation, while motor tics almost never interact with motor activity. Furthermore, in contrast with tics, myoclonus is a non-suppressible and simple movement, not preceded by an urge to move, and without relief after the movement. In contrast with tremor, myoclonus is generally arrhythmic. This can sometimes be difficult to discriminate in clinical practice and EMG registration might be required (9, 10). In dystonic jerks, the posture can often be influenced by a *geste antagonistique*, which is not seen in myoclonus. In chorea the individual movements can be myoclonic but the overall movements are more continuous and in a constant flow. Psychogenic movements can be a difficult diagnosis in jerky patients and will be discussed elsewhere in this chapter (see 'Aetiology and genetics', p.258). In general, it should be appreciated that myoclonic jerks regularly occur in combination with other movement disorders (1).

The identification and classification of myoclonus is important, with three generally accepted classifications: according to anatomical origin, based on clinical signs, and based on aetiology (1, 5, 11). The three classification systems are interrelated. In this chapter, the anatomical classification will be discussed first as it forms the basis of the approach towards the patient with myoclonus.

Anatomical classification

Myoclonus can originate from the cortex, subcortical areas (including brainstem), spinal cord, or peripheral nerves. Classification of the anatomical origin of myoclonus is based on electrophysiological characteristics and is additionally guided by clinical signs and the aetiological classification. It should be noted that different types of myoclonus can occur in a single patient. Here, a short overview will be given.

Cortical myoclonus originates from the cortex as a result of abnormal firing of the sensorimotor cortex (12). Body parts with the largest cortical representation, such as the hands and the mouth, are the most frequently involved (12, 13) (Video 25.1). The jerks are usually (multi)focal and are exacerbated by voluntary movements. Continuous frequent focal spontaneous jerks are also described as 'epilepsia partialis continua'. Reflex myoclonus is common; for example, the jerks can be elicited by touching the affected limb (12, 14). Electromyographic examination shows short bursts (usually <50 ms) (15). With EEG–EMG back-averaging a time-locked cortical spike preceding the jerk in the contralateral hemisphere can

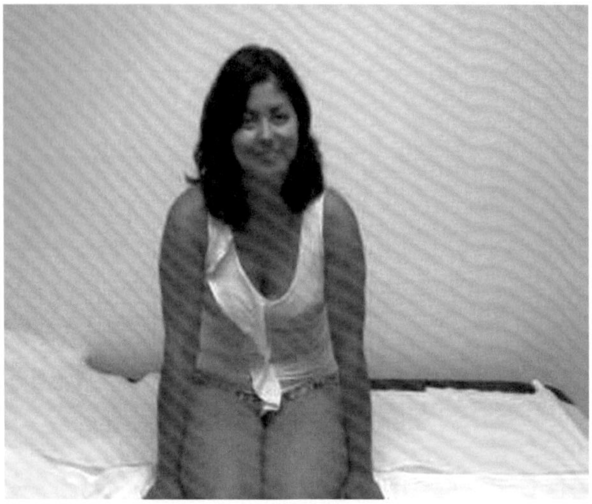

Video 25.1 The video shows a patient with cortical myoclonus. The body parts with the largest cortical representation, such as the hands and the mouth, are involved. The jerks are multifocal and are exacerbated due to voluntary movements. Tapping the fingers illustrates stimulus sensitivity.

be found (16). Examination of the somatosensory evoked potential (SSEP) shows an enlarged (giant) cortical amplitude (17).

In *subcortical myoclonus* the source of discharges leading to myoclonus is localized between the cortex and the spinal cord. The clinical and electrophysiological characteristics are variable between the different subtypes. In general, no signs of cortical hyperexcitability on EEG–EMG or SSEP can be detected.

Essential myoclonus or myoclonus–dystonia (MD) (see 'Aetiology and genetics', p.258, for more details) clinically consists of myoclonic jerks in the upper body often combined with mild to moderate dystonia. The myoclonus is not stimulus sensitive, but does increase with voluntary activity. On electrophysiology, no signs of cortical excitability can be detected and EMG studies show short bursts (25–256 ms) (18, 19). The exact origin of the myoclonus is unknown but is considered to be subcortical.

Brainstem myoclonus represents generalized, synchronized, and especially axial jerks and is very sensitive to external stimuli (12, 20). EMG polymyography shows simultaneous rostral and caudal activation of muscles (12, 21).

Spinal myoclonus is the result of abnormal discharges generated in the spinal cord and can be subdivided into segmental and propriospinal myoclonus.

Segmental myoclonus is a very rare disorder, inducing myoclonic jerks in muscles innervated by one or two contiguous spinal segments. The jerks are continuous, rhythmic, unaffected by voluntary movement or sensory stimulation, and often persist during sleep (22). On EMG recordings the frequency ranges from 1 to 200 per minute, with burst durations of up to 1000 ms.

Propriospinal myoclonus is characterized by generalized axial muscle contractions, often induced by lying down, without involvement of the facial muscles (23, 24). Jerks can be spontaneous and stimulus sensitive (23, 25). Polymyography shows a slow spreading of activity with repetitive bursts of EMG activity (frequency 1–7 Hz) and a long duration (up to several hudred milliseconds) (25).

Peripheral myoclonus is very rare and is limited to one segment of the body, usually the proximal part of a limb or the trunk. Bursts can be triggered by voluntary movement and the burst duration varies (26).

Epidemiology

Epidemiological studies of myoclonus are scarce. The main problem is that myoclonus has many different causes and a spectrum of clinical presentations, while epidemiological studies have mainly been performed for specific diagnoses. There is one study in a defined population in Olmsted County, Minnesota, showing that persistent and pathological myoclonus has a lifetime prevalence of 8.6 cases per 100 000 (27). In that study the most common aetiology for myoclonus was symptomatic (72%), followed by epileptic (17%) and then essential myoclonus (11%) (27). In a study in patients in the emergency room because of a movement disorder, 27.6% exhibited myoclonus, including patients with transient myoclonus (e.g. drug-induced) (28). Overall, myoclonus appears to be a relatively frequent cause of abnormal movement control.

Aetiology and genetics

Marsden was the first to classify myoclonus by aetiology, comprising four main groups (1, 5). The first group is physiological myoclonus, with examples such as sleep jerks and hiccoughs, which are common in healthy individuals. A second group is formed by 'essential' myoclonus, or myoclonus dystonia, which is usually hereditary (29, 30). Epileptic myoclonus forms the third group, dominated by epileptic seizures (31). The last group, symptomatic myoclonus, is by far the largest, with approximately 70% of cases. In this group myoclonus is a manifestation of an underlying disorder, with neurodegenerative disorders, hypoxia, drug-induced myoclonus, and toxic–metabolic myoclonus as the main causes (28, 32).

Physiological myoclonus

Physiological myoclonus occurs in the normal population under certain circumstances. Sleep jerks are the most frequent manifestations, but hiccoughs are also well known.

Essential myoclonus

In *essential myoclonus* or *myoclonus–dystonia (MD)*, myoclonic jerks in the upper body are often combined with mild to moderate dystonia. The myoclonus is multifocal, with 'twitching' jerks of variable amplitude and intensity increasing with action, and tends to be responsive to alcohol (18, 19) (Videos 25.2 and 25.3). Psychiatric symptoms such as depressed mood, anxiety or obsessive–compulsive disorder are frequently observed (33). In most patients, symptoms occur within the first two decades. MD is autosomal dominantly inherited, and a mutation in the epsilon-sarcoglycan gene (*SGCE*) on chromosome 7q21 (*DYT11*) is present in 30% of patients (34). If strict clinical criteria are applied, this number significantly increases up to 50% (35). Penetrance of MD is highly dependent on the parental origin of the disease allele, resulting from maternal imprinting (36). As *DYT11* mutations are absent in up to 50% of patients with the MD phenotype, the involvement of other genes or environmental factors is suggested (35). A second locus has been reported in one large MD family (DYT15, 18p11), but no gene has yet been identified (37, 38). SGCE is part of the sarcoglycan family which consists of *N*-glycosylated

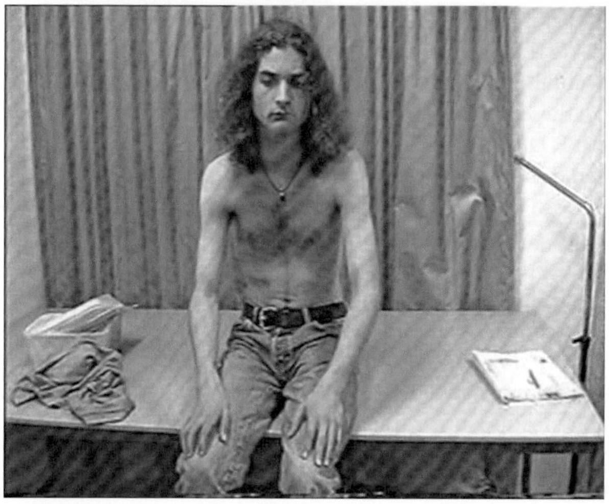

Video 25.2 The video shows a patient with myoclonus–dystonia (with a mutation in the *SGCE* gene). The typical features of 'twitching' jerks mainly in the upper part of the body are seen. The myoclonus is more prominent during voluntary action. In addition, mild cervical dystonia may be noted. Tijssen MAJ and Tijssen CC. Myoclonus. In: Parkinsonism and related disorders. Wolters E Ch, van Laar T, Berendse HW (eds). 2008. VU University Press. ISBN 9789086591503

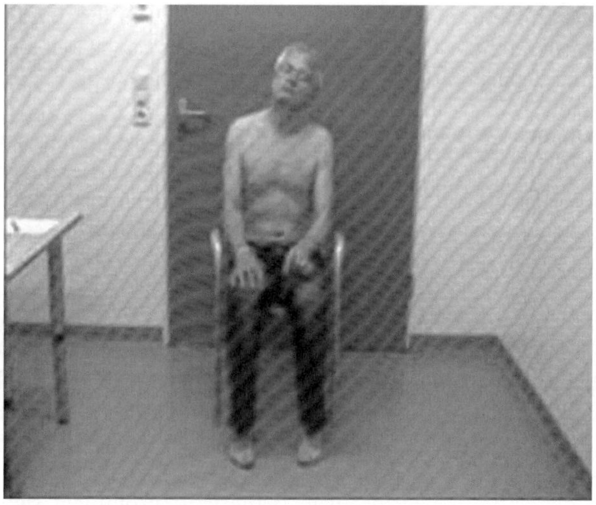

Video 25.3 The video shows a patient with myoclonus–dystonia (with a mutation in the *SGCE* gene). The patient has myclonic jerks in the upper part of the body, but also prominent disabling dystonic features. The patient was treated with stereotactic surgery (bilateral globus pallidus interna stimulation) with good effect. The second part of the video shows the patient several months after surgery.

transmembrane proteins (39), but little is known about its function in the brain. *SGCE* is highly homologous to α-sarcoglycan, but no muscle or myocardial muscle abnormalities have been identified in MD patients (40).

Epileptic myoclonus

Several forms of epilepsy can be accompanied by myoclonic jerks, such as isolated epileptic myoclonic jerks, photosensitive myoclonus, and myoclonic absences with petit mal (see Table 25.1). The EEG changes associated with epileptic myoclonus are usually spikes, polyspikes, and spike and slow-wave complexes. Movement disorders are the main issue of this book, and therefore epileptic

Table 25.1 Causes of myoclonus

Physiological myoclonus		Sleep jerks, hiccoughs
Essential myoclonus		Myoclonus dystonia
Epileptic myoclonus	Parts of epilepsy	Epileptic myoclonic jerks Photosensitive myoclonus Myoclonic absences with petit mal *Epilepsia partialis continua*
	Childhood myoclonic epilepsy	Benign 'myoclonus of infancy' Infantile spasms Lennox–Gastaut epilepsy Cryptogenic myoclonic epilepsy
	Benign familial myoclonic epilepsy	
	Familial cortical myoclonic tremor and epilepsy (FCMTE)	
Symptomatic myoclonus	Storage disease	Lafora body disease Sialidosis Lipidosis (GM1 and GM2 gangliosidosis, Krabbe disease) Tay–Sachs disease Neuronal ceroid-lipofuscinose
	Spinocerebellar degeneration	Unverricht–Lundborg disease Ataxia telangiectasia Friedreich's ataxia Spinocerebellar ataxias
	Degeneration basal ganglia	Multiple system atrophy Progressive supranuclear palsy Parkinson's disease Huntington's disease Corticobasal degeneration DRPLA Wilson disease Dystonia Pantothenate-kinase-associated neurodegeneration 2
	Mitochondrial encephalopathy	MERFF
	Dementia	Creutzfeldt–Jakob disease Alzheimer's disease Lewy body dementia Frontotemporal dementia
	Malabsorption syndrome	Whipple's disease Coeliac disease
	Infectious or postinfectious	SSPE Encephalitis lethargica Postinfectious encephalitis Arbovirus or herpes simplex virus encephalitis AIDS
	Metabolic encephalopathy	Hepatic failure Hyperthyroidism Renal failure Hypoglycaemia Hyponatraemia Vitamin E deficiency

(Continued)

Table 25.1 (Continued)

Toxic and drug induced (25, 59)
Physical encephalopathy
Paraneoplastic encephalopathy
Focal CNS lesions
Post-hypoxic

Modified from Caviness and Brown (20).

myoclonus in epilepsy syndromes will not be discussed further (for a review of epileptic myoclonic jerks and their treatment options, see ref. 31).

Familial cortical myoclonic tremor and epilepsy (FCMTE) is an example of a syndrome overlapping with movement disorders and should be discriminated from essential tremor. FCMTE presents with tremor-like myoclonus and epilepsy (41). It is a rare autosomal dominant inherited disorder characterized by late-onset intention-like tremor and distal myoclonus, myoclonic and generalized seizures, moderately progressive course, and good response to antiepileptic drugs. Electrophysiological studies reveal features of cortical reflex myoclonus, including giant somatosensory evoked potentials (gSSEP) and enhanced cortical reflexes (C-reflexes). Coherence analysis shows strong cortical and intermuscular coherence in the 8–30 Hz range (9). EEG may show polyspike–wave complexes. Genetic studies have revealed linkage to three loci (chromosomes 8q23.3-q24.1, 2p11.1-q12.2, and 5p15.31-p15) (42), but no gene has been identified yet.

Symptomatic myoclonus

Symptomatic myoclonic jerks are usually multifocal, occur spontaneously, and can be increased by action and external stimuli. In an attempt to help in clinical decision-making, symptomatic cases are divided according to their anatomical origin. Mental status abnormalities, seizures, ataxia, and other movement disorders are common clinical associations in symptomatic myoclonic syndromes. The various causes are outlined in Table 25.1.

Cortical

Cortical myoclonus forms the largest group within symptomatic myoclonus and can be subdivided into *progressive* myoclonic and *static* myoclonic encephalopathies.

Progressive myoclonic encephalopathy

Clinically, patients with progressive myoclonic encephalopathy suffer from action-induced stimulus-sensitive multifocal and generalized myoclonus. In general, it is often difficult to make the exact diagnosis. Further subgroups based on associated neurological symptoms, such as the presence or absence of epilepsy and/or dementia, help with classification (43).

If combined with both prominent epilepsy and dementia, the course is often progressive. Patients have intractable generalized tonic–clonic seizures and progressive dementia. The age at onset of these disorders is usually in early childhood, but occasionally late onset has been described. The differential diagnosis includes Lafora body disease, myoclonus epilepsy with ragged red fibres (MERRF), lipofuscinosis (Kuf's disease), sialidosis, and dentatorubral-pallidoluysian atrophy (DRPLA). New genes for several of these progressive myoclonus epilepsy syndromes, including MERFF, DRPLA, sialidosis, and neuronal ceroid lipofuscinosis, have been discovered in the last few years (44, 45) (see Table 25.2). The progressive nature of the illness and cognitive decline differentiate progressive myoclonic encephalopathy diagnoses from more benign epileptic myoclonic syndromes.

Without a prominent cognitive decline, but with epilepsy or ataxia, the course of the progression of myoclonic encephalopathy is usually slower. Clinically, patients exhibit a combination of action myoclonus, epilepsy, and ataxia. Depending on the most prominent feature other than myoclonus, two subgroups (43) can be recognized: progressive myoclonus epilepsy and progressive myoclonus ataxia. The cause of progressive myoclonus epilepsy is in most cases Unverricht–Lundberg (UL) disease, which usually manifests in the first years of life with action-induced and stimulus-sensitive multifocal myoclonus. Ataxia is usually mild. The associated generalized tonic–clonic seizures can be difficult to treat. Recently, the *CSTB* gene cystatin B has been implicated in UL (44, 45) (see Table 25.2).

In patients with progressive myoclonus ataxia, unsteadiness of gait is one of the most prominent signs next to the multifocal action-induced myoclonus. Occasional seizures can be well treated with antiepileptic drugs. Progressive myoclonic ataxia is usually sporadic, with age at onset ranging from childhood to age 70 years. Differential diagnosis includes Ramsay-Hunt syndrome, mitochondrial disorders (e.g. MERFF, POLG1), vitamin E deficiency, and coeliac disease (46, 47). If combined with nephropathy, action myoclonus renal failure syndrome (AMRFS) should be considered. AMRFS starts in the second or third decade with progressive action myoclonus associated with occasional seizures, cerebellar ataxia, and preserved cognition (48). Mutations in the gene coding for the lysosomal protein SCARB2 have been found in AMRFS (49). The combination of prominent ataxia and myoclonus together with other features can also point towards a spinocerebellar ataxia (SCA) (50). The myoclonus in SCAs can be cortical or subcortical (50, 51).

If dementia or parkinsonism is the most prominent sign in patients with progressive myoclonic encephalopathy who are not suffering from epilepsy, the differential diagnosis includes mainly late-onset neurodegenerative disorders. Examples include Alzheimer's disease, Parkinson's disease, and multiple system atrophy. Patients usually have irregular small jerks of the hand muscles ('poly-mini-myoclonus'). Cortical myoclonus can also occur in other neurodegenerative disorders such as Lewy body dementia and Huntington's disease. A characteristic type of myoclonus may be seen in corticobasal syndrome. The affected limb, especially the distal arm, shows irregular continuous jerks increasing with movement. Additional causes of severe cortical myoclonus include Creutzfeldt–Jakob disease, where the generalized myoclonus is commonly sensitive to sound. If the myoclonus is acute or subacute and accompanied by epilepsy and altered mental status, herpes simplex encephalitis and subacute sclerosing panencephalitis (SSPE), or NMDA encephalitis should be considered. Metabolic disorders, such as liver and kidney problems, usually lead to both positive and negative myoclonus (asterixis).

Table 25.2 Genetic abnormalities of progressive myoclonus epilepsies (45)

Disease	Inheritance	Chromosome	Gene	Protein
UL	AR	21q22.3	*CSTB*	Cystatin B
Lafora	AR	6q24	*EPM2A*	Laforin
MERRF	Mat.	mtDNA	*MTTK*	tRNALys
Sialidosis types 1 & 2	AR	6p21.3 & 20	*NEU1*	Sialidase 1
DRPLA	AD	12p13.31	*DRPLA*	Atrophin 1
NCL				
Late infantile	AR	11p15	*TPP1*	Tripeptidyl peptidase 1
Juvenile	AR	6p	*CLN3*	
Late infantile (Finnish)	AR	13q21–q32	*CLN5*	
Variant late infantile	AR	15q21–23	*CLN6*	

UL, Unverricht–Lundborg disease; MERRF, myoclonic epilepsy with ragged red fibres; DRPLA, dentatorubral-pallidoluysian atrophy; NCL, neuronal ceroid lipofuscinosis; AR, autosomal recessive; AD, autosomal dominant; CSTB, cystatin based on refs 44 and 45.

Drug-induced myoclonus (DIM) is frequent in clinical practice, and all drugs should be checked as potential culprits. DIM is considered to be cortical, but detailed electrophysiology is scarce. In lithium-induced myoclonus the origin is believed to be cortical as there are different clinical symptoms of motor cortex hyperexcitability (12), but some argue in favour of a subcortical origin as EEG recordings do not always show jerk-related abnormalities in DIM. In general, the jerks are usually reversible with discontinuation of the offending drug. Psychiatric medication is most commonly responsible, but a number of drugs can cause myoclonus, including anticonvulsants and propofol (20, 52).

Static myoclonic encephalopathy

Post-hypoxic myoclonus (PHM) is an important example of static myoclonic encephalopathy. Lance–Adams syndrome develops with a delay of a few days after the hypoxic episode. Disabling action myoclonus appears when moving a limb and is usually stimulus-sensitive, combined with negative myoclonus, resulting in postural lapses (53) (see Video 25.4). Patients may also suffer from brainstem myoclonus with generalized jerks. Acute PHM occurs shortly after a hypoxic episode with mainly generalized myoclonic jerks and has a poor prognosis.

Subcortical

Generalized reticular brainstem myoclonus can be caused by post-hypoxic encephalopathy, brainstem encephalitis, and metabolic disorders such as uraemia.

Excessive startle reflexes can be part of hyperekplexia, a hereditary mainly autosomal dominant disorder (54, 55). Patients with hyperekplexia also suffer from stiffness induced by the startle reflexes, and generalized stiffness in the neonatal period (56, 57). Clinically, an excessive head retraction reflex can be elicited (see Video 25.5). Hyperekplexia is a hereditary disorder with mutations in different parts of the inhibitory glycine receptor (GlyR) (21). The alpha-1 subunit of the glycine receptor (GLRA1) is the main gene for hyperekplexia. Dominant, recessive, and compound heterozygote mutations are identified. This gene is affected in about 80% of all hyperekplexia pedigrees, and can be regarded as the most

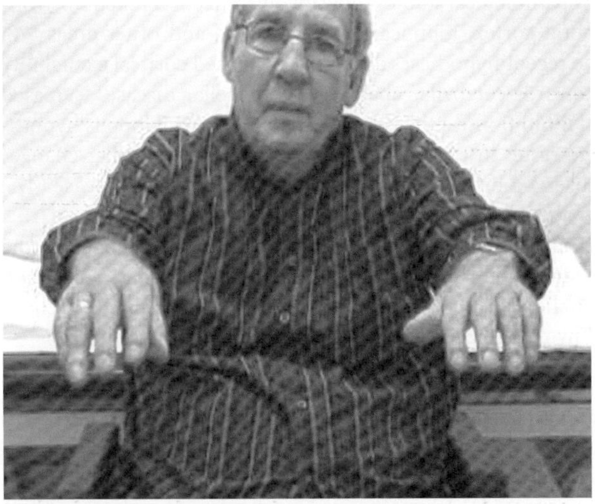

Video 25.4 The video shows a patient with post-anoxic encephalopathy (Lance–Adams syndrome) several years after the anoxic incident. Stretching of the arms shows an irregular jerky tremor. The patient's main problem is standing and walking. During standing between two subjects the postural lapses due to the negative myoclonus can be seen.

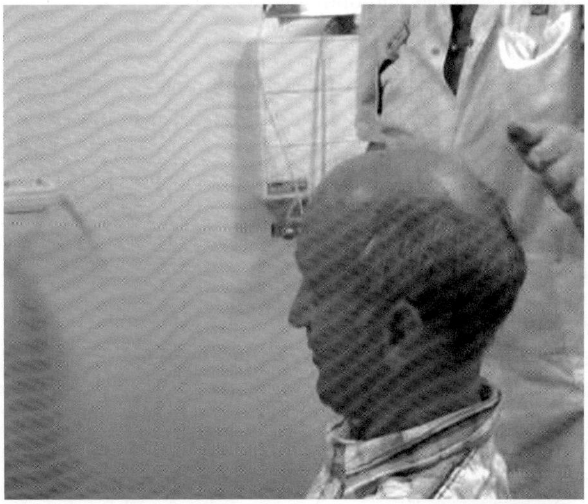

Video 25.5 The video shows a patient with hyperekplexia (mutation in the *GLRA1* gene). An excessive head retraction reflex is illustrated. *Mov Disord*. 2012 May;27(6):795-6. doi: 10.1002/mds.24917. Epub 2012 Jan 30. A new hyperekplexia family with a recessive frameshift mutation in the GLRA1 gene. Zoons E, Ginjaar IB, Bouma PA, Carpay JA, Tijssen MA.

important contributor to autosomal dominant hereditary hyperekplexia. The second most important gene, which accounts for hyperekplexia in about 20% of cases, is the GlyT2 (SCL6A5) encoding the presynaptic sodium- and chloride-dependent glycine transporter 2 (58). The mode of inheritance is recessive with compound heterozygosity in the majority of cases. Genetic heterogeneity has been confirmed in very rare sporadic cases of hyperekplexia with mutations affecting other postsynaptic glycinergic proteins, including the GlyR subunit (*GLRB*), gephyrin (*GPHN*), and RhoGEF collybistin (*ARHGEF9*). Other than hereditary hyperekplexia, excessive startle reflexes can also be symptomatic, usually due to lesions in the brainstem (21).

Orthostatic myoclonus is an irregular jerking of the legs induced or increased by an upright posture. Clinically, a slowly progressive unsteadiness of stance and gait is seen. EMG shows non-rhythmic short burst durations (20–100 ms) (59, 60). This type of myoclonus is not classified as yet, but is most likely of subcortical origin. It may occur in isolation, but is often associated with an underlying neurodegenerative disorder, particularly Parkinson's disease (59, 60). Orthostatic myoclonus has also been described in one family suffering from action-induced multifocal dystonia and generalized myoclonus. The most troublesome feature of their disorder was an orthostatic myoclonus in the lower limbs (61).

Spinal

Segmental myoclonus

Spinal segmental myoclonus is the result of spinal systems becoming hyperexcitable due to a spinal cord lesion such as a tumour, syringomyelia, myelitis, or ischaemia.

Propriospinal myoclonus

Occasionally, lesions in the spinal cord have been reported, but propriospinal myoclonus (PSM) is usually idiopathic (62). In idiopathic PSM a psychogenic origin might be considered. Recently, a *Bereitschaftspotential* was shown in 15 of 20 patients diagnosed with idiopathic spinal myoclonus (22). In another study, axial jerking closely resembling PSM had a psychogenic origin in 34 out of 35 patients (63). Further prospective studies of PSM are required (for more details see 'Pathophysiology').

Peripheral

Hemifacial spasm is the most frequent example of peripheral myoclonus (64). Jerks and tonic contractions occur in muscles innervated by the ipsilateral facial nerve. In two-thirds of 135 patients in one series, it was caused by vascular compression of the facial nerve at the exit zone (65). Other very rare examples include myoclonus after lesions of the brachial plexus and spinal root, and after amputation ('jumping stump').

Psychogenic myoclonus

An important cause of myoclonus not included in the current classifications is *psychogenic myoclonus*. Psychogenic myoclonus comprises around 15% of psychogenic movement disorders (66, 67). In a study of 212 patients with myoclonus, psychogenic myoclonus was diagnosed in 8.5% (68). The distribution of segmental myoclonus is most frequent, but generalized and focal presentations also occur. The myoclonus is seen at rest in all patients and increases with movement in most (68). There are some general features common to all functional movement disorders, such as an abrupt onset, fast progression, distractibility, and variability (66). Psychiatric co-morbidity, such as depression, anxiety, and panic disorders, occurs in 50–60% (68). Electrophysiological testing can be helpful in such cases. EMG registration shows variable and inconsistent muscle activity patterns. A premovement potential (*Bereitschaftspotential*) on the averaged EEG activity over several jerks (back-averaging) makes diagnosis of functional jerks likely, although absence of this potential does not exclude a psychogenic origin (67, 69, 70).

Pathophysiology

Cortical myoclonus

Cortical myoclonus is pathophysiologically related to epilepsy. It was first described by Ginker and colleagues (71) with EEG trains of spike and wave discharges correlating with myoclonus in familial myoclonus epilepsy. Shibasaki and Kuroiwa (72) were the first to report back-averaging of EEG time-locked to the myoclonic jerks on the EMG (jerk-locked back-averaging), showing contralateral cortical discharges preceding myoclonus by intervals consistent with conduction in corticospinal pathways (i.e. 15–25 ms when recorded from the upper limb, and 40 ms from the lower limb). Frequent myoclonic jerks do not allow back-averaging. Alternatively, coherence analysis can reveal the correlation between cortical and muscle activity and between muscles (73). In cortical myoclonus an exaggerated corticomuscular and intermuscular coherence in the alpha and beta bands can be found with a phase difference compatible with a cortical drive (9, 74, 75). Magnetoencephalography (MEG) studies suggest a generator in the primary motor cortex (76).

An EMG–fMRI study in FCMTE patients linked cortical myoclonus to parietal (sensory area) brain activation (77). This is in concordance with changes in sensory input that are likely to play an important role in the generation of the jerks. This is supported by clinical stimulus sensitivity and the electrophysiological signs of cortical hyperexcitability, as illustrated by a gSSEP and the presence of a C-reflex (see Fig. 25.1). With SSEP recordings the P25/P30 and N35 peak amplitudes are enlarged (77). The C-reflex response can be seen in the ipsilateral thenar muscle with a latency of around 45 ms (17).

Neuropathological studies show involvement of cerebellum, frontotemporal cortex, hippocampus, thalamus, and other areas (78, 79). The recent hypotheses about the increased cortical excitability point towards cerebellar changes. In cerebellar disease decreased cortical inhibition via the cerebellothalamocortical loop is hypothesized to result in cortical myoclonus. Primary cerebellar changes were observed by Hunt (80), in patients with coeliac disease (47), and in patients with FCMTE (79).

Cortical increased excitability due to intrinsic changes in the cortex cannot be ruled out. In the absence of structural changes, functional cortical changes may exist, for instance due to a channelopathy recognized in the inherited epilepsy syndromes.

Asterixis

Patients with cortical myoclonus usually manifest both positive and negative myoclonus (81). In postanoxic myoclonus, positive myoclonus correlated with an EEG spike, and negative myoclonus with an EEG slow wave (4). A hypothesized mechanism of cortical negative myoclonus is that stimulation of areas in the primary sensorimotor cortex produces a silent period in the corresponding muscle when electrically stimulated (82). The most frequent form is asterixis, or flapping tremor, with EMG registration highlighting brief periods

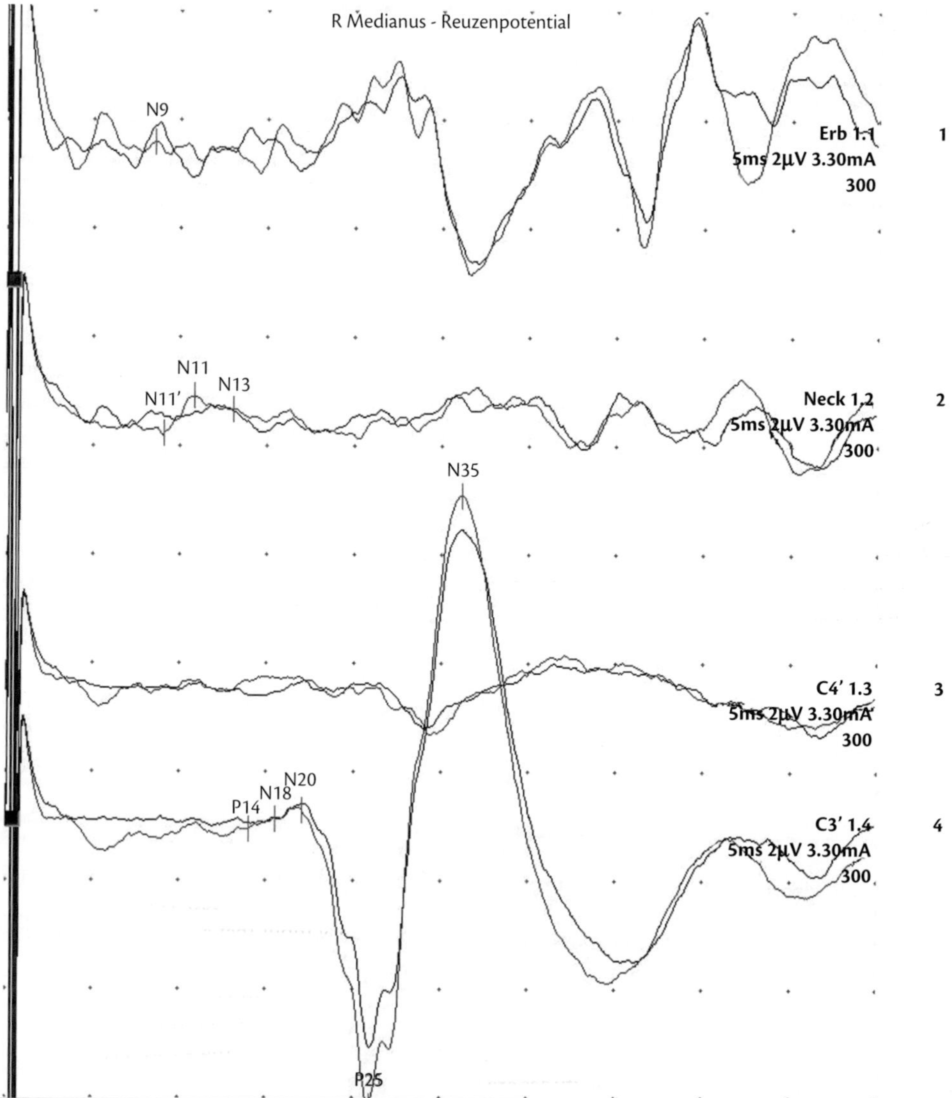

Run	N9 ms	N11 ms	N13 ms	P14 ms	N18 ms	N20 ms	P25 ms	N35 ms	onset R ms	top-top R ms	P14-N20 μV	N20-P25 μV	P25-N35 μV
1.1 Erb	8.6												
1.2 Nek		10.9	13.1										
1.3 C4'													
1.4 C3'				14.0	15.6	17.1	21.0	26.2	6.5	4.0	0.34	5.5	11.3

Fig. 25.1 A giant somatosensory evoked potential (gSSEP) is seen over C3 (trace 4) after stimulation of the right median nerve. Traces 1–3 show the right-sided response at Erb's point, the neck muscles, and C4.

(50–200 ms) of loss of EMG activity against gravity. Another form of negative myoclonus gives longer-lasting EMG silences (200–500 ms) in the axial and proximal lower limb muscles. Patients may lose postural stability during this type of negative myoclonus.

Subcortical myoclonus

Myoclonus–dystonia patients have variable but mainly short EMG bursts (25–750 ms) (18, 33), that are believed to originate from the basal ganglia. Local field potential recordings from the globus pallidus interna (GPi) in MD patients showed significant coherence between dystonic muscle activity and GPi (83). Reduced striatal D2 receptor binding was also detected in MD (84). Electrophysiological studies including (EMG-)EEG, SSEP, and transcranial magnetic stimulation (TMS) reveal no changes in cortical excitability (85, 86). Cortical functional changes have been described in a TMS study, showing polyphasic MEPs possibly reflecting central neuronal membrane instability. A functional MRI study revealed disorganized sensorimotor integration consistent with other types of dystonia (63, 85, 87). These cortical functional changes may be secondary to basal ganglia pathology. It is of interest that recent studies point towards the cerebellum in the pathophysiology of MD. Impaired saccadic adaptation in MD is compatible with cerebellar dysfunction (88). Even more convincingly, a major brain-specific *SGCE* isoform is differentially expressed in the human brain with a notably high expression in the cerebellum, namely in the Purkinje cells and neurons of the dentate nucleus (89). These findings illustrate that dysfunction of the cerebellum is involved in the pathogenesis of both cortical and subcortical myoclonus.

Brainstem reticular reflex myoclonus is characterized by abnormal activity starting in the brainstem and subsequently spreading in both rostral and caudal directions, producing generalized jerks due to the bilateral pathways involved. In reticular reflex myoclonus the pattern of spread resembles the startle reflex, but in contrast with reticular myoclonus in hyperekplexia the EMG responses in the intrinsic hand and foot muscles are relatively delayed (90). Furthermore, the latencies of muscle activity after an auditory stimulus in reticular reflex myoclonus are very short, compatible with the pyramidal tract, while startle reflex latencies are longer, travelling through slower corticospinal tracts (54, 90). The jerks in reticular reflex myoclonus are thought to originate from the reticular formation. The brainstem motor systems are closely related to subcortical reflex centres, possibly explaining the stimulus sensitivity (12, 13, 20).

Spinal myoclonus

Spinal myoclonus is the result of abnormal discharges generated in the spinal cord.

In *segmental myoclonus* the jerks are usually rhythmic with a frequency varying from 1 to 200 per minute. The duration of the EMG bursts can be up to 1000 ms. With nerve stimulation EMG discharges are found with different latencies, possibly reflecting involvement of polysynaptic pathways.

Propriospinal myoclonus (PSM) is characterized by both spontaneous and stimulus-sensitive jerks of the trunk and abdominal muscles, often induced by lying down (23, 24). PSM is presumed to originate from a spinal generator that elicits activity spreading up and down the spinal cord via intrinsic propriospinal pathways (24). Electrophysiological features include a fixed pattern of muscle activation, slow spinal cord conduction velocity (5–15 m/s), EMG burst duration of less than 1000 ms, and synchronous activation of agonist and antagonist muscles, without involvement of facial muscles (91). Diffusion tensor imaging showed associated microstructural abnormalities of the spinal cord in one study (92).

Clinical features

Classifying myoclonus according to clinical signs enables a clear description to be given of the characteristics of myoclonus in individual patients and to further categorize patients in an anatomical classification (Table 25.3). Different aspects are useful to determine the type of myoclonus.

The distribution of myoclonus can be focal, segmental, axial, or generalized (11). The temporal pattern of myoclonus is usually arrhythmic, but can also be rhythmic (as in segmental myoclonus) or oscillatory (11). Synchronized jerks (e.g. brainstem myoclonus) can be differentiated from asynchronous jerks (11). The relation to motor activity can be classified as myoclonus at rest or during voluntary activity, such as action or intention. Action myoclonus is frequently seen in patients with cortical myoclonus. Stimulus sensitivity means that the myoclonus can be triggered by sudden and unexpected tactile, visual, or auditory stimuli (as in cortical or brainstem myoclonus). Finally, myoclonus can present as muscular contractions (positive myoclonus) or as an interruption of a muscle contraction (negative myoclonus). Two forms have been described (6): asterixis or flapping tremor, and negative myoclonus in the axial and proximal lower limb muscles, resulting in patients losing their balance.

Diagnosis

The diagnostic procedure in patients with myoclonus starts with history, physical examination, and determination of the clinical syndrome classification (20). History taking includes mode of myoclonus, onset, presence of other neurological problems, history of

Table 25.3 The clinical and anatomical classification of myoclonus

	Anatomical classification				
	Cortical	Subcortical		Spinal	
		MD	BM	SM	PM
Clinical presentation					
Spontaneous	+	+	–	+	+
During activity	↑	↑	↑	+	–
Stimulus sensitivity	+	–	+	–	+
Distribution					
Focal	(multi)+	–	–	+/–	–
Segmental	–	–	–	+	–
Generalized	+	+/–	+	–	+
Synchronous	–	–	+	–	+
Temporal pattern					
Irregular	+	+	+	+/–	+
Rhythmic	+/–*	–	–	–	–
Negative myoclonus	+	–	–	–	–

The table correlates the clinical and anatomical classification of myoclonus.

+, likely to be a feature; +/–, can be a feature; –, not usually a feature; ↑, increase; MD, myoclonus dystonia; BM, brainstem myoclonus; SM, segmental myoclonus; PM, propriospinal myoclonus.

*Cortical tremor can clinically resemble a tremor (see text).

seizures, current and past drug or toxin exposure, past or current medical problems, and family history. During physical examination the features described under clinical diagnosis (Table 25.3) are determined. The combination of history and physical examination leads to the anatomical classification of myoclonus.

If the patient suffers from an acute or subacute form and the aetiological category can be determined with a relatively high degree of diagnostic certainty, basic and focused additional testing can subsequently be performed.

Basic ancillary testing includes electrolytes, glucose, renal and hepatic function tests, thyroid function, and, if history suggests it, a drug and toxin screen (20). An EEG is useful to identify both ictal and interictal patterns. Specific EEG spike patterns can point towards specific diagnosis. Loss of a normal EEG background rhythm and abnormal slow waves suggest diffuse encephalopathy. Imaging of the brain or spinal cord can be performed if focal lesions or metabolic disorders are suspected.

If the myoclonus is more chronic or if the anatomical type of myoclonus is unclear, clinical neurophysiology testing can be performed to confirm the anatomical classification. This includes, based on the history and physical examination, an EMG to determine the duration of the burst, an EEG, an EEG with back-averaging or coherence analysis, an SSEP, or a C-reflex.

Advanced testing for rare and specific diagnoses should be guided by the most prominent clinical features, age at onset, and the course of the myoclonic disorder (see 'Aetiology and genetics', p.258, and Table 25.1). Focused testing may comprise genetic testing, specific metabolic screening, lumbar puncture, and antibodies, including paraneoplastic antibodies (20).

Management

Therapy should first focus on cure of the underlying disorder, such as removal of a medication or toxin or reversal of an acquired abnormal metabolic state (93). Unfortunately, this approach is frequently impossible and symptomatic treatment is required. The treatment strategies for myoclonus are based on the anatomical classification. In general, treatment is often difficult, and several drug trials are required to find the best therapy for an individual patient. Drugs are usually partially beneficial and, because of the frequent side effects, initial low dosages with slow increase are advised.

Cortical myoclonus

The treatment for cortical myoclonus is based on treatment strategies for myoclonic epilepsy (31, 94, 95). Treatment strategies specific for cortical myoclonus are based on small observational studies and expert opinion as little evidence is available. Some evidence can be found for piracetam (96), a well-tolerated drug, but the daily dose is high (up to 24 g/day). Levetiracetam (2000–3000 mg/day), an analogue of piracetam, also has few side effects. The effect on epileptic myoclonus is positive, and the evidence in non-epileptic cortical myoclonus is based on case series. Levetiracetam is considered as the first choice of treatment for cortical myoclonus (see (Video 25.1). Based on a long history of clinical experience, but without evidence in the literature, valproic acid and clonazepam are also good therapeutic options. Clonazepam must be given in high doses in most cases (up to 14 mg/day), resulting in side effects such as drowsiness and sedation. In patients with post-hypoxic cortical myoclonus, valproic acid and clonazepam are equally effective and a combination may be best (93). In general, polytherapy is more effective than monotherapy in cortical myoclonus (93).

Subcortical myoclonus

Treatment options for different forms of subcortical myoclonus are largely based on small observational studies and case reports. Standard antiepileptic medication is usually not effective in subcortical myoclonus. In MD, L-5-HTP (a serotonin precursor) was effective in a few patients at the maximum dosage, but its use is often limited by side effects (14). Other small studies showed an effect of sodium oxybate, levodopa, or zolpidem on myoclonus. Clonazepam, piracetam, levetiracetam, and trihexyphenidyl are also prescribed for MD, but their effect is limited (93). In severe cases deep brain stimulation of the GPi can be considered, with a good effect reported for motor symptoms (see (Video 25.3). In brainstem myoclonus clonazepam is usually an effective drug. Furthermore, L-5-HTP may be effective, but is frequently not well tolerated. In hyperekplexia a double-blind placebo-controlled study has shown a favourable effect of clonazepam on the magnitude of motor startle reflexes and stiffness (97). Orthostatic myoclonus treatment options include clonazepam and gabapentin.

Spinal myoclonus

In spinal segmental myoclonus it is essential to treat the underlying cause first, before turning to symptomatic therapy. Clonazepam is considered the drug of choice for segmental myoclonus, although the evidence is very limited. Alternatively, carbamazepine, tetrabenazine, and botulinum toxin may also be beneficial. For propriospinal myoclonus, clonazepam is considered the drug of choice mainly based on clinical experience, while zonisamide may be an alternative (93).

Peripheral myoclonus

Botulinum toxin is the therapy of choice for hemifacial spasm, based on a randomized double-blind controlled trial in 11 patients (98) and on large observational studies with a good to excellent effect of botulinum toxin in most cases (93). Microsurgical vascular decompression is an alternative therapy, but the risk of complications is higher. Botulinum toxin may also be effective in other types of peripheral myoclonus.

Key advances

The major breakthroughs in myoclonus over the last 10 years have come from genetics. New genetic causes of myoclonus have been identified, and the molecular basis of several conditions has been discovered (45). Genetic counselling is now available for some patients. Finding new genes enables us to define and expand the phenotype of clinical syndromes. New genes for several disorders with cortical myoclonus include Unverricht–Lundborg disease and myoclonic epilepsy with ragged red fibres (45).

For subcortical myoclonus the *SGCE* gene was discovered in MD. Genetic testing showed that 30% of patients with the MD phenotype showed a mutation or deletion in the gene. A stricter definition of the phenotype increased this to 50% (35). A second gene *GLYT2* has been discovered for hyperekplexia (58). In about 20% of cases this gene shows a recessive or compound heterozygous mutation and has proved to be the main gene in sporadic cases of hyperekplexia.

Electrophysiological studies have always been of great value in defining the type and studying pathophysiological mechanisms in myoclonus. The major breakthroughs, such as EEG–EMG back-averaging and SSEP giant potentials for cortical myoclonus, were performed more than 10 years ago. More recent EMG, TMS, local field potential registrations after DBS, and MEG studies in both cortical and subcortical myoclonus have increased our understanding of the pathophysiology of myoclonus.

Recent electrophysiological and clinical studies in propriospinal myoclonus have shown that PSM has a psychogenic origin in many patients, shedding new light on this patient group (22, 99).

From pathological studies it is increasingly apparent that diseases of the cerebellum are particularly important in the genesis of myoclonus, although the precise mechanisms and origin of myoclonus in many situations remains uncertain. Cerebellar pathology has been detected in patients with cortical reflex myoclonus, such as FCMTE (100) and coeliac disease (47). However, MD patients with subcortical myoclonus also show alterations in the cerebellum (89), suggesting a common pathway in the mechanisms generating myoclonic jerks.

Future developments

The progress likely to be made in understanding and treating myoclonus in the next few years will come from further discovery of genetic mutations and from functional studies improving our understanding of neural networks. Effective treatment of myoclonus is still limited, and the challenge to develop more therapeutic options specifically designed for myoclonus rather than those intended for other disorders lies ahead.

Genetic information will yield more specific information with regard to the neurochemical and molecular pathophysiology of myoclonus which, in turn, will allow development of more specific treatments. Functional studies including electrophysiological and imaging studies, such as MEG, fMRI, and structural imaging studies, will improve our understanding of myoclonus. In particular, multimodality studies, combining concurrent spatial (imaging) and temporal (electrophysiology) information in patients, will delineate the neuronal networks that malfunction to produce myoclonus and this will also lead to identification of better therapeutic targets.

Current practice is mainly based on small observational studies and expert opinion. Double-blind randomized controlled trials in large homogeneous patient groups using a strict classification strategy are required to develop guidelines for treating myoclonus. Genetic and functional knowledge will also enable us to improve phenotyping and therefore to define homogenous groups of patients to study newly developed medical treatments. Not only new medications, but also the treatment options already used, should be tested in double-blinded randomized controlled studies. As most of the myoclonic disorders are rare, collaborative investigator groups will be required to systematically assess old and new drugs for the treatment of myoclonus.

Conclusion

Myoclonus is a relatively frequent movement disorder with a wide variety of causes. Based on clinical findings and electrophysiological testing, an anatomical classification can be made. Subsequent focused tests, guided by additional clinical features, enable an aetiological diagnosis to be made. In patients with progressive myoclonus epilepsies, it is not always possible to make a definite diagnosis. The finding of new genes in the future will improve this. Treatment options are also based on the anatomical classification of myoclonus. Polytherapy is often required, but the effects are still frequently disappointing. Current practice is mainly based on small observational studies and expert opinion. Double-blind randomized controlled trials in large homogeneous patient groups using a strict classification strategy are required to develop guidelines for treating myoclonus.

Key points

- Myoclonic jerks regularly occur in patients in combination with other movement disorders.
- Classification of the anatomical origin of myoclonus is based on clinical and electrophysiological characteristics.
- The aetiology of myoclonus is diverse and in 70% of cases is symptomatic.
- Always rule out drug-induced myoclonus.
- A diagnosis of psychogenic myoclonus should be considered ↓↔ 'idiopathic' propriospinal myoclonus.
- Treatment of cortical myoclonus is usually with polytherapy.

References

1. Fahn S, Marsden CD, Van Woert MH. Definition and classification of myoclonus. *Adv Neurol* 1986; 43: 1–5.
2. Rubboli G, Tassinari CA. Negative myoclonus: an overview of its clinical features, pathophysiological mechanisms, and management. *Neurophysiol Clin* 2006; 36: 337–43.
3. Friedreich N. Paramyoclonus multiplex. Neuropathologische Beobachtungen. *Arch Path Anat (Virchow Arch)* 1881; 86: 421–34.
4. Lance JW, Adams RD. The syndrome of intention or action myoclonus as a sequel to hypoxic encephalopathy. *Brain* 1963 Mar; 86: 111–36.
5. Marsden CD, Hallet M, Fahn S. The nosology and pathophysiology of myoclonus. In: Marsden CD, Fahn S (eds) *Movement disorders*, pp. 196–248. London: Butterworths, 1982.
6. Faught E. Clinical presentations and phenomenology of myoclonus. *Epilepsia* 2003; 44 (Suppl 11): 7–12.
7. Jankovic J. Treatment of hyperkinetic movement disorders. *Lancet Neurol* 2009; 8: 844–56.
8. Agarwal P, Frucht SJ. Myoclonus. *Curr Opin Neurol* 2003; 16: 515–21.
9. van Rootselaar AF, Maurits NM, Koelman JH, et al. Coherence analysis differentiates between cortical myoclonic tremor and essential tremor. *Mov Disord* 2006; 21: 215–22.
10. Obeso JA, Narbona J. Post-traumatic tremor and myoclonic jerking. *J Neurol Neurosurg Psychiatry* 1983; 46: 788.
11. Fahn S. Overview, history and classification of myoclonus. In: Fahn S, Frucht SJ, Hallet M, Truong DD (eds) *Myoclonus and paroxysmal dyskinesias*, pp. 13–17. Philadelphia, PA: Lippincott–Williams & Wilkins, 2002.
12. Caviness JN. Pathophysiology and treatment of myoclonus. *Neurol Clin* 2009; 27: 757–77, vii.
13. Tijssen MAJ, Tijssen CC. Myoclonus. In: Wolters ECh, van Laar T, Berendse HW (eds) *Parkinsonism and related disorders*, pp. 381–93. Amsterdam: VU University Press, 2007.
14. Obeso JA. Therapy of myoclonus. *Clin Neurosci* 1995; 3: 253–7.
15. Shibasaki H, Hallett M. Electrophysiological studies of myoclonus. *Muscle Nerve* 2005 Feb; 31(2): 157–74.

16. Shibasaki H, Yamashita Y, Kuroiwa Y. Electroencephalographic studies myoclonus. *Brain* 1978; 101: 447–60.
17. Shibasaki H, Yamashita Y, Neshige R, Tobimatsu S, Fukui R. Pathogenesis of giant somatosensory evoked potentials in progressive myoclonic epilepsy. *Brain* 1985; 108: 225–40.
18. Roze E, Apartis E, Clot F, et al. Myoclonus–dystonia: clinical and electrophysiologic pattern related to SGCE mutations. *Neurology* 2008; 70: 1010–16.
19. Kinugawa K, Vidailhet M, Clot F, Apartis E, Grabli D, Roze E. Myoclonus-dystonia: an update. *Mov Disord* 2009; 24: 479–89.
20. Caviness JN, Brown P. Myoclonus: current concepts and recent advances. *Lancet Neurol* 2004; 3: 598–607.
21. Bakker MJ, van Dijk JG, van den Maagdenberg AM, Tijssen MA. Startle syndromes. *Lancet Neurol* 2006; 5: 513–24.
22. Esposito M, Edwards MJ, Bhatia KP, Brown P, Cordivari C. Idiopathic spinal myoclonus: a clinical and neurophysiological assessment of a movement disorder of uncertain origin. *Mov Disord* 2009; 24: 2344–9.
23. Brown P, Thompson PD, Rothwell JC, Day BL, Marsden CD. Axial myoclonus of propriospinal origin. *Brain* 1991; 114: 197–214.
24. Brown P, Rothwell JC, Thompson PD, Marsden CD. Propriospinal myoclonus: evidence for spinal 'pattern' generators in humans. *Mov Disord* 1994; 9: 571–6.
25. Brown P, Rothwell JC, Thompson PD, Marsden CD. Propriospinal myoclonus: evidence for spinal 'pattern' generators in humans. *Mov Disord* 1994; 9: 571–6.
26. Jankovic J. Peripherally induced movement disorders. *Neurol Clin* 2009; 27: 821–32, vii.
27. Caviness JN, Alving LI, Maraganore DM, Black RA, McDonnell SK, Rocca WA. The incidence and prevalence of myoclonus in Olmsted County, Minnesota. *Mayo Clin Proc* 1999; 74: 565–9.
28. Yoon JH, Lee PH, Yong SW, Park HY, Lim TS, Choi JY. Movement disorders at a university hospital emergency room. An analysis of clinical pattern and etiology. *J Neurol* 2008; 255: 745–9.
29. Lang AE. Essential myoclonus and myoclonic dystonia. *Mov Disord* 1997; 12: 127.
30. Quinn NP. Essential myoclonus and myoclonic dystonia. *Mov Disord* 1996; 11: 119–24.
31. Andrade DM, Hamani C, Minassian BA. Treatment options for epileptic myoclonus and epilepsy syndromes associated with myoclonus. *Expert Opin Pharmacother* 2009; 10: 1549–60.
32. Caviness JN, Alving LI, Maraganore DM, Black RA, McDonnell SK, Rocca WA. The incidence and prevalence of myoclonus in Olmsted County, Minnesota. *Mayo Clin Proc* 1999; 74: 565–9.
33. Foncke EM, Cath D, Zwinderman K, Smit J, Schmand B, Tijssen M. Is psychopathology part of the phenotypic spectrum of myoclonus-dystonia?: a study of a large Dutch M-D family. *Cogn Behav Neurol* 2009; 22: 127–33.
34. Asmus F, Salih F, Hjermind LE, et al. Myoclonus–dystonia due to genomic deletions in the epsilon-sarcoglycan gene. *Ann Neurol* 2005; 58: 792–7.
35. Ritz K, Gerrits MC, Foncke EM, et al. Myoclonus–dystonia: clinical and genetic evaluation of a large cohort. *J Neurol Neurosurg Psychiatry* 2009; 80: 653–8.
36. Piras G, El KA, Kozlov S, et al. Zac1 (Lot1), a potential tumor suppressor gene, and the gene for epsilon-sarcoglycan are maternally imprinted genes: identification by a subtractive screen of novel uniparental fibroblast lines. *Mol Cell Biol* 2000; 20: 3308–15.
37. Grimes DA, Han F, Lang AE, George-Hyssop P, Racacho L, Bulman DE. A novel locus for inherited myoclonus–dystonia on 18p11. *Neurology* 2002; 59: 1183–6.
38. Han F, Racacho L, Lang AE, Bulman DE, Grimes DA. Refinement of the DYT15 locus in myoclonus dystonia. *Mov Disord* 2007; 22: 888–92.
39. Ozawa E, Mizuno Y, Hagiwara Y, Sasaoka T, Yoshida M. Molecular and cell biology of the sarcoglycan complex. *Muscle Nerve* 2005; 32: 563–76.
40. Hjermind LE, Vissing J, Asmus F, et al. No muscle involvement in myoclonus-dystonia caused by epsilon-sarcoglycan gene mutations. *Eur J Neurol* 2008; 15: 525–9.
41. van Rootselaar AF, van Schaik IN, van den Maagdenberg AM, Koelman JH, Callenbach PM, Tijssen MA. Familial cortical myoclonic tremor with epilepsy: a single syndromic classification for a group of pedigrees bearing common features. *Mov Disord* 2005; 20: 665–73.
42. Depienne C, Magnin E, Bouteiller D, et al. Familial cortical myoclonic tremor with epilepsy: the third locus (FCMTE3) maps to 5p. *Neurology* 2010; 74: 2000–3.
43. Obeso JA. Classification,clinical features, and treatment of myoclonus. In: Watts RL, Koller WC (eds) *Movement disorders: neurologic principles and practice*, pp. 532–50. New York: McGraw-Hil, 1997.
44. Shahwan A, Farrell M, Delanty N. Progressive myoclonic epilepsies: a review of genetic and therapeutic aspects. *Lancet Neurol* 2005; 4: 239–48.
45. Shibasaki H, Thompson PD. Milestones in myoclonus. *Mov Disord* 2011; 26: 1142–8.
46. Bhatia KP, Brown P, Gregory R, et al. Progressive myoclonic ataxia associated with coeliac disease. The myoclonus is of cortical origin, but the pathology is in the cerebellum. *Brain* 1995; 118: 1087–93.
47. Tijssen MA, Thom M, Ellison DW, et al. Cortical myoclonus and cerebellar pathology. *Neurology* 2000; 54: 1350–6.
48. Badhwar A, Berkovic SF, Dowling JP, et al. Action myoclonus–renal failure syndrome: characterization of a unique cerebro-renal disorder. *Brain* 2004; 127: 2173–82.
49. Berkovic SF, Dibbens LM, Oshlack A, et al. Array-based gene discovery with three unrelated subjects shows SCARB2/LIMP-2 deficiency causes myoclonus epilepsy and glomerulosclerosis. *Am J Hum Genet* 2008; 82: 673–84.
50. van GJ, Giunti P, van de Warrenburg BP. Movement disorders in spinocerebellar ataxias. *Mov Disord* 2011; 26: 792–800.
51. Foncke EM, Beukers RJ, Tijssen CC, Koelman JH, Tijssen MA. Myoclonus-dystonia and spinocerebellar ataxia type 14 presenting with similar phenotypes: trunk tremor, myoclonus, and dystonia. *Parkinsonism Relat Disord* 2010; 16: 288–9.
52. Gordon MF. Toxin and drug-induced myoclonus. In: Fahn S, Frucht SJ, Truong DD, Hallett M (eds). *Myoclonus and paroxysmal dyskinesias*, pp. 49–76. Philadelphia, PA: Lippincott–Williams & Wilkins, 2002.
53. Frucht S, Fahn S. The clinical spectrum of posthypoxic myoclonus. *Mov Disord* 2000; 15 (Suppl 1): 2–7.
54. Tijssen MA, Voorkamp LM, Padberg GW, van Dijk JG. Startle responses in hereditary hyperekplexia. *Arch Neurol* 1997; 54: 388–93.
55. Brown P, Rothwell JC, Thompson PD, Britton TC, Day BL, Marsden CD. The hyperekplexias and their relationship to the normal startle reflex. *Brain* 1991; 114: 1903–28.
56. Suhren O, Bruyn GW, Tuynman A. Hyperekplexia, a hereditary startle syndrome. *J Neurol Sci* 1966; 3: 577–605.
57. Tijssen MA, Shiang R, van Deutekom J, et al. Molecular genetic reevaluation of the Dutch hyperekplexia family. *Arch Neurol* 1995; 52: 578–82.
58. Rees MI, Harvey K, Pearce BR, et al. Mutations in the gene encoding GlyT2 (SLC6A5) define a presynaptic component of human startle disease. *Nat Genet* 2006; 38: 801–6.
59. Glass GA, Ahlskog JE, Matsumoto JY. Orthostatic myoclonus: a contributor to gait decline in selected elderly. *Neurology* 2007; 68: 1826–30.
60. Leu-Semenescu S, Roze E, Vidailhet M, et al. Myoclonus or tremor in orthostatism: an under-recognized cause of unsteadiness in Parkinson's disease. *Mov Disord* 2007; 22: 2063–9.
61. Groen J, van Rootselaar AF, van der Salm SM, Bloem BR, Tijssen M. A new familial syndrome with dystonia and lower limb action myoclonus. *Mov Disord* 2011; 26: 896–900.
62. Roze E, Bounolleau P, Ducreux D, et al. Propriospinal myoclonus revisited: clinical, neurophysiologic, and neuroradiologic findings. *Neurology* 2009; 72: 1301–9.

63. van der Salm SM, van Rootselaar AF, Foncke EM, et al. Normal cortical excitability in myoclonus–dystonia—a TMS study. *Exp Neurol* 2009; 216: 300–5.
64. Nilsen B, Le KD, Dietrichs E. Prevalence of hemifacial spasm in Oslo, Norway. *Neurology* 2004; 63: 1532–3.
65. Wang A, Jankovic J. Hemifacial spasm: clinical findings and treatment. *Muscle Nerve* 1998; 21: 1740–7.
66. Hinson VK, Haren WB. Psychogenic movement disorders. *Lancet Neurol* 2006; 5: 695–700.
67. Thomas M, Jankovic J. Psychogenic movement disorders: diagnosis and management. *CNS Drugs* 2004; 18: 437–52.
68. Monday K, Jankovic J. Psychogenic myoclonus. *Neurology* 1993; 43: 349–52.
69. Terada K, Ikeda A, Van Ness PC, et al. Presence of Bereitschaftspotential preceding psychogenic myoclonus: clinical application of jerk-locked back averaging. *J Neurol Neurosurg Psychiatry* 1995; 58: 745–7.
70. Shibasaki H, Hallett M. What is the Bereitschaftspotential? *Clin Neurophysiol* 2006; 117: 2341–56.
71. Ginker RR, SH, Stein SI. Myoclonic epilepsy. *Arch Neurol Psychiatry* 40; 1938: 968–80.
72. Shibasaki H, Kuroiwa Y. Electroencephalographic correlates of myoclonus. *Electroencephalogr Clin Neurophysiol* 1975; 39: 455–63.
73. Grosse P, Cassidy MJ, Brown P. EEG-EMG, MEG-EMG and EMG-EMG frequency analysis: physiological principles and clinical applications. *Clin Neurophysiol* 2002; 113: 1523–31.
74. Brown P, Farmer SF, Halliday DM, Marsden J, Rosenberg JR. Coherent cortical and muscle discharge in cortical myoclonus. *Brain* 1999; 122: 461–72.
75. Grosse P, Guerrini R, Parmeggiani L, Bonanni P, Pogosyan A, Brown P. Abnormal corticomuscular and intermuscular coupling in high-frequency rhythmic myoclonus. *Brain* 2003; 126: 326–42.
76. Mima T, Nagamine T, Ikeda A, Yazawa S, Kimura J, Shibasaki H. Pathogenesis of cortical myoclonus studied by magnetoencephalography. *Ann Neurol*; 43: 598–607.
77. van Rootselaar AF, Maurits NM, Renken R, et al. Simultaneous EMG-functional MRI recordings can directly relate hyperkinetic movements to brain activity. *Hum Brain Mapp* 2008; 29: 1430–41.
78. Cohen NR, Hammans SR, Macpherson J, Nicoll JA. New neuropathological findings in Unverricht–Lundborg disease: neuronal intranuclear and cytoplasmic inclusions. *Acta Neuropathol* 2011; 121(3): 241–7.
79. van Rootselaar AF, van der Salm SM, Bour LJ, et al. Decreased cortical inhibition and yet cerebellar pathology in 'familial cortical myoclonic tremor with epilepsy'. *Mov Disord* 2007; 22: 2378–85.
80. Hunt JR. Dyssynergia cerebellaris myoclonica, primary atrophy of the dentate system. *Brain* 1921; 44: 490–538.
81. Shibasaki H. Pathophysiology of negative myoclonus and asterixis. *Adv Neurol* 1995; 67: 199–209.
82. Ikeda A, Ohara S, Matsumoto R, Kunieda T, Nagamine T, Miyamoto S, et al. Role of primary sensorimotor cortices in generating inhibitory motor response in humans. *Brain* 2000; 123: 1710–21.
83. Foncke EM, Bour LJ, Speelman JD, Koelman JH, Tijssen MA. Local field potentials and oscillatory activity of the internal globus pallidus in myoclonus–dystonia. *Mov Disord* 2007; 22: 369–76.
84. Beukers RJ, Booij J, Weisscher N, Zijlstra F, van Amelsvoort TA, Tijssen MA. Reduced striatal D2 receptor binding in myoclonus–dystonia. *Eur J Nucl Med Mol Imaging* 2009; 36: 269–74.
85. Kinugawa K, Vidailhet M, Clot F, Apartis E, Grabli D, Roze E. Myoclonus–dystonia: an update. *Mov Disord* 2009; 24: 479–89.
86. Li JY, Cunic DI, Paradiso G, et al. Electrophysiological features of myoclonus-dystonia. *Mov Disord* 2008; 23: 2055–61.
87. Beukers RJ, Foncke EM, van der Meer JN, et al. Disorganized sensorimotor integration in mutation-positive myoclonus–dystonia: a functional magnetic resonance imaging study. *Arch Neurol* 2010; 67: 469–74.
88. Hubsch C, Vidailhet M, Rivaud-Pechoux S, et al. Impaired saccadic adaptation in DYT11 dystonia. *J Neurol Neurosurg Psychiatry* 2011; 82: 1103–6.
89. Ritz K, van Schaik BD, Jakobs ME, et al. SGCE isoform characterization and expression in human brain: implications for myoclonus–dystonia pathogenesis? *Eur J Hum Genet* 2011; 19: 438–44.
90. Brown P, Rothwell JC, Thompson PD, Britton TC, Day BL, Marsden CD. New observations on the normal auditory startle reflex in man. *Brain* 1991; 114: 1891–902.
91. Chokroverty S, Walters A, Zimmerman T, Picone M. Propriospinal myoclonus: a neurophysiologic analysis. *Neurology* 1992; 42: 1591–5.
92. Roze E, Apartis E, Vidailhet M, et al. Propriospinal myoclonus: utility of magnetic resonance diffusion tensor imaging and fiber tracking. *Mov Disord* 2007; 22: 1506–9.
93. Dijk JM, Tijssen MA. Management of patients with myoclonus: available therapies and the need for an evidence-based approach. *Lancet Neurol* 2010; 9: 1028–36.
94. Wheless JW, Sankar R. Treatment strategies for myoclonic seizures and epilepsy syndromes with myoclonic seizures. *Epilepsia* 2003; 44 (Suppl 11): 27–37.
95. Wallace SJ. Myoclonus and epilepsy in childhood: a review of treatment with valproate, ethosuximide, lamotrigine and zonisamide. *Epilepsy Res* 1998; 29: 147–54.
96. Brown P, Steiger MJ, Thompson PD, et al. Effectiveness of piracetam in cortical myoclonus. *Mov Disord* 1993; 8: 63–8.
97. Tijssen MA, Schoemaker HC, Edelbroek PJ, Roos RA, Cohen AF, van Dijk JG. The effects of clonazepam and vigabatrin in hyperekplexia. *J Neurol Sci* 1997; 149: 63–7.
98. Yoshimura DM, Aminoff MJ, Tami TA, Scott AB. Treatment of hemifacial spasm with botulinum toxin. *Muscle Nerve* 1992; 15: 1045–9.
99. van der Salm SM, Koelman JH, Henneke S, van Rootselaar AF, Tijssen MA. Axial jerks: a clinical spectrum ranging from propriospinal to psychogenic myoclonus. *J Neurol* 2010; 257: 1349–55.
100. van Rootselaar AF, Aronica E, Jansen Steur EN, Rozemuller-Kwakkel JM, de Vos RA, Tijssen MA. Familial cortical tremor with epilepsy and cerebellar pathological findings. *Mov Disord* 2004; 19: 213–17.

CHAPTER 26

Paroxysmal Movement Disorders

Melissa J. Armstrong and William Weiner

Summary

Paroxysmal movement disorders are characterized by distinct episodes of abnormal movements. These episodes have abrupt onset, variable duration, and a discrete conclusion on top of a normal or stable neurological baseline. Clinical phenomenology during the attacks is divided into dyskinesia—including chorea, athetosis, dystonia, and/or ballismus—or ataxia. By convention these are labelled paroxysmal dyskinesias and episodic ataxias. Because of the intermittent nature of these movement disorders, diagnosis is usually made from clinical and family history. Recent advances in genetics have identified causative mutations for many of these disorders.

Paroxysmal dyskinesias

Paroxysmal dyskinesias are rare disorders characterized by attacks of choreoathetosis, dystonia, and ballismus. Although phenomenology is diverse, six have received DYT designations (Table 26.1). Various clinical classification schemes have been proposed and revised over time, with four main subtypes—paroxysmal kinesigenic dyskinesia (PKD), paroxysmal non-kinesigenic dyskinesia (PNKD), paroxysmal exercise-induced dyskinesia (PED), and paroxysmal hypnogenic dyskinesia—each with idiopathic and secondary causes (1). Mixed forms are also described (2–4) with the suggestion that an additional classification of 'paroxysmal dyskinesias, mixed type' be considered (3). These categorizations based on clinically observed patterns are being further refined as genetic causes are identified.

Paroxysmal kinesigenic dyskinesia

PKD is the most common of the paroxysmal dyskinesias with an estimated prevalence of 1 in 150 000 (5). A series of 121 affected individuals evaluated in 2004 established the diagnostic criteria (Box 26.1) (6). Individuals affected by PKD have a normal interictal neurological examination. Dyskinetic episodes are triggered by activities such as standing up, walking, and running. Less common triggers include startle or focal movements such as stretching. Uncommon triggers include caffeine and fatigue. Anxiety often lowers attack threshold. Many PKD patients describe a non-specific and variable aura allowing them to minimize attack severity by stopping contributory movements (6).

PKD attacks generally last less than 30–60 seconds but can occur over 20 times daily. Episode phenomenology is dystonia in over half of cases; mixed hyperkinesias are present in another third. Chorea and ballism alone occur rarely. Involved limbs may be unilateral or bilateral. When unilateral, the affected limbs may be consistently on one side or variable (6).

Almost all PKD patients have their first attack before age 20 and 90% have episodes prior to age 15. Episodes stop or decrease in the majority of PKD patients in their twenties. While various antiepileptic drugs (AEDs) have been tried, 86% of PKD patients requiring medication responded to carbamazepine or phenytoin in one series (6). Similar benefits are seen in other PKD studies (7, 8). Oxcarbazepine may also be effective and has advantages given its different side-effect profile (9).

Familial PKD is more common than sporadic PKD, but clinical characteristics are similar (6). A small subset of familial PKD cases has an infantile-onset movement disorder with a mildly different phenotype (6). Patients with familial PKD are more likely to have a personal and family history of infantile convulsions. This is unsurprising given that the loci for benign infantile familial convulsions and paroxysmal choreoathetosis (ICCA) overlap with those for PKD (6, 7, 10). Adolescent- and adult-onset epilepsy (8, 10), migraine (6), and writer's cramp (6) are also described in PKD patients and families. It remains unclear if these relate to the same underlying pathophysiology.

Familial PKD shows autosomal dominant (AD) inheritance, but an associated gene has yet to be identified. Multiple studies link familial PKD to chromosome 16. Two different loci (EKD1 and EKD2) are known, with others still suspected (7, 8, 10, 11). Despite these linkages, screening for abnormal genes has been unsuccessful (12, 13). It is generally assumed that PKD is related to an ion-channel mutation, but this is yet to be shown. With no available genetic testing, diagnosis is based on clinical criteria (Box 26.1) supplemented by normal neurological examination, imaging, and electroencephalography (EEG).

Table 26.1 Paroxysmal dyskinesias assigned a DYT designation

Designation	Dystonia type	Mode of inheritance	Gene locus	Gene	OMIM number
DYT8	Paroxysmal non-kinesigenic dyskinesia (PNKD1)	AD	2q35	Myofibrillogenesis regulator 1 (*MR1*)	118800
DYT9	Paroxysmal choreoathetosis with episodic ataxia and spasticity	AD	1p	Unknown	601042
DYT10	Paroxysmal kinesigenic dyskinesia (PKD)	AD	16p11.2-q12.1	Unknown	128200
DYT18	Paroxysmal exertion-induced dyskinesia (PED) with or without epilepsy and/or haemolytic anaemia	AD	1p35-p31.3	Glucose transporter *SLC2A1*	612126
DYT19	Episodic kinesigenic dyskinesia 2 (EKD2) or PKD2	AD	16q13-q22.1	Unknown	611031
DYT20	Paroxysmal non-kinesigenic dyskinesia 2 (PNKD2)	AD	2q31	Unknown	611147

AD, autosomal dominant; OMIM, Online Mendelian Inheritance of Man.

Adapted from http://www.ncbi.nlm.nih.gov/omim.

Numerous reports hypothesize secondary causes for PKD presentations including cerebral palsy (14), peripheral trauma (2, 15), subcortical white matter ischaemia (16), cervical cord compression (17), primary central nervous system lymphoma (18), HIV (19), voltage-gated potassium channel (VGKC) complex protein antibody encephalitis (20), and hyperglycaemia (21). Whether these observations represent true causal links is unclear. Interestingly, several of these cases also respond to carbamazepine (2, 15, 17, 18). Phenytoin (14) and benzodiazepines (19) are beneficial in other cases. In the patient with VGKC-complex protein antibody encephalitis, PKD symptoms decreased after intravenous immunoglobulin infusions (20).

Paroxysmal non-kinesigenic dyskinesia

Attacks in PNKD are spontaneous rather than triggered by sudden movements as in PKD. PNKD attacks also tend to be longer (lasting minutes to hours) than those seen in PKD. With identification of causative mutations in the myofibrillogenesis regulator 1 (*MR-1*) gene, PNKD families are further divided into true PNKD (with the mutation) and 'PNKD-like' conditions without an identified mutation (22).

Box 26.1 Clinical diagnostic criteria for paroxysmal kinesigenic dyskinesia (PKD)

1. Dyskinetic attacks triggered by sudden movements.
2. Short duration attacks (<1 min).
3. No loss of consciousness or pain during attacks.
4. Antiepileptic drug responsiveness (particularly carbamazepine or phenytoin).
5. Exclusion of other organic diseases.
6. Age of onset between 1 and 20 years if there is no family history.

Adapted from Bruno MK, Hallett K, Gwinn-Hardy K, et al. Clinical evaluation of idiopathic paroxysmal kinesigenic dyskinesia: new diagnostic criteria. *Neurology* 2004; 63: 2280–7.

PNKD associated with *MR-1* mutations (DYT-8)

The PNKD phenotype is consistent across eight kindreds with different *MR-1* mutations. Attacks start at age 4 years on average (range 3 months to 12 years). PNKD attacks are superimposed on a normal baseline neurological examination. Positive and negative emotions can lower attack threshold. Caffeine and alcohol are almost universal triggers. Less common triggers include heat, exercise, fatigue, menstruation, and hunger. Sleep is commonly beneficial (22). Most patients experience attacks at least weekly, though rare attacks are also described. Typical attacks last from 10 minutes to 1 hour, ranging from several minutes to 12 hours (22). Aura occurs in approximately 40% of patients and may involve focal limb numbness, stiffening, or general anxiety. Attack phenomenology combines chorea and dystonia and can vary within an individual over time and between members of the same family. Less commonly reported phenomenology includes blepharospasm, risus sardonicus, and diplopia. Speech involvement occurs in just under half of patients. Attacks tend to decrease in frequency with age, although natural history varies (22). Headache and migraine are commonly reported in PNKD families (22). Based on these clinical findings and comparison with gene-negative PNKD patients (see further discussion in the next section), clinical diagnostic criteria for *MR-1* mutation PNKD have been proposed (Box 26.2) (22).

Non-benzodiazepine anticonvulsants are generally unsuccessful in preventing PNKD attacks. However, in a series of PNKD patients, 34 of 35 patients who tried benzodiazepines for either preventive or abortive therapy responded favourably (22). While benzodiazepines are the mainstay of treatment, individual PNKD cases improved with valproate (22), levetiracetam (23), oxcarbazepine (24), haloperidol (22), acetazolamide (22), and levodopa (22).

Familial PNKD follows an AD inheritance pattern. After linking PNKD to the long arm of chromosome 2 (2q32–36 locus), several studies identified causative *MR-1* mutations (25–28). Penetrance is high (22, 26–28). The function of *MR-1* remains unknown (26, 28), but it is predicted to be an enzyme in a stress response pathway (25).

PNKD-like phenotypes without *MR-1* mutations

Clinical features of six 'PNKD-like' kindreds without *MR-1*mutations have been compared with the gene-positive kindreds (22). Age of

Box 26.2 Clinical diagnostic criteria for *MR-1* mutation paroxysmal non-kinesigenic dyskinesia (PNKD)

1. Involuntary episodes of hyperkinetic movements (dystonia, chorea, or a combination).
2. Attack duration typically 10 minutes to 1 hour (up to 4 hours).
3. Normal interictal neurologic examination.
4. Exclusion of secondary causes.
5. Onset of attacks in infancy or early childhood.
6. Precipitation of attacks by caffeine and alcohol consumption.
7. Family history of movement disorder meeting criteria 1–6.

Adapted from Bruno MK, Lee H-Y, Auburger GWJ, et al. Genotype–phenotype correlation of paroxysmal nonkinesigenic dyskinesia. *Neurology* 2007; 68: 1782–9.

onset is later than in *MR-1*-positive patients (12.3 ± 10.8 years versus 4.0 ± 4.6 years). Aura is reported in 63%, and triggers include exercise, caffeine, fatigue, emotional stress, heat, and hunger. Exercise as a trigger is more common in these pedigrees (68% of patients) than in those with *MR-1* mutations (12%). Alcohol is not a trigger in PNKD-like patients, a notable distinction from *MR-1* mutation patients. Attack phenomenology includes dystonia, chorea, ballism, and combinations. Attack duration is similar to *MR-1*-positive PNKD attacks. Weekly attacks occur in a third of PNKD-like patients and are less frequent in the remainder. Of 22 PNKD-like patients, five also had epilepsy (two of whom had basal ganglia calcifications), two had mild ataxia on baseline examination, and single cases had migraine without aura, cluster headache, attention deficit hyperactivity disorder with autism, and a learning disability (22).

PNKD-like patients may partially improve with benzodiazepine therapy (22). Partial response with valproate, carbamazepine, topiramate, gabapentin, and acetazolamide has also been described in individual patients. Carbamazepine, phenytoin, and levodopa have worsened attacks (22).

Causative genes for familial PNKD-like disorders have yet to be identified. A Canadian family links to a locus at 2q31 without mutations in *MR-1* (29). Consistent with the PNKD-like phenotype identified by Bruno and colleagues (22), age at onset in this family was highly variable, attacks were not triggered by alcohol or caffeine, and there was no response to clonazepam (29). A genome-wide linkage scan of a family with AD generalized epilepsy and paroxysmal dyskinesia (GEPD) mapped to 10q22 with a mutation in *KCNMA1*. This mutation is in the alpha subunit of a calcium-sensitive potassium channel. While the movement disorder in this family was labelled PNKD, and described as episodic dystonia and chorea triggered by alcohol, fatigue, and stress but not movement, features unusual for PNKD included very brief episode duration (10 s to 2 min) and a strong association with familial epilepsy (30). A four-generation family with intracranial calcifications and PNKD has no linkage identified to date (31).

Secondary PNKD

Sporadic PNKD is rarely reported, but case reports and small series posit secondary causes including peripheral trauma (32), brachial plexus neuropathy (33), stroke (2), subcortical white matter ischaemia (16), intracerebral calcifications secondary to hypoparathyroidism (34), antiphospholipid syndrome (35), central trauma (2), kernicterus (2), HIV (19), cytomegalovirus encephalitis (2), streptococcal infection (36), multiple sclerosis (2), and migraine (2). Mixed PKD–PNKD phenotypes secondary to stroke, peripheral trauma, central trauma, and meningovascular syphilis are also proposed (2). Attack characteristics in these reports are not always consistent with PNKD or PNKD-like processes. Unsurprisingly, some patients with presumed secondary PNKD have abnormal neurological examinations at baseline (2, 19). Furthermore, attacks may be longer or shorter than those described in familial PNKD and PNKD-like processes (2, 34) and triggers other than stress are rare.

Pharmacological therapies described as effective in individuals with proposed secondary PNKD include anticonvulsants (e.g. carbamazepine, phenobarbital) (2), valproate (33), levetiracetam (34), clonazepam (2), tetrabenazine (2), biperiden (33), trihexyphenidyl (2), and botulinum toxin injections (33). Clonazepam and other agents have been of no reported benefit (2, 19, 33, 34). It is unclear whether treating the proposed underlying aetiology affects PNKD symptoms. Various functional stereotactic neurosurgical procedures have been utilized for refractory secondary PNKD cases with reported success, including deep brain stimulation (DBS) of the thalamus (33) and globus pallidus internus (GPi) (32). Bilateral GPi DBS also benefited a complicated patient with refractory PNKD of unknown aetiology (37).

Paroxysmal exercise-induced dyskinesia (PED)

The category paroxysmal exercise (or exertion)-induced dyskinesia (PED) is assigned when episodes of dyskinesia are trigged by prolonged exertion or exercise as opposed to simple movement. PED is less common than both PKD and PNKD. In 2008, mutations in *SLC2A1* were discovered in several families with PED and epilepsy. *SLC2A1* codes for glucose transporter 1 (GLUT1), a blood–brain barrier glucose transporter (38, 39). The gene is now labelled both *SLC2A1* and *GLUT1*. Familial PED demonstrates AD inheritance with incomplete penetrance (38).

Limited cases are available to establish a clinical picture of *SLC2A1–GLUT1* PED. In *SLC2A1–GLUT1* families, movement disorder onset tends to occur during childhood (median 8 years), though onset in individuals up to age 30 is described (38). By definition, the primary trigger is exertion, such as prolonged brisk walking. Typically, 15–60 minutes of exercise is required (39). Other triggers include stress, starvation, and sleep deprivation. Alleviating factors include eating (particularly something with glucose or sugar), rest, and avoidance or cessation of provoking activities (38). Aura, including autonomic and sensory symptoms, occurs in some patients (38). Phenomenology includes choreoathetosis, dystonia, ballism, and combinations (38, 39). Legs are more commonly affected than the face or arms (38–40), possibly representing preferential involvement of exercising limbs since attacks are common after walking. Localization can be consistent and focal or varied (38). Episode frequency ranges from weekly to yearly (38). Attacks generally last up to 15 min, but duration ranges from seconds to several hours (38, 39). Dyskinesias may stop immediately with exercise cessation or may resolve gradually over hours (39).

Box 26.3 Clinical diagnostic criteria for *SLC2A1–GLUT1* mutation paroxysmal exercise-induced dyskinesia (PED)

1. Childhood-onset intractable exercise-induced dyskinesias, sometimes with early-onset epilepsy.
2. Normal neurological examination between attacks.
3. Normal MRI.
4. Moderately low CSF glucose/serum glucose concentration (or demonstrated *SLC2A1–GLUT1* mutation).
5. Family history of PED and/or epilepsy is supportive, but sporadic mutations have been demonstrated.

Adapted from Suls A, Dedeken P, Goffin K, et al. Paroxysmal exercise-induced dyskinesia and epilepsy is due to mutations in SLC2A1, encoding the glucose transporter GLUT1. *Brain* 2008; 131: 1831–44.

As with the other paroxysmal dyskinesias, neurological examination between attacks is generally normal, though mildly reduced intelligence or cognitive impairments in some mutation carriers is reported (38, 39). Mild permanent neurological abnormalities are also described in some individuals (39). PED symptom severity may lessen with age (38, 39). Clinical features are summarized in Box 26.3.

Sporadic cases of PED with *SLC2A1–GLUT1* mutations have clinical features similar to those described in *SLC2A1–GLUT1* PED families including childhood onset, exercise-induced episodes, attack resolution with rest, and normal or only mildly abnormal neurological examination (41, 42). In four reported cases, two of whom were twins, writer's cramp, absence epilepsy, and migraine were each reported in three patients (41, 42).

Epilepsy can occur in PED patients or in family members with or without PED. Associated epilepsy syndromes include febrile, absence, generalized tonic–clonic, myoclonic, and simple and complex partial seizures (38, 39, 41). Epilepsy starts in childhood, sometimes earlier than the movement disorder (38). Haemolytic anaemia also occurs in PKD families with certain *SLC2A1–GLUT1* mutations (39).

MRI is described as normal (38, 39) or showing T_2 hypointensities in the caudal putamen (39). A PED case with a sporadic mutation showed mild cerebellar atrophy (41). Specialized imaging modalities are described in select individuals (38, 39). Studies suggest that mutation carriers have moderately reduced cerebrospinal fluid (CSF) glucose/serum glucose concentrations (range 0.37–0.59, normal >0.60). The reduction is generally less severe than that seen in patients with GLUT1 deficiency syndrome (<0.40) (38, 39, 42).

In severely affected patients, a ketogenic diet has helped PED, epilepsy, and migraine symptoms, but difficulty in adhering to the strict diet limits its usefulness (38, 39, 42). Carbohydrate-rich diets have been unsuccessful (38). Response to pharmacological agents is variable. AEDs may benefit patients who also suffer from epilepsy, but the effect on PED symptoms is less clear (38, 39, 41). Carbonic anhydrase inhibitors (e.g. acetazolamide, diclofenamide) are described as both beneficial (39, 41) and unhelpful (41). Similarly, levodopa is described as being mildly beneficial (41) and unhelpful (39). Haloperidol triggered an acute dystonic reaction in one patient with PED (41).

Numerous *SLC2A1–GLUT1* mutations are now identified in PED families and sporadic cases (38, 39, 41). PED attacks may result from reduced transport of glucose across the blood–brain barrier due to mutations affecting the GLUT1 transporter. It is hypothesized that because the basal ganglia are particularly sensitive to energy deficits, these areas may be preferentially affected (38, 39). Families with PED and epilepsy associated with *SLC2A1–GLUT1* mutations are distinct from the GLUT1 deficiency syndrome associated with microcephaly, motor and cognitive developmental delay, epilepsy, spasticity, dystonia, ataxia, and other severe impairments (38, 39).

While *SLC2A1–GLUT1* mutations are now identified in numerous families with a PED phenotype, at least two families with similar features have no *SLC2A1–GLUT1* mutations (39). The possibility of other gene involvement remains. Additionally, one family with PED and no mutation in *SLC2A1–GLUT1* had a mutation in GTP-cyclohydrolase 1. Patients in this family responded well to levodopa, consistent with a diagnosis of dopa-responsive dystonia (DRD). Clinical features differed slightly from the PED pattern described above; in addition to being levodopa-responsive, episodes were triggered more quickly than in *SLC2A1–GLUT1*-associated PED (requiring only a few minutes of exercise) and occurred more frequently (daily or several times weekly). In the index case, CSF glucose/plasma glucose ratio was borderline at 0.59, but the patient had abnormally low CSF neurotransmitter levels consistent with DRD (43). PED is also reported in the context of AD familial acanthocytosis with paroxysmal exertion-induced dyskinesias and epilepsy (FAPED), a rare neuroacanthocytosis syndrome associated with a glucose transporter mutation (44).

Rarely, alternative causes of non-familial PED are proposed. Exercise-induced dystonia is described as a presenting feature of young-onset Parkinson's disease, but these patients were older than in classic PED (45, 46). Exercise-induced dystonia is also reported in a case of atypical DRD (without gene confirmation) (47). Proposed secondary causes of PED include trauma (1, 48), moyamoya disease (49), and hypoglycaemia related to insulinomas (48, 49). Each of the proposed secondary causes occurred in adults (1, 48–51). Other features distinct from those in *SLC2A1–GLUT1*-associated PED exist; for example, episodes in the moyamoya disease case were triggered by working extra hours and occasionally by exercise, a different pattern from classic familial PED (49). One of the traumatic cases responded to low-dose baclofen (48), and both cases related to insulinoma responded to removal of the tumour (50, 51).

Paroxysmal hypnogenic dyskinesia/nocturnal paroxysmal dykinesia (nocturnal frontal lobe epilepsy)

Initially thought to be movement disorders or parasomnias, hyperkinesias previously termed nocturnal paroxysmal dyskinesias are now widely accepted as epileptic in nature. These are seen in nocturnal frontal lobe epilepsy (NFLE) and its inherited form, autosomal dominant nocturnal frontal lobe epilepsy (ADNFLE). While these episodes represent seizures they may come to the attention of the movement disorders specialist.

A series of 100 patients with NFLE (52) provides the most thorough description of these patients. Seizure onset occurred at a mean age of 14 years (±10 years), but with a broad range from 1 to

64 years. While patients complained of disrupted sleep, 72% were unaware of their nocturnal motor manifestations. Patients reported a mean of 20 ± 11 seizures per month. Over a quarter of patients experienced secondary generalized seizures at night; occasional daytime seizures also occurred. Various parasomnias (e.g. enuresis, sleepwalking) were described in a third of patients (52).

Hyperkinetic episodes seen in NFLE are classified into four types: paroxysmal arousals, hypermotor seizures, asymmetric bilateral tonic seizures, and epileptic nocturnal wanderings. Each pattern can have phenomenology consistent with movement disorders. Paroxysmal arousals represent brief seizures lasting seconds. Patients open their eyes and sometimes sit and appear frightened. These arousals may be associated with mild dystonic posturing or finger movements. They can recur every 20–30 seconds throughout long portions of non-rapid eye movement (non-REM) sleep. Hypermotor seizures consist of non-REM sleep attacks where patients appear to wake and perform complex movements, often appearing dystonic or choreoathetotic. Semi-purposeful movements such as rocking or cycling can also occur. Attacks may include vocalizations. Tachycardia and hypertension accompany episodes. The episodes tend to be highly stereotyped within an individual and can occur in a pulsatile manner throughout sleep, sometimes superimposed on other movements such as nocturnal myoclonus (53).

Asymmetric bilateral tonic seizures consist of several seconds of asymmetric tonic and dystonic posturing, often involving all four limbs and sometimes facial and oral muscles. Epileptic nocturnal wandering may start with one of the other seizure types but then progresses into a prolonged phase of complex semi-purposeful motor behaviours, including walking. Patients may display dystonic posturing during these events, which last for 1–2 minutes and may mimic sleepwalking (53).

Most NFLE patients have episodes superimposed on a normal neurological baseline, though various neuroradiological abnormalities are reported in 14% (52). Over half of patients have normal interictal waking and/or sleep scalp EEG. In patients where interictal epileptic activity is seen on sleep EEG, 20% require sphenoidal leads to detect the abnormality. Almost half of nocturnal ictal scalp EEG readings also fail to show epileptic activity, in part due to artefacts related to motor behaviours (52).

In the series of 100 NFLE patients, 25% had a family history of epilepsy and 8% were thought to have ADNFLE. Almost 40% of patients described at least one first-degree relative with a probable primary parasomnia (52). Genes implicated in ADNFLE include *CHRNA2*, *CHRNA4*, and *CHRNB2*, each encoding for subunits on neuronal acetylcholine (Ach) receptors. Other linkage loci are also known (54). The pathophysiological mechanism by which these mutations cause ADNFLE remains unclear, with different models showing different effects on ACh receptors. A positron emission tomography (PET) study in 2008 found reduced D1 receptor binding in patients with the α4-Ser248Phe mutation in *CHRNA4*, preliminarily suggesting that cholinergic-dopaminergic interactions may play a role in the paroxysmal motor manifestations in ADNFLE (55).

NFLE is non-progressive but rarely remits spontaneously. Carbamazepine is the first-line treatment, inducing complete episode remission in 20% and greater than 50% seizure reduction in another 48%. The remaining third of patients may be resistant to any antiepileptic drug (52). Oxcarbazepine may also be beneficial (56, 57). Both carbamazepine and oxcarbazepine affect nicotinic ACh receptors, possibly explaining their effectiveness for NFLE (58). Topiramate was also effective as single or add-on therapy in a small series (59).

Unsurprisingly, reports of possible secondary mechanisms are uncommon. In the NFLE series, 7% of patients reported perinatal events, 3% had febrile seizures, and 3% had mild head trauma preceding paediatric- and juvenile-onset seizures. It was unclear whether these histories related to the NFLE (52). A case of posttraumatic paroxysmal nocturnal right hemidystonia was described in a teenager with right hemiplegia after a severe head injury. MRI revealed small left putaminal lesions and episodes improved with acetazolamide therapy (60). Similarly, baclofen-responsive paroxysmal nocturnal dystonia related to stroke is described (2). No epileptic correlates were reported in either of these cases.

Other paroxysmal dyskinesias

While the most common clinical and genetic patterns of paroxysmal dyskinesias are detailed in the preceding sections, other paroxysmal dyskinesias have also been reported. Paroxysmal dystonic episodes triggered by sensory stimuli or passive movements were reported in a small series of boys with severe global retardation and thyroid abnormalities associated with X-linked mutations in the thyroid hormone transporter gene *MCT8* (61). AD paroxysmal choreoathetosis/spasticity (CSE) (DYT9) is a disorder where episodic dyskinesia is triggered by exercise, stress, lack of sleep, or alcohol. Episodes range from daily to annually and last approximately 20 minutes. Acetazolamide or phenytoin benefit some patients. Patients may have a normal baseline or spastic paraplegia. Genetic studies demonstrate linkage to chromosome 1p near a cluster of potassium-channel genes (62).

Psychogenic paroxysmal dyskinesia is described with cases often showing key atypical features (6, 63, 64). Psychogenic movement disorders and methods for making this diagnosis are covered in Chapter 31.

Transient and benign paroxysmal paediatric dyskinesias are also described in the literature, but are beyond the scope of this chapter. Examples include benign paroxysmal torticollis of infancy (65) and paroxysmal dystonic posturing seen in the context of gratification behaviour (masturbation) in children between 3 months and 3 years old (66).

Episodic ataxias

Unlike the paroxysmal dyskinesias which are historically categorized by clinical characteristics, the episodic ataxias (EAs) are channelopathies categorized by genetic mutations, although different mutations are associated with specific clinical phenotypes. Seven EA designations have been assigned to date (Table 26.2).

Episodic ataxia type 1 (EA1)

The phenotype of EA1 was a recognized clinical entity even prior to identification of the causative gene in 1994 (67). The two cardinal features of EA1 are episodic ataxia and interictal myokymia present on examination or electromyography (EMG). With the discovery of pathological mutations in *KCNA1*, the associated clinical

Table 26.2 Episodic ataxias with EA designation

Designation	Episodic ataxia type	Mode of inheritance	Gene locus	Gene	OMIM number
EA1	Episodic ataxia type 1	AD	12p13	KCNA1	160120
	Episodic ataxia with myokymia				176260
EA2	Episodic ataxia type 2	AD	19p13	CACNA1A	108500
	Episodic ataxia with nystagmus, acetazolamide-responsive				
EA3	Episodic ataxia type 3	AD	1q42	Unknown	606554
	Episodic ataxia with vertigo and tinnitus				
EA4	Episodic ataxia type 4	AD	Unknown	Unknown	606552
	Periodic vestibulocerebellar ataxia (PATX)				
EA5	Episodic ataxia type 5	AD	2q22-q23	CACNB4	601949
EA6	Episodic ataxia type 6	AD	5p13	SLC1A3	612656
EA7	Episodic ataxia type 7	AD	19q13	Unknown	611907

AD, autosomal dominant; OMIM, Online Mendelian Inheritance of Man.

Adapted from http://www.ncbi.nlm.nih.gov/omim

phenotypes have broadened beyond EA and myokymia. The prevalence is estimated at 1 in 500 000 (68).

EA1 classically presents in childhood, usually before age 10, although early adolescent onset is reported. Patients experience attacks of cerebellar dysfunction including imbalance, wide-based gait with or without falls, truncal and limb ataxia, tremor, jerking, head titubation, dysarthria, and visual disturbances including blurring and oscillopsia (69–75). Dizziness, nausea, and headache may also occur (70, 75). Conditions that can trigger or lower the threshold for episodes include startle, exertion, emotional stress, menstruation, illness, fever, heat, hunger, caffeine, alcohol, and fatigue (69–72, 74–76). While no distinct aura is described, some patients may have a feeling of general discomfort or weakness prior to attack onset (71, 73). Choosing to rest or sleep at attack onset may help. Episode duration ranges from seconds to minutes. Frequency varies and ranges from multiple times daily to a few attacks per year (70–74). Descriptions of changes in episodes over time and with age have been conflicting.

The second cardinal feature of EA1 is myokymia—spontaneous skeletal muscle contractions—which may produce clinically visible rippling of the muscles or which may be detectable only by EMG. Myokymia may be associated with neuromyotonia (muscle cramps and stiffness). Unlike the ataxia, the myokymia is not episodic in nature. When visible or palpable, myokymia may be identified in the face (e.g. around the eyes and mouth) or the limbs. When present in the fingers, myokymia produces small-amplitude pseudo-choreiform movements when the hands are outstretched or in a relaxed prone position. Myokymia is detected by EMG even when subclinical (67, 69–73, 75). Other neuromuscular features may also be observed in EA1. For example, calf hypertrophy and shortened Achilles tendons are described (70, 72, 76). Patients may also develop fixed postures in the hands which can worsen during attacks (70, 71). Sometimes abnormal hand and foot posturing is described as being present since birth (71, 72). Apart from these generally mild neuromuscular abnormalities, the neurological examination in EA1 is usually normal (70, 73), although mild interictal cerebellar features are described (74, 76). A single patient is reported to have a progressive interictal cerebellar syndrome (75).

With identification of associated *KCNA1* mutations, the phenotype of EA1 has broadened beyond the cardinal features. One family with classic EA1 also has paroxysmal dyspnoea both alone and in association with the ataxic episodes (77). Epilepsy was mentioned in one of the earliest cases of EA1 (70), and was later described in two EA families (75, 78). Additionally, a family with a G724C mutation had epilepsy and myokymia but no episodic ataxia (76). Isolated myokymia was described in a family with a C731A mutation (76) and a Brazilian family had a *KCNA1* mutation associated with hypomagnesaemia, tremor, muscle cramps, tetanic episodes, and limb weakness (79). Presentations without the classic ataxia seen in EA1 are considered allelic disorders. It is postulated that the phenotypic diversity seen with EA1 and allelic disorders may be related to the nature and degree of potassium channel dysfunction with different mutations (80). While genotype–phenotype correlations may explain some differences, affected individuals within the same family or with identical mutations may also exhibit substantial heterogeneity. A recent description of markedly different presentations in pairs of identical twins with EA1 suggests that environmental factors may play a role (75).

Pharmacological effects are described in individual cases without formal clinical trials. Early reports describe improvement with phenytoin (69, 70, 72, 73), but worsening with phenytoin is also described (72). Carbamazepine is variably reported as helpful or ineffective (74–76). While often presumed to be the treatment of choice, acetazolamide and diclofenamide, both carbonic anhydrase inhibitors, are ineffective (69, 72, 73, 81) or only transiently beneficial (76). Sulthiame, another carbonic anhydrase inhibitor, halved attack frequency in one patient (73). Flunarazine was also helpful for one patient (69). Agents reported as ineffective include vigabatrin (76) and clonazepam (73, 76). Lamotrigine worsened attack frequency in one case (76). It is suggested that drug-resistant EA1 may be associated with certain genotypes (76), but this has yet to be confirmed. Depending on attack characteristics, patients and families should be counselled regarding particular care or avoidance of potentially dangerous activities—one EA1 patient almost drowned during an attack (73).

EA1is a monogenic potassium channelopathy associated with *KCNA1*. It has AD inheritance and incomplete penetrance. Over

20 pathogenic mutations of *KCNA1* have been described, primarily missense mutations. Mutations are identified via sequence analysis (68). *KCNA1* encodes the potassium channel subunit Kv1.1. It is theorized that mutations result in different effects on channel function, including changing potassium currents and affecting neurotransmitter release (68, 82, 83).

Episodic ataxia type 2 (EA2)

The most common of the EAs (80), episodic ataxia type 2 (EA2), is related to mutations in *CACNA1A*. Different mutations in *CACNA1A* lead to familial hemiplegic migraine (FHM) and spinocerebellar ataxia type 6 (SCA6). Additionally, families and individuals with phenotypes similar to *CACNA1A*-related EA2 are described without an identified mutation.

The clinical phenotype of EA2 related to *CACNA1A* mutations can vary even within families (84), but a general pattern is still clear. Attack onset almost always begins before age 20 (84–86), although presentations as delayed as the late sixties are described (87, 88). Episodes of truncal and limb ataxia usually last hours, though episodes of shorter duration (minutes) and longer duration (days) are also described (84–86, 89). Episodes may occur several times per day or only occasionally during a lifetime (84, 86). Triggers include physical exertion, emotional stress, heat, fever, alcohol, and coffee (84, 86, 89, 90). Episodes of ataxia may be accompanied by vertigo, nausea and vomiting, dysarthria, headache, and fluctuating generalized weakness (84–86, 89, 90). During attacks, spontaneous nystagmus may be seen (85) and patients may complain of double or blurred vision (84, 86). Rarely, dystonia is observed in addition to ataxia (80, 85). Clinical features of classic *CACNA1A*-associated EA2 are summarized in Box 26.4.

Unlike most other paroxysmal movement disorders, the interictal neurological examination in EA2 patients is usually abnormal. Most patients have gaze-evoked nystagmus. Primary position downbeat nystagmus may also be present. Additionally, over half of EA2 patients display gradually progressive ataxia on interictal neurological examination. Rare EA2 family members may have progressive ataxia without superimposed attacks. Interictal dysarthria can be present (84–86, 89–91). Strabismus and cranial nerve palsies affecting extra-ocular movements are described in some EA2 cases (84, 92).

Box 26.4 Clinical features of *CACNA1A* mutation episodic ataxia type 2 (EA2)

1. Onset before age 20.
2. Episodes of ataxia lasting hours to days, often triggered by emotional stress and physical exertion. Ataxia may be accompanied by vertigo, generalized weakness, and dystonia.
3. Associated symptoms may include migraine or hemiplegic migraine and seizures.
4. Interictal neurological examination demonstrates gaze-evoked and rebound nystagmus. Interictal ataxia and dysarthria may also be seen.
5. Family history of a similar movement disorder is supportive but not required.

Adapted from Jen J, Kim GW, Baloh RW. Clinical spectrum of episodic ataxia type 2. *Neurology* 2004; 62: 17–22.

Over half of EA2 patients have migraine and a small number have symptoms suggestive of FHM, consistent with the fact that both EA2 and FHM are due to mutations in *CACNA1A* (85, 86, 89). Extreme alcohol sensitivity is characteristic (89, 90). Epilepsy, dystonia, and learning disabilities have each been reported (separately and in combination) in EA2 families (84, 85, 88, 91, 93, 94). A recent paper highlights psychiatric disorders in three patients with EA2 (91), but psychiatric disturbance is not commonly described in prior reports. Phenomenology and associated symptoms vary widely between and within families. One family had different individuals exhibiting EA2, FHM, and SCA6 phenotypes, despite the fact that these typically reflect different *CACNA1A* mutations (95).

Abnormalities are present in some children with *CACNA1A* mutations prior to the EA onset. Bertholon and colleagues (92) described early onset of episodic imbalance in one child (suggestive of benign paroxysmal vertigo of childhood) and permanent imbalance, strabismus, hyperactivity, and delayed cognitive milestones in another child, both of whom had family histories of EA2 and later developed EA themselves. Paroxysmal torticollis of infancy is reported in many families with *CACNA1* mutations (91). Three reported individuals with *CACNA1* mutations, two of whom were brothers, exhibited early childhood ataxia and mental retardation without superimposed ataxic episodes (84).

MRI in EA2 may be normal or show cerebellar atrophy (84, 86, 89, 91, 95, 96). In one study, the presence of cerebellar atrophy correlated with interictal limb ataxia and impaired tandem gait (91). Half the patients in one series had abnormal EEGs (91). Another study showed varied EEG findings among family members (95). Quantitative eye-movement testing and formal posturography can reveal interictal abnormalities not detected clinically (86). A preliminary study investigated the use of nerve excitability studies to assist in the diagnosis of EA2 (97), but the results require further confirmation.

The majority of EA2 patients describe decreased severity and frequency of ataxic episodes with acetazolamide (84, 85, 89), and abnormal interictal oculomotor findings respond to acetazolamide in some patients (98). In a series of EA2 patients, 71% (15/21) improved with acetazolamide at doses of 250–1000 mg daily (85). Response can differ across family members carrying the same mutation. Given that over a quarter of EA2 patients will not respond to acetazolamide, lack of treatment effect should not exclude the possibility of *CACNA1A* mutations (85). One patient with late-onset EA2 and a confirmed *CACNA1A* mutation experienced a dramatic dose-dependent worsening with acetazolamide, but subsequently responded to therapy with 4-aminopyridine (96). The potassium-channel blocker 4-aminopyridine is another therapeutic option for EA2, with complete resolution of episodes described in three patients at a dose of 5 mg three times daily (99). Improvement in interictal ataxia with 4-aminopyridine in a patient with clinically diagnosed late-onset EA2 is also described (100). Treatment with 4-aminopyridine is generally considered if acetazolamide therapy has been ineffective, or has lost effectiveness, or is associated with adverse effects. One patient who experienced side effects with acetazolamide benefited from topiramate (92) and another patient with an incomplete response to acetazolamide benefited from the addition of valproic acid (94).

EA2 related to *CACNA1A* mutations is inherited in an AD manner with incomplete penetrance, but *de novo* mutations are also described. Thus patients with an EA2-like presentation should be screened for *CACNA1A* mutations regardless of family history (84, 85). Over 50 different *CACNA1A* mutations producing an EA2 phenotype are identified throughout the gene, so a full sequence analysis must be performed in patients in whom a mutation is suspected (80, 85). Families linking to 19p but without identifiable mutations in *CACNA1A*, and patients and families with an EA2-like picture but without identifiable linkages, are described (84, 85). In recent years, large deletions in *CACNA1A* have been identified in EA2 patients in whom point mutation screening was negative (101–103). A genetic study in 2010 found deletions in *CACNA1A* in 4/27 patients (14%) with an EA2-like clinical picture but no point mutation in *CACNA1A* (101). One family with a duplication in *CACNA1A* is also described (103). These reports suggest that *CACNA1A* deletion and duplication analysis should be considered in EA2 patients, particularly if routine sequence analysis is negative. Caution should be used in assigning a diagnosis of EA2 clinically without genetic confirmation as numerous patients and families with EA2-like presentations are negative for *CACNA1A* mutations, including individuals later categorized as EA6 and EA7. This distinction may become increasingly important as therapies targeting mutated channels become available.

A comparison in 2010 of EA2 patients with *CACNA1A* mutations and mutation-negative patients suggests that *CACNA1A* mutation carriers may present at a younger age, have more frequent attacks, respond more frequently to acetazolamide, and demonstrate more interictal abnormalities in pursuit and saccades but less interictal ataxia than the mutation-negative patients (though screening for deletions and duplications was not performed). Only age at onset and the presence of pursuit and saccade abnormalities remained statistically significant after Bonferroni correction (91).

CACNA1A codes for the Cav2.1 subunit of P/Q type voltage-gated calcium channels, which has roles including pore-forming and voltage-sensing. These channels are expressed in the cerebellum and presynaptically at the neuromuscular junction. The mechanism underpinning the episodic attacks in EA2 remains unknown (80). A full discussion of the evolving understanding of the pathophysiology of EA2 is complicated, but a summary of the current knowledge regarding changes in Cav2.1 channels with *CACNA1A* mutations is available (104). The role of abnormally prolonged hyperexcitability is also under investigation as an explanation of the paroxysmal nature of EA2 attacks (105). Further studies are required to elucidate the pathophysiology of this disease.

Other episodic ataxias

The other EAs, while labelled through to EA7 (see Table 26.2), are substantially less common than EA1 and EA2. Each is only reported in three or fewer families. Rare late-onset EAs without an official designation are also described.

EA3 was described in a large Canadian Mennonite kindred. Ataxic episodes in the family occurred daily and lasted for 10–30 minutes (106). Median age of onset was 13 (107). Triggers included exertion, certain movements, stress, fatigue, and arousal from sleep. The episodic ataxia was frequently accompanied by falls. Ataxic episodes commonly included vertigo, tinnitus, headache, and visual blurring or diplopia (106). Almost half the affected individuals described episodes of myokymia (106), but EMG did not reveal abnormalities (107). A few individuals demonstrated mild cerebellar findings on examination, but only one patient—with congenital nystagmus—displayed interictal oculomotor abnormalities. One EA3 patient and two siblings without EA had epilepsy. Acetazolamide reduced attack frequency (106). Genome-wide screening of this family with AD inheritance links EA3 to 1q42, but the affected gene remains unknown (107).

EA4 is an AD disorder described in three North Carolina kindreds with suspected common ancestry (108). It is also termed PATX (periodic ataxia). Unlike other EAs, attack onset is in adulthood (23–60 years) (108, 109). Attack frequency ranges from daily to rarely, with years separating episodes. Attack duration is generally minutes, but attacks lasting for months are described (109). Triggers include sudden changes in head position or objects moving across one's vision (108, 109). Ataxia, vertigo, and diplopia form the characteristic episode triad. Tinnitus, oscillopsia, nausea, and vomiting are also reported. One family experienced decreased episode frequency and severity with the antihistamine dimenhydrinate (109). Acetazolamide is ineffective (110) or not tolerated (108). Lying quietly with the eyes closed helps episodes resolve (108). Tinnitus occurs between attacks in some patients. Interictal nystagmus is common, and over half of patients with serial examinations develop interictal cerebellar ataxia of varying degrees, sometimes severe (109). Formal ocular motility testing shows gaze-evoked nystagmus, abnormal smooth pursuits, and inability to suppress the vestibulo-ocular reflex (108). Linkage to several AD ataxias and EAs has been excluded, but the genetic basis of EA4 remains unknown (110).

EA associated with mutations in *CACNB4* on chromosome 2q22–23, designated *EA5*, was identified in one family when 71 families with EA were screened for this mutation. Limited clinical data for this French Canadian family suggest that episodes of vertigo and ataxia began in adulthood (around 20–30 years old) and lasted for hours to days. Interictal neurological examination may reveal mild ataxia, dysarthria, and nystagmus. Acetazolamide prevents attacks (111). The same *CACNB4* missense mutation was identified in a family with generalized epilepsy and no ataxia (111).

EA6 relates to mutations in *SLC1A3* which encodes the glutamate transporter EAAT1. An *SLC1A3* mutation was initially identified in a child with sporadic disease. This 10-year-old boy had a severe clinical phenotype, including motor developmental delay, progressive ataxia, superimposed episodic ataxia and slurred speech starting at age 6 months, alternating hemiplegia and migraine starting at age 6 years, and seizures (112). Subsequent screening of 20 additional EA patients identified a novel EAAT1 mutation in the proband of a Dutch family. The clinical phenotype in this family was similar to that seen in EA2. Attacks started in childhood (3–14 years old) and were triggered by exercise, stress, fatigue, alcohol, and caffeine. Attack frequency ranged from monthly to every few months and most episodes lasted hours. Ataxia, vertigo, nausea, vomiting, dysarthria, photophobia, and phonophobia occurred during attacks, but not headache. Acetazolamide markedly reduced attack frequency. Interictal neurological examination showed horizontal gaze-evoked nystagmus in the proband (113). In both studies, the mutant EAAT1 demonstrated varying degrees of reduced uptake of glutamate (112, 113).

A single report described the EA designated *EA7* (114). The affected family had attack onset in childhood. Episodes lasted for hours to days but were infrequent, ranging from monthly to every few years. Triggers included excitement and exercise, and episodes were characterized by ataxia, weakness, and dysarthria. Associated vertigo was variable and migraines, apart from attacks, occurred in some family members. Attack frequency tended to decrease with age. Baseline neurological examination was normal. Affected family members linked to chromosome 19q13, but sequencing of the suspected genes *KCNC3* and *SLC17A7* showed no mutations (114).

Late-onset episodic ataxias without official designations are also reported. Julien and colleagues (115) describe four unrelated patients with onset of episodic ataxia after age 60. Episodes occurred daily to several times per week, lasted for minutes to hours, and were unresponsive to acetazolamide (500 mg daily). Nystagmus and slowly progressive ataxia were noted on examination (115). Four families with late-onset (40–64 years) episodic oscillopsia were reported with progressive gait ataxia but without clear episodic ataxia. Probands shared some features with EA phenotypes, such as triggers including exertion, alcohol, and caffeine, interictal nystagmus, and development of slowly progressive ataxia. Response to acetazolamide was generally poor. A linkage to chromosome 13 was suggested in two of the families (116). Most recently, a two-generation French family with late-onset (between 48 and 56 years) EA was reported. Attacks in this family lasted minutes to hours and were triggered by exertion, stress, alcohol, and coffee. Ataxia, dysarthria, and nystagmus characterized attacks, sometimes with associated vertigo and diplopia. Slowly progressive interictal ataxia occurred in some family members. Acetazolamide was unhelpful when tried. Known EA mutations were excluded (117).

Conclusion

Because of the intermittent nature of these disorders, appropriate diagnosis of paroxysmal dyskinesias and episodic ataxias relies on the neurologist's ability to elicit a thorough history and recognize the phenotypes associated with different diagnoses. As genetic advances continue, further refinement of phenotypes related to different causative mutations will be identified. Improved recognition of pathological mutations and associated physiological changes may allow more specific targeting of therapeutic agents in the future.

Top clinical tips

- Given that neurological examination is typically normal in paroxysmal movement disorders, obtaining a detailed clinical and family history is essential.
- Paroxysmal dyskinesias are divided into the clinical categories of paroxysmal kinesigenic dyskinesia (PKD), paroxysmal non-kinesigenic dyskinesia (PNKD), paroxysmal exertion-induced dyskinesia (PED), and paroxysmal nocturnal dyskinesia, though the last represents an epilepsy rather than a movement disorder.
- Specific mutated genes are known for many PNKD (*myofibrillogenesis regulator 1*) and PED (*SLC2A1–GLUT1*) presentations.
- Episodic ataxias are categorized by mutation and phenomenology, with seven designations formally assigned.
- Episodic ataxia type 1 (EA1) is characterized by episodic ataxia and interictal myokymia and is related to mutations in *KCNA1*.
- Episodic ataxia type 2 (EA2) is characterized by acetazolamide-responsive episodic ataxia and interictal nystagmus and is related to mutations in *CACNA1*.

References

1. Demirkiran M, Jankovic J. Paroxysmal dyskinesias: clinical features and classification. *Ann Neurol* 1995; 38: 571–9.
2. Blakeley J, Jankovic J. Secondary paroxysmal dyskinesias. *Mov Disord* 2002; 17: 726–34.
3. Pourfar MH, Guerrini R, Parain D, Frucht SJ. Classification conundrums in paroxysmal dyskinesias: a new subtype or variations on classic themes? *Mov Disord* 2005; 20: 1047–51.
4. Prakash S, Mathew C, Bhagat S, Dholakia SY, Shah ND. A case of mixed type of paroxysmal dyskinesia: is there an overlap between two clinical categories of paroxysmal dyskinesia? *Neurol Sci* 2011; 32: 143–5.
5. van Rootselaar AF, van Westrum SS, Velis DN, Tijssen MA. The paroxysmal dyskinesias. *Pract Neurol* 2009; 9: 102–9.
6. Bruno MK, Hallett M, Gwinn-Hardy K, et al. Clinical evaluation of idiopathic paroxysmal kinesigenic dyskinesia: new diagnostic criteria. *Neurology* 2004; 63: 2280–7.
7. Tomita H, Nagamitsu S, Wakui K, et al. Paroxysmal kinesigenic choreoathetosis locus maps to chromosome 16p11.2-q12.1. *Am J Hum Genet* 1999; 65: 1688–97.
8. Spacey SD, Valente EM, Wali GM, et al. Genetic and clinical heterogeneity in paroxysmal kinesigenic dyskinesia: evidence for a third EKD gene. *Mov Disord* 2002; 17: 717–25.
9. Chillag KL, Deroos ST. Oxcarbazepine use in paroxysmal kinesigenic dyskinesia: report on four patients. *Pediatr Neurol* 2009; 40: 295–7.
10. Swoboda KJ, Soong BW, McKenna C, et al. Paroxysmal kinesigenic dyskinesia and infantile convulsions: clinical and linkage studies. *Neurology* 2000; 55: 224–30.
11. Bennett LB, Roach ES, Bowcock AM. A locus for paroxysmal kinesigenic dyskinesia maps to human chromosome 16. *Neurology* 2000; 54: 125–30.
12. Kikuchi T, Nomura M, Tomita H, et al. Paroxysmal kinesigenic choreoathetosis (PKC): confirmation of linkage to 16p11-q21, but unsuccessful detection of mutations among 157 genes at the PKC-critical region in seven PKC families. *J Hum Genet* 2007; 52: 334–41.
13. Ono S, Yoshiura KI, Kurotaki N, Kikuchi T, Niikawa N, Kinoshita A. Mutation and copy number analysis in paroxysmal kinesigenic dyskinesia families. *Mov Disord* 2011; 26: 762–4.
14. Bonakis A, Papageorgiou SG, Potagas C, Karahalios G, Kalfakis N. A case of refractory secondary paroxysmal kinesigenic dyskinesia with high sensitivity to phenytoin monotherapy. *Parkinsonism Relat Disord* 2009; 15: 68–70.
15. Chiesa V, Tamma F, Gardella E, Caputo E, Canger R, Canevini MP. Possible post-traumatic paroxysmal kinesigenic dyskinesia. *Mov Disord* 2008; 23: 2428–30.
16. Norlinah MI, Shahizon AM. Paroxysmal dyskinesia as an unusual and only presentation of subcortical white matter ischaemia: a report of two cases. *Med J Malaysia* 2008; 63: 410–12.
17. Yulug B, Bakar M, Ozer H, Yilmaz M, Unlü B. Paroxysmal kinesigenic dyskinesia and cervical disc prolapse with cord compression: more than a coincidence? *J Neuropsychiatry Clin Neurosci* 2008; 20: 237–9.
18. Rollnik JD, Winkler T, Ganser A. A case of symptomatic paroxysmal kinesigenic dyskinesia with primary central nervous system lymphoma. *Nervenarzt* 2003; 74: 362–5.
19. Mirsattari SM, Berry ME, Holden JK, Ni W, Nath A, Power C. Paroxysmal dyskinesias in patients with HIV infection. *Neurology* 1999; 52: 109–14.
20. Aradillas E, Schwartzman RJ. Kinesigenic dyskinesia in a case of voltage-gated potassium channel-complex protein antibody encephalitis. *Arch Neurol* 2011; 68: 529–32.
21. Saiki M, Saiki S, Gondo Y, Murata KY, Sakai K, Hirose G. Ictal alteration of 99mTc ECD SPECT imaging in a patient with secondary paroxysmal

kinesigenic dyskinesia caused by hyperglycemia. *Rinsho Shinkeigaku* 2005; 45: 312–16.

22. Bruno MK, Lee HY, Auburger GW, et al. Genotype-phenotype correlation of paroxysmal nonkinesigenic dyskinesia. *Neurology* 2007; 68: 1782–9.
23. Szczaluba K, Jurek M, Szczepanik E, et al. A family with paroxysmal nonkinesigenic dyskinesia: genetic and treatment issues. *Pediatr Neurol* 2009; 41: 135–8.
24. Szekely AM, Jabbari B. Oxcarbazepine is exceptionally effective in treating a genetic form of paroxysmal non-kinesigenic dyskinesia (Abstract). *Neurology* 2011; 76 (Suppl 4).
25. Lee HY, Xu Y, Huang Y, et al. The gene for paroxysmal non-kinesigenic dyskinesia encodes an enzyme in a stress response pathway. *Hum Mol Genet* 2004; 13: 3161–70.
26. Chen DH, Matsushita M, Rainier S, et al. Presence of alanine-to-valine substitutions in myofibrillogenesis regulator 1 in paroxysmal nonkinesigenic dyskinesia: confirmation in 2 kindreds. *Arch Neurol* 2005; 62: 597–600.
27. Hempelmann A, Kumar S, Muralitharan S, Sander T. Myofibrillogenesis regulator 1 gene (MR-1) mutation in an Omani family with paroxysmal nonkinesigenic dyskinesia. *Neurosci Lett* 2006; 402: 118–20.
28. Rainier S, Thomas D, Tokarz D, et al. Myofibrillogenesis regulator 1 gene mutations cause paroxysmal dystonic choreoathetosis. *Arch Neurol* 2004; 61: 1025–9.
29. Spacey SD, Adams PJ, Lam PCP, et al. Genetic heterogeneity in paroxysmal nonkinesigenic dyskinesia. *Neurology* 2006; 66: 1588–90.
30. Du W, Bautista JF, Yang H, et al. Calcium-sensitive potassium channelopathy in human epilepsy and paroxysmal movement disorder. *Nat Genet* 2005; 37: 733–8.
31. Yeghiazaryan NS, Striano P, Accorsi P, et al. Familial nonkinesigenic paroxysmal dyskinesia and intracranial calcifications: a new syndrome? *Mov Disord* 2010; 25: 2468–70.
32. Yamada K, Goto S, Soyama N, et al. Complete suppression of paroxysmal nonkinesigenic dyskinesia by globus pallidus internus pallidal stimulation. *Mov Disord* 2006; 21: 576–9.
33. Loher TJ, Krauss JK, Burgunder JM, Taub E, Siegfried J. Chronic thalamic stimulation for treatment of dystonic paroxysmal nonkinesigenic dyskinesia. *Neurology* 2001; 56: 268–70.
34. Alemdar M, Iseri P, Selekler M, Komsuoğlu SS. Levetiracetam-responding paroxysmal nonkinesigenic dyskinesia. *Clin Neuropharmacol* 2007; 30: 241–4.
35. Engelen M, Tijssen MA. Paroxysmal non-kinesigenic dyskinesia in antiphospholipid syndrome. *Mov Disord* 2005; 20: 111–13.
36. Senbil N, Yapici Z, Gürer YK. Paroxysmal non-kinesigenic and hypnogenic dyskinesia associated with streptococcal infection. *Pediatr Int* 2008; 50: 255–6.
37. Kaufman CB, Mink JW, Schwalb JM. Bilateral deep brain stimulation for treatment of medically refractory paroxysmal nonkinesigenic dyskinesia. *J Neurosurg* 2010; 112: 847–50.
38. Suls A, Dedeken P, Goffin K, et al. Paroxysmal exercise-induced dyskinesia and epilepsy is due to mutations in SLC2A1, encoding the glucose transporter GLUT1. *Brain* 2008; 131: 1831–44.
39. Weber YG, Storch A, Wuttke TV, et al. GLUT1 mutations are a cause of paroxysmal exertion-induced dyskinesias and induce hemolytic anemia by a cation leak. *J Clin Invest* 2008; 118: 2157–68.
40. Afawi Z, Suls A, Ekstein D, et al. Mild adolescent/adult onset epilepsy and paroxysmal exercise-induced dyskinesia due to GLUT1 deficiency. *Epilepsia* 2010; 51: 2466–9.
41. Schneider SA, Paisan-Ruiz C, Garcia-Gorostiaga I, et al. GLUT1 gene mutations cause sporadic paroxysmal exercise-induced dyskinesias. *Mov Disord* 2009; 24: 1684–8.
42. Urbizu A, Cuenca-León E, Raspall-Chaure M, et al. Paroxysmal exercise-induced dyskinesia, writer's cramp, migraine with aura and absence epilepsy in twin brothers with a novel SLC2A1 missense mutation. *J Neurol Sci* 2010; 295: 110–13.
43. Dale RC, Melchers A, Fung VS, Grattan-Smith P, Houlden H, Earl J. Familial paroxysmal exercise-induced dystonia: atypical presentation of autosomal dominant GTP-cyclohydrolase 1 deficiency. *Dev Med Child Neurol* 2010; 52: 583–6.
44. Walker RH, Jung HH, Dobson-Stone C, et al. Neurologic phenotypes associated with acanthocytosis. *Neurology* 2007; 68: 92–8.
45. Bozi M, Bhatia KP. Paroxysmal exercise-induced dystonia as a presenting feature of young-onset Parkinson's disease. *Mov Disord* 2003; 18: 1545–7.
46. Lees AJ, Hardie RJ, Stern GM. Kinesigenic foot dystonia as a presenting feature of Parkinson's disease. *J Neurol Neurosurg Psychiatry* 1984; 47: 885.
47. O'Sullivan JD, Costa DC, Gacinovic S, Lees AJ. SPECT imaging of the dopamine transporter in juvenile-onset dystonia. *Neurology* 2001; 56: 266–7.
48. Lim EC, Wong YS. Post-traumatic paroxysmal exercise-induced dystonia: case report and review of the literature. *Parkinsonism Relat Disord* 2003; 9: 371–3.
49. Lyoo CH, Kim DJ, Chang H, Lee MS. Moyamoya disease presenting with paroxysmal exercise-induced dyskinesia. *Parkinsonism Relat Disord* 2007; 13: 446–8.
50. Shaw C, Haas L, Miller D, Delahunt J. A case report of paroxysmal dystonic choreoathetosis due to hypoglycaemia induced by an insulinoma. *J Neurol Neurosurg Psychiatry* 1996; 61: 194–5.
51. Tan NC, Tan AK, Sitoh YY, Loh KC, Leow MK, Tjia HT. Paroxysmal exercise-induced dystonia associated with hypoglycaemia induced by an insulinoma. *J Neurol* 2002; 249: 1615–16.
52. Provini F, Plazzi G, Tinuper P, Vandi S, Lugaresi E, Montagna P. Nocturnal frontal lobe epilepsy: a clinical and polygraphic overview of 100 consecutive cases. *Brain* 1999; 122: 1017–31.
53. Tinuper P, Provini F, Bisulli F, Lugaresi E. Hyperkinetic manifestations in nocturnal frontal lobe epilepsy: semeological features and physiopathological hypothesis. *Neurol Sci* 2005; 26 (Suppl 3): S210–14.
54. Tinuper P, Bisulli F, Provini F, Lugaresi E. Familial frontal lobe epilepsy and its relationship with other nocturnal paroxysmal events. *Epilepsia* 2010; 51 (Suppl 1): 51–3.
55. Fedi M, Berkovic SF, Scheffer IE, et al. Reduced striatal D1 receptor binding in autosomal dominant nocturnal frontal lobe epilepsy. *Neurology* 2008; 71: 795–8.
56. Raju GP, Sarco DP, Poduri A, Riviello JJ, Bergin AM, Takeoka M. Oxcarbazepine in children with nocturnal frontal-lobe epilepsy. *Pediatr Neurol* 2007; 37: 345–9.
57. Romigi A, Marciani MG, Placidi F, et al. Oxcarbazepine in nocturnal frontal-lobe epilepsy: a further interesting report. *Pediatr Neurol* 2008; 39: 298 (author reply).
58. Di Resta C, Ambrosi P, Curia G, Becchetti A. Effect of carbamazepine and oxcarbazepine on wild-type and mutant neuronal nicotinic acetylcholine receptors linked to nocturnal frontal lobe epilepsy. *Eur J Pharmacol* 2010; 643: 13–20.
59. Oldani A, Manconi M, Zucconi M, Martinelli C, Ferini-Strambi L. Topiramate treatment for nocturnal frontal lobe epilepsy. *Seizure* 2006; 15: 649–52.
60. Biary N, Singh B, Bahou Y, al Deeb SM, Sharif H. Posttraumatic paroxysmal nocturnal hemidystonia. *Mov Disord* 1994; 9: 98–9.
61. Brockmann K, Dumitrescu AM, Best TT, Hanefeld F, Refetoff S. X-linked paroxysmal dyskinesia and severe global retardation caused by defective MCT8 gene. *J Neurol* 2005; 252: 663–6.
62. Auburger G, Ratzlaff T, Lunkes A, et al. A gene for autosomal dominant paroxysmal choreoathetosis spasticity (CSE) maps to the vicinity of a potassium channel gene cluster on chromosome 1p, probably within 2 cM between D1S443 and D1S197. *Genomics* 1996; 31: 90–4.
63. Morgan JC, Hughes M, Figueroa RE, Sethi KD. Psychogenic paroxysmal dyskinesia following paroxysmal hemidystonia in multiple sclerosis. *Neurology* 2005; 65: E12.

64. Baik JS, Han SW, Park JH, Lee MS. Psychogenic paroxysmal dyskinesia: the role of placebo in the diagnosis and management. *Mov Disord* 2009; 24: 1244–5.

65. Rosman NP, Douglass LM, Sharif UM, Paolini J. The neurology of benign paroxysmal torticollis of infancy: report of 10 new cases and review of the literature. *J Child Neurol* 2009; 24: 155–60.

66. Yang ML, Fullwood E, Goldstein J, Mink JW. Masturbation in infancy and early childhood presenting as a movement disorder: 12 cases and a review of the literature. *Pediatrics* 2005; 116: 1427–32.

67. Browne DL, Gancher ST, Nutt JG, et al. Episodic ataxia/myokymia syndrome is associated with point mutations in the human potassium channel gene, KCNA1. *Nat Genet* 1994; 8: 136–40.

68. Pessia M, Hanna MG. Episodic ataxia type 1. In: Pagon RA, Bird TD, Dolan CR, Stevens K (eds). *GeneReviews* [Internet]. Seattle, WA: University of Washington, 2010.

69. Vaamonde J, Artieda J, Obeso JA. Hereditary paroxysmal ataxia with neuromyotonia. *Mov Disord* 1991; 6: 180–2.

70. VanDyke DH, Griggs RC, Murphy MJ, Goldstein MN. Hereditary myokymia and periodic ataxia. *J Neurol Sci* 1975; 25: 109–18.

71. Hanson PA, Martinez LB, Cassidy R. Contractures, continuous muscle discharges, and titubation. *Ann Neurol* 1977; 1: 120–4.

72. Gancher ST, Nutt JG. Autosomal dominant episodic ataxia: a heterogeneous syndrome. *Mov Disord* 1986; 1: 239–53.

73. Brunt ER, van Weerden TW. Familial paroxysmal kinesigenic ataxia and continuous myokymia. *Brain* 1990; 113: 1361–82.

74. Hand PJ, Gardner RJ, Knight MA, Forrest SM, Storey E. Clinical features of a large Australian pedigree with episodic ataxia type 1. *Mov Disord* 2001; 16: 938–9.

75. Graves TD, Rajakulendran S, Zuberi SM, et al. Nongenetic factors influence severity of episodic ataxia type 1 in monozygotic twins. *Neurology* 2010; 75: 367–72.

76. Eunson LH, Rea R, Zuberi SM, et al. Clinical, genetic, and expression studies of mutations in the potassium channel gene KCNA1 reveal new phenotypic variability. *Ann Neurol* 2000; 48: 647–56.

77. Shook SJ, Hafsa M, Jen JC, Baloh RW, Zhou L. Novel mutation in KCNA1 causes episodic ataxia with paroxysmal dyspnea. *Muscle Nerve* 2008; 37: 399–402.

78. Zuberi SM, Eunson LH, Spauschus A, et al. A novel mutation in the human voltage-gated potassium channel gene (Kv1.1) associates with episodic ataxia type 1 and sometimes with partial epilepsy. *Brain* 1999; 122: 817–25.

79. Glaudemans B, van der Wijst J, Scola RH, et al. A missense mutation in the Kv1.1 voltage-gated potassium channel-encoding gene KCNA1 is linked to human autosomal dominant hypomagnesemia. *J Clin Invest* 2009; 119: 936–42.

80. Jen JC, Graves TD, Hess EJ, Hanna MG, Griggs RC, Baloh RW. Primary episodic ataxias: diagnosis, pathogenesis and treatment. *Brain* 2007; 130: 2484–93.

81. Lee H, Wang H, Jen JC, Sabatti C, Baloh RW, Nelson SF. A novel mutation in KCNA1 causes episodic ataxia without myokymia. *Hum Mutat* 2004; 24: 536.

82. Heeroma JH, Henneberger C, Rajakulendran S, Hanna MG, Schorge S, Kullmann DM. Episodic ataxia type 1 mutations differentially affect neuronal excitability and transmitter release. *Dis Model Mech* 2009; 2: 612–19.

83. Rajakulendran S, Schorge S, Kullmann DM, Hanna MG. Episodic ataxia type 1: a neuronal potassium channelopathy. *Neurotherapeutics* 2007; 4: 258–66.

84. Denier C, Ducros A, Vahedi K, et al. High prevalence of CACNA1A truncations and broader clinical spectrum in episodic ataxia type 2. *Neurology* 1999; 52: 1816–21.

85. Jen J, Kim GW, Baloh RW. Clinical spectrum of episodic ataxia type 2. *Neurology* 2004; 62: 17–22.

86. Subramony SH, Schott K, Raike RS, et al. Novel CACNA1A mutation causes febrile episodic ataxia with interictal cerebellar deficits. *Ann Neurol* 2003; 54: 725–31.

87. Imbrici P, Eunson LH, Graves TD, et al. Late-onset episodic ataxia type 2 due to an in-frame insertion in CACNA1A. *Neurology* 2005; 65: 944–6.

88. Cuenca-León E, Banchs I, Serra SA, et al. Late-onset episodic ataxia type 2 associated with a novel loss-of-function mutation in the CACNA1A gene. *J Neurol Sci* 2009; 280: 10–14.

89. Kaunisto MA, Harno H, Kallela M, et al. Novel splice site CACNA1A mutation causing episodic ataxia type 2. *Neurogenetics* 2004; 5: 69–73.

90. Jen J, Yue Q, Nelson SF, et al. A novel nonsense mutation in CACNA1A causes episodic ataxia and hemiplegia. *Neurology* 1999; 53: 34–7.

91. Mantuano E, Romano S, Veneziano L, et al. Identification of novel and recurrent CACNA1A gene mutations in fifteen patients with episodic ataxia type 2. *J Neurol Sci* 2010; 291: 30–6.

92. Bertholon P, Chabrier S, Riant F, Tournier-Lasserve E, Peyron R. Episodic ataxia type 2: unusual aspects in clinical and genetic presentation: special emphasis in childhood. *J Neurol Neurosurg Psychiatry* 2009; 80: 1289–92.

93. Spacey SD, Materek LA, Szczygielski BI, Bird TD. Two novel CACNA1A gene mutations associated with episodic ataxia type 2 and interictal dystonia. *Arch Neurol* 2005; 62: 314–16.

94. Scoggan KA, Friedman JH, Bulman DE. CACNA1A mutation in a EA-2 patient responsive to acetazolamide and valproic acid. *Can J Neurol Sci* 2006; 33: 68–72.

95. Romaniello R, Zucca C, Tonelli A, et al. A wide spectrum of clinical, neurophysiological and neuroradiological abnormalities in a family with a novel CACNA1A mutation. *J Neurol Neurosurg Psychiatry* 2010; 81: 840–3.

96. Melzer N, Classen J, Reiners K, Buttmann M. Fluctuating neuromuscular transmission defects and inverse acetazolamide response in episodic ataxia type 2 associated with the novel CaV2.1 single amino acid substitution R2090Q. *J Neurol Sci* 2010; 296: 104–6.

97. Krishnan AV, Bostock H, Ip J, Hayes M, Watson S, Kiernan MC. Axonal function in a family with episodic ataxia type 2 due to a novel mutation. *J Neurol* 2008; 255: 750–5.

98. Harno H, Hirvonen T, Kaunisto MA, et al. Acetazolamide improves neurotological abnormalities in a family with episodic ataxia type 2 (EA-2). *J Neurol* 2004; 251: 232–4.

99. Strupp M, Kalla R, Dichgans M, Freilinger T, Glasauer S, Brandt T. Treatment of episodic ataxia type 2 with the potassium channel blocker 4-aminopyridine. *Neurology* 2004; 62: 1623–5.

100. Lohle M, Schrempf W, Wolz M, Reichmann H, Storch A. Potassium channel blocker 4-aminopyridine is effective in interictal cerebellar symptoms in episodic ataxia type 2: a video case report. *Mov Disord* 2008; 23: 1314–16.

101. Riant F, Lescoat C, Vahedi K, et al. Identification of CACNA1A large deletions in four patients with episodic ataxia. *Neurogenetics* 2010; 11: 101–6.

102. Riant F, Mourtada R, Saugier-Veber P, Tournier-Lasserve E. Large CACNA1A deletion in a family with episodic ataxia type 2. *Arch Neurol* 2008; 65: 817–20.

103. Labrum RW, Rajakulendran S, Graves TD, et al. Large scale calcium channel gene rearrangements in episodic ataxia and hemiplegic migraine: implications for diagnostic testing. *J Med Genet* 2009; 46: 786–91.

104. Pietrobon D. CaV2.1 channelopathies. *Pflugers Arch* 2010; 460: 375–93.

105. Helmich RC, Siebner HR, Giffin N, Bestmann S, Rothwell JC, Bloem BR. The dynamic regulation of cortical excitability is altered in episodic ataxia type 2. *Brain* 2010; 133: 3519–29.

106. Steckley JL, Ebers GC, Cader MZ, McLachlan RS. An autosomal dominant disorder with episodic ataxia, vertigo, and tinnitus. *Neurology* 2001; 57: 1499–502.

107. Cader MZ, Steckley JL, Dyment DA, McLachlan RS, Ebers GC. A genome-wide screen and linkage mapping for a large pedigree with episodic ataxia. *Neurology* 2005; 65: 156–8.

108. Small KW, Pollock SC, Vance JM, Stajich JM, Pericak-Vance M. Ocular motility in North Carolina autosomal dominant ataxia. *J Neuroophthalmol* 1996; 16: 91–5.
109. Farmer TW, Mustian VM. Vestibulocerebellar ataxia: a newly defined hereditary syndrome with periodic manifestations. *Arch Neurol* 1963; 8: 471–80.
110. Damji KF, Allingham RR, Pollock SC, et al. Periodic vestibulocerebellar ataxia, an autosomal dominant ataxia with defective smooth pursuit, is genetically distinct from other autosomal dominant ataxias. *Arch Neurol* 1996; 53: 338–44.
111. Escayg A, De Waard M, Lee DD, et al. Coding and noncoding variation of the human calcium-channel beta4-subunit gene CACNB4 in patients with idiopathic generalized epilepsy and episodic ataxia. *Am J Hum Genet* 2000; 66: 1531–9.
112. Jen JC, Wan J, Palos TP, Howard BD, Baloh RW. Mutation in the glutamate transporter EAAT1 causes episodic ataxia, hemiplegia, and seizures. *Neurology* 2005; 65: 529–34.
113. de Vries B, Mamsa H, Stam AH, et al. Episodic ataxia associated with EAAT1 mutation C186S affecting glutamate reuptake. *Arch Neurol* 2009; 66: 97–101.
114. Kerber KA, Jen JC, Lee H, Nelson SF, Baloh RW. A new episodic ataxia syndrome with linkage to chromosome 19q13. *Arch Neurol* 2007; 64: 749–52.
115. Julien J, Denier C, Ferrer X, et al. Sporadic late onset paroxysmal cerebellar ataxia in four unrelated patients: a new disease? *J Neurol* 2001; 248: 209–14.
116. Cha YH, Lee H, Jen JC, Kattah JC, Nelson SF, Baloh RW. Episodic vertical oscillopsia with progressive gait ataxia: clinical description of a new episodic syndrome and evidence of linkage to chromosome 13q. *J Neurol Neurosurg Psychiatry* 2007; 78: 1273–5.
117. Damak M, Riant F, Boukobza M, Tournier-Lasserve E, Bousser MG, Vahedi K. Late onset hereditary episodic ataxia. *J Neurol Neurosurg Psychiatry* 2009; 80: 566–8.

CHAPTER 27

Hereditary and Acquired Cerebellar Ataxias

George Koutsis and Nicholas W. Wood

Summary

'Cerebellar ataxia' refers to a clinical syndrome caused by damage to the cerebellum and its connections and characterized by lack of coordination most evident in gait, use of the extremities, speech, and ocular movement. Although individual ataxic disorders are relatively rare, the ataxias as a whole represent a common clinical problem. Acquired ataxias are the most frequent, but heredoataxias also contribute a substantial proportion of cases. Over the past two decades, neuroimaging and molecular genetics have revolutionized the field, shedding light on the aetiology of these diverse disorders.

The differential diagnosis of cerebellar ataxia is complex and consists of an extensive list of acquired and an ever-expanding list of recognized hereditary causes. Acquired causes include viral cerebellitis, space-occupying lesions, multiple sclerosis, alcoholic cerebellar degeneration, drug toxicity, paraneoplastic cerebellar degeneration, superficial siderosis, multiple system atrophy, and idiopathic late-onset cerebellar ataxia. Hereditary causes include inborn errors of metabolism, episodic ataxias, autosomal recessive cerebellar ataxias, autosomal dominant cerebellar ataxias (also known as spinocerebellar ataxias), X-linked ataxias, and mitochondrial ataxias. A systematic approach based on relatively straightforward clinical rules can be a useful guide to the diagnostic process. Determining the age of onset can limit the differential to congenital, early-onset (<25 years), and late-onset (>25 years) causes. Clarifying the mode of onset can further narrow down the list to acute-onset, subacute-onset, and insidious-onset causes. The presence of a non-progressive, intermittent, or progressive course can focus the diagnosis further. Deciding whether an acquired or hereditary cause should be sought reduces the differential to a manageable list. Finally, specific information gathered from the history, the examination (including extracerebellar and extraneural findings), and routine or directed investigations allows the correct diagnosis to be made in most cases.

Unfortunately, the treatment of cerebellar ataxia, both disease-modifying and symptomatic, remains poor. Among the multitude of disorders which are at present untreatable, it is important to promptly identify those ataxias which are amenable to treatment. Hopefully, as we gain insights into the molecular pathogenesis of ataxias effective disease-modifying therapies for some of the currently untreatable disorders will be identified.

Introduction

'Ataxia', a Greek word meaning lack of order, refers to a clinical syndrome characterized by disturbance of coordination most evident in gait, use of the extremities, speech, and ocular movement. 'Cerebellar ataxia' refers to ataxia caused by damage to the cerebellum and its connections. Ataxia can also result from sensory dysfunction due to lesions of the dorsal columns or proprioceptive peripheral neurons (sensory ataxia). In the present chapter, hereditary and acquired cerebellar ataxias are discussed in some detail. Clinically 'pure' cerebellar ataxia is a relatively rare phenomenon. Most disorders causing cerebellar ataxia also cause dysfunction of other neurological systems, and the extent to which other systems are involved varies. An attempt has been made to limit this chapter to disorders in which cerebellar ataxia can be the most prominent clinical feature.

Epidemiology

Data are lacking on the overall prevalence of ataxia in the general population. This is partly due to ataxia's being a clinical syndrome rather than a disease. Additionally, in the case of acquired ataxias some of the most common conditions, such as viral cerebellitis or acute drug toxicity, are of short duration and less suited to prevalence estimations. Epidemiological data on the hereditary ataxias are generally more comprehensive.

Acquired ataxias are far more frequent than hereditary ataxias, although an overall prevalence figure has not been reported. Quoting the frequency of some of the most common acquired ataxias should give a feel for their general prevalence in the population. Alcoholic cerebellar degeneration (ACD) is present in 11–27% of chronic alcohol users (1). Cerebellar infarction represents 3% of all infarcts (2). Acute cerebellitis represents 0.4% of children with neurological problems (3). Prevalence of multiple system atrophy (MSA) and idiopathic late-onset cerebellar ataxia (ILOCA) has been estimated at 4.4 and 8.4 in 100 000, respectively (4, 5).

The overall prevalence of heredoataxias is around 1 in 10 000. The autosomal recessive cerebellar ataxias (ARCAs) have a prevalence of 7 in 100 000, with Friedreich's ataxia (FRDA) being the most common followed by ataxia telangiectasia (AT) (6). The autosomal dominant cerebellar ataxias (ADCAs), also known as spinocerebellar ataxias (SCAs), have a prevalence of 3 in 100 000 (7). SCA3 is the most common, followed by SCA2, SCA6, SCA1, and SCA7 in approximate descending order of frequency (8). X-linked cerebellar ataxias are rare, with fragile X-associated tremor–ataxia syndrome (FXTAS) representing around 2% of patients in ataxia series (9). Mitochondrial ataxias are also rare, with no figure for their overall prevalence reported to date. The prevalence of congenital ataxias has been estimated at around 1.3 in 10 000 in the 6–22 age group (10).

The age of onset of cerebellar ataxias varies widely and covers the entire lifespan. In some cases, such as the congenital ataxias or AT, symptoms may develop in the first years of life. At the other end of the spectrum, certain ataxias can present in late adult life. Examples include MSA-C, FXTAS, and SCA6. Table 27.1 broadly divides ataxias based on the age of onset.

Table 27.1 Classification of cerebellar ataxias based on age of onset, mode of onset, disease course, and inheritance

Age of onset	Mode of onset and course		
Congenital	*Relatively non-progressive*		
	Non-hereditary		
	Chiari malformation		
	Dandy–Walker syndrome		
	Ataxic cerebral palsy		
	Hereditary		
	Joubert syndrome		
	Gillespie syndrome		
Early onset (<25 years)	*Acute onset with or without intermittent course*	*Subacute onset with or without progression*	*Insidious onset with chronic progression*
	Acquired	*Acquired*	*Acquired*
	Viral cerebellitis	Posterior fossa tumours (primary)	Chronic drug toxicity
	ADEM	Vascular malformations	Heavy metal poisoning
	Vascular causes	Relapsing MS	*Hereditary*
	Acute drug toxicity	SSPE	*Autosomal recessive*
	Trauma/hypoxia	Cerebellar abscess	FRDA
	Miller Fisher syndrome	Opsoclonus–myoclonus syndrome	AVED
	Basilar migraine		AT and AT-like disorder
	Conversion reaction		AOA 1 and 2
	Hereditary		WD
	Autosomal dominant		MSS
	Episodic ataxias		ARSACS
	Autosomal recessive		Ataxia CoQ10 deficiency
	Inborn errors of metabolism		GM2 gangliosidosis
	Urea cycle disorders		ABL
	Aminoacidopathies		RD
	Organic acidopathies		CTX
	PDH deficiency		NPC
			MLD
			VWMD
			PMEs
			X-linked
			Adrenoleucodystrophy
			PMD
			Mitochondrial disease
Late onset (>25 years)	*Acquired*	*Acquired*	*Acquired*
	Vascular causes	Relapsing MS	Alcoholic CD
	Acute drug toxicity	Posterior fossa tumours (metastatic)	Primary progressive MS
	Trauma/hypoxia/heat stroke	Vascular malformations	Chronic drug toxicity

(Continued)

Table 27.1 (Continued)

Age of onset	Mode of onset and course		
	Wernicke's encephalopathy	Paraneoplastic CD	Heavy metal poisoning
	Miller Fisher syndrome	Inflammatory diseases/vasculitides	Vitamin deficiency
		Cerebellar abscess	Superficial siderosis
		HIV infection	Gluten ataxia
		Whipple's disease	Anti-GAD ataxia
		Sporadic CJD	Hypothyroidism
		Hashimoto encephalopathy	CANVAS
			MSA
			ILOCA
			Hereditary
			Autosomal dominant
			Type I ADCAs
			Type II ADCAs
			Type III ADCAs
			GSS
			X-linked
			FXTAS
			Mitochondrial disease

ADEM, acute disseminated encephalomyelitis; PDH, pyruvate dehydrogenase; MS, multiple sclerosis; SSPE, subacute sclerosing panencephalitis; FRDA, Friedreich's ataxia; AVED, ataxia with vitamin E deficiency; AT, ataxia telangiectasia; AOA, ataxia with oculomotor apraxia; WD, Wilson disease; MSS, Marinesco–Sjögren syndrome; ARSACS, autosomal recessive ataxia of Charlevoix-Saguenay; ABL, abetalipoproteinaemia; RD, Refsum's disease; CTX, cerebrotendinous xanthomatosis; NPC, Niemann–Pick disease type C; MLD, metachromatic leucodystrophy; VWMD, vanishing white matter disease; PMEs, progressive myoclonic epilepsies; PMD, Pelizaeus–Merzbacher disease; CD, cerebellar degeneration; CJD, Creutzfeldt–Jakob disease; GAD, glutamic acid decarboxylase; MSA, multiple system atrophy; ILOCA, idiopathic late-onset cerebellar ataxia; ADCAs, autosomal dominant cerebellar ataxias; GSS, Gerstmann–Sträussler–Scheinker disease; FXTAS, fragile X-associated tremor–ataxia syndrome.

Aetiology and genetics

The potential causes of cerebellar ataxia comprise an extensive list of diverse entities which are summarized in Table 27.1. Although this table includes the common and most of the rarer causes of ataxia, it is by no means exhaustive.

Congenital ataxias can result from sporadic developmental anomalies, such as Chiari malformation and Dandy–Walker complex, or hereditary conditions which are often genetically heterogeneous, such as Joubert syndrome and Gillespie syndrome.

Acquired ataxias can have a wide range of causes including chronic alcohol use, drug toxicity, immune-mediated inflammation ranging from post-infectious cerebellitis to paraneoplastic syndromes, stroke, tumours, vitamin deficiency, endocrine abnormalities, CNS infection, and leptomeningeal iron deposition leading to superficial siderosis. MSA is a sporadic degenerative disease classified pathologically as an alpha-synucleinopathy, whose cause at present remains unknown. ILOCA, as the name suggests, is essentially a diagnosis of exclusion (1).

The specific genetic mutations underlying different heredoataxias are discussed in more detail in the relevant sections and summarized in Tables 27.5, 27.6, 27.7, and 27.8. In the case of episodic ataxias (Table 27.5), conventional mutations in ion channels are responsible for the disease manifestations (11). The ARCAs (Table 27.6) are a heterogeneous group of disorders caused by mutations in genes involved in mitochondrial function, metabolic pathways and DNA repair. With the exception of FRDA, which is caused by an intronic GAA expansion, ARCAs are caused by conventional mutations (6, 12). The ADCAs (Table 27.7) can be caused by mutations in diverse genes, ranging from ion channels to genes involved in transcription regulation, mitochondrial function, or protein phosphorylation. Three types of mutations are found: exonic CAG-repeat expansions (SCA1, 2, 3, 6, 7, 17, DRPLA), intronic trinucleotide or pentanucleotide expansions (SCA8, 10, 12, 31), and conventional mutations (SCA5, 11, 13, 14, 15/16, 27, 28, 35) (8, 13). Mitochondrial ataxias (Table 27.8) can be caused by conventional mutations in mitochondrial genes coding for transfer RNAs, ribosomal RNAs, and respiratory chain subunits, or in nuclear genes coding for respiratory chain subunits and assembly factors, proteins involved in intergenomic signalling, and mitochondrial transport machinery (14).

Topography and pathophysiology

All cerebellar ataxias are ultimately caused by dysfunction of the cerebellum itself or its connections. From a clinical viewpoint, lesions affecting midline cerebellar structures (vermis) primarily affect stance and gait, whereas lesions affecting the lateral hemispheres cause limb ataxia. As a general rule, appendicular motor impairment is ipsilateral to the side of the cerebellar lesion. Dysarthria is often caused by lesions in the paravermal regions, whereas oculomotor abnormalities can result from lesions in the so-called oculomotor vermis, which includes the inferiorly placed flocculonodular lobe (15).

The topography of cerebellar deficits becomes relevant in understanding the pathogenesis of specific cerebellar symptoms in ataxias resulting from focal damage. The pathophysiological mechanisms involved reflect the underlying causes, which include stroke, inflammation, tumours, and abscesses. However, most cerebellar ataxias result from diffuse damage to the cerebellum and lesion topography is less relevant.

Ataxia caused by diffuse cerebellar dysfunction can be divided from a pathophysiological perspective into conditions which affect the function of cerebellar neurons without causing neurodegeneration and conditions which affect structure and function concomitantly, resulting in cerebellar degeneration and atrophy. In the case of acquired ataxias, examples of conditions causing purely transitory functional effects include acute drug toxicity and basilar migraine. Acute ethanol-induced cerebellar ataxia may result from temporary inhibition of granule cell sensory responses (16). In basilar migraine the possibility of spreading depression affecting the cerebellar cortex has been raised (17). Paraneoplastic cerebellar disease may also cause functional loss without degeneration in the early stages. In cerebellar ataxia associated with Lambert–Eaton myasthenic syndrome, antibodies against voltage-gated calcium channels are thought to reduce transmission at the parallel fibre–Purkinje cell synapse (11). In the case of hereditary ataxias, transitory functional effects without neuronal loss are seen in some episodic ataxias (EAs). The ion channel mutations observed in EAs cause dominant-negative effects by affecting multimeric channel assembly, which impairs channel function (11).

Conditions which affect function through diffuse cerebellar neurodegeneration represent the majority of cerebellar ataxias. Cerebellar neurons are particularly vulnerable to oxidative stress, NMDA-mediated excitotoxicity, DNA repair/transcriptional dysregulation, or toxic protein accumulation (18). In the case of acquired ataxias, examples of conditions causing diffuse cell loss include ACD and MSA. In ACD a combination of ethanol with vitamin B_1 deficiency leads to diffuse cerebellar neuronal cell loss through mechanisms including excitotoxicity, oxidative stress, and apoptosis (1, 19, 20). In MSA, glial cytoplasmic and neuronal nuclear inclusions containing alpha-synuclein are thought to underlie the neurodegeneration observed primarily in the olives, pons, and cerebellum in cases of MSA-C (21). In the case of hereditary ataxias, different mechanisms underlie the neuronal loss seen in ARCAs and ADCAs. In ARCAs, loss-of-function mutations in genes involved in mitochondrial function, metabolic pathways, and DNA repair lead to neuronal cell death (6, 12). For example, in FRDA an intronic GAA repeat expansion in the gene coding for frataxin disturbs iron homeostasis and mitochondrial function (22). In ADCAs, three pathophysiological mechanisms are observed. Exonic CAG-repeat expansions lead to polyglutamine-containing inclusion bodies which cause toxic gain of function through aberrant protein aggregation. Intronic repeat expansions also cause toxic gain of function, but via RNA mechanisms. In the case of conventional mutation SCAs, haploinsufficiency (SCA5, 11, 15), or dominant-negative effects (SCA 13, 27) can underlie the pathogenesis of neuronal cell loss (8, 11, 23, 24).

Classification

Arriving at the correct diagnosis in a patient with cerebellar ataxia can be a daunting task, given the multitude of acquired causes and the ever-expanding list of recognized hereditary causes. A clinically useful classification is often the first step to a correct diagnosis. Classifying cerebellar ataxias according to the age of onset, mode of onset of symptoms, and course of the disease is a good starting point (Table 27.1) (25). Determining the age of onset, although not always straightforward, can narrow the differential diagnosis down by pointing to congenital early-onset (defined as <25 years for ataxias) or late-onset causes (25). The mode of onset, whether acute, subacute, or insidious, can also significantly limit the spectrum of potential causes. The presence of a non-progressive, intermittent, or progressive course can further focus the diagnostic process.

Dividing cerebellar disorders into non-hereditary and hereditary can be the next step in the diagnostic algorithm. A three-generation pedigree will allow adequate assessment of the family history, assisting in the identification of any hereditary ataxias. Autosomal dominant inheritance is suggested by affected members in consecutive generations, and it is always worth looking for evidence of male–male transmission which excludes X-linked and mitochondrial DNA inheritance. Autosomal recessive inheritance may be suggested by the presence of multiple affected members in a single generation or by evidence of consanguinity. X-linked transmission is characterized by affected males in the maternal line. Mitochondrial disease can be caused by mitochondrial or nuclear gene mutations. Mitochondrial mutations follow maternal inheritance. Nuclear mutations can be dominant or recessive. However it should be noted that up to 15% of apparently sporadic cases can have a hereditary cause (26).

Once the ataxic disorder has been broadly classified, the presence of characteristic constellations of extracerebellar and extraneural findings may allow the clinician to reach a specific diagnosis.

Clinical features

The patient with cerebellar ataxia may complain of gait unsteadiness, frequent falls, 'dizziness', clumsiness, slurring of speech, or blurring of vision. Features of the past medical history that may prove useful in the differential diagnosis include alcohol abuse, past episodes of optic neuritis, recent febrile illness, known malignancy, headache or vomiting, recent trauma, diarrhoea, diabetes, seizures, dysautonomic symptoms, symptoms of connective tissue disease, cardiac involvement, or deafness (Table 27.2).

On examination, the ataxic patient may have wide-based gait, difficulty in tandem gait, truncal ataxia, titubation, intention tremor, dysmetria, dysdiadochokinesis, hypotonia or slurring, and scanning dysarthria. Oculomotor assessment may reveal square-wave jerks, saccadic pursuit, dysmetric saccades, skew deviation, or gaze-evoked nystagmus. Oculomotor apraxia may be seen in disorders such as AT and ataxia with oculomotor apraxia (AOA). A cognitive cerebellar syndrome has been reported, but signs are very subtle and from a clinical viewpoint less relevant. Deficits may be more detectable in cases of acute cerebellar dysfunction, such as stroke (15). Careful examination of other neurological systems should be carried out to determine the presence of pigmentary retinopathy, ophthalmoplegia, hearing loss, pyramidal signs, extrapyramidal signs, myoclonus, sensory neuropathy, amyotrophy, areflexia, postural hypotension, or cognitive impairment. A careful general examination should also be carried out in order to reveal signs including Kayser–Fleischer rings, cataracts, oculocutaneous telangiectasias, skin rashes, dysmorphic features, short stature, scoliosis, pes cavus, tendon xanthomas, or hepatomegaly (Table 27.2).

Table 27.2 Clinical features that can aid in the differential diagnosis of cerebellar ataxia

Clinical feature	Possible diagnosis
From the history	
Alcohol abuse	Alcoholic CD, Wernicke's encephalopathy
Drug use and abuse	Drug toxicity, solvent toxicity, HIV
Recent or current infection	Viral/postviral cerebellitis, ADEM, Miller Fisher syndrome
Past optic neuritis	MS
Fever	Cerebellar abscess, viral cerebellitis, Whipple's disease
Hypertension	Vascular causes, cerebellar haemangioblastomas and phaeochromocytoma in VHL
Diabetes	Vascular causes, FRDA, anti-GAD ataxia, mitochondrial disease
Seizures	Tumours, inborn errors of metabolism, mitochondrial disease, PMEs, ADCAs (DRPLA, SCA17, SCA10, SCA14), GM2 gangliosidosis, NPC
Intermittent ataxia	Basilar migraine, inborn errors of metabolism, EAs
Hearing loss	Superficial siderosis, mitochondrial disease, RD, NPC
Dysautonomic symptoms	MSA, FXTAS
Headache and vomiting	Haemorrhage, abscess, tumour, basilar migraine, EA2
Diarrhoea	Gluten ataxia, Whipple's disease, deficiency states due to malabsorption
Hair loss	Hypothyroidism
Dry eyes-mouth, venous thrombosis, photosensitivity	Sjögren's syndrome, APS, SLE
Known malignancy	Paraneoplastic CD, metastatic disease, AT
Heavy metal exposure	Lead, mercury, or thallium ataxia
Precipitant infection or high protein load	Inherited metabolic disorders, VWMD
From the examination	
Extracerebellar findings	
Sensory neuropathy	Alcoholic CD, paraneoplastic CD, connective tissue disease, Miller Fisher syndrome, vitamin deficiency, heavy metal poisoning, CANVAS, ARCAs (including FRDA, AOA, AT, AVED, ABL), FXTAS, ADCAs
Amyotrophy	ARCAs, ADCAs, GM2 gangliosidosis
Reduced reflexes	Miller Fisher syndrome, paraneoplastic CD, ARCAs, SCA2
Ophthalmoplegia	MS, Wernicke's encephalopathy, Miller Fisher syndrome, mitochondrial disease, Whipple's disease, AOA1, ADCAs, NPC
Oculomotor apraxia	AT, ATLD, AOA1, AOA2
Lateralized brainstem signs	Vascular causes, posterior fossa tumours, MS
Pyramidal features	MS, ADEM, superficial siderosis, FRDA, AVED, GM2 gangliosidosis, CTX, ARSACS, mitochondrial disease, AT, AOA2, ADCAs, ALD, MLD, PMD
Myoclonus	CJD, gluten ataxia, Hashimoto encephalopathy, hypoxia, paraneoplastic CD, SSPE, MSA, PMEs, inborn errors of metabolism, GM2 gangliosidosis, CTX, mitochondrial disease, AT, AOA2, SCA14
Extrapyramidal features	MSA, ADCAs, FXTAS, GM2 gangliosidosis, CTX, AT, ATLD, AOA1, AOA2, WD, NPC
Cognitive impairment/mental retardation	Alcoholic CD, CJD, Hashimoto encephalopathy, MS, SSPE, hypothyroidism, ADCAs (DRPLA, SCA17, SCA13), GSS, FXTAS, GM2 gangliosidosis, CTX, mitochondrial disease, AOA1, AOA2, ARSACS, MSS, Gillespie syndrome, inborn errors of metabolism, NPC
Psychiatric disturbances	Alcoholic CD, paraneoplastic CD, CJD, Hashimoto encephalopathy, ADCAs (DRPLA, SCA17), GM2 gangliosidosis, CTX, mitochondrial disease, hypothyroidism, NPC, MLD
Retinitis pigmentosa	AVED, ABL, RD, mitochondrial disease
Degenerative maculopathy	ADCAII (SCA7)
Extraneural findings	
Short stature	Mitochondrial disease, MSS
Scoliosis	FRDA, AOA1, AOA2, MSS
Dysmorphic features	PDH deficiency, RD, MSS
Pes cavus	FRDA, other ARCAs
Cataracts	MSS, CTX
Aniridia	Gillespie syndrome
Kayser–Fleischer rings	WD

(Continued)

Table 27.2 (Continued)

Clinical feature	Possible diagnosis
Telangiectasias	AT, ACD
Skin rash	SLE, Lyme disease, Hartnup disease
Tendon xanthomas	CTX
Cervical lipomas	Mitochondrial disease
Arthritis	SLE, Whipple's disease
Cardiomyopathy	Alcoholic CD, vascular causes, FRDA, AVED, ABL, RD
Hepatomegaly	Urea cycle disorders, NPC

CD, cerebellar degeneration; ADEM, acute disseminated encephalomyelitis; MS, multiple sclerosis; VHL, von Hippel–Lindau disease; FRDA, Friedreich's ataxia; GAD, glutamic acid decarboxylase; PMEs, progressive myoclonic epilepsies; ADCA, autosomal dominant cerebellar ataxia; SCA, spinocerebellar ataxia; DRPLA, dentatorubral–pallidoluysian atrophy; NPC, Niemann–Pick disease type C; EA, episodic ataxia; RD, Refsum's disease; MSA, multiple system atrophy; FXTAS, fragile X tremor–ataxia syndrome; APS, antiphospholipid syndrome; SLE, systemic lupus erythematosus; AT, ataxia telangiectasia; VWMD, vanishing white matter disease; CANVAS, cerebellar ataxia with neuropathy and bilateral vestibular areflexia syndrome; ARCAs, autosomal recessive cerebellar ataxias; AOA, ataxia with oculomotor apraxia; AVED, ataxia with vitamin E deficiency; ABL, abetalipoproteinaemia; ATLD, ataxia telangiectasia-like disorder; CTX, cerebrotendinous xanthomatosis; ARSACS, autosomal recessive spastic ataxia of Charlevoix-Saguenay; ALD, adrenoleucodystrophy; MLD, metachromatic leucodystrophy; PMD, Pelizaeus–Merzbacher disease; CJD, Creutzfeldt–Jakob disease; SSPE, subacute sclerosing panencephalitis; GSS, Gerstmann–Sträussler–Scheinker disease; WD, Wilson disease; MSS: Marinesco–Sjögren syndrome; PDH, pyruvate dehydrogenase.

Investigations

Magnetic resonance imaging

The advent of MRI has revolutionized the diagnosis of cerebellar ataxias. A large number of acquired causes can be diagnosed with its assistance. These include tumours, abscesses, demyelinating lesions, other inflammatory lesions, infarcts, haemorrhages, or superficial siderosis. Gradient-echo T_2^* sequences are particularly sensitive for picking up superficial siderosis. MRI can also assist in the diagnosis of sporadic degenerative ataxias, such as Creutzfeldt–Jakob disease (CJD), MSA, and ILOCA, as well as many of the hereditary degenerative ataxias. However, it should be noted that in such cases MRI findings are often non-specific, consisting of cerebellar and/or brainstem atrophy (25).

The absence of findings on MRI can also be helpful in the diagnosis of cerebellar ataxia, with paraneoplastic CD (in its early stages) and FRDA being characteristic examples.

Congenital ataxias, including Chiari malformation, Dandy–Walker syndrome and Joubert syndrome, also have characteristic MRI appearances.

Other tests including genetic testing

A multitude of other diagnostic tests can shed light on the patient with cerebellar ataxia. These include electrophysiological tests (nerve conduction studies, EMG, EEG, visual evoked potentials, somatosensory evoked potentials, and central motor conduction time), CSF analysis, and numerous routine and more specialized blood tests. Such tests may steer the diagnosis towards more specific disorders (Table 27.3).

Regarding specific genetic testing, guidelines have been recently published by a European task force (27). In the case of ADCAs, testing should include SCA1, 2, 3, 6, and 7. These tests are widely available. For episodic ataxias (EAs), testing for EA1 and EA2, available in specialist and research laboratories, is recommended. Concerning ARCAs, testing for FRDA (widely available) should be initially requested. Testing for AT, AOA1 and AOA2 should be done in patients with positive biochemical findings, such as hypoalbuminaemia, hypercholesterolaemia or elevated alpha-fetoprotein (AFP). For the X-linked ataxias, testing for FXTAS, which is widely available, is recommended. Testing for other rarer hereditary ataxias is currently only performed within research settings.

Management

The treatment of cerebellar ataxia, both disease-modifying and symptomatic, remains poor. Significant advances made on pathogenesis have not yet been translated into successful disease-modifying therapy. However, among numerous cerebellar disorders which are at present untreatable, it is important to identify those ataxias which are amenable to disease modification. Within the acquired ataxias, these include disorders due to toxic effects, vitamin deficiencies, vascular pathology, immune-mediated inflammation and neurodegeneration, tumours or endocrine abnormalities. Among the hereditary ataxias, conditions amenable to modification include some autosomal recessive metabolic disorders, such as ataxia with vitamin E deficiency (AVED), Wilson disease (WD), Refsum's disease (RD), cerebrotendinous xanthomatosis (CTX), ataxia with co-enzyme Q10 deficiency and Niemann–Pick disease type C (NPC). In the EAs carbonic anhydrase inhibitors can reduce the frequency of attacks and may have an effect on disease progression (25). More details on specific disease-modifying treatments are given in the corresponding paragraphs on different ataxias.

In the case of FRDA, data implicating oxidative stress in its pathogenesis have led to therapeutic trials involving antioxidant agents such as vitamin E, co-enzyme Q10, and idebenone. No definitive improvement in ataxia was clearly demonstrated in these trials. A potentially significant cardioprotective effect of idebenone reported initially has not been borne out by more recent larger trials (28, 29).

Regarding symptomatic treatment, several approaches have been tried with very limited success. Findings implicating the cholinergic system in cerebellar ataxia led to trials involving physostigmine, choline, and choline derivatives. Overall, results were disappointing (30). Attempts at manipulating the serotoninergic and dopaminergic systems were also largely ineffective. Minor effects were reported for buspirone and amantadine (30, 31). Clonazepam, propranolol, and primidone, used in action tremor, have also been tried in cerebellar tremor with limited success (29). Aminopyridines may have some effect in cerebellar oculomotor disturbances (32).

Table 27.3 Investigating the patient with cerebellar ataxia (more widely used tests are displayed first, and blood and CSF tests are grouped together)

Investigation	Purpose	Notes
Imaging, electrophysiology, specialist assessment, biopsies		
Brain MRI	Vascular causes, MS, ADEM, inflammatory disease, tumours, infection, trauma, congenital malformations, superficial siderosis, CJD, cerebellar atrophy in hereditary and acquired degenerative ataxias, molar tooth sign in Joubert syndrome	Can exclude common causes of sporadic ataxia Can also assist in hereditary and degenerative ataxias
Spinal cord MRI	MS, ADEM, inflammatory disease, Chiari malformations, superficial siderosis, vitamin deficiency, ARCAs	
ECG, echocardiography	Vascular causes, FRDA, AVED, RD	
Nerve conduction studies, EMG	ACD, paraneoplastic CD, inflammatory disease, MFS, ARCAs, ADCAs, RD, MSA	Abnormal anal sphincter EMG in MSA
EEG	CJD, mitochondrial disease, DRPLA, SCA17, SCA10, SCA14, PMEs, inborn errors of metabolism, SSPE, NPC	
Ophthalmology, VEP, ERG	WD, MS, ADCA II, AVED, mitochondrial diseases, ABL, RD	Kayser–Fleischer rings (WD), SCA7 retinal degeneration
SSEP	MS, ADEM, ARCAs, ADCAs, vitamin deficiency, superficial siderosis	
TMS	MS, ADEM, ARCAs, ADCAs, vitamin deficiency, superficial siderosis	
Chest and abdominal CT, pelvic US, mammography, testicular US, PET, gallium scan	Tumours, paraneoplastic CD, sarcoidosis	
ENT examination	Mitochondrial disease, FRDA, RD, superficial siderosis	
Autonomic function tests	MSA, FXTAS	
Muscle biopsy	Mitochondrial disease	
Small bowel biopsy	Coeliac disease, Whipple's disease	
Skin biopsy	NPC (fibroblast culture), PMEs (Lafora body disease)	
Blood and urine tests		
U&E, glucose, LFTs, FBC, ESR	Systemic disease, inflammatory disease, infection, ACD, inborn errors of metabolism, AOA1	Low albumin in AOA1
TFTs, anti-thyroid antibodies	Hypothyroidism, Hashimoto encephalopathy	
HbA1c	Vascular causes, FRDA, mitochondrial disease, anti-GAD ataxia	
Arterial blood gases	Inherited metabolic disorders	
ANA, antiDNA, antiENA, ACL	Inflammatory disease (SLE, Sjögren's syndrome, APS)	
SACE	Neurosarcoidosis	
Serum immunoglobulins	Inflammatory disease, AT	
Cholesterol, lipoprotein electrophoresis	Vascular causes, ABL, AOA1, AOA2	
Viral serology	Viral/postviral cerebellitis	
Tumour markers	Tumours, paraneoplastic CD	
Antigliadin and antiendomysial antibodies	Gluten ataxia	Not very specific
Antineuronal antibodies	Paraneoplastic CD	Most commonly with SCLC, breast, ovarian, lymphoma
Anti-GAD antibodies	Ataxia with anti-GAD antibodies	Association with stiffperson syndrome
Anti-GQ1b antibodies	MFS	
Ethanol and drug levels	Ethanol and drug toxicity	
Vitamin E	AVED, ABL, other deficiency states	
Vitamin B_1, B_{12}	ACD, ABL, other deficiency states	
Serum alpha-fetoprotein	AT, AOA2, malignancy	
Serum caeruloplasmin, 24hr urine copper	WD	
Plasma ammonia, lactate and pyruvate	Urea cycle disorders, disorders of amino acid and organic acid metabolism, mitochondrial disease, PDH deficiency	Consider in early-onset acute or intermittent phenotypes
Genetic testing *FRDA, ATXN1,2,3,7, CACNA1A, TBP, FMR1, ATM, APTX, SNTX, KCNA1*	FRDA, SCA1,2,3,6,7,17, FXTAS, AT, AOA1, AOA2, EAs	Consider also in undiagnosed sporadic ataxias

(Continued)

Table 27.3 (Continued)

Investigation	Purpose	Notes
Serum and urine amino acids, urine organic acids	Disorders of amino acid and organic acid metabolism, PDH deficiency	Consider in early-onset acute or intermittent phenotypes
Blood film for acanthocytes	ABL	
Serum cholestanol	CXT	
Serum phytanic acid	RD	
Blood VLCFA	Adrenoleucodystrophy	
White cell enzymes (hexosaminidase A, arylsulfatase A, PDH, chitotriosidase)	GM2 gangliosidosis, MLD, PDH deficiency, NPC	
Serum biotinidase	Biotinidase deficiency	
Serum heavy metals	Heavy metal toxicity	
CSF analysis		
CSF analysis including OCB	Viral cerebellitis, MS, ADEM, paraneoplastic CD, inflammatory disease, MFS, HIV, CJD, RD	
CSF ACE	Neurosarcoidosis	
CSF antineuronal antibodies	Paraneoplastic CD	
CSF analysis for protein 14–3-3	CJD	

MS, multiple sclerosis; ADEM, acute disseminated encephalomyelitis; CJD, Creutzfeldt–Jakob disease; ARCAs, autosomal recessive cerebellar ataxias; FRDA, Friedreich's ataxia; AVED, ataxia with vitamin E deficiency; RD, Refsum's disease; CD, cerebellar degeneration; MFS, Miller Fisher syndrome; ADCAs, autosomal dominant cerebellar ataxias; MSA, multiple system atrophy; DRPLA, dentatorubral-pallidoluysian atrophy; SCA, spinocerebellar ataxia; PMEs, progressive myoclonic epilepsies; SSPE, subacute sclerosing panencephalitis; NPC, Niemann–Pick disease type C; WD, Wilson disease; VEP, visual evoked potentials; ERG, electroretinogram; ABL, abetalipoproteinaemia; SSEP, somatosensory evoked potentials; TMS, transcranial magnetic stimulation; FXTAS, fragile X tremor–ataxia syndrome; AOA, ataxia with oculomotor apraxia; TFTs, thyroid function tests; GAD, glutamic acid decarboxylase; ANA, antinuclear antibodies; ENA, extractable nuclear antigen; ACL, anticardiolipin antibodies; SLE, systemic lupus erythematosus; APS, antiphospholipid syndrome; SACE, serum angiotensin-converting enzyme; AT, ataxia telangiectasia; SCLC, small-cell lung cancer; PDH, pyruvate dehydrogenase; EA, episodic ataxia; CTX, cerebrotendinous xanthomatosis; VLCFA, very long chain fatty acids; MLD, metachromatic leucodystrophy; OCB, oligoclonal bands; ACE, angiotensin-converting enzyme.

Rehabilitation measures are particularly important in patients with ataxia to help them maintain as good a functional status as possible and cope with activities of daily living. Regular physiotherapy, if possible, and occupational therapy are recommended (18). Speech therapy can be helpful with cerebellar dysarthria. Assistive devices including orthoses, sticks, or strollers should be used to improve ambulation. Wheelchair and bed-bound patients require specific care to avoid complications (33).

Specific ataxic disorders

In the analysis that follows, non-hereditary and hereditary causes of cerebellar ataxia are discussed separately in order to ensure a more coherent presentation.

The non-hereditary congenital and acquired cerebellar ataxias

Congenital non-hereditary ataxias

Congenital ataxias are due to anomalies present at birth. They are, by definition, relatively non-progressive. Because the cerebellar system is functionally incomplete at birth, they can initially manifest with non-specific hypotonia and developmental delay. More typical ataxic symptoms are usually recognized after the first year of life (34). The demonstration of non-progression against the background of a child acquiring new motor skills can be difficult. In general, the combination of severe cerebellar hypoplasia on imaging with a child who is not profoundly ataxic can point towards a congenital ataxia (25). Certain congenital ataxias, such as Chiari malformation, can present much later in life.

Chiari malformation

Chiari type I malformation is a common condition (prevalence 1 in 1000 in the general population) characterized by cerebellar tonsillar herniation through the foramen magnum. A proportion of children with Chiari type I can present with ataxia (35). Other manifestations include suboccipital headache, vertigo, blurred vision, lower cranial nerve involvement, and long tract signs. Symptom onset is usually in the second or third decade. MRI establishes the diagnosis. Surgical decompression is recommended in symptomatic patients (36).

Dandy–Walker syndrome

This is a relatively common malformation occurring in 1 in 5000 infants. The key components include hypoplasia of the cerebellar vermis and cystic dilatation of the fourth ventricle, diagnosed on MRI. It can be associated with macrocephaly and hydrocephalus. Many patients have ataxia and nystagmus as a prominent feature (37).

Ataxic cerebral palsy

A small percentage of children with cerebral palsy present with 'ataxic cerebral palsy' (38). It is believed that a significant proportion of congenital genetic ataxias may be masked under this umbrella term (25).

Acute-onset acquired ataxias with or without intermittent course

Vascular causes

Cerebellar infarction is a cause of acute-onset ataxia that can be unilateral and is usually associated with other brainstem symptoms.

Surgical treatment may be necessary in a subset of these patients to avoid brainstem compression (2). Cerebellar haemorrhage, often associated with reduced level of consciousness, may require emergency neurosurgical evacuation (39).

Acute drug toxicity

The direct toxic effect of several drugs, including ethanol, antiepileptics, and lithium, is a common cause of acute cerebellar ataxia (19, 40, 41). Immediate cessation of exposure is often therapeutic (1).

Acute viral/postviral cerebellitis

An acute-onset ataxia can often result from viral/postviral cerebellitis in childhood. A large number of viruses has been implicated, including varicella, measles, mumps, and rubella (most common), as well as influenza, para-influenza, Coxsackie virus, herpes simplex virus, cytomegalovirus, Epstein–Barr virus, paramyxovirus, and poliovirus (42). *Mycoplasma pneumoniae*, *Borrelia burgdoferi*, *Bordetella pertussis*, *Coxiella burnetii*, and *Salmonella typhi* have also been associated with cerebellitis (43). MRI often shows diffuse increased signal on T_2 images in the cerebellar hemispheres (44). Antivirals, antibiotics, and steroids are recommended in the management of acute cerebellitis (3).

Acute disseminated encephalomyelitis

Ataxia can be a prominent symptom of acute disseminated encephalomyelitis (ADEM), a postinfectious demyelinating disease most commonly observed in children. Up to 75% of patients report an antecedent infection or vaccination (45). Characteristic MRI findings and the usual absence of oligoclonal bands (OCBs) in the CSF can assist in making the diagnosis (46). Steroids, intravenous immunoglobulin (IVIG), and plasma exchange are used therapeutically (45).

Traumatic brain injury/hypoxia/heat stroke

Acute ataxia may occasionally develop following traumatic brain injury (47) or acute hypoxia, and sometimes as a component of acute mountain sickness (48) or as a result of acute heat stroke (49). Management of posterior fossa trauma is initially directed to stabilizing vital functions and controlling intracranial pressure. Steroids are not recommended (50). Steroids are used in acute mountain sickness (48).

Wernicke's encephalopathy

Acute-onset ataxia is a prominent symptom of Wernicke's encephalopathy, which is characterized by the 'classic triad' of confusional state, ataxia, and eye signs (nystagmus and ophthalmoplegia). It is caused by thiamine deficiency, often, but not always, associated with alcohol abuse. Intravenous thiamine should be given without delay to avoid long-term complications (51).

Miller Fisher syndrome

An acute-onset ataxia is one of the three classic features comprising Miller Fisher syndrome (MFS), the other two being ophthalmoplegia and areflexia (52). The presence of anti-GQ1B anti-ganglioside antibodies characterizes MFS, which is thought to be part of a spectrum including Bickerstaff's encephalitis. Brain MRI is usually unremarkable. Treatment is with IVIG or plasma exchange. The outcome is usually good (53).

Basilar migraine

Acute ataxia is often a prominent symptom of basilar-type migraine, which can also include other brainstem manifestations, such as dysarthria, vertigo, tinnitus, diplopia, and bilateral paraesthesias, without motor deficit. It is more commonly seen in adolescent girls (17). Treatment is as for more typical migraine. Labyrinthine sedative drugs can also be used symptomatically (54).

Conversion reaction

Ataxia is a common conversion reaction in children, particularly in the 5–10-year-old age group. Psychosocial stressors can be identified in most cases (55).

Subacute-onset acquired ataxias

Relapsing multiple sclerosis

Subacute-onset ataxia can develop within the context of a multiple sclerosis (MS) attack. Previous episodes of optic neuritis, often undetected, can shed light on the diagnosis. A 'pure' cerebellar ataxia is the presenting symptom of MS in less than 3% of cases (56). Much more often other brainstem or long-tract signs accompany the ataxia. Characteristic findings on MRI, delayed visual evoked potentials, and the presence of OCBs in the CSF assist in the diagnosis. Steroids are used to treat the attacks.

Tumours

Posterior fossa tumours can be a relatively common cause of subacute-onset cerebellar ataxia, which is often accompanied by headache and vomiting (57). They are more common in children. Primary tumours, such as cystic cerebellar astrocytoma, medulloblastoma, and ependymoma, predominate in childhood. Metastatic tumours are more common in adults (58). Cerebellar haemangioblastomas are vascular, and cystic tumours of the posterior fossa often found in patients with von Hippel–Lindau disease. These patients require a multidisciplinary approach to management (59).

Vascular malformations

Rarely, a vascular anomaly in the posterior fossa, such as a dural fistula or an arteriovenous malformation, can cause a subacute to chronic cerebellar syndrome. Surgical or endovascular approaches to treatment are recommended when appropriate (60, 61).

Paraneoplastic cerebellar degeneration

Paraneoplastic cerebellar degeneration (PCD) is an immune-mediated disorder characterized by degeneration of the cerebellar cortex, which occurs most frequently in association with small cell lung cancer, breast and ovarian cancer, and Hodgkin's lymphoma (62). The most commonly detected antineuronal antibodies in PCD and their associated tumours are shown in Table 27.4 (62, 63). At presentation, MRI is often unremarkable in patients with PCD, although atrophy develops over time (1). In children with an underlying neuroblastoma, cerebellar ataxia may accompany the classic opsoclonus–myoclonus syndrome (64). In general, treatment of the underlying tumour and immunosuppressive therapy may be helpful in PCD if given early on. However, more often than not the clinical picture is unresponsive to therapy (1).

Infectious causes

HIV infection has been associated with cerebellar ataxia, typically resulting from lesions caused by opportunistic infections such as toxoplasmosis and progressive multifocal leucoencephalopathy. Primary cerebellar degeneration associated with HIV infection can also result in a more insidious-onset ataxia (65). Specific treatment

Table 27.4 Autoantibodies and associated malignancies in paraneoplastic cerebellar degeneration

Autoantibody	Associated malignancy	Associated paraneoplastic syndromes
Anti-Yo	Ovarian, breast	
Anti-Hu	SCLC	PEM, sensory neuronopathy
Anti-Ri	SCLC, NSCLC, breast	Opsoclonus–myoclonus
Anti-Tr	Hodgkin's lymphoma	
Anti-Ma	NSCLC, breast, colonic	Brainstem dysfunction
Anti-CV2/CRMP5	SCLC, thymoma	PEM, sensory neuronopathy
Anti-Ta/Ma2	Testicular	Limbic encephalopathy
Anti-VGCC	SCLC	LEMS
Anti-mGluR1	Hodgkin's lymphoma	
Anti-ZIC4	SCLC	

SCLC, small-cell lung cancer; NSCLC, non-small-cell lung cancer; PEM, paraneoplastic encephalomyelitis; LEMS, Lambert–Eaton myasthenic syndrome.

against opportunistic infections and highly active antiretroviral therapy should be instituted (66).

Cerebellar ataxia of subacute onset is a prominent CNS manifestation in patients with Whipple's disease. Systemic symptoms of Whipple's disease include fever, weight loss, arthralgia, nausea, and diarrhoea. Other neurological manifestations include altered conscious level, hallucinations, ophthalmoplegia, nystagmus, myoclonus, and oculomasticatory myorrhythmia (highly characteristic, if not pathognomonic) (67). Patients often have multiple enhancing lesions on MRI. Several antibiotic combinations have been used to treat these patients (68).

A cerebellar abscess can also be the cause of a subacute ataxia and will often need neurosurgical drainage (69).

Subacute sclerosing panencephalitis

Cerebellar ataxia can be a prominent symptom in some patients with subacute sclerosing panencephalitis (SSPE). SSPE is caused by persistent infection of the brain by an aberrant measles virus and is a disorder of childhood. It is extremely rare in developed countries with widespread vaccination, but more common in developing countries. The EEG may show characteristic periodic complexes and MRI, although normal in the initial stages, may later show diffuse T_2 signal increase especially in the periventricular and subcortical white matter (70). Isoprinosine, alpha-interferon, and ribavirin have been used therapeutically in SSPE but results have overall been disappointing (70).

Inflammatory diseases/vasculitides

Cerebellar ataxia has been reported as a rare finding in patients with systemic lupus erythematosus (SLE) (71), primary Sjögren's syndrome (72), and antiphospholipid syndrome (73). Multifocal lesions are usually present on MRI (73). Ataxia is also a common symptom in patients with neurosarcoidosis (74). Patients with CNS vasculitides, such as Behçet's disease, may also feature cerebellar ataxia as a prominent symptom (75). Corticosteroids and other immunosuppressive drugs have been used with good response.

Sporadic Creutzfeldt–Jakob disease

A subacute-onset ataxia is often the first symptom of the ataxic variant of sporadic Creutzfeldt–Jakob disease (sCJD) (1). As the disease progresses dementia becomes prominent. The EEG may show characteristic periodic discharges (76). MRI reveals basal ganglia hyperintensities and the CSF shows increased concentration of 14-3-3 proteins (77). No effective treatments are known at present.

Hashimoto encephalopathy

Hashimoto encephalopathy is characterized by cognitive changes accompanied by ataxia, tremor, and myoclonus in the presence of anti-thyroid antibodies. It can mimic the ataxic variant of sCJD. It responds well to steroid therapy (78).

Insidious-onset acquired ataxias with chronic progression

Alcoholic cerebellar degeneration (ACD)

ACD is thought to be one of the most common forms of chronic cerebellar ataxia and occurs primarily in middle-aged men with a history of chronic alcohol abuse (1). The pathogenesis is complex and is thought to involve both the toxic action of alcohol and the sequelae of thiamine deficiency (1). MRI characteristically reveals vermal cerebellar atrophy (79). Strict abstinence and vitamin B_1 supplementation are recommended and can lead to symptomatic improvement (1).

Chronic drug and solvent toxicity/heavy metal poisoning

Apart from the acute toxic effect of drugs on the cerebellum, an insidious cerebellar syndrome can ensue following chronic use in certain cases. Such cases include phenytoin (80), lithium (81), amiodarone (82), anticancer drugs such as 5-fluorouracil (83), and solvents such as toluene (84). Poisoning with heavy metals including organo-lead compounds, mercury, and thallium can also cause insidious cerebellar ataxia (1). The most important therapeutic measure for chronic toxicity is immediate discontinuation of exposure (1).

Primary progressive multiple sclerosis

Primary progressive multiple sclerosis (PPMS) manifests in 10–15% of patients as a chronic progressive ataxic syndrome with prominent cerebellar features (85). Such a presentation is seen in only about 1% of MS patients. Given the often scarce MRI findings in PPMS, positive OCB can be central to the diagnosis. PPMS responds poorly to disease-modifying treatment (85).

Vitamin B and E deficiency

An insidious-onset cerebellar ataxia can occur following deficiency in vitamin E (86), thiamine (87), or cobalamin (88), often within the context of malabsorption in gastrointestinal disease. Vitamin supplementation can arrest or even improve the neurological picture.

Superficial siderosis of the CNS

Superficial siderosis of the CNS is caused by deposition of haemosiderin in the leptomeninges and subpial layers of the brain and spinal cord. The clinical syndrome is characterized by insidious onset cerebellar ataxia, sensorineural deafness, and pyramidal tract signs (89). The underlying cause is repeated subarachnoid bleeding from various sources (90). Characteristic rim hyperintensities on T_2* imaging are seen on MRI. The CSF is usually xanthocromic with a high protein content. If the cause of chronic bleeding can be identified and surgically removed, patients may stabilize (89).

Ataxia associated with anti-GAD antibodies

A cerebellar ataxia of insidious onset, suggesting a degenerative process, has been reported in patients with anti-glutamic acid decarboxylase (anti-GAD) antibodies. It is associated with cerebellar atrophy on MRI in half of the cases (91). Many of these patients also have type 1 diabetes (92). IVIG and other immunosuppressive regimes have been tried in anti-GAD ataxia with variable results (1, 92).

Gluten ataxia

A cerebellar ataxia of insidious onset, occasionally associated with myoclonus, has been reported to be the most common neurological manifestation in patients with coeliac disease. This association has been termed 'gluten ataxia' and is often found in patients with antigliadin antibodies and silent enteropathy (93). Patients also have one or more types of transglutaminase antibody. Sixty% of patients have cerebellar atrophy on MRI (94). A gluten-free diet should be started without delay, but response depends on the duration of ataxia. IVIG has also been used to treat gluten ataxia in conjunction with dietary measures (94).

Hypothyroidism

Hypothyroidism has long been recognized as a subacute to chronic cause of cerebellar ataxia. Thyroxine treatment can reverse the symptoms (95).

Cerebellar ataxia with neuropathy and bilateral vestibular areflexia syndrome (CANVAS)

CANVAS is a late-onset ataxia characterized by the triad of insidious-onset cerebellar dysfunction, bilateral vestibulopathy, and sensory neuronopathy. Initially described in the early 1990s, it was recognized as a distinct syndrome in 2004. Patients characteristically have an impaired visually enhanced vestibulo-ocular reflex. Brain MRI shows cerebellar atrophy in most cases. The identification of two affected sibling pairs has raised the possibility of a late-onset recessive disorder (96).

Multiple system atrophy (see also Chapter 13)

Multiple system atrophy (MSA) is a late-onset (usually sixth decade) progressive neurodegenerative disease characterized by severe dysautonomia, parkinsonism, and cerebellar ataxia. In around 20% of European patients the cerebellar component is initially predominant (MSA-C), and the other manifestations only become obvious with time (1). MSA represents around 30% of adult-onset cerebellar ataxias (26). It is associated with severe brainstem and cerebellar atrophy, as well as pontine and middle cerebellar peduncle hyperintensity (1). Consensus criteria that assist in the diagnosis of MSA have recently been published by an international task force (97). Treatment of the cerebellar component of MSA is disappointing (21).

Idiopathic late-onset ataxia

Idiopathic late-onset ataxia (ILOCA) is the most common late-onset cerebellar ataxia (5). As with MSA, onset is in the sixth decade. However, although slowly progressive, it is a more benign condition and the lasting absence of dysautonomia differentiates it from MSA-C. It is characterized by a relatively pure cerebellar ataxia with mild sensory and pyramidal signs (1). Diagnosis can only be made following the exclusion of acquired and inherited causes of ataxia. MRI shows cerebellar atrophy without associated brainstem atrophy (98). Treatment, as in all degenerative ataxias, is disappointing.

The hereditary cerebellar ataxias

Congenital hereditary ataxias

Rare developmental anomalies associated with vermal or cerebellar agenesis or hypoplasia may give rise to congenital ataxia. Most of them are now thought to be genetic and follow autosomal recessive inheritance. Two of the most widely recognized are the Joubert and Gillespie syndromes (99). Others include the pontocerebellar hypoplasias and congenital disorders of glycosylation.

Joubert syndrome

Joubert syndrome is a rare genetically heterogeneous inherited congenital ataxia. It is characterized by hypotonia evolving into ataxia and developmental delay, neonatal respiratory disturbances, and oculomotor abnormalities. It is defined by the presence of a characteristic MRI finding in the posterior fossa known as the 'molar tooth' sign (100).

Gillespie syndrome

Gillespie syndrome is a rare inherited congenital ataxia characterized by the triad of ataxia, aniridia, and mental retardation. The genetic causes have not been fully elucidated. MRI reveals cerebellar, and especially vermal, hypoplasia (101).

Acute-onset hereditary ataxias with or without intermittent course

Episodic ataxias (EAs)

The EAs are an expanding group of dominantly inherited disorders characterized by intermittent episodes of acute cerebellar dysfunction, with more subtle residual neurological dysfunction between episodes. They belong to the large family of hereditary channelopathies. Seven EAs have been recognized to date with four genes identified (Table 27.5), but the main forms are EA1 and EA2 (6, 102).

Episodic ataxia 1

EA1 is an autosomal dominant potassium channelopathy caused by mutations in the *KCNA1* gene. It is characterized by brief attacks of ataxia (lasting seconds to minutes), often triggered by emotional stress, fatigue, postural changes or startle, and interictal myokymia. Onset is in childhood. It may respond to antiepileptic medications or acetazolamide (103).

Episodic ataxia 2

EA2, the most common EA, is an autosomal dominant calcium channelopathy caused by mutations in the *CACNA1A* gene. It is characterized by more prolonged attacks of ataxia (lasting hours to days), often triggered by exercise, emotional stress, caffeine, or alcohol, and interictal residual ataxia with nystagmus. Onset, as in EA1, is in childhood. Acute attacks respond well to acetazolamide. EA2 is allelic to familial hemiplegic migraine (FHM) and SCA6 (104).

Inborn errors of metabolism

Inborn errors of metabolism can present with acute or intermittent ataxia often due to metabolic decompensation in response to dietary intake or intercurrent illness. Inheritance is usually autosomal recessive. An early-onset ataxia with intermittent course, associated

Table 27.5 The hereditary episodic ataxias (all autosomal dominant)

Episodic ataxia	Gene/locus	Frequency	Duration of attacks	Other manifestations	Interictal manifestations	Clinical notes
EA1	*KCNA1*/12q13	Relatively common	Seconds to minutes	None	Myokymia	
EA2	*CACNA1A*/19p13	Most common	Hours to days	Vertigo, nausea, vomiting, headache	Ataxia, nystagmus	Progressive ataxia
EA3	1q42	Rare	Minutes to hours	Vertigo, tinnitus, myokymia	None	
EA4	NK	Rare	Brief	Vertigo, diplopia	Ataxia, nystagmus	Later onset, progressive ataxia
EA5	*CACNB4beta*/ 2q22–23	Rare	Hours	Vertigo	Ataxia, nystagmus, seizures	Progressive ataxia
EA6	*SLC1A3*/p13	Rare	Hours	Cognitive impairment	Ataxia, seizures	Progressive ataxia
EA7	19q13	Rare	Hours to days	Vertigo, dysarthria	None	

EA, episodic ataxia; NK, not known

encephalopathy, seizures, and developmental delay should raise the possibility of inherited metabolic ataxia, especially urea cycle disorders (including ornithine transcarbamylase deficiency, which is X-linked), amino acidopathies (including Hartnup and maple syrup urine disease), organic acidopathies (including biotinidase deficiency), and pyruvate dehydrogenase deficiency. Screening for these disorders might include a full blood count, liver function tests, arterial blood gases, blood ammonia, lactate, pyruvate, and ketone, plasma and urinary amino acids, urinary organic acids, and serum biotinidase (Table 27.3) (105). Therapeutic management includes dietary restrictions and vitamin administration, such as biotin in the case of biotinidase deficiency (106).

Insidious-onset hereditary ataxias with chronic progression

Autosomal recessive cerebellar ataxias

Most ARCAs are early-onset disorders, although exceptions to this rule are well documented. They are characterized by spinocerebellar ataxia, involving both the cerebellum and the dorsal columns, with associated peripheral neuropathy, often leading to areflexia, and common involvement outside the nervous system (12). The prototype and most common ARCA is FRDA. MRI can help distinguish between the ARCAs by revealing the presence or absence of cerebellar atrophy. FRDA, AVED, abetalipoproteinaemia (ABL), and RD are characterized by the absence of cerebellar atrophy. The remaining ARCAs show cerebellar atrophy (12). Table 27.6 summarizes the most widely recognized ARCAs.

The progressive myoclonic epilepsies (PMEs), which include Unverricht–Lundborg disease and Lafora body disease, are characterized by myoclonus, tonic–clonic seizures, progressive cerebellar ataxia, and cognitive decline. They are briefly mentioned here because they are mostly autosomal recessive disorders. A more detailed discussion of the PMEs is beyond the scope of this chapter.

Friedreich's ataxia

FRDA is the most common hereditary ataxia with a prevalence of around 2–3 in 100 000 (107). Age at onset is usually between 5 and 25 years. It is characterized neurologically by progressive gait and limb ataxia, dysarthria, loss of position and vibration sense, areflexia, and extensor plantars. Cardiomyopathy, diabetes, scoliosis, and pes cavus are common non-neurological manifestations. MRI may show some cord but no cerebellar atrophy. The disease is caused by a triplet GAA expansion in the *FRDA* gene coding for frataxin (12). Antioxidants, such as vitamin E, co-enzyme Q10, and idebenone have been used in FRDA with very limited therapeutic success (12).

Ataxia with vitamin E deficiency (AVED)

The clinical phenotype of AVED is very similar to FRDA. However, cardiomyopathy and diabetes are much more common in FRDA, whereas titubation and dystonia appear to be specific for AVED. Very low levels of vitamin E are characteristically found in AVED, and this allows the correct diagnosis. Administration of vitamin E supplements can arrest disease progression. The disease is caused by a mutation in the *ATPP* gene coding for alpha-tocopherol transfer protein, but genetic diagnosis is usually unnecessary (108).

Ataxia telangiectasia and ataxia telangiectasia-like disorder

AT is the second most common ARCA with a prevalence of 1–2.5 per 100 000 (99). Onset is usually by the age of 2 years (109). It is characterized by progressive ataxia, oculomotor apraxia, oculocutaneous telangiectasias, immunodeficiency, and a predilection for malignancy, especially leukaemia and lymphoma. Most patients have elevated AFP levels. MRI reveals cerebellar atrophy (99). AT is caused by mutations in the *ATM* gene which is involved in the DNA damage response pathway (109). AT-like disorder is clinically similar to AT but with later onset, slower progression, no telangiectasias, and normal AFP. It is caused by mutations in the meiotic recombination 11 gene (*MRE11*) (12).

Ataxia with oculomotor apraxia 1 (AOA1)

AOA1 has a clinical phenotype that is similar to AT, although onset is usually a few years later and patients do not develop telangiectasias or have a predilection for malignancy. Oculomotor apraxia is often the first symptom, and chorea may also be common at onset. Most patients have a degree of cognitive impairment (110). Laboratory studies reveal normal AFP, hypoalbuminaemia, and hypercholesterolaemia (111). AOA1 is common in Portugal and Japan (18). It is caused by mutations in the *APTX* gene coding for aprataxin (112).

Ataxia with oculomotor apraxia 2 (AOA2)

AOA2 is the third most common ARCA and represents around 8% of non-FRDA ARCAs (113). It has a neurological phenotype

Table 27.6 A clinically oriented classification of the autosomal recessive cerebellar ataxias (ARCAs) and X-linked cerebellar ataxias, based on disease frequency data*

Inheritance	Disease	Frequency (% of ARCAs)	Gene/locus	Genetic basis	Clinical pointers/notes
Autosomal recessive	FRDA	40%	*FRDA*/9q13	GAA repeat	Cardiomyopathy, diabetes
	AT	10%	*ATM*/11q22–23	CM	Telangiectasias not always identifiable, oculomotor apraxia, immunodeficiency
	AOA2	4–5%	*SETX*/9q34	CM	50% have oculomotor apraxia
	AOA1	Common in Portugal and Japan	*APTX*/9p13	CM	Chorea, cognitive impairment
	WD	Not rare	*ATP7B*/13q14.3	CM	Parkinsonism, dystonia, tremor, Kayser–Fleischer rings, treatable
	AVED	Rare	*TTPA*/8q13.1–13.3	CM	Titubation, cardiomyopathy, treatable
	AT-like disorder	Rare	*MRE11*/11q21	CM	Oculomotor apraxia
	ARSACS	Rare	*SACS*/13q11	CM	Common in Quebec province
	MSS	Rare	*SIL1*/5q31	CM	Cataracts and mental retardation
	ABL	Rare	*MTP*/4q22–24	CM	Retinitis pigmentosa, treatable
	RD	Rare	*PHYH*/10pter-11.2 *PEX7*/6q21–22.2	CM	Anosmia, retinitis pigmentosa, treatable
	GM2 gangliosidosis	Rare	*HEXA*/15q23–24	CM	Amyotrophy, psychiatric symptoms
	CTX	Rare	*CYP27*/2q33-ter	CM	Spasticity, tendon xanthomas, treatable
	Ataxia with co-enzyme Q10 deficiency	Rare	Variable		Seizures, areflexia, treatable
	NPC	Rare	*NPC1*/18p11 *NPC2*/14q24	CM	Vertical gaze palsy, dystonia, psychiatric symptoms, treatable
	MLD	Rare	*ARSA*/22q13.33	CM	Spasticity, cognitive impairment
	VWMD	Rare	*EIF2B1–5*/5 loci	CM	Rapid deterioration following infection
X-linked	FXTAS	Uncommon	*FMR1*/Xq27.3	CGG repeat	Late-onset, pre-mutation
	ADL	Rare	*ABCD1*/Xq28	CM	Spasticity
	PMD	Rare	*PLP*/Xq22	CM	Spasticity

*ARCAs have an overall prevalence of 7 in 100 000.

FRDA, Friedreich's ataxia; AT, ataxia telangiectasia; CM, conventional mutations; AOA, ataxia with oculomotor apraxia; WD, Wilson disease; AVED, ataxia with vitamin E deficiency; ARSACS, autosomal recessive ataxia of Charlevoix-Saguenay; MSS, Marinesco–Sjögren syndrome; ABL, abetalipoproteinaemia; RD, Refsum's disease; CTX, cerebrotendinous xanthomatosis; NPC, Niemann–Pick disease type C; MLD, metachromatic leucodystrophy; VWMD, vanishing white matter disease; FXTAS, fragile X tremor–ataxia syndrome; ALD, adrenoleucodystrophy; PMD, Pelizaeus–Merzbacher disease.

that is very similar to AT and AOA1, although only about 50% of patients have oculomotor apraxia. Onset is later than in either AT or AOA1 (usually the second decade). Laboratory studies reveal elevated AFP and hypercholesterolaemia (113). AOA2 is caused by mutations in the *SETX* gene coding for senataxin (114).

Wilson disease (see also Chapter 23)

WD has a prevalence of 1–3 in 100 000. It usually presents in the second or third decade. It has hepatic, neurological, ophthalmic, and psychiatric manifestations. Around 40–50% of patients present with CNS symptoms. In a minority of these patients, cerebellar ataxia can be a prominent symptom, often associated with postural tremor. Patients with WD have Kayser–Fleischer rings on slit-lamp examination, reduced serum caeruloplasmin, and high urinary copper. Treatment with copper chelating agents should be started as soon as possible to prevent neurological deterioration. WD is caused by mutations in the *APT7B* gene coding for a copper-dependent ATPase. Although systematic genetic testing for WD remains difficult, it can be valuable in confirming the diagnosis in unusual cases and can also allow presymptomatic screening of relatives and early treatment before the onset of complications (115).

Marinesco–Sjögren syndrome (MSS)

MSS is a rare ARCA characterized by cerebellar ataxia, cataracts, mental retardation, hypogonadotrophic hypogonadism, short stature, and skeletal abnormalities (116). In a recent epidemiological study in France, it was found to be as common as AOA1 (117). MSS is caused by mutations in the *SIL* gene coding for the BiP-associated protein (116).

Autosomal recessive spastic ataxia of Charlevoix-Saguenay

Autosomal recessive spastic ataxia of Charlevoix-Saguenay (ARSACS) is characterized by progressive cerebellar ataxia, pyramidal signs, and a sensorimotor neuropathy (mixed demyelinating–axonal) with amyotrophy. It was originally described and is commonly found in the province of Quebec in Canada (118). However, more recently it has been found in several other regions.

ARSACS is caused by mutations in the *SACS* gene coding for sacsin (12).

Ataxia with co-enzyme Q10 deficiency

Ataxia with co-enzyme Q10 deficiency is a rare genetically heterogeneous disorder with phenotypic variability. The ataxic variant is the most common and is characterized by cerebellar ataxia, nystagmus, pyramidal signs, absent reflexes, and seizures. Diagnosis is based on reduced co-enzyme Q10 levels in muscle (119). Disease progression may be arrested by treatment with co-enzyme Q10 (120).

GM2 gangliosidosis

GM2 gangliosidosis in its classic infantile form is characterized by hypotonia, developmental delay, seizures, blindness, the presence of a 'cherry-red spot' on fundoscopy, and early death (121). However, late-onset disease often presents as a cerebellar syndrome with areflexia, amyotrophy, and psychiatric features (122). The disease is caused by mutations in the *HEXA* gene coding for the enzyme beta-hexosaminidase A. In the late-onset form at least one allele with a less severe mutation results in some residual enzyme activity (122).

Abetalipoproteinaemia (ABL)

ABL is a rare disorder with a frequency of less than 1 in 100 000. The fundamental biochemical defect is absence of apolipoprotein-B-containing lipoproteins. All patients have fat malabsorption, acanthocytosis, hypocholesterolaemia, and absent apoB. Lipid-soluble vitamin malabsorption results in cerebellar ataxia. The neurological picture of ABL can resemble FRDA with additional retinitis pigmentosa. ABL is caused by mutations in the *MTP* gene coding for microsomal triglyceride transfer protein. Treatment includes dietary modification and vitamin supplementation, which may prevent or improve neurological complications (123).

Refsum's disease (RD)

RD is a rare disorder that usually presents in late childhood with anosmia and visual deterioration caused by retinitis pigmentosa. With progression, cerebellar ataxia, demyelinating polyneuropathy, ichthyosis, and cardiomyopathy are added to the picture. The pathognomonic finding is a highly elevated plasma phytanic acid. RD is caused by mutations in the *PHYH* gene coding for the peroxisomal enzyme phytanoyl-CoA hydroxylase, and less commonly in the *PEX7* gene coding for peroxin 7 receptor protein. Treatment is by dietary restriction of phytanic acid, which can gradually improve neurological complications (124).

Cerebrotendinous xanthomatosis (CTX)

CTX is a rare disorder of bile acid metabolism which results in abnormal deposition of cholestanol and cholesterol in multiple tissues. It is characterized by premature cataracts, tendon xanthomas, cerebellar ataxia, pyramidal signs, peripheral neuropathy, and dementia. It is diagnosed by finding elevated serum cholestanol (125). CTX is caused by mutations in the *CYP27* gene coding for the mitochondrial enzyme sterol 27-hydroxylase. Treatment is by administration of chenodeoxycholic acid, which can prevent or improve the neurological symptoms (126).

Niemann–Pick disease type C (NPC)

NPC is a neurovisceral lysosomal lipid storage disorder characterized by intracellular accumulation of cholesterol, sphingomyelin, and glycolipids. It is rare, with a frequency of less than 1 in 100 000. Characteristic clinical features include hepatosplenomegaly, vertical gaze palsy, ataxia, dystonia, seizures, and neuropsychiatric impairment. Cerebellar ataxia is prominent in late-onset forms (127). Diagnosis is by demonstrating impaired intracellular cholesterol transport and homeostasis in cultured fibroblasts, followed by genetic testing. NPC is caused by mutations in *NPC1* and *NPC2*, coding for a membrane glycoprotein and a lysosomal protein, respectively. Miglustat, an inhibitor of glycosylceramide synthase, has recently been shown to have significant disease-modifying effects in NPC (127).

Metachromatic leucodystrophy

Late-onset metachromatic leucodystrophy (MLD) can present with cerebellar ataxia associated with pyramidal signs, cognitive or psychiatric disturbances, and a demyelinating neuropathy (128). It is caused by deficiency of the enzyme arylsulfatase A as a result of mutations in the *ASA* gene. Patients with late-onset MLD are often homozygous for an allele which allows low enzyme expression (129).

Vanishing white matter disease

Vanishing white matter disease (VWMD) is a childhood-onset cerebellar ataxia, accompanied by spasticity and mild mental decline. Characteristically, the clinical picture can rapidly deteriorate following infection or minor trauma. MRI is pathognomonic, revealing progressive rarefaction and cystic degeneration of white matter. VWMD is caused by mutations in the *EIF2B 1–5* genes coding for the five subunits of a eukaryotic translation initiation factor (130).

Autosomal dominant cerebellar ataxias

The ADCAs, referred to as SCAs in the genetic nomenclature, are a rare cause of cerebellar ataxia with an overall prevalence around half that of ARCAs (7). Onset is usually in the third or fourth decade, although exceptions to this rule with onset in childhood or old age are well documented (8). The list of SCAs is ever-expanding, currently standing at 30, including dentatorubral-pallidoluysian atrophy (DRPLA) (8, 13, 131).

Several SCAs are caused by coding CAG repeat expansions and are known as 'polyglutamine expansion SCAs' (SCA1, 2, 3, 6, 7, 17 and DRPLA). With the notable exception of SCA6, these SCAs are prone to the phenomenon of genetic anticipation, with successive generations having larger CAG expansions, younger disease onset, and more severe disease course. This is particularly true for DRPLA and SCA7 (8).

Before the era of molecular diagnostics, Harding (132) suggested a way of classifying these disorders, which is still clinically useful. Type I ADCAs are 'complicated ataxias' characterized by cerebellar ataxia plus optic atrophy, ophthalmoplegia, dementia, pyramidal signs, extrapyramidal features, and amyotrophy. Type II ADCAs include only SCA7, which is a complicated ataxia like type I ADCAs, but in addition features visual loss due to pigmentary retinal degeneration. Type III ADCAs are relatively 'pure ataxias', possibly with mild pyramidal signs.

The ADCAs are characterized by brainstem and cerebellar atrophy. In general, MRI reveals predominant brainstem atrophy with lesser cerebellar atrophy in ADCA I and II and cerebellar atrophy without brainstem atrophy in ADCA III (8). However, overlap exists and it remains unclear how useful this distinction is clinically (7).

Only the most common SCAs are discussed briefly in this chapter. The rest are included for reference in Table 27.7. To aid the clinician, SCAs have been classified in order of descending frequency in the table.

Gerstmann–Sträussler–Scheinker disease is discussed briefly in this section as it is an autosomal dominant trait, although it is not part of the SCAs.

Type I autosomal dominant cerebellar ataxias

SCA1

SCA1 represents around 10% of SCAs (7). It is characterized by cerebellar ataxia, dysarthria, oculomotor abnormalities evolving into ophthalmoplegia, pyramidal signs, extrapyramidal signs, amyotrophy, peripheral neuropathy, and cognitive impairment (133, 134). Onset is usually in the fourth decade. SCA1 is caused by an exonic CAG repeat expansion in the *ATXN1* gene coding for ataxin-1 (8).

SCA2

SCA2 represents around 15% of SCAs (6). It is similar clinically to SCA1 but might be differentiated by the prominence of saccadic slowing, hyporeflexia, tremor, and titubation (135). SCA2 is caused by an exonic CAG repeat expansion in the *ATXN2* gene coding for ataxin-2 (8).

Table 27.7 A clinically oriented classification of the autosomal dominant cerebellar ataxias (ADCAs) based on Harding's scheme and disease frequency data*

Harding classification	SCA class	Frequency (% of ADCAs)	Gene/locus	Genetic basis	Clinical pointers/notes
ADCA I (ataxia ± optic atrophy, ophthalmoplegia, dementia, extrapyramidal features, amyotrophy)	SCA3	20–50%	*ATXN3/14q24.3–31*	CAG repeat	Prominent extrapyramidal features
	SCA2	15%	*ATXN2/12q24*	CAG repeat	Slow saccades, reduced reflexes
	SCA1	10%	*ATXN1/6p23*	CAG repeat	
	SCA17	3%	*TBP/6q27*	CAG repeat	HD-like features, seizures
	SCA12	7% in India	*PPP2R2B/5q31–33*	CAG repeat	Arm tremor
	DRPLA	Common in Japan	*ATN1/12p13.31*	CAG repeat	HD-like features, myoclonus
	SCA28	<1%	*AFG3L2/18p11.22q11.2*	CM	
	SCA8	Probably rare	*ATXN8* and *ATXN8OS/13q21*	CTG repeat	Uncertain pathogenicity
	SCA9	Probably rare	NK	NK	
	SCA10	Probably rare	*ATXN10/22q13*	ATTCT repeat	Seizures
	SCA13	Probably rare	*KCNC3/19q13.3-q13.4*	CM	Cognitive impairment
	SCA18	Probably rare	7q31	NK	
	SCA19	Probably rare	1p21-q21	NK	
	SCA20	Probably rare	11q12	NK	Dysphonia
	SCA21	Probably rare	7p21	NK	Extrapyramidal features
	SCA25	Probably rare	2p11-p21	NK	Severe sensory neuropathy
	SCA27	Probably rare	*FGF14/13q34*	CM	
	SCA35	Probably rare	*TGM6/20p13*	CM	
ADCA II (as ADCA I + pigmentary retinal degeneration)	SCA7	3–5%	*ATXN7/3p21.1-p12*	CAG repeat	Visual loss
ADCA III (pure cerebellar ataxia ± mild pyramidal signs)	SCA6	15%	*CACNA1A/19p13*	CAG repeat	Late onset, allelic to EA2
	SCA31	Common in Japan	*BEAN-TK2/ 16q22*	TGGAA repeat	
	SCA4	Probably rare	16q22	NK	
	SCA5	Probably rare	*SPTBN2/11q13*	CM	
	SCA11	Probably rare	*TTBK2/15q14-q21.3*	CM	
	SCA14	Probably rare	*PRKCG/19q13.4-qter*	CM	Myoclonus
	SCA15/16	Probably rare	*ITPR1/3p26-p25*	CM	
	SCA22	Probably rare	1p21-q23	NK	Allelic to SCA 19
	SCA23	Probably rare	*PDYN/20p13*	CM	
	SCA26	Probably rare	19p13	NK	
	SCA30	Probably rare	4q34	NK	

*ADCAs have an overall prevalence of around 3 in 100,000 but this, along with the frequency of individual SCAs, can vary considerably according to country of origin.

ADCA, autosomal dominant cerebellar ataxia; SCA, spinocerebellar ataxia; DRPLA, dentatorubral-pallidoluysian atrophy; CM, conventional mutations; HD, Huntington's disease; NK, not known.

SCA3

SCA3, also known as Machado–Joseph disease, is the most common SCA with a frequency of 20–50% among SCAs (6). Its phenotype is amongst the most variable of SCA phenotypes, but typical type I ADCA signs are found in most patients (7). Dystonic–rigid extrapyramidal features can be prominent. SCA3 is caused by an exonic CAG repeat expansion in the *ATXN3* gene coding for ataxin-3 (8).

SCA17

SCA17 is a rare SCA, with a frequency of around 3% in some ADCA populations (136). It has a highly variable disease phenotype. A proportion of patients have a predominantly ataxic phenotype, but others may present with a Huntington's disease-like phenotype (137). SCA17 is caused by an exonic CAG repeat expansion in the *TBP* gene coding for a TATA-binding protein (8).

SCA12

SCA12 is rare in the West, but is relatively common in India, representing 7% of SCAs (138). In addition to the more typical clinical features of type I ADCAs, it is characterized by a postural tremor of the upper limbs (6). SCA12 is caused by a non-coding CAG repeat expansion in the *PPP2R2B* gene coding for protein phosphatase 2 (8).

Dentatorubral-pallidoluysian atrophy

DRPLA is rare worldwide, but is particularly prevalent in Japan (7). Myoclonic epilepsy is a typical feature of these patients, as is a neurological presentation resembling Huntington's disease (139). DRPLA is caused by an exonic CAG repeat expansion in the *ATN1* gene coding for atrophin-1 (8).

Type II autosomal dominant cerebellar ataxias

SCA7

SCA7 represents around 3% of SCAs (7). It is the only type II ADCA and is characterized by the presence of visual loss secondary to pigmentary macular degeneration (132). The first signs of retinal involvement are reduced central visual acuity and dyschromatopsia in the blue–yellow axis. SCA7 displays pronounced expanded repeat instability with prominent anticipation, and children sometimes develop symptoms before their parents (7). SCA7 is caused by an exonic CAG repeat expansion in the *ATXN7* gene coding for ataxin-7 (8).

Type III autosomal dominant cerebellar ataxias

SCA6

SCA6 represents around 15% of SCAs (7). It is the prototype type III ADCA, characterized by relatively 'pure' cerebellar ataxia, although mild pyramidal signs and peripheral neuropathy may develop. Another characteristic feature of SCA6 is its late onset, with 60% of patients developing symptoms after age 50 (7). It is thus commonly found in patients with apparently sporadic cerebellar ataxia. SCA6 is caused by an exonic CAG repeat expansion in the *CACNA1A* gene coding for a calcium channel subunit (8). It is therefore a channelopathy allelic to FHM and EA2 (104).

SCA31

SCA31 has only recently been identified and is thought to rank as the third most common SCA in Japan, after SCA3 and SCA6 (140). It is a type III ADCA, presenting as 'pure' cerebellar ataxia. SCA31 is caused by a non-coding TGGAA repeat expansion in the *BEAN* and *TK2* genes (140).

Gerstmann–Sträussler–Scheinker disease

Gerstmann–Sträussler–Scheinker disease (GSS) is an autosomal dominant hereditary prion disease which classically presents as a chronic cerebellar ataxia with associated pyramidal signs. Dementia develops later in the course of the disease. The EEG in these patients lacks the typical periodic discharges seen in sCJD. GSS is caused by mutations in the *PRNP* gene, usually a Pro102Leu amino acid substitution (76).

X-linked cerebellar ataxias

X-linked cerebellar ataxias were traditionally thought to be very rare. However, with the delineation of FXTAS, they now form a small but significant part of neurodegenerative cerebellar disease (Table 27.6) (9, 141).

Fragile X-associated tremor–ataxia syndrome

FXTAS is characterized by limb and gait ataxia associated with parkinsonian features, cognitive impairment, neuropathy, and dysautonomia (141). It is seen in males carrying a pre-mutation (55–200 CGG repeats) in the *FMR1* gene. Full mutation in the *FMR1* gene (>200 repeats) causes fragile-X-associated mental retardation (142). Penetrance of FXTAS increases with age, and about 50% of males carrying the pre-mutation will develop symptoms by age 60. The frequency of males carrying the pre-mutation in the general population (1 in 800) should make FXTAS a relatively common cause of late-onset cerebellar ataxia. However, in ataxia series the percentage of FXTAS cases has been only around 2% and in MSA series only around 1% (9, 143). FXTAS has a very characteristic MRI appearance of hyperintense signal changes lateral to the dentate nuclei and into the middle cerebellar peduncle (141).

Adrenoleucodystrophy

Adrenoleucodystrophy (ALD) can rarely present as a spinocerebellar variant with predominant ataxic features, usually associated with pyramidal signs (144). ALD is diagnosed by the presence of very-long-chain fatty acids in peripheral blood. MRI abnormalities in some of these patients may be restricted to the brainstem and cerebellum and resemble patients with ADCAs (145). ALD is caused by mutations in the *ABCD1* gene, which codes for a peroxisomal ATP-binding cassette transporter (144).

Pelizaeus–Merzbacher disease

Pelizaeus–Merzbacher disease is another rare X-linked leucodystrophy with cerebellar ataxia and nystagmus as prominent features, in addition to spastic paraparesis. It is caused by mutations, usually duplications, in the *PLP* gene and is allelic to type 2 X-linked hereditary spastic paraplegia (146).

Mitochondrial cerebellar ataxias

Mitochondrial disorders (MIDs) encompass an ever-expanding spectrum of disease. They can be caused by defects of mitochondrial or nuclear DNA and hence can follow autosomal, X-linked, or maternal patterns of inheritance or be sporadic. MIDs are multisystem disorders. They can include involvement of the peripheral and central nervous systems, endocrine glands, heart, eyes, inner ears, gastrointestinal tract, kidney, bone marrow, and skin. One of the most prevalent CNS manifestations of MIDs is cerebellar ataxia (14).

Ataxia can be a prominent manifestation of both syndromic and non-syndromic MIDs (14). Mitochondrial syndromes associated

Table 27.8 Mitochondrial syndromes associated with cerebellar ataxia

Mitochondrial syndrome	Other extracerebellar manifestations	Gene
Mutations in mitochondrial DNA		
MELAS	Stroke-like episodes, lactic acidosis, dementia, deafness, seizures, myopathy	*tRNALeu, tRNASer*
MERRF	Myoclonus, seizures, deafness, myopathy	*tRNALys*
LHON	Optic neuropathy, peripheral neuropathy	RC subunits
NARP	Neuropathy, retinitis pigmentosa, dementia, seizures	*ATP6*
MILS	Developmental delay, pyramidal signs, extrapyramidal signs, lactic acidosis, neuropathy	*ND1–6, ATP6, COXIII, tRNALys*
PS	Pancytopenia, developmental delay, hepatic involvement, kidney failure	Deletions in mitochondrial DNA
KSS	Ophthalmoplegia, retinitis pigmentosa, arrhythmias, elevated CSF protein	Deletions in mitochondrial DNA
MIDD	Diabetes, sensorineural deafness	*tRNALeu, tRNALys*
MSL	Multiple lipomas, PEO, myopathy, neuropathy	*tRNALys*
Mutations in nuclear DNA		
LS	Developmental delay, pyramidal signs, extrapyramidal signs, respiratory failure, seizures, lactic acidosis	*SURF1, NDUFS1–8, NDUFV1–2*
PEO	Ophthalmoplegia, myopathy, deafness, neuropathy	*POLG1, C10orf2* (Twinkle), *ANT1*
SANDO	Neuropathy, ophthalmoplegia, myopathy	*POLG1, C10orf2*
SCAE	Seizures	*POLG1, C10orf2, ANT1*
AS	Developmental delay, seizures, stroke-like episodes, hepatic failure	*POLG1*
MNGIE	Nausea, vomiting, diarrhoea, ophthalmoplegia, neuropathy, myopathy	*TYMP*
ADOAD	Optic atrophy, deafness, neuropathy, ophthalmoplegia, myopathy	*OPA1*
IOSCA	Seizures, extrapyramidal signs, deafness, ophthalmoplegia, hypogonadism, neuropathy	*C10orf2*
MIRAS	Mild cognitive impairment, involuntary movements, psychiatric symptoms, seizures	*POLG1*
MEMSA	Seizures, myopathy, neuropathy	*POLG1*
XLSA/A	Sideroblastic anaemia	*ABC7*

MELAS, mitochondrial encephalomyopathy, lactic acidosis, stroke-like episodes; MERRF, myoclonic epilepsy with ragged red fibres; LHON, Leber's hereditary optic neuropathy; NARP, neurogenic muscle weakness, ataxia, retinitis pigmentosa; MILS, maternally inherited Leigh syndrome; PS, Pearson syndrome; KSS, Kearns–Sayre syndrome; MIDD, mitochondrial diabetes and deafness; MSL, multiple systemic lipomatosis; LS, Leigh syndrome; PEO, progressive external ophthalmoplegia; SANDO, sensory ataxic neuropathy, dysarthria, ophthalmoplegia; SCAE, juvenile-onset spinocerebellar ataxia and epilepsy; AS, Alpers syndrome; MNGIE, mitochondrial neuro-gastrointestinal encephalomyopathy; ADOAD, autosomal dominant optic atrophy and deafness; IOSCA, infantile onset spinocerebellar ataxia; MIRAS, mitochondrial recessive ataxia syndrome; MEMSA, myoclonus epilepsy myopathy and sensory ataxia; XLSA/A, X-linked sideroblastic anaemia with ataxia.

with ataxia are shown in Table 27.8 (14, 18). An ataxic syndrome caused by mutations in the *POLG1* gene is increasingly recognized as a common form of autosomal recessive ataxia in European populations (147).

Mitochondrial recessive ataxia syndrome (MIRAS) due to POLG mutations

MIRAS is a common form of autosomal recessive ataxia. It is characterized by cerebellar ataxia, dysarthria, mild cognitive impairment, involuntary movements, psychiatric symptoms, and seizures (147). It is caused by homozygous or compound heterozygous mutations in the *POLG1* gene coding for the mitochondrial DNA polymerase gamma catalytic subunit (14). It should be noted that mutations in *POLG1* can cause, beyond MIRAS, extensively heterogeneous phenotypes (148).

Key advances

Advances in the genetic aetiology of heredoataxias have dominated the ataxia field over the past 10 years. New knowledge has been accumulating at an impressive rate and numerous dominant, recessive, X-linked, and mitochondrial ataxic syndromes have been characterized at the molecular level. In the case of SCAs, the causative genes for SCA5, 10, 11, 13, 14, 15/16, 27, 28, 31, and 35 have recently been identified (8, 13). It is primarily the group of conventional-mutation SCAs that has been rapidly growing in recent years. In fact, the causative gene for SCA35 was the first to be identified through exome sequencing (13). Among the ARCAs, genes for MSS, AOA1, and AOA2 have also been identified in the past decade (14). The clinical delineation of FXTAS was also one of the major recent breakthroughs in the ataxia field (141). Finally, mitochondrial ataxias caused by nuclear genes such as *POLG1*, Twinkle, and *ANT1* have only recently been adequately recognized and diagnosed (14).

Advances in immunology have also added new knowledge to the field through the identification of novel antineuronal antibodies associated with paraneoplastic CD, such as mGluR1, Zic4, and PKCgamma (62).

In the case of polyglutamine expansion disorders, knowledge of the genetic aetiology has allowed the development of cell and animal models. These have been used in the past decade for the development of potential disease-modifying therapies. Strategies explored include the use of RNA interference to silence gene expression, the administration of histone deacetylase inhibitors to counteract the inhibitory action of mutant polyglutamine proteins on histone acetyltransferases, and the overexpression of chaperone proteins such as HSP70 that prevent protein misfolding and aggregation (6, 149).

Future developments

Over the next few years the genetic characterization of heredoataxias is likely to expand further. More genes will be identified and novel disease mechanisms will be uncovered. The proportion of genetically uncharacterized SCAs and ARCAs will gradually diminish. The use of new-generation sequencing techniques, such as exome sequencing, will allow the discovery of new genes that are difficult to identify using more traditional genetic methodology.

Advances are also likely to be made in the development of potential disease-modifying therapies through the continuing use of cell and animal models of polyglutamine disease. It is not inconceivable that the first phase I trials in human subjects may commence. The ability to identify pathogenic mutations early, in presymptomatic individuals, provides an invaluable window of opportunity for the administration of agents that may prevent disease development. There is every reason to be optimistic that in the more distant future such debilitating diseases may be preventable.

Conclusions

The cerebellar ataxias represent one of the most complex areas of clinical neurology. The diversity of potential causes can seem daunting to any physician. Over the past two decades, neuroimaging and molecular genetics have revolutionized the field, delineating numerous distinct well-characterized syndromes. Although individual ataxic disorders are relatively rare, the ataxias as a whole represent a common clinical problem.

The differential diagnosis of cerebellar ataxia is long and complicated, given the multitude of acquired and recognized hereditary causes. However, a systematic approach based on relatively straightforward clinical rules can be a useful guide. Determining the age of onset of the ataxia, along with the mode of onset and the subsequent disease course, can substantially focus the diagnostic process. Deciding next whether a hereditary or acquired cause should be sought further limits the differential to a manageable number of diseases. Specific information from the past medical history can then be combined with specific findings from the neurological and general examination to further narrow down the possible causes. Finally, routine and directed investigations allow the clinician to home in on the specific cause of ataxia.

Among the large number of cerebellar disorders which are at present untreatable, prompt identification of those ataxias which can be modified or cured by treatment is important. It is hoped that in the not too distant future, insights into the molecular pathogenesis of ataxias will lead to effective disease-modifying therapies for some of the currently untreatable disorders.

Key points

- Cerebellar ataxia can be caused by an extensive list of congenital, acquired, and hereditary disorders.
- Classifying ataxias according to the age of onset, the mode of onset, the disease course, and the presence of family history can assist in making a correct diagnosis.
- MRI and molecular genetics have revolutionized the diagnosis of congenital, acquired and hereditary ataxias.
- Regarding genetic testing:
  - In early-onset ARCAs, testing for FRDA is recommended. Positive biochemical findings should guide testing for AT, AOA1, and AOA2. AVED should be excluded.
  - In ADCAs, testing for SCA1, 2, 3, 6, and 7 should be offered. In the case of EAs testing for EA1 and 2 should be offered if available.
  - If X-linked inheritance is suspected, testing for FXTAS is recommended.
  - The possibility of a mitochondrial ataxia should always be borne in mind, especially disorders caused by nuclear genes such as *POLG1*.
- Prompt identification of ataxic disorders which are amenable to disease-modifying treatment is very important.
- The symptomatic and disease-modifying treatment of ataxias remains poor.

References

1. Klockgether T. Sporadic ataxia with adult onset: classification and diagnostic criteria. *Lancet Neurol* 2010; 9: 94–104.
2. Edlow JA, Newman-Toker DE, Savitz SI. Diagnosis and initial management of cerebellar infarction. *Lancet Neurol* 2008; 7: 951–64.
3. Sawaishi Y, Takada G. Acute cerebellitis. *Cerebellum* 2002; 1: 223–8.
4. Schrag A, Ben-Shlomo Y, Quinn NP. Prevalence of progressive supranuclear palsy and multiple system atrophy: a cross-sectional study. *Lancet* 1999; 354: 1771–5.
5. Muzaimi MB, Thomas J, Palmer-Smith S, et al. Population based study of late onset cerebellar ataxia in south east Wales. *J Neurol Neurosurg Psychiatry* 2004; 75: 1129–34.
6. Finsterer J. Ataxias with autosomal, X-chromosomal or maternal inheritance. *Can J Neurol Sci* 2009; 36: 409–28.
7. Schöls L, Bauer P, Schmidt T, Schulte T, Riess O. Autosomal dominant cerebellar ataxias: clinical features, genetics, and pathogenesis. *Lancet Neurol* 2004; 3: 291–304.
8. Durr A. Autosomal dominant cerebellar ataxias: polyglutamine expansions and beyond. *Lancet Neurol* 2010; 9: 885–94.
9. Berry-Kravis E, Abrams L, Coffey SM, et al. Fragile X-associated tremor/ataxia syndrome: clinical features, genetics, and testing guidelines. *Mov Disord* 2007; 22: 2018–30.
10. Esscher E, Flodmark O, Hagberg G, Hagberg B. Non-progressive ataxia: origins, brain pathology and impairments in 78 Swedish children. *Dev Med Child Neurol* 1996; 38: 285–96.
11. Shakkottai VG, Paulson HL. Physiologic alterations in ataxia: channeling changes into novel therapies. *Arch Neurol* 2009; 66(10): 1196–201.
12. Fogel BL, Perlman S. Clinical features and molecular genetics of autosomal recessive cerebellar ataxias. *Lancet Neurol* 2007; 6: 245–57.
13. Wang JL, Yang X, Xia K, et al. TGM6 identified as a novel causative gene of spinocerebellar ataxias using exome sequencing. *Brain* 2010; 133: 3510–18.
14. Finsterer J. Mitochondrial ataxias. *Can J Neurol Sci* 2009; 36(5): 543–53.
15. Grimaldi G, Manto M. Topography of cerebellar deficits in humans. *Cerebellum* 2012; 11: 336–51.

16. Huang C, Huang RH. Ethanol inhibits the sensory responses of cerebellar granule cells in anaesthetized cats. *Alcohol Clin Exp Res* 2007; 31: 336–44.
17. Vincent M, Hadjikhani N. The cerebellum and migraine. *Headache* 2007; 47: 820–33.
18. Manto M, Marmolino D. Cerebellar ataxias. *Curr Opin Neurol* 2009; 22: 419–29.
19. Jaatinen P, Rintala J. Mechanisms of ethanol-induced degeneration in the developing, mature and aging cerebellum. *Lancet Neurol* 2008; 7: 332–47.
20. Yokota O, Tsuchiya K, Terada S, et al. Alcoholic cerebellar degeneration: a clinicopathological study of six Japanese autopsy cases and proposed potential progression pattern in the cerebellar lesion. *Neuropathology* 2007; 27: 99–113.
21. Stefanova N, Bücke P, Duerr S, Wenning GK. Multiple system atrophy: an update. *Lancet Neurol* 2009; 8: 1172–8.
22. Pandolfo M. Friedreich ataxia. *Arch Neurol* 2008; 65: 1296–303.
23. Houlden H. Spinocerebellar ataxia type 11. In: Pagon RA, Bird TC, Dolan CR, Stephens K (eds) *GeneReviews* (Internet). Seattle, WA: University of Washington, 1993. Available online at http: //www.ncbi.nlm.nih.gov/ bookshelf/ (posted 22 July 2008).
24. Storey E. Spinocerebellar ataxia type 15. In: Pagon RA, Bird TC, Dolan CR, Stephens K (eds) *GeneReviews* (Internet). Seattle, WA: University of Washington, 1993. Available online at http: //www.ncbi.nlm.nih.gov/ bookshelf/ (last updated 21 April 2011).
25. Wood M. Cerebellar ataxias and related conditions. In: Clarke C, Howard R, Rossor M, Shorvon S (eds) *Neurology*, pp. 629–43. London: Wiley–Blackwell, 2009.
26. Abele M, Bürk K, Schöls L, et al. The aetiology of sporadic adult-onset ataxia. *Brain* 2002; 125: 961–8.
27. Gasser T, Finsterer J, Baets J, et al. EFNS guidelines on the molecular diagnosis of ataxias and spastic paraplegias. *Eur J Neurol* 2010; 17: 179–88.
28. Mariotti C, Solari A, Torta D, Marano L, Fiorentini C, Di Donato S. Idebenone treatment in Friedreich patients: one-year-long randomized placebo-controlled trial. *Neurology* 2003; 60: 1676–9.
29. Lagedrost SJ, Sutton MS, Cohen MS, et al. Idebenone in Friedreich ataxia cardiomyopathy: results from a 6-month phase III study (IONIA). *Am Heart J* 2011; 161: 639–45.
30. Ogawa M. Pharmacological treatment of cerebellar ataxia. *Cerebellum* 2004; 3: 107–11.
31. Perlman SL. Cerebellar ataxia. *Curr Treat Options Neurol* 2000; 2: 215–24.
32. Strupp M, Kalla R, Glasauer S. *Am Heart J* Aminopyridines for the treatment of cerebellar and ocular motor disorders. *Prog Brain Res* 2008; 171: 535–41.
33. Manto M. Overview of the general management of cerebellar disorders. In: Manto M (eds) *Cerebellar disorders. A practical approach to diagnosis and management*, pp.75–7. Cambridge: Cambridge University Press, 2010.
34. Steinlin M. Non-progressive congenital ataxias. *Brain Dev* 1998; 20: 199–208.
35. Vannemreddy P, Nourbakhsh A, Willis B, Guthikonda B. Congenital Chiari malformations. *Neurol India* 2010; 58: 6–14.
36. Fernandez AA, Guerrero AI, Martinez MI, et al. Malformations of the craniocervical junction (chiari type I and syringomyelia: classification, diagnosis and treatment. *BMC Muskuloskel Dis* 2009; 10(Suppl 1): S1.
37. Parisi MA, Dobyns WB. Human malformations of the midbrain and hindbrain: review and proposed classification scheme. *Mol Genet Metab* 2003; 80: 36–53.
38. O'Shea TM. Diagnosis, treatment, and prevention of cerebral palsy. *Clin Obstet Gynecol* 2008; 51: 816–28.
39. Broderick J, Connolly S, Feldmann E, et al. Guidelines for the management of spontaneous intracerebral hemorrhage in adults: 2007 update. *Stroke* 2007; 116: e391–413.
40. Camfield P, Camfield C. Acute and chronic toxicity of antiepileptic medications: a selective review. *Can J Neurol Sci* 1994; 21: S7–11.
41. Roy M, Stip E, Black DN, Lew V, Langlois R. [Neurologic sequelae secondary to acute lithium poisoning.] *Can J Psychiatry* 1999; 44: 671–9.
42. Kamate M, Chetal V, Hattiholi V. Fulminant cerebellitis: a fatal, clinically isolated syndrome. *Pediatr Neurol* 2009; 41: 220–2.
43. Shkalim V, Amir J, Kornreich L, Scheuerman O, Straussberg R. Acute cerebellitis presenting as tonsillar herniation and hydrocephalus. *Pediatr Neurol* 2009; 41: 200–3.
44. De Bruecker Y, Claus F, Demaerel P, et al. MRI findings in acute cerebellitis. *Eur Radiol* 2004; 14: 1478–83.
45. Tenembaum S, Chitnis T, Ness J, Hahn JS. Acute disseminated encephalomyelitis. *Neurology* 2007; 68 (Suppl 2): S23–36.
46. Marchioni E, Tavazzi E, Minoli L, et al. Acute disseminated encephalomyelitis. *Neurol Sci* 2008; 29 (Suppl 2): S286–8.
47. Fumeya H, Hideshima H. Cerebellar concussion—three case reports. *Neurol Med Chir (Tokyo)* 1994; 34: 612–15.
48. Hackett PH, Roach RC. High altitude cerebral edema. *High Alt Med Biol* 2004; 5: 136–46.
49. Ookura R, Shiro Y, Takai T, Okamoto M, Ogata M. Diffusion-weighted magnetic resonance imaging of a severe heat stroke patient complicated with severe cerebellar ataxia. *Intern Med* 2009; 48: 1105–8.
50. Manto M. Trauma of the posterior fossa. In: Manto M (ed) *Cerebellar disorders. A practical approach to diagnosis and management*, pp. 149–56. Cambridge: Cambridge University Press, 2010.
51. Thomson AD, Cook CC, Guerrini I, Sheedy D, Harper C, Marshall EJ. Wernicke's encephalopathy: 'Plus ça change, plus c'est la même chose'. *Alcohol Alcoholism* 2008; 43: 180–6.
52. Snyder LA, Rismondo V, Miller NR. The Fisher variant of Guillain–Barré syndrome (Fisher syndrome). *J Neuroophthalmol* 2009; 29: 312–24.
53. Yuki N. Fisher syndrome and Bickerstaff brainstem encephalitis (Fisher–Bickerstaff syndrome). *J Neuroimmunol* 2009; 215: 1–9.
54. Davies R, Luxon L, Bamiou DE, Shorvon S. Neuro-otology: problems of dizziness, balance and hearing. In: Clarke C, Howard R, Rossor M, Shorvon S (eds) *Neurology*, pp. 533–83. London: Wiley–Blackwell, 2009.
55. Gupta V, Singh A, Upadhyay S, Bhatia B. Clinical profile of somatoform disorders in children. *Indian J Pediatr* 2011 ; 78: 283–6.
56. Koutsis G, Evangelopoulos ME, Andreadou E, et al. The onset of multiple sclerosis in Greece: a single-center study of 1,034 consecutive patients. *Eur Neurol* 2010; 63: 350–6.
57. Wilne S, Collier J, Kennedy C, Koller K, Grundy R, Walker D. Presentation of childhood CNS tumours: a systematic review and meta-analysis. *Lancet Oncol* 2007; 8: 685–95.
58. Eichler AF, Loeffler JS. Multidisciplinary management of brain metastases. *Oncologist* 2007; 12: 884–98.
59. Lonser RR, Glenn GM, Walther M, et al. Von Hippel–Lindau disease. *Lancet* 2003; 361: 2059–67.
60. Batjer H, Samson D. Arteriovenous malformations of the posterior fossa: clinical presentation, diagnostic evaluation and surgical treatment. *Neurosurg Rev* 1986; 9: 287–96.
61. Lee SK, Willinsky RA, Montanera W, terBrugge KG. MR imaging of dural arteriovenous fistulas draining into cerebellar cortical veins. *Am J Neuroradiol* 2003; 24: 1602–6.
62. Dalmau J, Rosenfeld MR. Paraneoplastic syndromes of the CNS. *Lancet Neurol* 2008; 7: 327–40.
63. Shams'ili S, Grefkens J, de Leeuw B, et al. Paraneoplastic cerebellar degeneration associated with antineuronal antibodies: analysis of 50 patients. *Brain* 2003; 126: 1409–18.
64. Gosalakkal JA. Ataxias of childhood. *Neurologist* 2001; 7: 300–6.
65. Tagliati M, Simpson D, Morgello S, Clifford D, Schwartz RL, Berger JR. Cerebellar degeneration associated with human immunodeficiency virus infection. *Neurology* 1998; 50: 244–51.

66. Howard R, Manji H. Infections of the nervous system. In: Clarke C, Howard R, Rossor M, Shorvon S (eds), *Neurology*, pp. 289–335. Chichester: Wiley–Blackwell, 2009.
67. Matthews BR, Jones LK, Saad DA, Aksamit AJ, Josephs KA. Cerebellar ataxia and central nervous system Whipple disease. *Arch Neurol* 2005; 62: 618–20.
68. Panegyres PK, Edis R, Beaman M, Fallon M. Primary Whipple's disease of the brain: characterization of the clinical syndrome and molecular diagnosis. *Q J Med* 2006; 99: 609–23.
69. Pandey P, Umesh S, Bhat D, et al. Cerebellar abscesses in children: excision or aspiration? *J Neurosurg Pediatr* 2008; 1: 31–4.
70. Garg RK. Subacute sclerosing panencephalitis. *J Neurol* 2008; 255: 1861–71.
71. Appenzeller S, Cendes F, Costallat LT. Cerebellar ataxia in systemic lupus erythematosus. *Lupus* 2008; 17: 1122–6.
72. Collison K, Rees J. Asymmetric cerebellar ataxia and limbic encephalitis as a presenting feature of primary Sjögren's syndrome. *J Neurol* 2007; 254: 1609–11.
73. Mayer M, Cerovec M, Rados M, Cikes N. Antiphospholipid syndrome and central nervous system. *Clin Neurol Neurosurg* 2010; 112: 602–8.
74. Joseph FG, Scolding NJ. Neurosarcoidosis: a study of 30 new cases. *J Neurol Neurosurg Psychiatry* 2009; 80: 297–304.
75. Ashjazadeh N, Borhani Haghighi A, Samangooie SH, Moosavi H. Neuro-Behçet's disease: a masquerader of multiple sclerosis. A prospective study of neurologic manifestations of Behçet's disease in 96 Iranian patients. *Exp Mol Pathol* 2003; 74: 17–22.
76. Brown K, Mastrianni JA. The prion diseases. *J Geriatr Psychiatry Neurol* 2010; 23: 277–98.
77. Collins SJ, Sanchez-Juan P, Masters CL, et al. Determinants of diagnostic investigation sensitivities across the clinical spectrum of sporadic Creutzfeldt–Jakob disease. *Brain* 2006; 129: 2278–87.
78. Castillo P, Woodruff B, Caselli R, et al. Steroid-responsive encephalopathy associated with autoimmune thyroiditis. *Arch Neurol* 2006; 63: 197–202.
79. Maschke M, Weber J, Bonnet U, et al. Vermal atrophy of alcoholics correlate with serum thiamine levels but not with dentate iron concentrations as estimated by MRI. *J Neurol* 2005; 252: 704–11.
80. De Marcos FA, Ghizoni E, Kobayashi E, Li LM, Cendes F. Cerebellar volume and long-term use of phenytoin. *Seizure* 2003; 12: 312–15.
81. Niethammer M, Ford B. Permanent lithium-induced cerebellar toxicity: three cases and review of literature. *Mov Disord* 2007; 22: 570–3.
82. Orr CF, Ahlskog JE. Frequency, characteristics, and risk factors for amiodarone neurotoxicity. *Arch Neurol* 2009; 66: 865–9.
83. Pirzada NA, Ali II, Dafer RM. Fluorouracil-induced neurotoxicity. *Ann Pharmacother* 2000; 34: 35–8.
84. Win-Shwe TT, Fujimaki H. Neurotoxicity of toluene. *Toxicol Lett* 2010; 198: 93–9.
85. Miller DH, Leary SM. Primary-progressive multiple sclerosis. *Lancet Neurol* 2007; 6: 903–12.
86. Harding AE, Muller DP, Thomas PK, Willison HJ. Spinocerebellar degeneration secondary to chronic intestinal malabsorption: a vitamin E deficiency syndrome. *Ann Neurol* 1982; 12: 419–24.
87. Mulholland PJ. Susceptibility of the cerebellum to thiamine deficiency. *Cerebellum* 2006; 5: 55–63.
88. Morita S, Miwa H, Kihira T, Kondo T. Cerebellar ataxia and leukoencephalopathy associated with cobalamin deficiency. *J Neurol Sci* 2003; 216: 183–4.
89. Kumar K, Cohen-Gadol AA, Wright RA, Miller GM, Piepgras DG, Ahlskog JE. Superficial siderosis. *Neurology* 2006; 66: 1144–52.
90. Fearnley JM, Stevens JM, Rudge P. Superficial siderosis of the central nervous system. *Brain* 1995; 118: 1051–66.
91. Honnorat J, Saiz A, Giometto B, et al. Cerebellar ataxia with anti-glutamic acid decarboxylase antibodies: study of 14 patients. *Arch Neurol* 2001; 58: 225–30.
92. Manto MU, Laute MA, Aguera M, Rogemond V, Pandolfo M, Honnorat J. Effects of anti-glutamic acid decarboxylase antibodies associated with neurological diseases. *Ann Neurol* 2007; 61: 544–51.
93. Hadjivassiliou M, Grünewald RA, Chattopadhyay AK, et al. Clinical, radiological, neurophysiological, and neuropathological characteristics of gluten ataxia. *Lancet* 1998; 352: 1582–5.
94. Hadjivassiliou M, Sanders DS, Grünewald RA, Woodroofe N, Boscolo S, Aeschlimann D. Gluten sensitivity: from gut to brain. *Lancet Neurol* 2010; 9: 318–30.
95. Edvardsson B, Persson S. Subclinical hypothyroidism presenting with gait abnormality. *Neurologist* 2010; 16: 115–16.
96. Szmulewicz DJ, Waterston JA, Macdougall HG, et al. Cerebellar ataxia, neuropathy, vestibular areflexia syndrome (CANVAS): a review of the clinical features and video-oculographic diagnosis. *Ann NY Acad Sci* 2011; 1233: 139–47.
97. Gilman S, Wenning GK, Low PA, et al. Second consensus statement on the diagnosis of multiple system atrophy. *Neurology* 2008; 71: 670–6.
98. Klockgether T, Schroth G, Diener HC, Dichgans J. Idiopathic cerebellar ataxia of late onset: natural history and MRI morphologhy. *J Neurol Neurosurg Psychiatry* 1990; 53: 297–305.
99. Palau F, Espinós C. Autosomal recessive cerebellar ataxias. *Orphanet J Rare Dis* 2006; 1: 47.
100. Brancati F, Dallapiccola B, Valente EM. Joubert Syndrome and related disorders. *Orphanet J Rare Dis* 2010; 5: 20.
101. Mariën P, Brouns R, Engelborghs S, et al. Cerebellar cognitive affective syndrome without global mental retardation in two relatives with Gillespie syndrome. *Cortex* 2008; 44: 54–67.
102. Tomlinson SE, Hanna MG, Kullmann DM, Tan SV, Burke D. Clinical neurophysiology of the episodic ataxias: insights into ion channel dysfunction *in vivo*. *Clin Neurophysiol* 2009; 120: 1768–76.
103. Pessia M, Hanna MG. Episodic ataxia type 1. In: Pagon RA, Bird TC, Dolan CR, Stephens K (eds) *GeneReviews* (Internet). Seattle, WA: University of Washington, 1993. Available online at http: //www.ncbi.nlm.nih.gov/bookshelf/ (posted 9 Feb 2010).
104. Spacey S. Episodic Ataxia Type 2. 2003 Feb 24 (updated 2009 Jun 30). In: Pagon RA, Bird TC, Dolan CR, Stephens K (ed) *GeneReviews* (Internet). Seattle, WA: University of Washington, Seattle; 1993. Available from http: //www.ncbi.nlm.nih.gov/bookshelf/
105. Ryan MM, Engle EC. Acute ataxia in childhood. *J Child Neurol* 2003; 18: 309–16.
106. Sedel F, Lyon-Caen O, Saudubray JM. Therapy insight: inborn errors of metabolism in adult neurology—a clinical approach focused on treatable diseases. *Nat Clin Pract Neurol* 2007; 3: 279–90.
107. Schöls L, Amoiridis G, Przuntek H, Frank G, Epplen JT, Epplen C. Friedreich's ataxia. Revision of the phenotype according to molecular genetics. *Brain* 1997; 120: 2131–40.
108. Di Donato I, Bianchi S, Federico A. Ataxia with vitamin E deficiency: update of molecular diagnosis. *Neurol Sci* 2010; 31: 511–15.
109. Taylor AM, Byrd PJ. Molecular pathology of ataxia telangiectasia. *J Clin Pathol* 2005; 58: 1009–15.
110. Le Ber I, Moreira MC, Rivaud-Péchoux S, et al. Cerebellar ataxia with oculomotor apraxia type 1: clinical and genetic studies. *Brain* 2003; 126: 2761–72.
111. Liu W, Narayanan V. Ataxia with oculomotor apraxia. *Semin Pediatr Neurol* 2008; 15: 216–20.
112. Moreira MC, Barbot C, Tachi N, et al. The gene mutated in ataxia-ocular apraxia 1 encodes the new HIT/Zn-finger protein aprataxin. *Nat Genet* 2001; 29: 189–93.
113. Le Ber I, Bouslam N, Rivaud-Péchoux S, et al. Frequency and phenotypic spectrum of ataxia with oculomotor apraxia 2: a clinical and genetic study in 18 patients. *Brain* 2004; 127: 759–67.
114. Moreira MC, Klur S, Watanabe M, et al. Senataxin, the ortholog of a yeast RNA helicase, is mutant in ataxia-ocular apraxia 2. *Nat Genet* 2004; 36: 225–7.

115. Ala A, Walker AP, Ashkan K, Dooley JS, Schilsky ML. Wilson's disease. *Lancet* 2007; 369: 397–408.
116. Anttonen AK, Mahjneh I, Hämäläinen RH, et al. The gene disrupted in Marinesco–Sjögren syndrome encodes SIL1, an HSPA5 cochaperone. *Nat Genet* 2005; 37: 1309–11.
117. Anheim M, Fleury M, Monga B, et al. Epidemiological, clinical, paraclinical and molecular study of a cohort of 102 patients affected with autosomal recessive progressive cerebellar ataxia from Alsace, Eastern France: implications for clinical management. *Neurogenetics* 2010; 11: 1–12.
118. Bouchard JP, Richter A, Mathieu J, et al. Autosomal recessive spastic ataxia of Charlevoix-Saguenay. *Neuromuscul Disord* 1998; 8: 474–9.
119. Montero R, Pineda M, Aracil A, et al. Clinical, biochemical and molecular aspects of cerebellar ataxia and coenzyme Q10 deficiency. *Cerebellum* 2007; 6: 118–22.
120. Pineda M, Montero R, Aracil A, et al. Coenzyme Q(10)-responsive ataxia: 2-year-treatment follow-up. *Mov Disord* 2010; 25: 1262–8.
121. Montalvo AL, Filocamo M, Vlahovicek K, et al. Molecular analysis of the HEXA gene in Italian patients with infantile and late onset Tay–Sachs disease: detection of fourteen novel alleles. *Hum Mutat* 2005; 26: 282.
122. Neudorfer O, Pastores GM, Zeng BJ, Gianutsos J, Zaroff CM, Kolodny EH. Late-onset Tay–Sachs disease: phenotypic characterization and genotypic correlations in 21 affected patients. *Genet Med* 2005; 7: 119–23.
123. Zamel R, Khan R, Pollex RL, Hegele RA. Abetalipoproteinemia: two case reports and literature review. *Orphanet J Rare Dis* 2008; 3: 19.
124. Wierzbicki AS. Peroxisomal disorders affecting phytanic acid alpha-oxidation: a review. *Biochem Soc Trans* 2007; 35: 881–6.
125. Verrips A, Hoefsloot LH, Steenbergen GCH, et al. Clinical and molecular characteristics of patients with cerebrotendinous xanthomatosis. *Brain* 2000; 123: 908–19.
126. Gallus GN, Dotti MT, Federico A. Clinical and molecular diagnosis of cerebrotendinous xanthomatosis with a review of the mutations in the CYP27A1 gene. *Neurol Sci* 2006; 27: 143–9.
127. Vanier MT. Niemann–Pick disease type C. *Orphanet J Rare Dis* 2010; 5: 16.
128. Rauschka H, Colsch B, Baumann N, et al. Late-onset metachromatic leukodystrophy: genotype strongly influences phenotype. *Neurology* 2006; 67: 859–63.
129. Gieselmann V, Krägeloh-Mann I. Metachromatic leukodystrophy–an update. *Neuropediatrics* 2010; 41: 1–6.
130. van der Knaap MS, Pronk JC, Scheper GC. Vanishing white matter disease. *Lancet Neurol* 2006; 5: 413–23.
131. Bird TD. Hereditary ataxia overview. In: Pagon RA, Bird TC, Dolan CR, Stephens K (eds) *GeneReviews* (Internet). Seattle, WA: University of Washington, 1993. Available online at http: //www.ncbi.nlm.nih.gov/bookshelf/ (last updated 11 February 2011).
132. Harding AE. Classification of the hereditary ataxias and paraplegias. *Lancet* 1983; 1: 1151–5.
133. Sasaki H, Fukazawa T, Yanagihara T, et al. Clinical features and natural history of spinocerebellar ataxia type 1. *Acta Neurol Scand* 1996; 93: 64–71.
134. Bürk K, Globas C, Bösch S, et al. Cognitive deficits in spinocerebellar ataxia type 1, 2, and 3. *J Neurol* 2003; 250: 207–11.
135. Giunti P, Sabbadini G, Sweeney MG, et al. The role of the SCA2 trinucleotide repeat expansion in 89 autosomal dominant cerebellar ataxia families. Frequency, clinical and genetic correlates. *Brain* 1998; 121: 459–67.
136. Rolfs A, Koeppen AH, Bauer I, et al. Clinical features and neuropathology of autosomal dominant spinocerebellar ataxia (SCA17). *Ann Neurol* 2003; 54: 367–75.
137. Mariotti C, Alpini D, Fancellu R, et al. Spinocerebellar ataxia type 17 (SCA17): oculomotor phenotype and clinical characterization of 15 Italian patients. *J Neurol* 2007; 254: 1538–46.
138. Srivastava AK, Choudhry S, Gopinath MS, et al. Molecular and clinical correlation in five Indian families with spinocerebellar ataxia 12. *Ann Neurol* 2001; 50: 796–800.
139. Koide R, Onodera O, Ikeuchi T, et al. Atrophy of the cerebellum and brainstem in dentatorubral pallidoluysian atrophy. Influence of CAG repeat size on MRI findings. *Neurology* 1997; 49: 1605–12.
140. Sato N, Amino T, Kobayashi K, et al. Spinocerebellar ataxia type 31 is associated with 'inserted' penta-nucleotide repeats containing (TGGAA)*n*. *Am J Hum Genet* 2009; 85: 544–57.
141. Jacquemont S, Hagerman RJ, Leehey M, et al. Fragile X premutation tremor/ataxia syndrome: molecular, clinical, and neuroimaging correlates. *Am J Hum Genet* 2003; 72: 869–78.
142. Baba Y, Uitti RJ. Fragile X-associated tremor/ataxia syndrome and movement disorders. *Curr Opin Neurol* 2005; 18: 393–8.
143. Kamm C, Healy DG, Quinn NP, et al. The fragile X tremor ataxia syndrome in the differential diagnosis of multiple system atrophy: data from the EMSA Study Group. *Brain* 2005; 128: 1855–60.
144. Li JY, Hsu CC, Tsai CR. Spinocerebellar variant of adrenoleukodystrophy with a novel ABCD1 gene mutation. *J Neurol Sci* 2010; 290: 163–5.
145. Vianello M, Manara R, Betterle C, Tavolato B, Mariniello B, Giometto B. X-linked adrenoleukodystrophy with olivopontocerebellar atrophy. *Eur J Neurol* 2005; 12: 912–14.
146. Hudson LD. Pelizaeus–Merzbacher disease and spastic paraplegia type 2: two faces of myelin loss from mutations in the same gene. *J Child Neurol* 2003; 18: 616–24.
147. Hakonen AH, Heiskanen S, Juvonen V, et al. Mitochondrial DNA polymerase W748S mutation: a common cause of autosomal recessive ataxia with ancient European origin. *Am J Hum Genet* 2005; 77: 430–41.
148. Milone M, Massie R. Polymerase gamma 1 mutations: clinical correlations. *Neurologist* 2010; 16(2): 84–91.
149. Manto M. Dominant ataxias. In: Manto M (ed.) *Cerebellar disorders. A practical approach to diagnosis and management*, pp. 242–83. Cambridge: Cambridge University Press.

CHAPTER 28

Drug-Induced Movement Disorders

Shyamal H. Mehta, John C. Morgan, and Kapil D. Sethi

Movement disorders due to dopamine-receptor blocking agents (DBAs)

Antipsychotic agents, also commonly referred to as neuroleptics, are used not only to treat psychiatric disorders but also in neurological diseases such as Tourette's syndrome, Huntington's disease, and psychosis in advanced Parkinson's disease. The introduction of chlorpromazine in the early 1950s was a great advance in the treatment of psychosis, but it was soon realized that significant neurological side effects are associated with this class of drugs. In fact, in the 1950s when it was noted that both chlorpromazine and reserpine induced extrapyramidal side effects (EPS), despite being distinct chemical entities, it was thought that induction of EPS was integral to their clinical antipsychotic efficacy. Recent advances in drug development have revealed that this is not true and evidence implicates D2 receptor antagonism and the speed of dissociation of the drug from the receptor in the development of these EPS (DBAs with less D2 affinity and more rapid dissociation are less likely to produce EPS). Over the last several decades, cumulative experience with the older (typical) and newer (atypical) neuroleptics has highlighted the wide range of acute to more delayed movement disorders that may be caused by these agents (Table 28.1) (1).

Acute dystonia

Acute dystonia occurs shortly after the introduction of the DBA and occasionally after a dose increase. Estimates of incidence of acute dystonia from DBAs depend on several factors, such as patient population being studied, type and dosage of DBA used, and concurrent medications (2). Studies in patients with a first episode of psychosis treated with DBAs have reported a 34–60% risk of developing drug-induced acute dystonia (2–4) and ~50% of patients experience the first signs of dystonia within 48 hours of drug intake (5).

Some of the risk factors for developing acute dystonia after exposure to DBAs are young age, male sex, previous dystonic reaction, higher dose and high potency of DBAs, familial predisposition, underlying psychiatric illness, mental retardation, and a history of electroconvulsive therapy (2, 6). Interestingly, a retrospective study also showed a 2.4-fold higher risk of DBA-induced EPS in AIDS patients compared with age-matched psychotic patients without AIDS (7). Cocaine abuse may predispose to acute dystonic reactions (8). Also, in contrast with other antidepressant medications, selective serotonin-reuptake inhibitors (SSRIs) have been known to induce acute dystonic reactions, mostly early in the course of treatment or after a dose increase (2). These reactions have also been reported with the dopamine depletor tetrabenazine, perhaps because of its partial dopamine blocking activity.

Although the pathophysiology of acute dystonia due to DBAs is unclear, it is well known that the propensity of any DBA to cause acute dystonia strongly correlates with its ability to block the D2 receptor in the striatum. It is through this D2-receptor mediated signalling that the DBA influences the intricate neuronal circuitry and modulates the cholinergic, GABAergic, and NO-synthase-positive interneurons in the striatum (2). As far as modulation of cholinergic signalling is concerned, one hypothesis is that dopaminergic hypofunction results in a relative overactivity of cholinergic mechanisms (9). This hypothesis is supported by a consistent response of acute dystonia to anticholinergic drugs. Another hypothesis proposes that DBAs induce paradoxical dopaminergic hyperfunction by blockade of presynaptic dopamine receptors. As the level of the DBA decreases, postsynaptic receptors are exposed to the natural release of dopamine from presynaptic terminals (10) which may precipitate the dystonia.

Clinical features

Drug-induced dystonia can affect various regions of the body and can be very painful. Based on several prospective studies, Mazurek and Rosebush (2) reported that ~42% of acute dystonic reactions involved torticollis or retrocollis as a clinical feature. Involvement of the facial muscles, which may range from grimacing and tightness to masseter spasm, is another common finding. Although rare, other facial muscles causing blepharospasm or lip curling may also be involved. Similarly, the limb muscles may also be involved, although less frequently.

Some of the more severe clinical manifestations involve the throat musculature (~19%) causing swallowing difficulties or

Table 28.1 Movement disorders induced by dopamine blocking agents

I. Acute
Acute dystonia
Acute akathisia
Drug-induced parkinsonism
II. Chronic
Tardive dyskinesia/stereotypy
Tardive myoclonus
Tardive tics
Tardive tremor
Tardive dystonia
Tardive akathisia
III. Miscellaneous
Withdrawal emergent syndrome
Neuroleptic malignant syndrome

laryngospasm, which can be potentially life-threatening. Oculogyric crises (upward deviation of the eyes) and opisthotonus (back arching) are a striking presentation of acute drug-induced dystonia. These represent ~6–15% and ~3.5–12% of dystonic reactions, respectively, and are seen in acute as well as tardive dystonia (2).

Management

Acute dystonia responds well to injectable anticholinergic drugs such as benztropine (11) or antihistaminic agents such as diphenhydramine (12). Benzodiazepines such as diazepam or lorazepam are equally efficacious. The response to anticholinergics is so consistent that if a patient with suspected DBA-induced acute dystonia fails to respond, clinicians should suspect phencyclidine-induced dystonia (13). If an episode of acute dystonia persists after an initial parenteral dose, another dose should be repeated in ~30 minutes. At times, acute dystonic reactions such as laryngeal dystonia are severe enough to warrant life-saving measures (tracheostomy). The acute dystonic reaction may recur after an initial response even without exposure to a subsequent dose of DBA and repeated therapeutic intervention may be necessary.

There is some evidence to suggest that acute dystonic reactions may be prevented by the use of anticholinergic drugs (14, 15). It is recommended that patients at high risk of acute dystonia (young patients, cocaine abusers, and AIDS patients) or in specific situations (i.e. first exposure to DBA) receive prophylactic anticholinergics (15). Since the increased risk of developing a dystonic reaction to DBAs is in the first week of initiating treatment, the prophylactic medication can be withdrawn thereafter.

Acute akathisia

The term 'akathisia' (from Greek, literally 'inability to sit') was introduced by Haskovec in 1902, who thought that the symptoms had a psychological cause (16). The first case report of drug-induced akathisia was by Sigwald in 1947, prior to the introduction of neuroleptics, who noticed it in association with promethazine (17). There are two aspects of akathisia:

- a subjective report of restlessness or inner tension, mostly in the legs, with a consequent inability to maintain a posture for several minutes and anxiety;
- the objective manifestations of restlessness in the form of movements of the limbs, a tendency to shift body position in the chair while sitting, or marching while standing.

Recent studies using large databases clearly indicate that akathisia occurs with the newer DBAs, although the frequency is not as high as with conventional antipsychotics. These symptoms have also been associated with the administration of SSRIs. Other drugs that can cause acute akathisia are listed in Table 28.2.

The temporal association with drug administration is a very important feature in the diagnosis of acute akathisia. Acute akathisia usually starts within the first 2 weeks and almost always within the first 6 weeks (18, 19). The appearance of akathisia is also dose dependent, with higher dosages of DBAs more likely to precipitate symptoms (18, 19). Other risk factors include use of conventional or higher-potency antipsychotics, bipolar depression, palliative care settings, and co-morbid substance abuse in psychosis (20).

The reported prevalence of neuroleptic-induced akathisia varies widely depending on the DBAs used. With older neuroleptics it is typically around 20% (18, 19). With the advent of newer atypical neuroleptics the incidence of akathisia has decreased, although has not completely disappeared. A study of quetiapine across a dose range 75–750 mg/day found an akathisia prevalence of 0–2% versus 8% and 15% for patients randomized to placebo and haloperidol, respectively (21).

A variety of conditions should be considered in the differential diagnosis of acute drug-induced akathisia. Agitation and restlessness can be seen as a part of generalized anxiety disorder, mania, or depression, and patients with acute psychosis may have agitated pacing similar to akathisia (22). Movement disorders such as restless legs syndrome and pseudo-akathisia (movements as seen in akathisia without the subjective complaints of restlessness) may also be difficult to distinguish from acute akathisia (22).

Although the exact mechanism of drug-induced akathisia remains unknown, the increased frequency of acute akathisia with high-potency D2 blocking DBAs suggests that D2 receptor antagonism plays an integral role. Two studies using positron emission tomography (PET) demonstrated an association between D2 occupancy in the striatum and the development of akathisia, with the authors suggesting a threshold for D2 receptor occupancy of 74–82% for the production of EPS including akathisia (23, 24). Evidence also suggests that reduced activity of dopaminergic projections from the midbrain to the ventral striatum may lead to the development of akathisia (25). In addition to the dopaminergic systems, the serotonergic system may also be involved as SSRIs are a common cause of acute akathisia. A recent double-blind placebo-controlled study showed improvement of akathisia with trazodone, most likely through its property of serotonin 2A postsynaptic receptor antagonism (26).

Table 28.2 Other drugs that can cause acute akathisia

Antiepileptics	Carbamazepine, ethosuximide
Antidepressants:	Lithium
	SSRIs: fluoxetine, sertraline, citalopram, etc.
	Tricyclic and heterocyclic antidepressants
Calcium-channel blockers	Diltiazem, flunarizine, cinnarizine
Dopamine depleters	Tetrabenazine and reserpine
5-HT receptor ligands	Buspirone, methysergide

Management

The drugs most commonly used to treat drug-induced akathisia include beta-blockers, anticholinergics, amantadine, benzodiazepines, and newer agents such as serotonergic (5-HT) antagonists (27).

Propranolol (40–80 mg/day), a non-selective lipophilic beta-adrenergic antagonist, has been used as a first-line anti-akathisia agent for decades. Studies with propranolol have shown significant overall improvement in both subjective and objective measures of akathisia (28, 29). Anticholinergics used to treat akathisia include biperiden (2–6 mg/day), benztropine (1.5–8 mg/day), or trihexyphenidyl (2–10 mg/day). However, many clinicians feel that these are only partially effective and their use is limited by anticholinergic side effects. It is recommended that these agents are only used in patients with akathisia who have associated parkinsonism (27).

Commonly used benzodiazepines include lorazepam (1–2 mg/day), clonazepam (0.5–1 mg/day), and diazepam (5–15 mg/day). Placebo-controlled studies with clonazepam and diazepam showed benefit in patients with akathisia (22). Improvements occurred after the first week of treatment, with minimal additional benefit after the second week of treatment (22).

Agents with marked 5-HT_{2A} receptor antagonism such as mirtazapine, mianserin, and cyproheptadine are anti-akathisia therapies based on their potential to counteract antipsychotic-induced dopamine D2 receptor blockade by increasing dopaminergic neurotransmission (27). Clinical studies attest to the utility and efficacy of this class of compounds as an alternative to beta-adrenergic blockers for the treatment of acute akathisia.

Drug-induced parkinsonism

Drug-induced parkinsonism (DIP) may result from a variety of prescribed medications. Drugs that either block the dopamine receptors or deplete dopamine stores produce a functional dopaminergic deficiency and signs/symptoms akin to idiopathic Parkinson's disease (PD). The most common offending drugs are DBAs, such as neuroleptics; however, there are other non-neuroleptic drugs which may also cause DIP. From a review of 17 years' experience of 261 drugs suspected of causing DIP, most involved central dopaminergic antagonists (49%), followed by antidepressants (8%), calcium-channel blockers (5%), peripheral dopaminergic antagonists (5%), and H1 antihistamines (5%). Cases with lithium, valproic acid, amiodarone, anticholinesterases, or trimetazidine were also found (30). Table 28.3 lists the drugs that can cause or exacerbate parkinsonism.

Since the advent of atypical neuroleptics and increasing awareness (i.e. litigation) regarding medications such as metoclopramide, the incidence of DIP has now decreased. However, clinically it remains a challenge as it is often missed and also misinterpreted as idiopathic PD.

Epidemiology and pathophysiology

DIP is a common complication of antipsychotic drug use, occurring in 15–60% of patients treated with DBAs (18). In one study, 51% of 95 patients referred for evaluation had parkinsonism associated with prescribed drugs (31). Another study found that in a general neurology practice, 56.8% of 306 cases with parkinsonism were either induced or aggravated by drugs (32). Frequently, these patients are misdiagnosed as idiopathic PD and treated with dopaminergic drugs without benefit. In a community study, 18% of all cases initially thought to have idiopathic PD were subsequently diagnosed as DIP (33).

Table 28.3 Drugs that can cause or exacerbate drug-induced parkinsonism

Neuroleptics	Typical neuroleptics:
	Phenothiazines such as chlorpromazine, promethazine, etc.
	Butyrophenones such as haloperidol, droperidol, triperidol, etc.
	Thioxanthenes such as thiothexene, zuclopenthixol, flupenthixol, etc.
	Atypical neuroleptics:
	Risperidone, olanzapine, clozapine, ziprasidone, etc.
Dopamine depleters	Tetrabenazine, reserpine
Substituted benzamides	Metoclopramide, cisapride, sulpiride, clebopride, etc.
Vestibular sedatives	Flunarizine, cinnarizine, etc.
Calcium-channel blockers	Amiodarone, verapamil, diltiazem, nifedipine, etc.
Immunosuppressants	Cyclophosphamide, cytosine arabinoside, cyclosporin, etc.
Antidepressants	SSRIs (fluoxetine etc.), lithium, phenelzine, etc.
Others	Valproic acid, amphotericin B, disulfiram, molindone, etc.

Numerous retrospective analyses and epidemiologic studies have been performed to reliably identify risk factors for DIP. However, all studies have demonstrated one unambiguous fact—there is enormous individual variation in susceptibility to develop movement disorders secondary to the DBAs (34). Ayd (18) was the first to identify female sex, old age, and high-potency neuroleptics as potential risk factors for DIP. Based on current research, only neuroleptic potency and dose are unequivocal risk factors for DIP. Others, such as increasing age, female sex, pre-existing EPS, dementia, brain injury, family history of PD, and severe psychiatric illness, are best regarded as possible predisposing factors (34).

DIP appears to develop in almost all patients given high doses of high-potency DBAs sufficient to block ~80% of central dopaminergic receptors, especially D2 receptors (35). In addition, comparative ratios between antagonism of different receptors may play an important role: high acetylcholine/dopamine receptor antagonism, and a favourable ratio of 5-HT_2 to D2 receptor antagonism have a lower propensity to result in movement disorders (36).

Clinical features

Clinically, DIP may present with rest tremor, bradykinesia, and rigidity. Patients with DIP are less likely to have prominent gait freezing and postural instability. Other manifestations include speech disturbance, micrographia, and facial hypomimia. Thus, DIP cannot be distinguished clinically from idiopathic PD as the features can be similar (34). Also, asymmetry is common in DIP and should not be misconstrued as a sign against the diagnosis. In general, patients with DIP are less likely to exhibit tremor, but this is not helpful in the individual patient in differentiating DIP from IPD (37). The relative lack of tremor may either reflect a younger patient population afflicted with DIP or an intrinsic, as yet unrealized, pathophysiological difference between the two conditions (34). The co-existence of a hyperkinetic movement disorder, such as oro-buccal-lingual dyskinesia, in the absence of levodopa treatment supports a diagnosis of DIP rather than idiopathic PD.

In a survey of 3775 patients, Ayd (18) found that DIP usually occurs later than akathisia and dystonia, and 90% of cases developed within the first 72 days. Another study reported that the time of onset of DIP from haloperidol was dose related, with higher doses producing symptoms within 2 weeks (38). Not much is known regarding the natural progression of DIP with continued neuroleptic exposure. Fernandez and colleagues (39) studied 53 patients who remained on neuroleptics over a 14-year period; these subjects experienced a decrease in tardive dyskinesia symptoms but a significant increase in DIP, suggesting that DIP progresses over time. Upon cessation of the offending agent, DIP may ameliorate with time as patients with DIP who are treated with antiparkinsonian drugs can often have these discontinued without a recurrence of symptoms (34). Even though data are limited, evidence suggests that severe long-term DIP is uncommon and chronic antiparkinsonian therapy is rarely required (40).

In older patients and for those with more protracted and chronic symptoms it is possible that DIP may unmask subclinical PD. This is supported by the persistence of parkinsonism in some patients after discontinuing DBA. In addition, a pathological study revealed cell loss and Lewy bodies in the substantia nigra of two patients who died some time after their parkinsonism had resolved following discontinuation of DBA. Clinically, it is difficult to distinguish DIP from idiopathic PD, and functional imaging has been used to clarify this issue. One study examined ^{18}F-dopa PET scans in thirteen DIP patients. In four out of thirteen DIP patients there was evidence of significant reduction of ^{18}F-dopa uptake in the putamen within the PD range, and in three of these four patients there was continuing or worsening parkinsonism. However, all nine patients with normal scans recovered from their DIP symptoms (41). In another study, twenty patients who developed parkinsonism while on neuroleptics underwent a [^{123}I]-FP-CIT SPECT scan. Nine patients had normal scans and eleven showed significantly diminished striatal binding, suggesting underlying nigrostriatal dysfunction. Notably, there were no differences in clinical features between patients with normal and abnormal scans (42).

Management

Ideally, prevention of DIP would be best. Some authorities suggest using antiparkinsonian drugs at the onset of neuroleptic therapy. Since anticholinergics and amantadine also have side effects, a more prudent approach might be to institute prophylactic therapy to cover high-risk patients such as those with a family history of PD, elderly subjects, and female subjects (43).

The treatment of clinically manifest DIP is difficult. In most cases, DIP is reversible once the offending drug is withdrawn. However, in some cases this may not be possible; decreasing the dose of the neuroleptic or switching to an atypical neuroleptic such as clozapine or quetiapine may be beneficial. Mild DIP can be left untreated. When symptoms of DIP are more troublesome, several studies have shown improvement with amantadine. Anticholinergics have also been used with some success in the treatment of DIP. However, the evidence for amantadine remains less conflicting than for anticholinergics, and this drug also seems to be better tolerated (34, 44). Limited experience exists for other therapeutic modalities, such as dopamine agonists, levodopa, propranolol and electroconvulsive therapy (34).

Chronic/delayed movement disorders caused by dopamine receptor blocking agents

Tardive dyskinesia

Tardive dyskinesia (TD) refers to abnormal excessive involuntary movements related to exposure to at least one DBA. The onset of symptoms should be within 6 months of the last DBA use and persist for at least a month after cessation of the offending drug (45). In 1980 the American Psychiatric Association Task Force defined TD as an abnormal involuntary movement following a minimum of 3 months of neuroleptic treatment in a patient with no other identifiable aetiology for movement disorders (46). However, the DSM-IV criteria require only one month of exposure to neuroleptics in individuals aged 60 and older (47).

The term dyskinesia refers to any abnormal, involuntary, repetitive, co-ordinated movements, regardless of aetiology. Stereotypy is the most common manifestation of classic TD. Other forms of tardive movements include tics, dystonia, akathisia, and myoclonus, among others. However, most often patients clinically manifest classic TD as a combination of orofacial stereotypy with choreic movements of hands, fingers, and lower extremities or dystonia (48). Rarely, when diaphragm and chest muscles are involved, these are called 'respiratory dyskinesias' or referred to as 'copulatory dyskinesias' when the involvement of abdominal or pelvic muscles produces pelvic rocking type movements (49, 50). Sometimes hyperkinetic (stereotypy, chorea, etc.) and hypokinetic (parkinsonism) movements co-exist (51). The symptoms of TD may first emerge upon a reduction in or cessation of a DBA. The term 'withdrawal-emergent dyskinesia' refers to emergence of dyskinesia upon discontinuation of the DBA. It may manifest as generalized chorea, especially in children, and resolves within 90 days. Persistence beyond this is called covert dyskinesia.

Epidemiology and risk factors

It has been over 50 years since the first reports of TD associated with neuroleptic exposure. However, it was not until the 1970s that there was general acceptance of the association of TD with long-term neuroleptic use (52). The frequency of TD has changed over the past several decades, driven by one important factor—the transition from typical to atypical (second-generation) neuroleptics. The pharmacological profile of the newer atypical neuroleptics is shown in Table 28.4.

A detailed literature review by Smith and colleagues (53, 54) provides an insight into the prevalence of TD in an earlier neuroleptic era. In 56 studies involving nearly 35 000 typical neuroleptic-treated patients, the overall prevalence of dyskinesia averaged 20%. Large-scale prospective studies indicate an average rate of developing TD of ~5% per year for the first several years of treatment with typical neuroleptics and a cumulative 5-year incidence rate of 20–26% (54, 55). Glazer and colleagues (56) suggested risk increases in a linear fashion with continued exposure (49% at 10 years and 25-year risk estimated at 68%). However, with the advent of second-generation neuroleptics, prevalence

Table 28.4 Receptor binding profile of atypical neuroleptics

Receptor binding	Atypical neuroleptic						Typical neuroleptic
	Risperidone	Olanzapine	Quetiapine	Ziprasidone	Aripiprazole	Clozapine	Haloperidol
D1	–	+++	+	+	–	++	+++
D2	+++	+++	++	+++	+++	++	++++
5-HT_2	++++	++++	+++	++++	++	++++	+
α_1	+++	+++	++++	++	+	+++	++
α_2	+++	–	+	–	+	+++	–
EPS	+++	++	+	++	+	+	++++

of both acute EPS and TD declined over months of treatment in patients changed from traditional to modern neuroleptics (57). In mid-2003, the Hillside Hospital group analysed several clinical trials with ~2700 patients on modern neuroleptics, with an average duration of exposure of 301 days. They found the annual incidence of TD associated with second-generation neuroleptics (weighted by numbers of subjects exposed) averaged 2.1% overall: 0.8% in adults aged <50 years versus 5.3% among patients aged >50 years (58). Thus the risk of TD is significantly lower (by two- to threefold) with most modern neuroleptics compared with older neuroleptics (57). However, TD risks associated with modern antipsychotics may be similar to those of older antipsychotics of low to moderate potency. Risperidone (and its active metabolite paliperidone), at high doses, may carry a high TD risk, whereas TD risk is intrinsically low with clozapine, and perhaps quetiapine and aripiprazole (59).

Epidemiological studies have identified several putative risk factors which may increase the chance of developing TD. Demographic risk factors include increased age, diagnosis of mood disorders, and gender. The gender effect is complicated: earlier studies suggested a higher risk in the female population, whereas more recent controlled studies show a higher risk in females only over age 65 and increased severity in younger males (60). Other risk factors include total cumulative drug exposure, diabetes, alcohol consumption, cocaine abuse, persistence of drug exposure after development of TD, and a history of electroconvulsive therapy (60).

Pathophysiology of tardive dyskinesia

The pathophysiology of TD is complicated and poorly understood. Concisely put, most accepted theories suggest that chronic exposure to neuroleptics result in a combination of postsynaptic dopamine receptor hypersensitivity, abnormalities of striatal GABA-containing neurons, and degeneration of striatal cholinergic interneurons (61). It seems plausible that dopamine receptor hypersensitivity may create a condition simulating dopaminergic excess in the striatum, leading to the development of TD. Observations which support this theory include reduction of DBA dose which can precipitate TD (withdrawal-emergent syndrome or covert dyskinesia). Similarly, increasing the DBA dose can temporarily mask TD symptoms. Also, dyskinesias induced by levodopa in PD patients may closely resemble the movements seen in TD (1). Another hypothesis implicates GABA depletion as a cause. This is based on animal studies which showed decreased GABA turnover and upregulation of receptors in animals with significant TD (62). A small human post-mortem study showed significantly decreased glutamic acid decarboxylase activity (the rate-limiting enzyme in GABA synthesis) in patients with TD compared with patients without (63).

Clinical features

Tardive stereotypy/dyskinesias

The term tardive dyskinesia denotes repetitive, co-ordinated, and seemingly purposeful movements, affecting mainly the orofacial area, which are induced by chronic exposure to neuroleptics. Classic TD is characterized by stereotypic movements affecting the orolinguobuccal muscles. Some prefer to use the term 'tardive stereotypy', since that is the predominant movement disorder. It manifests as repetitive movements of the tongue, lips, and mouth causing tongue protrusion and retraction, lip smacking, and chewing movements. The diaphragm and chest muscles are frequently involved in respiratory dyskinesias, resulting in noisy and difficult breathing. The abdominal and pelvic muscles may also be involved producing truncal or pelvic movements known as copulatory dyskinesia (1). Most commonly, TD patients exhibit a combination of movement disorders. Frequently, the stereotypy of classic TD is combined with choreic movements of the hands, fingers, arms, and feet or with akathisia, which involves restlessness, pacing, rubbing of hands together, etc. Other causes of orofacial dyskinesias should also be considered in the differential diagnosis, and these are outlined in Table 28.5.

Tardive tourettism

Tardive tourettism is an acquired form of tourettism, with onset of abnormal movements and vocalizations following chronic neuroleptic exposure. The first case was reported by Golden in 1974 (64) and was named 'tardive tourettism' by Stahl in 1980 (65). Clinically, the symptoms of tardive tourettism are indistinguishable

Table 28.5 Differential diagnosis of orofacial dyskinesias

1. Spontaneous dyskinesia of elderly (usually dystonic)
2. Neuroacanthocytosis
3. Hereditary chorea (Huntington's disease etc.)
4. Basal ganglia strokes
5. Edentulous dyskinesia
6. Drugs other than neuroleptics causing dyskinesias: levodopa amphetamines cocaine tricyclic antidepressants cimetidine flunarizine antihistamines phenytoin toxicity

from classic Tourette's syndrome, with most motor tics occurring in the craniocervical region and vocalizations involving barking, sniffing, coprolalia, etc. (66). To make a diagnosis of tardive tourettism, it is imperative that the patient has no previous history of tics (motor or vocal) prior to neuroleptic exposure (1). Usually patients also have other associated movements (such as orofacial dyskinesia etc.), and their presence strengthens the association between the occurrence of tics and neuroleptic exposure (66).

Tardive myoclonus

Myoclonus is characterized by abrupt, brisk, jerky, and repetitive involuntary movements caused by asynchronous or synchronous contractions of muscles. Tardive myoclonus with or without other associated movements has been reported as a complication of neuroleptic exposure (67, 68). Other drugs that can worsen or cause myoclonus are listed in Table 28.6. Improvement of tardive myoclonus with clonazepam has been reported.

Tardive tremor

Tardive syndromes rarely manifest as a pure tremor. Stacy and Jankovic (69) reported a small series of patients who developed a 3–5 Hz rest and action tremor, which developed during the course of neuroleptic treatment and worsened after neuroleptic withdrawal (69). The symptoms improved after treatment with the dopamine-depleting agent tetrabenazine. These features, along with the absence of other parkinsonian symptoms and lack of response to traditional medications used to treat tremor, distinguish tardive tremor from other typical causes of tremor. Table 28.7 lists most of the common drugs and drugs of abuse which can cause resting, postural/action, and intention tremors.

Tardive dystonia

Tardive dystonia (TDt) is defined as sustained muscle contractions causing twisting and repetitive movements or abnormal postures in the setting of chronic DBA therapy (70). The diagnostic criteria for TDt, first outlined by Burke and colleagues (71), are as follows:

- the dystonia must be present for more than a month and may occur during ongoing neuroleptic treatment or within 3 months of its discontinuation;
- there must be a negative family history of dystonia;
- other known causes of secondary dystonia must be excluded;
- it is not necessary for other movements to be absent (i.e. tardive dyskinesia or tardive akathisia), as long as dystonia is present and is the dominant movement disorder.

Table 28.6 Other drugs that worsen or cause myoclonus

Drug class	Examples
Anaesthetics	Etomidate, enflurane, propofol
	Spinal anaesthetics
Antibiotics/antimalarials	Cephalosporins, fluoroquinolones, imipenem, mefloquine, penicillins
Antiepileptics	Carbamazepine, gabapentin, lamotrigine, phenytoin, valproate, vigabatrin
Antidepressants	MAOIs, SSRIs, tricyclics
Antineoplastic drugs	Chlorambucil, ifosfamide
Calcium-channel antagonists	Diltiazem, nifedipine, verapamil
Contrast agents	
Dopaminergics	Levodopa, dopamine agonists and antagonists
Drugs of abuse	MDMA
Gastrointestinal drugs	Bismuth salts
Narcotics	Methadone, meperidine, morphine, oxycodone
Other drugs	γ-hydroxybutyrate, tranexamic acid

MAOI, monoamine oxidase inhibitor; MDMA, 3,4-methylenedioxymethamphetamine ('ecstasy').

Table 28.7 Major drugs known to cause postural, intention, and resting tremors

Major category	Typical examples
Postural	
Antiarrhythmics	Amiodarone, mexiletine, procainamide
Antidepressants/mood stabilizers	Amitriptyline, lithium, SSRIs
Antiepileptics	Valproate
Bronchodilators	Albuterol, salmeterol
Chemotherapeutics	Tamoxifen, Ara-C, ifosfamide
Drugs of abuse	Cocaine, ethanol, MDMA ('ecstasy'), nicotine
Gastrointestinal drugs	Metoclopramide, cimetidine
Hormones	Thyroxine, calcitonin, medroxyprogesterone
Immunosuppressants	Tacrolimus, cyclosporine, α-interferon
Methylxanthines	Theophylline, caffeine
Neuroleptics/dopamine depleters	Haloperidol, thioridazine, cinnarizine, reserpine, tetrabenazine
Intention	
Antibiotics/antivirals/antimycotics	Ara-A
Antidepressants/mood stabilizers	Lithium
Bronchodilators	Albuterol, salmeterol
Chemotherapeutics	Ara-C, ifosfamide
Drugs of abuse	Ethanol
Hormones	Adrenaline
Immunosuppressants	Tacrolimus, cyclosporin
Resting	
Antibiotics/antivirals/antimycotics	Trimethoprim/sulfa, amphotericin B
Antidepressants/mood stabilizers	SSRIs, lithium
Antiepileptics	Valproate
Chemotherapeutics	Thalidomide
Drugs of abuse	Cocaine, ethanol, MDMA, MPTP
Gastrointestinal drugs	Metoclopramide
Hormones	Medroxyprogesterone
Neuroleptics/dopamine depleters	Haloperidol, thioridazine, cinnarizine, reserpine, tetrabenazine

MDMA, 3,4-methylenedioxymethamphetamine ('ecstasy'); MPTP, 1-methyl-4-phenyl-1,2,3-tetrahydropyridine; SSRIs, selective serotonin reuptake inhibitors; Ara-A; vidarabine; Ara-C, cytarabine.

Reproduced with permission from Morgan JC, Sethi KD. *Lancet Neurol* 2005; 4: 866–76.

Based on a review of eleven cross-sectional studies involving psychiatric patients, the prevalence of TDt ranged from 0.5 to 21.6% with a mean of 2.7% in a total of over 4000 patients exposed to DBAs (72). All classes of DBAs are implicated, and even atypical neuroleptics can produce TDt. Clozapine appears to be the least likely to produce TDt. Children and young adults are more likely to develop TDt, and increasing age decreases the likelihood of developing generalized dystonia (72).

The onset of TDt is often insidious, developing over weeks to months. It usually starts with one body part and can become segmental or even generalized. Craniocervical areas are the most common sites of onset and are involved in ~80% (72). Presentation with arm, trunk, or leg involvement is less common. Younger patients tended to have a more rapid spread than older patients with TDt. In a study by Kiriakakis and colleagues (73) the mean age of onset in TDt patients with rapid spread (<1 year) was 32 years compared with 42 years for patients in whom the dystonia spread more slowly (>1 year) (73). TDt may be difficult to distinguish from idiopathic dystonia, although Molho and colleagues (74) reported that torticollis, laterocollis, and sensory tricks were less common in TDt than in idiopathic dystonia. In a study of oromandibular dystonia (OMD), Tan and Jankovic (75) found that oro-buccal-lingual stereotypies were more common in the tardive group when compared with idiopathic OMD (74). Also, lateral flexion of the trunk and Pisa syndrome can occur in TDt and are less common in idiopathic dystonia (76).

TDt is a rather persistent disorder and remissions are uncommon. A review highlighted a low remission rate of ~10% in TDt patients after a mean follow-up period of 6.6 years (73). However, our personal experience suggests that remission may occur if intervention is early in the course of TDt. Prompt discontinuation of the offending DBA seems to be the only factor relevant to influencing remission. From a treatment perspective, it is important to distinguish TDt from tardive dyskinesia as anticholinergic drugs tend to worsen classic tardive dyskinesia but are beneficial in tardive dystonia.

Tardive akathisia

Akathisia is characterized by a subjective aversion to remaining still which is relieved by moving. The movements may be simple or complex and are stereotyped. Neuroleptic drug exposure is a common cause of chronic akathisia; some of the other causes include restless legs syndrome and parkinsonism. Tardive akathisia (TA) frequently seems to evolve from acute akathisia (which is clearly a complication of neuroleptic exposure). TA, rather than TDt, is more commonly associated with tardive dyskinesia (66). Multiple studies suggest a high prevalence of TA in patients with long-term neuroleptic exposure, ranging from 20 to 30% (66, 77). Like other tardive syndromes, TA has been reported with both typical and atypical neuroleptics; case reports of TA induced by clozapine also exist, although they are rare (78).

As mentioned above, clinically akathisia comprises both a subjective component of restlessness (which is often described as jitteriness or nervousness) and an objective component of increased frequency of movement which may be complex and stereotyped. However, in TA the subjective component becomes less severe and sometimes may evolve into a state of 'pseudo-akathisia' (79). Patients with TA can temporarily suppress the abnormal movements, but it is associated with an increasing sense of tension or restlessness and there is a sense of relief when carrying out the movements. A study of patients with TA showed that the legs were the most frequently involved body part, with patients either marching in place while standing or crossing/uncrossing their legs while sitting, etc. (80). Truncal movements with rocking back and forth were also commonly noted. A variety of less common movements such as face rubbing, folding/unfolding arms, respiratory irregularities (e.g. panting), and moaning have also been reported (80).

As far as prognosis is concerned, a large proportion of TA patients continue to have symptoms for years, even after the neuroleptics have been discontinued. True remissions are infrequent, although they can occur. It seems that younger patients or early age of onset of TA may have a more reversible course and favourable prognosis (66).

Management of tardive syndromes

Tardive stereotypy/dyskinesias

The optimal management of TD is to prevent it in the first place by not using DBAs unless absolutely necessary or, if they have to be used, choosing an atypical neuroleptic at the lowest possible dose. However, when symptoms of TD first appear an important decision involves whether to continue neuroleptic therapy or not. Data compiled from multiple studies showed that 36% of patients improved after drug withdrawal (81). Ideally, the neuroleptic drug should be discontinued; however, if the risk for relapse of the psychiatric condition is high, other options such as dose reduction, switching to high-potency atypical neuroleptics, or adding other medications to treat the symptoms should be considered.

Often, additional medications to treat the symptoms of TD are needed. Dopamine-depleting agents such as tetrabenazine and reserpine are considered to be the most effective treatment for severe TD. Both of these medications should be introduced at low doses (tetrabenazine at 25 mg/day and reserpine at 0.25 mg/day) and then slowly titrated upwards at weekly intervals until adequate therapeutic benefit or side effects occur. The dose of tetrabenazine needed for adequate control of TD symptoms is ~75–100 mg/day, and that for reserpine is ~3–6 mg/day. Reserpine has been used in combination with α-methyl para-tyrosine, another dopamine-depleting agent, with significant benefit (82).

Drugs with GABAergic properties have also been used to treat TD. Among these, clonazepam has been successfully used to treat milder forms of TD. A common practice is to start with 0.5 mg at bedtime and increase the dose by 0.5 mg every week until a therapeutic effect is achieved. Caution needs to be exercised in combining clonazepam with antipsychotic medication as it can lead to respiratory depression (83). Other GABAergic drugs such as sodium valproate and vigabatrin have been reported to have some efficacy in a small number of patients (84) but, given their unfavourable risk–benefit profile, they are not commonly used in clinical practice.

For patients who must be treated with antipsychotics, an atypical neuroleptic such as clozapine may be used. Clozapine has the lowest risk of causing TD and symptoms often improve once patients are switched to this drug. This may in part be due to the preferential blockade of D4 over D2 receptors by clozapine (60). Treatment is initiated at 25 mg/day and slowly titrated (range, 100–500 mg/day) until therapeutic benefit or side effects occur. With clozapine, weekly blood counts are required for 6 months to monitor for leucopenia, and then every 2 weeks for the next 6 months, and then monthly, as it can cause agranulocytosis (60).

Some other drugs that have shown limited success, either in a limited number of patients or small clinical trials, include the following. Amantadine showed efficacy in a small study of ~20 patients with TD when compared with placebo (85). This drug should be used carefully in the elderly as it can cause or worsen confusion. Calcium-channel blockers have produced varying results, with nifedipine and verapamil demonstrating efficacy (86), and diltiazem being ineffective (87).

Clonidine, at doses ranging from 0.15 to 0.45 mg/day, has shown moderate improvement of symptoms in 75% of patients and complete resolution of abnormal movements in 50% of treated patients (88). Much attention has also been focused on vitamin E whose use is based on the belief that it may reverse the toxic effect of free radicals produced via DBAs (89). The doses employed range from 1200 to 1600 mg/day in three divided doses. Mixed results have been reported, making its usefulness unclear. A Cochrane review of eight small studies with poor randomization suggested that vitamin E does improve symptoms of TD (89), but a large prospective randomized 2-year trial of vitamin E versus matching placebo in patients with TD failed to show any benefit (90).

Other drugs, such as propranolol, and antiepileptics such as levetiracetam have also been reported to have some benefit in the treatment of TD based on anecdotal reports or small studies (89).

Botulinum toxin injections have been used for the treatment of orofacial TD, with injections into the lingual and masticatory muscles. Treatment should be initiated with low doses and then gradually increased as tolerated, as side effects such as dysphagia may occur (91). Rarely, deep brain stimulation of the globus pallidus internus has been used with some benefit to treat severe symptoms of orofacial TD, but more often in tardive dystonia (92).

Tardive tourettism, myoclonus, and tremor

In general, the principles of treatment of tardive tourettism, myoclonus, and tremor are similar to those outlined in the section on tardive dyskinesias.

Tardive akathisia

The principles of treating tardive akathisia are similar to those for treating TD. Whenever possible, the offending neuroleptic should be stopped. It is important to note that TA differs significantly from acute akathisia. Opiates and propranolol, which are effective in acute akathisia, are not useful in treating TA, whereas dopamine blockers, which worsen acute akathisia, have the opposite effect in TA (66).

Although there are few studies focused on treatments for tardive akathisia, evidence suggests that dopamine blockers (tetrabenazine and reserpine) are most effective in managing these patients (66).

Tardive dystonia

As with other tardive syndromes, discontinuation of the offending drug is the first step. If the offending DBA cannot be discontinued and the involuntary movements are disabling, additional medications may have to be added. The dopamine-depleting agents tetrabenazine and reserpine are the most effective drugs for the treatment of TDt. Unlike tardive dyskinesia, tardive dystonia responds well to anticholinergic therapies such as trihexyphenidyl. Since it is unclear which patients will respond to either of these classes of medications, the decision to use dopamine-depleting agents versus anticholinergics is driven by their side-effect profile (66). Anticholinergics should be avoided in elderly patients prone to cognitive impairment, and patients with a history of depression should avoid dopamine-depleting agents. Benzodiazepines such as clonazepam may also be useful in treating TDt and they are often used in combination with the dopamine depleters or anticholinergics mentioned above. Other drugs, such as bromocriptine, clonidine, verapamil, amantadine, carbamazepine, and valproate, may be helpful in some patients (93).

In addition to systemic pharmacological approaches to management, focal tardive dystonias affecting the craniocervical region have been successfully treated with botulinum toxin injections (94, 95). Select patients with severe, irreversible tardive dystonia can show improvement after bilateral globus pallidus (GPi) deep brain stimulation (92).

Other tardive phenomena

Withdrawal emergent syndrome

The withdrawal emergent syndrome is typically seen following the abrupt withdrawal of drugs from children who have been on long-standing DRBA (96). In contrast with classic TD, the movements in withdrawal emergent syndrome are choreic in nature and more generalized. They tend to involve the neck, limbs, and trunk, and seldom involve the orofacial region (unlike classic TD). These movements have also been called 'withdrawal dyskinesias' and reported to occur rarely in adults with sudden cessation of an antipsychotic agent (60, 66). The withdrawal emergent syndrome is usually self-limiting and typically disappears within 3 months. Another term encountered in the literature is 'covert dyskinesias'. These occur upon reduction of neuroleptic therapy and persist for longer periods. However, this distinction is arbitrary, as some covert dyskinesias will disappear after prolonged follow-up (1). Another strategy to eliminate the abnormal movements is to reinstitute the offending DRBA and then slowly taper it off (60, 66).

Neuroleptic malignant syndrome

Neuroleptic malignant syndrome (NMS), first recognized in 1960 by Delay and colleagues (97), is an iatrogenic disorder associated with (but not limited to) exposure to neuroleptics. Some of the other causes of NMS are listed in Table 28.8. The overall incidence of NMS is quite low, at around 0.2%, although other reports of

Table 28.8 Causes of neuroleptic malignant syndrome

Use of neuroleptics	At any time during its use (from initiation to being on stable dose)
Withdrawal of dopaminergic therapy in PD	Associated with stopping amantadine, levodopa, or dopamine agonists suddenly in PD patients
	Can occur during levodopa OFF periods
	Rarely, with dopaminergic medication dose adjustments
Use of tetrabenazine	
Cocaine abuse	
Combining TCA + MAOI	Can lead to NMS-like syndrome.

TCA, tricyclic antidepressant; MAO-I, monoamine oxidase inhibitor.

higher incidence exist (98, 99). Even though a uniform consensus regarding the definition and criteria are lacking, most experts agree that NMS is a clinical syndrome comprising fever, rigidity, mental status changes, autonomic dysfunction, and other movement disorders (tremor, dystonia, and myoclonus) (100). Prominent laboratory abnormalities include leucocytosis and elevated serum creatine kinase. Additionally, acute-phase reactants, including albumin and serum iron levels, may be decreased (100). NMS typically occurs with exposure to DBAs, such as neuroleptics (both typical and atypical), and dopamine depleters, such as reserpine or tetrabenazine, and following withdrawal of dopaminergic agents in Parkinson's disease (in the absence of neuroleptic exposure it has also been called parkinsonism–hyperpyrexia syndrome) (60). NMS may occur within days to months of initiating neuroleptics, although only around 3% develop the syndrome after 6 months of stable neuroleptic medication (101). Risk factors include young age, male sex, potency of the neuroleptics, and rate of dose increase. Duration of NMS symptoms is significantly shorter with atypical neuroleptics than with the older typical agents (102).

NMS has to be distinguished from the serotonin syndrome that is caused by SSRI plus MAO-I and some other drugs. Primary management of NMS comprises prevention through conservative use of antipsychotics and cautious dose increases. Given the high mortality (5–20%), clinical vigilance and a high index of suspicion are necessary to make an early diagnosis which may be termed 'pre-malignant' NMS. Immediate withdrawal of the offending antipsychotic agent is key. After this, supportive care and careful observation may suffice for mild cases. In more severe cases, intensive care unit monitoring, treatment with pharmacological agents such as benzodiazepines, dantrolene, or bromocriptine, or electroconvulsive therapy in refractory cases, may be necessary (103).

References

1. Sethi KD, Morgan JC. Drug-induced movement disorders. In Jankovic J, Tolosa E (eds) *Parkinson's disease and movement disorders* (5th edn). Philadelphia, PA: Lippincott, Williams & Wilkins, 2007.
2. Mazurek MF, Rosebush PI. Acute drug-induced dystonia. In: Factor SA, Lang AE and Weiner W (eds), *Drug induced movement disorders* (2nd edn) pp. 72–102. Boston, MA: Blackwell, 2005.
3. Aguilar EJ, Keshavan MS, Martínez-Quiles MD, et al. Predictors of acute dystonia in first-episode psychotic patients. *Am J Psychiatry* 1994; 151: 1819–21.
4. Chakos MH, Mayerhoff DI, Loebel AD, et al. Incidence and correlates of acute extrapyramidal symptoms in first episode of schizophrenia. *Psychopharmacol Bull* 1992; 28: 81–6.
5. Keepers GA, Clappison VJ, Casey DE. Initial anticholinergic prophylaxis for neuroleptic-induced extrapyramidal syndromes. *Arch Gen Psychiatry* 1983: 40: 492–6.
6. Priori A, Bertolasi L, Berardelli A, Manfredi M. Predictors of acute dystonia in first-episode psychotic patients. *Am J Psychiatry* 1994; 151: 1819–21.
7. Hriso E, Kuhn T, Masdeu JC, et al. Extrapyramidal symptoms due to dopamine-blocking agents in patients with AIDS encephalopathy. *Am J Psychiatry.* 1991; 148: 1558–61.
8. van Harten PN, van Trier JC, Horwitz EH, Matroos GE, Hoek HW. Cocaine as a risk factor for neuroleptic-induced acute dystonia. *Am J Psychiatry* 1986; 143: 706–10.
9. Nealer R, Gerhardt S, Liebman JM. Effects of dopamine agonists, catecholamine depletors, and cholinergic and GABAergic drugs on acute dyskinesia in the squirrel monkeys. *Psychopharmacology (Berl)* 1984; 82: 20–6.
10. Marsden CD, Jenner P. the pathophysiology of extrapyramidal side effects of neuroleptic drugs. *Psychol Med* 1980; 10: 55–72.
11. KeepersGA,CaseyDE.Clinicalmanagementofacuteneuroleptic-inducedextrapyramidal syndromes. In: Masserman JH (ed.) *Current psychiatric therapies*, pp. 139–57. New York: Grune & Stratton, 1986.
12. Waugh WH, Metts JC. Severe extrapyramidal motor activity induced by prochlorperazine: its relief by the intravenous injection of diphenhydramine. *N Engl J Med* 1960; 262: 353–4.
13. Piecuch S, Thomas U, Shah BR. Acute dystonic reactions that fail to respond to diphenhydramine: think of PCP. *J Emerg Med* 1999; 17: 527.
14. Keepers GA, Clappison VJ, Casey DE. Initial anticholinergic prophylaxis for neuroleptic-induced extrapyramidal syndromes. *Arch Gen Psychiatry* 1983; 40: 492–6.
15. World Health Organization. Prophylactic use of anticholinergics in patients on long term neuroleptic treatment: a consensus statement. *Br J Psychiatry* 1990; 156: 412.
16. Haskovec L. Akathisie. *Arch Bohemes Med Clin* 1902; 17: 704–8.
17. Sigwald J, Grossiord A, Duriel P, et al. Le traitement de la maladie de Parkinson et des manifestations extrpyramidales par le diethyl aminoethynthiodiphenylamine (2987 RP) resultats d'une annee d'application. *Rev Neurol (Paris)* 1947; 79: 683–7.
18. Ayd FJ, Jr. A survey of drug-induced extrapyramidal reactions. *JAMA* 1961; 175: 1054–60.
19. Braude WM, Barnes TR, Gore SM. Clinical characteristics of akathisia: a systematic investigation of acute psychiatric inpatient admissions. *Br J Psychiatry* 1983; 143: 139–50.
20. Kumar R, Sachdev PS. Akathisia and second-generation antipsychotic drugs. *Curr Opin Psychiatry* 2009; 22: 293–9.
21. Arvanitis LA, Miller BG. Multiple fixed doses of 'Seroquel' (quetiapine) in patients with acute exacerbation of schizophrenia: a comparison with haloperidol and placebo. The Seroquel Trial 13 Study Group. *Biol Psychiatry* 1997; 42: 233–46.
22. Adler LA, Rotrosen J, Angrist B. Acute drug-induced akathisia. In: Factor SA, Lang AE, Weiner W (eds) *Drug induced movement disorders* (2nd edn), pp. 140–73. Boston, MA: Blackwell, 2005.
23. Nordström AL, Farde L, Halldin C. Time course of D2-dopamine receptor occupancy examined by PET after single oral doses of haloperidol. *Psychopharmacology (Berl)* 1992; 106: 433–8.
24. Farde L, Nordström A, Weisel F, et al. Positron emission tomographic analysis of central D1 and D2 dopamine receptor occupancy in patients treated with classical neuroleptics and clozapine. *Arch Gen Psychiatry* 1992; 49: 539–44.
25. Stahl SM, Lonnen AJ. The mechanism of drug-induced akathisia. *CNS Spectr* 2011 [Epub ahead of print].
26. Stryjer R, Rosenzcwaig S, Bar F, et al. Trazodone for the treatment of neuroleptic-induced acute akathisia: a placebo-controlled, double-blind, crossover study. *Clin Neuropharmacol* 2010; 33: 219–22.
27. Poyurovsky M. Acute antipsychotic-induced akathisia revisited. *Br J Psychiatry* 2010; 196: 89–91.
28. Adler L, Angrist B, Peselow E, et al. A controlled assessment of propranolol in the treatment of neuroleptic-induced akathisia. *Br J Psychiatry* 1986; 149: 42–5.
29. Adler L, Angrist B, Peselow E, et al. Efficacy of propranolol in neuroleptic-induced akathesia. *J Clin Psychopharmacol* 1985; 5: 164–6.
30. Bondon-Guitton E, Perez-Lloret S, Bagheri H, et al. Drug-induced parkinsonism: a review of 17 years' experience in a regional pharmacovigilance center in France. *Mov Disord* 2011; 26: 2226–31.
31. Stephen PJ, Williams J. Drug induced parkinsonism in the elderly. *Lancet* 1984; ii: 1082–3.
32. Masso JF, Poza JJ. Drug-induced or aggravated parkinsonism: clinical signs and the changing pattern of implicated drugs. *Neurologia* 1996; 11: 10–15.
33. Mutch WJ, Dingwall-Fordyce I, Downie AW, et al. Parkinson's disease in a Scottish city. *Br Med J* 1986; 292: 534–6.

34. Friedman JH, Trieschmann ME, Fernandez HH. Drug-induced parkinsonism. In: Factor SA, Lang AE and Weiner W (eds) *Drug induced movement disorders* (2nd edn), pp. 103–39. Boston, MA: Blackwell, 2005.
35. Farde L, Wiesel FA, Halldin C, et al. Central D2-dopamine receptor occupancy in schizophrenic patients treated with antipsychotic drugs. *Arch Gen Psychiatry* 1988; 45: 71–6.
36. Meltzer HY, Matsubara S, Lee JC. Classification of typical and atypical antipsychotic drugs on the basis dopamine D1, D2 and serotonin pKi values. *Pharmacol Exp Ther* 1989; 251: 238–46.
37. Hardie R, Lees A. Neuroleptic-induced Parkinson's syndrome: clinical features and results of treatment with levodopa. *J Neurol Neurosurg Psychiatry* 1988; 51: 850–4.
38. Levinson DF, Simpson GM, Singh H, et al. Fluphenazine dose, clinical response, and extrapyramidal symptoms during acute treatment. *Arch Gen Psychiatry* 1990; 47: 761–8.
39. Fernandez HH, Krupp B, Friedman J. The course of tardive dyskinesia and parkinsonism in psychiatric inpatients: 14-year follow-up. *Neurology* 2001; 56: 805–7.
40. DiMascio A, Demergian E. Antiparkinson drug overuse. *Psychosomatics* 1970; 11: 596–601.
41. Burn DJ, Brooks DJ. Nigral dysfunction in drug-induced parkinsonism: an ^{18}F-dopa PET study. *Neurology* 1993; 43: 552–6.
42. Lorberboym M, Treves TA, Melamed E, et al. [^{123}I]-FP/CIT SPECT imaging for distinguishing drug-induced parkinsonism from Parkinson's disease. *Mov Disord* 2006; 21: 510–14.
43. Chaudhuri KR, Nott J. Drug-induced parkinsonism. In: Sethi KD (ed.) *Drug-induced movement disorders*, pp. 61–75. New York: Marcel Dekker, 2005.
44. Fann WE, Lake CR. Amantidine versus trihexiphenidyl in the treatment of neuroleptic induced parkinsonism. *Am J Psychiatry* 1976; 133: 940–3.
45. Fahn S. The tardive dyskinesias. In Matthews WB, Glaser GH (ed.) *Recent advances in clinical neurology*,Vol, 4, pp. 229–60. Edinburgh: Churchill Livingstone.
46. Baldessarini RJ, Cole JO, Davis JM, et al. Tardive dyskinesia: summary of a Task Force Report of the American Psychiatric Association. *Am J Psychiatry* 1980; 137: 1163–72.
47. Jeste DV, Lacro JP, Palmer B, et al. Incidence of tardive dyskinesia in early stages of low-dose treatment with typical neuroleptics in older patients. *Am J Psychiatry* 1999; 156: 309–11.
48. Klawans HL, Tanner CM, Goetz CG. Epidemiology and pathophysiology of tardive dyskinesia. *Adv Neurol* 1988; 49: 185–7.
49. Faheem AD, Brightwell DR, Burton GC, et al. Respiratory dyskinesia and dysarthria from prolonged neuroleptic use: tardive dyskinesia? *Am J Psychiatry* 1982; 139: 517–18.
50. Alentorn A, Palasí A, Campdelacreu J, et al. Pelvic dyskinesia with an outstanding response to tetrabenazine. *Prog Neuropsychopharmacol Biol Psychiatry* 2009; 33: 847–8.
51. Jankovic J, Casabona J. Coexistent tardive dyskinesia and parkinsonism. *Clin Neuropharmacol* 1987; 10: 511–21.
52. Tarsy D. History and definition of tardive dyskinesia. *Clin Neuropharmacol* 1983; 6: 91–9.
53. Smith JM, Baldessarini RJ. Changes in prevalence, severity, and recovery in tardive dyskinesia with age. *Arch Gen Psychiatry* 1980; 37: 1368–73.
54. Kane JM, Smith JM. Tardive dyskinesia: prevalence and risk factors, 1959 to 1979. *Arch Gen Psychiatry* 1982; 39: 473–81.
55. Morgenstern H, Glazer WM. Identifying risk-factors for tardive dyskinesia among long-term outpatients maintained with neuroleptic medications. *Arch Gen Psychiatry* 1993; 50: 723–33.
56. Glazer WM, Morgenstern H, Doucette JT. Predicting the long-term risk of tardive dyskinesia in out patients maintained on neuroleptic medications. *J Clin Psychiatry* 1993; 54: 133–9.
57. Tarsy D, Baldessarini RJ. Epidemiology of tardive dyskinesia: is risk declining with modern antipsychotics? *Mov Disord* 2006; 21: 589–98.
58. Correll CU, Leucht S, Kane JM. Lower risk for tardive dyskinesia associated with second generation antipsychotics: systematic review of one-year studies. *Am J Psychiatry* 2004; 161: 414–25.
59. Tarsy D, Lungu C, Baldessarini RJ. Epidemiology of tardive dyskinesia before and during the era of modern antipsychotic drugs. *Handb Clin Neurol* 2011; 100: 601–16.
60. DeLeon M, Jankovic J. Clinical features and management of classic tardive dyskinesia, tardive myoclonus, tardive tremor and tardive tourettism. In: Sethi KD (ed.) *Drug-induced movement disorders*, pp. 77–109. New York: Marcel Dekker, 2005.
61. Margolese HC, Chouinard G, Kolivakis TT, et al. Tardive dyskinesia in the era of typical and atypical antipsychotics. Part 1: pathophysiology and mechanisms of induction. *Can J Psychiatry* 2005; 50: 541–7.
62. Gunne LM, Häggström JE, Sjöquist B. Association with persistent neuroleptic-induced dyskinesia of regional changes in brain GABA synthesis. *Nature* 1984; 309: 347–9.
63. Andersson U, Häggström JE, Levin ED, et al. Reduced glutamate decarboxylase activity in the subthalamic nucleus in patients with tardive dyskinesia. *Mov Disord* 1989; 4: 37–46.
64. Golden GS. Gilles de la Tourette's syndrome following methylphenidate administration. *Dev Med Child Neurol* 1974; 16: 76–8.
65. Stahl SM. Tardive Tourette syndrome in an autistic patient after long-term neuroleptic administration. *Am J Psychiatry* 1980; 137: 1267–9.
66. Skidmore F, Weiner WJ, Burke R. Neuroleptic-induced tardive dyskinesia variants. In: Factor SA, Lang AE and Weiner W (eds) *Drug induced movement disorders* (2nd edn), pp. 257–84. Boston, MA: Blackwell, 2005.
67. Little JT, Jankovic J. Tardive myoclonus: a case report. *Mov Disord* 1987; 2: 307–11.
68. Tominaga H, Fukuzako H, Izumi K, et al. Tardive myoclonus. *Lancet* 1987; i: 322.
69. Stacy M, Jankovic J. Tardive tremor. *Mov Disord* 1992; 7: 53–7.
70. Fahn S. Concept and classification of dystonia. *Adv Neurol* 1988; 50: 2–8.
71. Burke RE, Fahn S, Jankovic J, et al. Tardive dystonia: late-onset and persistent dystonia caused by antipsychotic drugs. *Neurology* 1982; 32: 1335–46.
72. Bhatt M, Sethi KD, Bhatia K. Acute and tardive dystonia. In: Sethi KD (ed.) *Drug-induced movement disorders*, pp. 111–28. New York: Marcel Dekker, 2005.
73. Kiriakakis V, Bhatia KP, Quinn NP, et al. The natural history of tardive dystonia: a long-term follow-up study of 107 cases. *Brain* 1998; 121: 2053–66.
74. Molho ES, Feustel PJ, Factor SA. Clinical comparison of tardive and idiopathic cervical dystonia. *Mov Disord* 1998; 13: 486–9.
75. Tan EK, Jankovic J. Tardive and idiopathic oromandibular dystonia: a clinical comparison. *J Neurol Neurosurg Psychiatry* 2000; 68: 186–90.
76. Suzuki T, Matsuzaka H. Drug-induced Pisa syndrome (pleurothotonus): epidemiology and management. *CNS Drugs* 2002; 16: 165–74.
77. Halstead SM, Barnes TR, Speller JC. Akathisia: prevalence and associated dysphoria in an in-patient population with chronic schizophrenia. *Br J Psychiatry* 1994; 164: 177–83.
78. Gogtay N, Sporn A, Alfaro CL, et al. Clozapine-induced akathisia in children with schizophrenia. *J Child Adolesc Psychopharmacol* 2002; 12: 347–9.
79. Braude WM, Barnes TRE. Late-onset akathisia—an incident of covert dyskinesias: two case reports. *Am J Psychiatry* 1983; 140: 611–12.
80. Burke RE, Kang UK, Jankovic J, et al. Tardive akathisia: an analysis of clinical features and response to open therapeutic trials. *Mov Disord* 1989; 4: 157–75.
81. Jeste DV, Wyatt RJ. In search of treatment of tardive dyskinesia: review of the literature. *Schizophr Bull* 1979; 5: 253–93.
82. Fahn S. Long term treatment of tardive dyskinesia with presynaptically acting dopamine-depleting agents. *Adv Neurol* 1983; 37: 267–76.

83. Egan MF, Apud J, Wyatt RJ. Treatment of tardive dyskinesia. *Schizophr Bull* 1997; 23: 583–603.
84. Srinivasan J, Richens A. A risk-benefit assessment of vigabatrin in the treatment of neurological disorders. *Drug Saf* 1994; 10: 395–405.
85. Pappa S, Tsouli S, Apostolou G, et al. Effects of amantadine on tardive dyskinesia: a randomized, double-blind, placebo-controlled study. *Clin Neuropharmacol* 2010; 33: 271–5.
86. Duncan E, Adler L, Angrist B, Rotrosen J. Nifedipine in the treatment of tardive dyskinesia. *J Clin Pharmacol* 1990; 10: 414–16.
87. Loonen AJ, Verwey HA, Roels PR, et al. Is diltiazem effective in treating the symptoms of (tardive) dyskinesia in chronic psychiatric inpatients? *J Clin Psychopharmacol* 1992; 12: 39–42.
88. Nishikawa T, Tanaka M, Tsuda A, et al. Clonidine therapy for tardive dyskinesia and related syndromes. *Clin Neuropharmacol* 1984; 7: 239–45.
89. Aia PG, Revuelta GJ, Cloud LJ, et al. Tardive dyskinesia. *Curr Treat Options Neurol* 2011; 13: 231–41.
90. Adler LA, Rotrosen J, Edson R, et al. Vitamin E treatment for tardive dyskinesia. Veterans Affairs Cooperative Study #394 Study Group. *Arch Gen Psychiatry* 1999; 56: 836–41.
91. Slotema CW, van Harten PN, Bruggeman R, et al. Botulinum toxin in the treatment of orofacial tardive dyskinesia: a single blind study. *Prog Neuropsychopharmacol Biol Psychiatry* 2008; 32: 507–9.
92. Welter ML, Grabli D, Vidailhet M. Deep brain stimulation for hyperkinetics disorders: dystonia, tardive dyskinesia, and tics. *Curr Opin Neurol* 2010; 23: 420–5.
93. Fahn S. The tardive syndromes: phenomenology, concepts on pathophysiology and treatment. A comprehensive review of movement disorders for the clinical practitioner. 2003, 181–265.
94. Tarsy D, Kaufman D, Sethi KD, et al. An open-label study of botulinum toxin A for treatment of tardive dystonia. *Clin Neuropharmacol* 1997; 20: 90–3.
95. Hennings JM, Bötzel KE, Wetter TC. Successful treatment of tardive lingual dystonia with botulinum toxin: case report and review of the literature. *Prog Neuropsychopharmacol Biol Psychiatry* 2008; 32: 1167–71.
96. Gardos G, Cole JO, Tarsy D. Withdrawal syndromes associated with antipsychotic drugs. *Am J Psychiatry* 1978; 135: 1321–4.
97. Delay J, Pichot P, Lemperiere T, Elissalde B, Peigne F. [A non-phenothiazine and non-reserpine major neuroleptic, haloperidol, in the treatment of psychoses.] *Ann Med Psychol (Paris)* 1960; 118: 145–52.
98. Naganuma H, Fujii I. Incidence and risk factors in neuroleptic malignant syndrome. *Acta Psychiatr Scand* 1994; 90: 424–6.
99. Caroff SN, Mann SC. Neuroleptic malignant syndrome. *Med Clin North Am* 1993; 77: 185–202.
100. Robottom BJ, Weiner WJ, Factor SA. Movement disorders emergencies. Part 1: Hypokinetic disorders. *Arch Neurol* 2011; 68: 567–72.
101. Pearlam CA. Neuroleptic malignant syndrome: a review of the literature. *J Clin Psychopharmacol* 1986; 6: 257–73.
102. Neuhut R, Lindenmayer JP, Silva R. Neuroleptic malignant syndrome in children and adolescents on atypical antipsychotic medication: a review. *J Child Adolesc Psychopharmacol* 2009; 19: 415–22.
103. Strawn JR, Keck PE, Jr, Caroff SN. Neuroleptic-malignant syndrome. *Am J Psychiatry* 2007; 164: 870–6.

CHAPTER 29

Systemic Disease and Movement Disorders

Leslie J. Cloud and Joseph Jankovic

Summary

Systemic illness is often complicated by the development of movement disorders, and the spectrum of movement disorders occurring in systemic diseases is as diverse as the spectrum of diseases eliciting them. While movement disorders often develop in patients with a known systemic illness, they can sometimes be the presenting feature of a systemic disease (1). Although pregnancy is not considered an 'illness', there are many movement disorders associated with this condition (2). Recognition and treatment of the underlying condition or a systemic disorder is essential for the optimal management of associated abnormal movements. Therefore, when evaluating patients with movement disorders, clinicians should carefully consider all medical historical details, associated symptoms and signs, and risk factors for systemic diseases, as these may provide important clues to the underlying aetiology of both the systemic and the associated movement disorders. The information presented in this chapter should serve as a guide not only to movement disorder clinicians but also to general and primary care physicians. Recognizing the movement disorder phenomenology is the first step that eventually leads to the aetiological diagnosis.

This chapter reviews movement disorders occurring in conjunction with several broad categories of systemic disease, including paraneoplastic, autoimmune, endocrine, metabolic, nutritional, and infectious diseases.

Paraneoplastic syndromes

Paraneoplastic neurological syndromes are a heterogeneous group of disorders caused by an immune response to an underlying malignancy. Paraneoplastic antibodies simultaneously target antigens expressed by tumour cells and cellular components of the central and/or peripheral nervous system(s), thereby producing neurological symptoms that are not due to direct invasion of the affected tissue by the primary tumour or metastasis. The underlying cancer is often occult and the paraneoplastic neurological syndrome may be the presenting complaint. Fortunately, paraneoplastic neurological syndromes are rare, occurring in <1% of all cancer patients (3). A subset of paraneoplastic neurological syndromes presents with movement disorders. The classical paraneoplastic neurological syndromes that cause movement disorders are cerebellar degeneration, stiff person syndrome (SPS), and opsoclonus–myoclonus syndrome. Much less commonly, paraneoplastic chorea, tremors, and parkinsonism can occur. Recently, antibodies to the *N*-methyl-D-aspartate (NMDA) subtype of the glutamate receptor have been associated with a neuropsychiatric syndrome, dystonia, and other dyskinesias, typically observed in young women with ovarian teratomas.

Paraneoplastic ataxia

Paraneoplastic cerebellar degeneration presents subacutely with onset of cerebellar ataxia, asymmetric in many cases, over a few weeks or months. The ataxia can present as a pure cerebellar syndrome or may be associated with signs and symptoms of a more widespread encephalomyelitis, limbic encephalitis, sensory neuropathy, or Lambert–Eaton myasthenic syndrome (3). Patients may experience dizziness, oscillopsia, vertigo, diplopia, dysarthria, dysphagia, gait dysfunction, and truncal and/or appendicular ataxia. A number of eye movement abnormalities can occur such as nystagmus, ocular dysmetria, slow saccades, jerkiness of smooth pursuits, square-wave jerks, opsoclonus, and saccadic oscillations (4). After a subacute onset and progression, patients eventually stabilize at a severe level of disability. The differential diagnosis for subacute cerebellar ataxia is wide and is summarized in Table 29.1. The malignancies most commonly associated with paraneoplastic cerebellar degeneration are breast and ovarian cancer, small-cell lung cancer, and Hodgkin's disease (5). Paraneoplastic cerebellar degeneration is associated with many different antibodies (Table 29.2), and more than one antibody may be present in the same individual (5). In the early stages, brain imaging can be normal, though cerebellar atrophy occurs as the disorder advances. Cerebrospinal fluid (CSF) analysis may reveal mildly elevated protein or oligoclonal bands (6, 7). Histopathologically, diffuse loss of Purkinje cells with inflammatory infiltrates in the cerebellar cortex, deep cerebellar nuclei, and inferior olivary nuclei are seen (3). Prognosis depends on the antibody and cancer type. Earlier detection is associated with an improved prognosis. Figure 29.1 shows an MRI scan of a patient with paraneoplastic cerebellar degeneration with anti-Yo antibodies associated with her underlying breast cancer.

Table 29.1 Differential diagnosis of subacute cerebellar ataxia

Endocrine	Hypothyroidism, Hashimoto's thyroiditis
Infectious	Infections and postinfectious cerebellitis
Toxic and nutritional	Alcohol-related cerebellar ataxia, vitamin B_{12} or folate deficiency, medications
Malignancy	Posterior fossa tumours (primary and metastatic)

Table 29.2 Antibodies associated with paraneoplastic cerebellar degeneration

Antineuronal antibody	Clinical syndromes	Associated tumours
Anti-Hu/ANNA-1	PCD	SCLC
Anti-Yo/PCA-1	PCD	Breast, ovarian
Anti-Ri/ANNA-2	PCD, OM	Breast, gynaecological, SCLC
Anti-Tr	PCD	Hodgkin's lymphoma
Anti-P/Q type VGCC	PCD, LEMS	SCLC
Anti-Ma	PCD	Many
Anti-Ta/Ma2	PCD, limbic encephalitis	Testis
Anti-CRMP5/CV2	PCD	SCLC, thymoma, gynaecological
Anti-mGluR1	PCD	Hodgkin's lymphoma

PCD, paraneoplastic cerebellar degeneration; OM, opsoclonus–myoclonus; LEMS, Lambert–Eaton myasthenic syndrome; SCLC, small-cell lung cancer

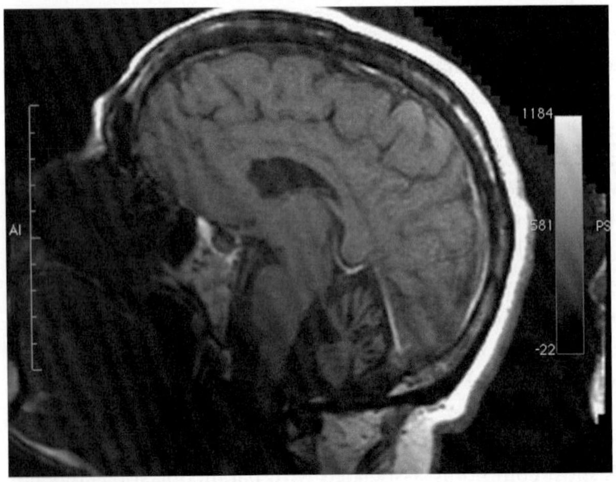

Fig. 29.1 Diffuse cerebellar atrophy on T_1 sagittal MRI in a woman presenting with subacute cerebellar ataxia. A paraneoplastic antibody panel revealed anti-Yo antibodies, which ultimately led to the diagnosis of previously occult breast cancer. (MRI courtesy of Dr George Wilmot)

Paraneoplastic stiff person syndrome

Paraneoplastic SPS clinically resembles non-paraneoplastic SPS, presenting with prominent axial muscle rigidity and intermittent painful spasms. The condition fluctuates, with spasms often being exacerbated by emotion, activity, or sensory stimulation. Only about 5% of all cases of SPS are associated with an underlying malignancy (3). Although there is no clinically reliable way to distinguish paraneoplastic from non-paraneoplastic forms, a paraneoplastic aetiology should be considered when SPS only affects one or both upper extremities, has a very rapid onset, responds poorly to benzodiazepines, occurs at an advanced age, or occurs as part of an encephalomyeloneuropathy (8). While the non-paraneoplastic form is usually associated with glutamic acid decarboxylase (GAD) antibodies, the paraneoplastic form is most frequently associated with amphiphysin antibodies, although anti-gephyrin antibodies have also been described (9). Adenocarcinoma of the breast is the most commonly associated malignancy, though SPS may also be associated with underlying thymoma, Hodgkin's lymphoma, renal cell carcinoma, myeloma, and lung cancer (10–12). Although SPS is a clinical diagnosis supported by the presence of appropriate autoantibodies, electromyography (EMG) can also be used to support the diagnosis. Surface EMG reveals an initial burst of myoclonic activity followed by continuous muscle activity and prolonged tonic muscle contraction in response to cutaneous stimulation. This pattern is virtually diagnostic of SPS. CSF analysis may demonstrate oligoclonal bands. MRI of the brain is usually normal. Pathologically, the disorder involves inhibitory interneurons in the spinal cord, vacuolar degeneration of anterior horn motor neurons, and inflammatory infiltrates (13). Benzodiazepines, drugs that enhance GABAergic inhibition (e.g. baclofen), and steroids may relieve spasms, but they do not usually influence the natural course.

Paraneoplastic opsoclonus–myoclonus syndrome

Paraneoplastic opsoclonus–myoclonus syndrome presents with chaotic but conjugate eye movements which consist of involuntary arrhythmic high-amplitude saccades in all directions (opsoclonus), in conjunction with sudden jerky movements of the body (myoclonus). It is clinically indistinguishable from non-paraneoplastic forms of opsoclonus–myoclonus (OM), listed in Table 29.3. In children, paraneoplastic OM accounts for roughly 50% of all OM cases and is most frequently associated with underlying neuroblastoma (14). Antibodies are rarely identified in children with paraneoplastic OM (15). In adults, roughly 20% of cases of OM are paraneoplastic, with breast and lung cancer being the most commonly associated malignancies (16). In patients with breast cancer, paraneoplastic OM may be associated with anti-Ri antibodies. CSF studies and brain MRI are normal in most cases. Pathologically, there may be no abnormalities, although cases with cerebellar atrophy and perivascular lymphocytic cuffing have been reported (17). Treatment of paediatric paraneoplastic OM involves treating the underlying tumour along with administration of adjunctive immunotherapy. Steroids, intravenous immunoglobulin (IVIG), plasmapheresis, rituximab, and adrenocorticotrophic hormone (ACTH) are commonly employed as adjunctive treatments in the paediatric population. In adults, treatment is targeted against

Table 29.3 Non-paraneoplastic causes of opsoclonus–myoclonus

Postinfectious (poststreptococcal and postviral)
Drug-induced (lithium, amitriptyline overdose, cyclosporin toxicity)
Midbrain or thalamic haemorrhage or neoplasm
Diabetic hyperosmolar coma
Connective tissue and inflammatory disorders
Idiopathic

the underlying malignancy without the use of adjunctive immunotherapy. Eye movements and myoclonus can be symptomatically treated with benzodiazepines and baclofen.

Other paraneoplastic movement disorders

Paraneoplastic chorea, hemiballismus, dyskinesia, dystonia, tremor, and parkinsonism have all been reported, although they are thought to be exceptionally rare (3, 18). Paraneoplastic chorea is the best characterized of these movement disorders (Video 29.1). Paraneoplastic chorea is most frequently associated with CV2/CRMP-5 antibodies and small-cell lung cancer; however, it has also been reported to occur with thymoma, lymphoma, and renal and testicular cancer (3). In one series of 16 patients with paraneoplastic chorea, 11 had small-cell carcinoma; the others had renal cell carcinoma, lymphoma, and other cancers. All had CRMP-5-IgG; six also had ANNA-1 (anti-Hu), including one without evident cancer. Chorea was the initial and most prominent symptom in 11 patients and was asymmetric or unilateral in five patients. MRI or autopsy provided evidence for perivascular inflammation and microglial activation in the basal ganglia. In some patients, chemotherapy and intravenous methylprednisolone were associated with improvement in the chorea (19).

Paraneoplastic choreiform movements are usually part of a more widespread neurological syndrome which may include peripheral neuropathy, autonomic neuropathy, ataxia, dementia, neuromuscular junction problems, cranial neuropathy, limbic encephalitis, and optic neuritis (3). Most patients with paraneoplastic chorea have non-specific basal ganglia changes on MRI. CSF is normal or shows mild leucocytosis with elevated protein or possibly oligoclonal bands (3).

Recently, antibodies to the NMDA subtype of the glutamate receptor have been associated with encephalopathy in young women with ovarian teratomas. Patients may present with psychiatric symptoms, memory problems, seizures, and can ultimately develop dystonia, dyskinesias, opsoclonus–myoclonus syndrome, autonomic instability, unresponsiveness, and hypoventilation (2, 20, 21). The dyskinesia has a predilection for the orofacial-lingual region and may be initially misdiagnosed as tardive dyskinesia (Video 29.2) (22). Rarely, a similar syndrome can occur in young men with testicular teratoma. NMDA receptor encephalitis may be slightly more common in black than in white women (21). Initially, CSF analysis reveals pleocytosis and may ultimately reveal oligoclonal bands (23). Brain MRI may be normal or may show abnormalities in the white matter and hippocampi (23). Principal pathological features include microgliosis and IgG deposits with rare inflammatory infiltrates in the hippocampus, forebrain, basal ganglia, and spinal cord (24). Once diagnosed with a teratoma, patients are treated with tumour resection and immunotherapy (steroids, IVIG, plasmapheresis), and symptoms improve as antibody titres fall (25).

When presenting with any of the aforementioned classic paraneoplastic neurological syndromes, patients should be evaluated for an underlying malignancy with a CT scan of the chest, abdomen, and pelvis. A paraneoplastic antibody panel should be performed and may point towards a specific underlying malignancy. If the aforementioned tests fail to identify malignancy, a whole-body fluoro-2-deoxy-glucose (FDG) positron emission tomography (PET) scan may be useful. One study of patients with paraneoplastic neurological syndromes and positive paraneoplastic antibodies found the sensitivity of FDG-PET for detecting malignancy to be 90%, which was significantly higher than the 30% sensitivity reported for CT ($p < 0.01$) (26). Identification and treatment of the malignancy may lead to improvement or even remission of the paraneoplastic neurological syndrome. As discussed previously, immunosuppressive treatments can be useful in some cases.

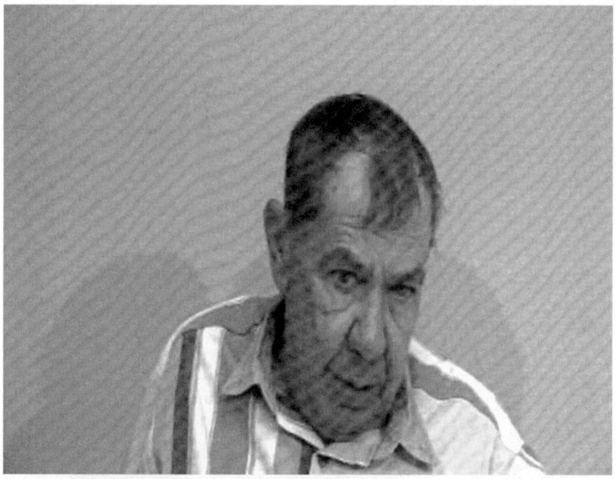

Video 29.1 This 60-year-old right-handed man presented with generalized seizure 4 years earlier and was found to have hyponatraemia but no specific cause was identified. Three years later he was admitted to the hospital for evaluation of recent weight loss and acute confusion. He had marked hyponatraemia (Na = 116 mEq/L). While in the hospital he was also noted to have involuntary movements, initially in the shoulders, but gradually progressing to involve his legs as well, and he began to stumble when walking. He has a 60-pack-year smoking history. On his initial examination at the Movement Disorders Clinic, his Montreal Cognitive Assessment (MoCA) score was 20/30 and he was noted to have generalized chorea which was temporarily suppressible. MRI showed hyperintensity in the striatum on T_2-weighted images. He was found to have positive titre (1:245 760) of collapsin response-mediator protein-5 (CRMP-5) IGG (by immunofluorescence). All other tests were negative. He was found to have lung cancer and died within 3 months after evaluation.

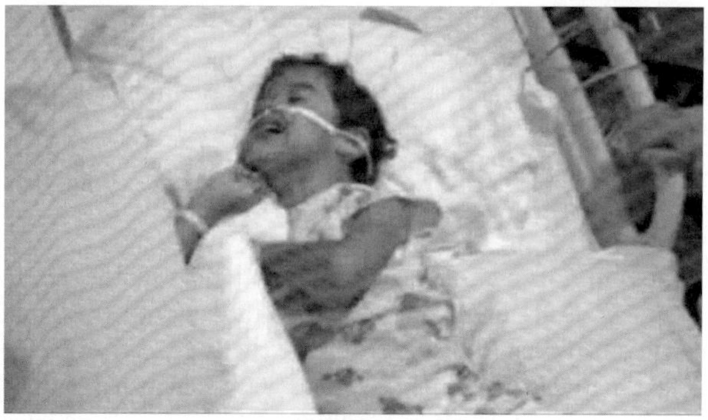

Video 29.2 This 3 year old boy was initially admitted to the Children's Hospital after a 2–3 day history of progressive lethargy and emesis. While in the emergency room he was noted to have abnormal involuntary movements manifested by orofacial stereotypies and generalized chorea. MRI of the head was normal on two occasions, as was extensive infectious work-up. His chorea markedly improved within 1–2 days after starting tetrabenazine, but when later tetrabenazine was lowered and eventually discontinued his chorea worsened and dystonic posturing emerged. Further autoimmune and metabolic testing was normal except for the presence of high titre of anti-NMDA receptor antibodies. The patient was started on monthly IVIG and mycophenolate and his mental and neurological status gradually improved. The tetrabenazine was eventually discontinued without recurrence of the involuntary movements.

The widespread commercial availability of gender-specific paraneoplastic antibody panels represents a key advance in the management of paraneoplastic disease, and future developments are likely to include the identification and characterization of additional paraneoplastic antibodies. The increasing availability of PET scans represents another key advance in the diagnosis and management of both paraneoplastic and neoplastic disease, and future developments will almost certainly include improved imaging modalities for the early detection of occult malignancy.

Autoimmune diseases

Autoimmune diseases, which arise from an overactive immune response against normal body tissues, are frequently the cause of movement disorders (27). Autoimmune disease can be restricted to certain organs or tissue types, or can occur in a more widespread distribution, making this a very heterogeneous group of diseases. Key advances in the field of autoimmune disease include the development of newer immunosuppressant drugs. These newer agents can be used in combination with steroids, thereby enabling the use of lower doses of both agents and reducing the potential for serious medication-related side effects. For example, a recent report suggested that adalimumab may be associated with parkinsonism and dystonia (28).

This section highlights the autoimmune diseases that are most often associated with movement disorders.

Autoimmune thyroid disease

In Hashimoto's thyroiditis, also referred to as steroid-responsive encephalopathy associated with autoimmune thyroiditis (SREAT) or Hashimoto's encephalopathy, anti-thyroperoxidase and anti-thyroglobulin antibodies disrupt thyroid function, resulting in encephalopathy that is often accompanied by involuntary movements and ataxia. All of this can occur despite a biochemically euthyroid state. Chorea, tremor, multifocal myoclonus, and ataxia are the most common movement disorders occurring in Hashimoto's thyroiditis; however, opsoclonus, akinetic–rigid syndromes, palatal tremor, and myorhythmias have also been reported (1). Brain MRI is usually normal (1). Prominent EEG changes (slowing and epileptiform activity) are common (1). Elevated CSF protein is common, and both mild pleocytosis and oligoclonal clonal bands can also occur (29). High-dose intravenous steroids usually lead to prompt resolution (1).

Coeliac disease

Ataxia is a common neurological manifestation of gluten enteropathy (30, 31). Anti-gliadin antibodies are thought to be responsible for the ataxia, via direct cerebellar toxicity (32). Cerebellar involvement may also occur in individuals with coeliac disease and resultant low vitamin E levels, a condition discussed in detail later in this chapter (33). Symptoms can include eye-movement abnormalities, dysarthria, limb ataxia, and gait disturbance. Occasionally, biopsy-confirmed coeliac disease is found; however, there is often no evidence of intestinal disease (32). MRI usually reveals cerebellar atrophy. Co-morbid sensorimotor axonal neuropathy is common (32). Pathologically, there is perivascular cuffing with both CD4 and CD8 cells in the white matter of the cerebellum and often significant Purkinje cell loss (34). The ataxia, for the most part, is not responsive to treatment. Some reports suggest that IVIG and gluten-restricted diets may be of benefit (35).

Systemic lupus erythematosus

Neurological manifestations of systemic lupus erythematosus (SLE) are diverse and can include psychosis, seizures, encephalopathy, neuropathy, transverse myelitis, and movement disorders. While spasmodic torticollis, hemiballismus, tremor, parkinsonism, and stiff person syndrome have all been reported, chorea is the most common movement disorder in SLE, occurring in up to 4% of patients (36, 37) (Video 29.3). It is usually accompanied by other neurological manifestations of the disease, although it can be the presenting feature, sometimes occurring years before other manifestations (38). Most patients who develop chorea are young women. Chorea is often unilateral or asymmetrical, but usually evolves into a generalized chorea that interferes with speech, balance, and activities of daily living. While it usually spontaneously resolves after several days or weeks, rarely it can be permanent. Some cases have occurred in association with hormonal shifts, such as during pregnancy, in the postpartum period, or after starting or stopping oral contraceptives (39–41). Although the pathology is inconsistent, widespread microinfarcts are the classic hallmark of neurolupus. Antiphospholipid antibodies, which predispose patients to recurrent thrombotic events, are strongly associated with chorea in SLE; however, the mechanism whereby these antiphospholipid antibodies cause chorea and other features of the antiphospholipid syndrome (see below) is unclear. Neuroimaging in patients with SLE and chorea is usually normal, although ischaemic lesions in the basal ganglia may be found (42). The chorea of SLE may respond to low doses of haloperidol or to tetrabenazine (43, 44) (Video 29.3). IVIG and plasma exchange have also been used to successfully treat refractory chorea in SLE (45).

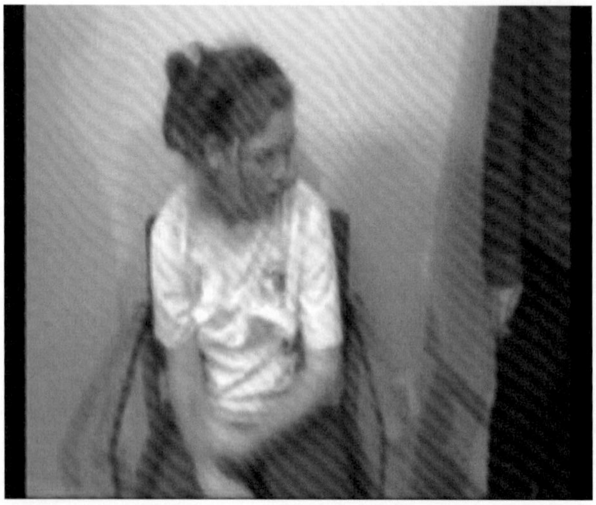

Video 29.3 This 19-year-old college student was diagnosed with SLE meningoencephalitis at age 10 years. She subsequently had intermittent paroxysmal abdominal complaints, myalgias, and arthralgias, and at age 18 years had an episode of pericarditis. All these SLE-related conditions generally responded to brief courses of prednisone. About 10 days before her initial evaluation at the Movement Disorders Clinic she noted rapidly progressive difficulties with fine dexterity, progressing to generalized uncontrolled movements, slurred speech, and gait and balance problems. The video shows marked generalized chorea. She was initially treated with prednisone and subsequently switched to mycophenylate. Her chorea markedly improved within a few days after starting tetrabenazine.

Although parkinsonism has been described, it is a rare manifestation of SLE. Antiphospholipid antibodies are not consistently reported in SLE parkinsonism as they are with SLE chorea. MRI scanning may show hyperintensities in the thalamus or basal ganglia on T_2-weighted images (46). CSF may reveal mild pleocytosis and protein elevation. Successful treatment has been reported with corticosteroids, other immunosuppressants, and levodopa, although the clinical response to treatment varies considerably.

Cerebellar syndromes with an abrupt or subacute onset have been noted in less than 2% of patients with SLE. Truncal and appendicular ataxia, dysarthria, and nystagmus have been noted. Isolated cases of tremor, hemiballismus, spasmodic torticollis, blepharospasm, and stiff person syndrome have been reported.

Antiphospholipid antibody syndrome

Primary antiphospholipid syndrome is characterized by recurrent thrombosis and miscarriages in the setting of high titres of antibodies, either anticardiolipin IgG or IgM, lupus anticoagulant, or anti-B2-glycoprotein 1 ('Sapporo criteria') (47). Chorea has been reported in 1.3% of patients (48). The clinical presentation resembles that of patients with SLE chorea. Imaging studies may be normal or may reveal non-specific changes that fail to explain the chorea. Thus, a functional, immunologically mediated mechanism, rather than an ischaemic one, is suspected. Successful treatment has occurred with corticosteroids, anticoagulants, aspirin, and dopamine antagonists. Hemidystonia, writer's cramp, and parkinsonism have also been reported in primary antiphospholipid syndrome.

Sjögren's syndrome

Sjögren's syndrome is associated with a wide range of neurological disorders, including rare movement disorders. Parkinsonism has been well described in association with Sjögren's syndrome. Clinically, patients have features of atypical parkinsonism with very slow progression over time (49). A symmetric akinetic–rigid syndrome, gait disorder, postural instability, and minimal tremor are typical (49). Lack of levodopa responsiveness is also typical (49). MRI may be normal or may reveal multiple T_2 hyperintense lesions in periventricular, subcortical, and deep locations involving both grey and white matter (49). Pathophysiology is unclear, and response to immunosuppressive therapy is unpredictable. Other movement disorders reported to occur in Sjögren's syndrome include cerebellar degeneration, chorea, and dystonia (50–52).

Behçet's disease

Behçet's disease can cause a variety of neurological symptoms including, rarely, movement disorders. Tremor, palatal myoclonus, chorea, oromandibular dystonia, and parkinsonism have also been reported (53–56). CSF pleocytosis and elevated protein levels are common (56). MRI may be normal, or may reveal focal lesions throughout the brain (56). Pathologically, there may be scattered foci of necrosis, demyelination, and scarring throughout the CNS (56). Response to immunosuppressive therapy is mixed.

Sarcoidosis

Sarcoidosis is a systemic granulomatous disease that involves the CNS in approximately 5% of cases (57). However, as many as 15% of autopsy cases may have evidence of neurosarcoidosis (57). While basilar meningitis is the most common neurological presentation of neurosarcoidosis, parenchymal lesions can also occur, producing a variety of neurological symptoms (58). Parkinsonism, hemidystonia, chorea, and hemiballismus have all been described when the granulomatous process infiltrates the basal ganglia (58). These movement disorders often improve or resolve with administration of corticosteroids or other immunosuppressants (59, 60). The diagnosis of neurosarcoidosis can be challenging because no test, apart from biopsy, is completely reliable. Parenchymal lesions often show gadolinium enhancement on MRI. CSF protein is usually elevated, and pleocytosis and oligoclonal bands may be present (59). Additional tests such as CSF ACE levels are of little added value.

Endocrine and metabolic disorders

Thyroid disease

Hyperkinetic movement disorders occur with hyperthyroid states, and the movement disorder usually presents and remits in parallel with other symptoms of hyperthyroidism. Enhanced physiological tremor is by far the most commonly seen movement disorder in hyperthyroidism, occurring in as many as 97% of hyperthyroid patients (61). Changes in peripheral beta-adrenergic receptor tone may be the pathophysiological basis, a theory supported by the fact that beta-blockers effectively suppress the tremor. Chorea is a much less common manifestation of hyperthyroid states, occurring in less than 2% of patients with thyrotoxicosis (61). The distal extremities are most affected, although the neck and tongue may also be involved. Movements are usually continuous, although paroxysmal choreoathetosis has been reported (62). The pathophysiology is not well understood, and no cerebral lesions have been identified via MRI or post-mortem pathological studies (36). The chorea is reversible with treatment of the underlying hyperthyroidism. It also responds to dopamine receptor blocking agents which, in conjunction with the fact that there are decreased concentrations of the dopamine metabolite homovanillic acid in the CSF of hyperthyroid patients, seems to suggest that altered dopamine turnover or increased dopamine receptor sensitivity may be responsible (63).

Hypothyroid states can lead to ataxia. Truncal ataxia is generally more prominent than appendicular ataxia (64). The ataxia improves as the patient becomes euthyroid.

Parathyroid disease

Hypoparathyroid states, both primary hypoparathyroidism and pseudo-hypoparathyroidism, are associated with movement disorders. Associated hypocalcaemia is responsible for the more common neurological complications such as tetany and neuromuscular irritability, manifest as carpopedal spasm and Chvostek's sign (65). Calcifications occur in the basal ganglia in most patients with primary hypoparathyroidism, but they do not correlate well with the presence of movement disorders (66, 67). Chorea, paroxysmal dystonias and choreoathetosis, and parkinsonism can all occur in hypoparathyroid states (67–69). The pathophysiology is not well understood. In all the aforementioned movement disorders, improvement occurs with treatment of the underlying hypoparathyroidism and associated electrolyte abnormalities.

Diabetes mellitus

Both hyperglycaemia and hypoglycaemia are rare causes of choreoathetosis (70, 71). When the cause is hypoglycaemia, the chorea usually resolves as blood sugar normalizes; however, recurrent episodes of hypoglycaemia have resulted in permanent bilateral chorea (72). There is a well-recognized syndrome of hemiballism–hemichorea (HB–HC) that occurs in diabetics with acute non-ketotic hyperosmolar hyperglycaemia in the range of 400–1000 mg/dl. This syndrome can sometimes be the presenting feature of diabetes. Most reported cases have occurred in elderly women (73–76). The HB–HC may resolve shortly after resolution of the hyperglycaemia, may improve slowly over months, or may be permanent (72–76). Brain MRI often reveals contralateral putaminal hyperintensity on T_1-weighted images (73). The pathophysiology of this disorder is uncertain, although dopamine hypersensitivity in postmenopausal women, co-existence of lacunar infarction in the contralateral basal ganglia, and increased blood flow in the contralateral striatum and thalamus have all been suggested as pathogenic factors (75, 76). If needed, treatment with dopamine receptor antagonists or tetrabenazine can be effective (73, 77). Figure 29.2 and Video 29.4 feature a typical case.

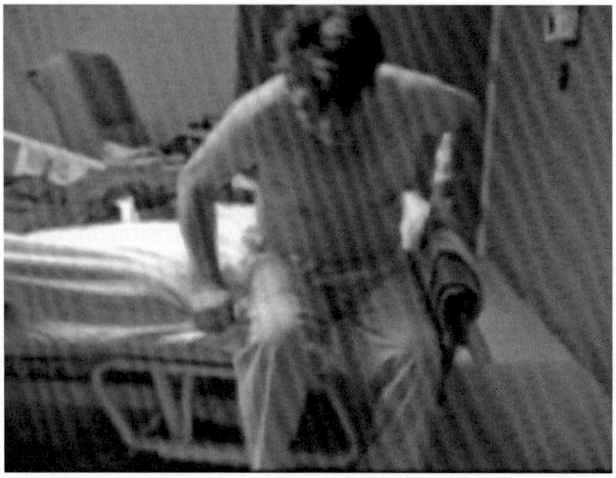

Video 29.4 This 58-year-old man, who had not seen a physician in more than 30 years, was hospitalized for acute onset of right-sided hemichorea that began 4 weeks prior to admission. It started in the right arm but then disappeared for a week. The movement then recurred and spread to involve both the right arm and leg. Upon admission, he was found to be in a hyperglycaemic non-ketotic state. Hospital work-up demonstrated a haemoglobin A1C of 14.8, with serum glucose as high as 401. CSF glucose was 113. An MRI scan showed hyperintensity of the left striatum (Fig. 29.2). While in the hospital, he was started on treatment for his type 2 diabetes, and he was placed on risperidone for the involuntary movements. Movements diminished dramatically and the risperidone was eventually discontinued without recurrence. (Video courtesy of Dr Stewart Factor)

Renal disease

Multiple movement disorders, including tremor, ataxia, asterixis, myoclonus, and restless legs syndrome (RLS), can occur in the setting of renal failure and uraemic encephalopathy. Tremor usually manifests before asterixis and is coarse, irregular, absent at rest, and most evident in the fingers of the outstretched hands. It may respond partially to beta-blockers (78). Multifocal myoclonus is common in uraemic encephalopathy, and both action myoclonus and stimulus-sensitive myoclonus can occur (78–80). Myoclonus can often be treated effectively with benzodiazepines. Asterixis, or negative myoclonus, is a common sensitive early indication of uraemic encephalopathy (81). RLS occurs in 15–20% of patients with chronic kidney disease (82). It can also occur in association with iron deficiency, which is common in patients with renal disease. In addition to correcting the renal metabolic abnormality, dopamine agonists and levodopa are the first-line treatments, followed by second-line agents such as benzodiazepines, gabapentin, clonidine, and opioids. It may also be useful to utilize a lower-temperature dialysate, correct iron deficiency, and treat anaemia when present. RLS may improve dramatically after kidney transplantation (83, 84).

Advances in transplant medicine have made kidney transplant a safer, more effective, and more widespread treatment option for patients with renal disease and therefore represent a key advance in the field of renal disease.

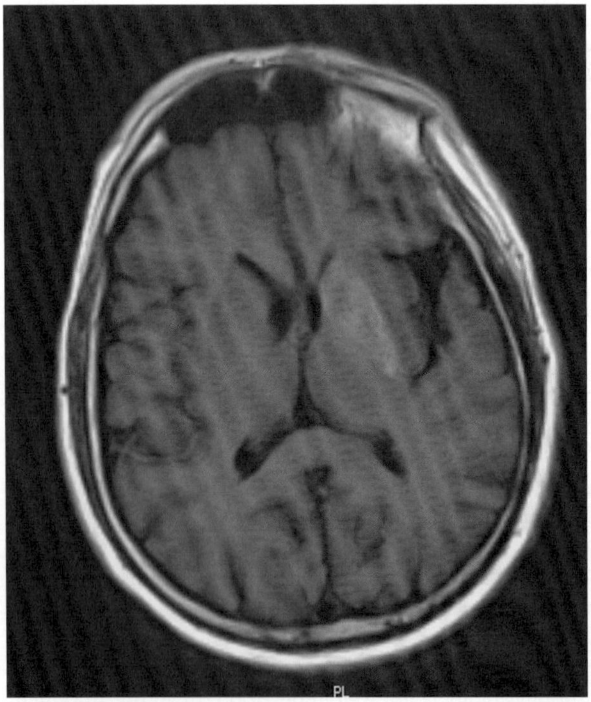

Fig. 29.2 T_1 axial MRI from a diabetic man presenting with right hemichorea in the context of acute non-ketotic hyperosmolar hyperglycaemia. Note the abnormal signal in the left striatum. (Image courtesy of Dr Stewart Factor)

Liver disease

Cirrhosis can lead to a variety of neurological complications, the most common being hepatic encephalopathy. Although movement disorders are uncommon in hepatic encephalopathy, tremor, asterixis, and myoclonus can occur (85). More often, movement disorders occur in patients with acquired hepatocerebral degeneration (AHD), which is a chronic progressive neurological syndrome, characterized by parkinsonism, ataxia, and other movement disorders. AHD may occur in patients with advanced liver disease from any cause, especially those with portosystemic shunts. Rare cases have been reported in patients with portosystemic shunting in the absence of underlying hepatocellular disease, such as those with portal vein thrombosis (86). Portosystemic shunting may lead to AHD by allowing neurotoxins to bypass hepatic metabolism and enter the brain via the systemic circulation. While a precise neurotoxin has not been identified, ammonia, aromatic amino acids, and manganese are candidates (87). Pathologically, there is patchy degeneration of neurons, with microcavitation and pseudo-laminar necrosis in the deep cortical layers and basal ganglia (87, 88). In contrast with hepatic encephalopathy, the movement disorders occurring in AHD are not associated with a depressed level of consciousness (85). The exact prevalence of AHD is not known, but movement disorders are estimated to occur in 20–90% of patients awaiting liver transplantation (89). AHD arises subacutely, and its course is highly variably, often not paralleling other features of liver disease. Parkinsonism, ataxia, dystonia, chorea, and orobuccolingual stereotypy, mimicking tardive dyskinesia, can occur in AHD (89). In contrast with Parkinson's disease, the parkinsonism associated with AHD tends to be symmetric, more rapidly progressive, and is more likely to be associated with cognitive impairment and postural instability early in the disease course (90). Also, action tremor is far more common than resting tremor in AHD (90). Response to levodopa is inconsistent (89, 91). The differential diagnosis of AHD is broad and includes hepatic encephalopathy, central pontine myelinolysis, alcoholic cerebellar degeneration, Wilson disease, and Wernicke's encephalopathy. Brain MRI reveals very characteristic changes, including increased T_1 signal in the pallidal nuclei. T_2 and postcontrast images are usually normal (85, 89). In contrast with hepatic encephalopathy, movement disorders in AHD typically do not respond to ammonia-lowering agents. Hyperkinetic movements such as chorea and orobuccolingual stereotypies can be treated with dopamine receptor antagonists, although these agents carry the risk of inducing tardive dyskinesia (TD). Tetrabenazine, a dopamine-depleting agent, can be used without the risk of TD (44). Levodopa and dopamine agonists may be useful in some patients with parkinsonism. AHD and its characteristic movement disorders may improve dramatically during the months following liver transplantation (92).

Advances in transplant medicine have made liver transplant a safer, more effective, and more widespread treatment option for patients with liver failure and therefore represent a key advance in the field.

Toxic and nutritional deficiencies

Vitamin E malabsorption

Any disease causing fat malabsorption (e.g. cystic fibrosis) can lead to tocopherol (vitamin E) deficiency, which may produce neurological dysfunction after several years. A syndrome of spinocerebellar ataxia and peripheral neuropathy is typical. Dysarthria, oculomotor abnormalities, ataxia, and loss of vibratory and position sense occur. Loss of myelinated nerve fibres in the posterior columns and CNS are seen pathologically (93). Oral or parenteral vitamin E supplementation should be initiated to prevent ongoing neurological decline.

Ethanol

Although alcohol may have some beneficial effects on movement disorders such as essential tremor and myoclonus–dystonia syndrome, when abused it can lead to a variety of movement disorders (94). Abrupt ethanol withdrawal in physically dependent individuals is associated with a tremor that is promptly relieved by alcohol ingestion or benzodiazepines. This tremor is distal, coarse, irregular, rapid, and worse with movement. If left untreated, delirium tremens may ensue (95). Alcohol withdrawal has also been reported to cause transient parkinsonism in older individuals. The parkinsonism remits spontaneously in a few days or weeks (96). Transient orolingual dyskinesias, sometimes involving neck and arm muscles, have also been reported in the setting of alcohol withdrawal (97).

Tremor can also be found in alcoholics who are not actively drinking or withdrawing. This tremor is usually a mild asymmetric postural tremor with a higher frequency than essential tremor. Beta-blocking drugs can also be effective in suppressing this tremor. A 3 Hz tremor of the legs that is slow and rhythmic, involving flexion and extension of the hip girdle muscles, can also be seen in alcoholics. This tremor may affect gait (97).

Long-standing alcohol abuse can lead to alcohol liver disease, which can ultimately cause acquired hepatic encephalopathy and/or hepatocerebral degeneration, both of which are associated with movement disorders discussed earlier.

Cerebellar ataxia is a feature of acute alcohol intoxication, and chronic alcohol dependence can be associated with vermal degeneration and a syndrome of truncal ataxia. Pathologically, there is degeneration of the anterior superior aspect of the vermis. In severe cases, there may be atrophy of the cerebellar hemispheres. There is often a striking loss of Purkinje cells (98).

Infectious diseases

Viruses

Movement disorders such as hemichorea–hemiballismus, myoclonus, dystonia, tremor, parkinsonism, and akathisia have been identified in 5–44% of HIV/AIDS patients in prospective studies (99). Several pathogenic mechanisms are possible. HIV can directly involve the basal ganglia, thereby causing significant motor dysfunction (100). Immunocytochemistry studies have revealed high viral loads in the basal ganglia and substantia nigra, and SPECT and PET studies lend further support to this mechanism by demonstrating abnormal metabolic activity of the basal ganglia in HIV patients (101, 102). Alternatively, movement disorders can result from the presence of opportunistic infections (e.g. toxplasmosis), primary CNS lymphoma, progressive multifocal leucoencephalopathy, or AIDS dementia complex (ADC). Lastly, HIV patients are significantly more susceptible to the development of extrapyramidal reactions when exposed to neuroleptics (103). Autopsy studies reveal severe neuronal loss in the basal ganglia, along with reactive gliosis, and macrophage and multinucleated giant cell infiltration, particularly in the putamen, caudate, and substantia nigra (102). Table 29.4 summarizes the common movement disorders reported in association with HIV/AIDs. Key advances in antiretroviral therapy have reduced the frequency of ADC and severe opportunistic infections such as CNS toxoplasmosis, both of which are common causes of movement disorders in HIV/AIDS. Future developments are likely to include improvements in the efficacy and tolerability of antiretroviral therapy and the development and widespread availability of a vaccine to prevent HIV infection.

Many other viruses can lead to movement disorders, but a detailed discussion of each one is beyond the scope of this chapter.

Table 29.4 Movement disorders occurring in association with HIV/AIDS

Movement disorder	Aetiology	Clinical features and comments
Parkinsonism	HIV infection, ADC, opportunistic infections (CNS toxoplasmosis or tuberculosis, Whipple's disease, PML), drug-induced (neuroleptics)	Often atypical with symmetric signs, lack of rest tremor, and early postural instability
Tremor	HIV infection, ADC, CNS tuberculosis, drug-induced (neuroleptics and TMP–SMX)	Usually mild bilateral postural tremor, though other types of tremor have been described
Hemichorea–ballism	Opportunistic infections (CNS toxoplasmosis, cryptococcus, PML), ADC, HIV encephalitis	Toxoplasma abscess in subthalamic nucleus is the most common cause; most common MD in HIV/AIDS
Dystonia	CNS toxoplasmosis, ADC, drug-induced (neuroleptics)	Rare
Myoclonus	HIV infection, ADC, opportunistic infections (CNS toxoplasmosis, tuberculosis, herpes zoster, PML)	Rare reports of spinal, segmental, and generalized myoclonus
Tic disorder	CNS toxoplasmosis	Single report of a dystonic tic involving ocular oral and cervical movements
Paroxysmal dyskinesias	ADC	Rare reports of both kinesigenic and non-kinesigenic forms

HIV, human immunodeficiency virus; ADC, AIDS dementia complex; CNS, central nervous system; PML, progressive multifocal leucoencephalopthy, TMP–SMX, trimethoprim–sulfamethoxazole; MD, movement disorder.

Adapted from Tse W, Cersosimo MG, Gracies JM, et al. Movement disorders and AIDS: a review. *Parkinsonism Relat Disord* 2004; 10: 323–34.

Table 29.5 Viruses known to cause movement disorders

Virus	Movement disorder
Japanese encephalitis	Parkinsonism, dystonia, chorea, tremor
Encephalitis lethargica	Parkinsonism, myoclonus, chorea, oculogyric crisis
Influenza	Parkinsonism, chorea, dystonia, tremor
Arbovirus	Parkinsonism
Enterovirus	Parkinsonism, chorea
Epstein–Barr virus	Chorea, opsoclonus–myoclonus
Varicella-zoster virus	Parkinsonism, chorea, opsoclonus–myoclonus
Cytomegalovirus	Chorea
Paramyxovirus	Chorea
Rubella virus	Chorea
Measles virus	Parkinsonism, chorea, myoclonus (subacute sclerosing panencephalitis)
Herpes simplex virus	Tics, chorea

Adapted from Cardoso F. Infectious and transmissible movement disorders. In: Jankovic J, Tolosa E (eds) *Parkinson's disease and movement disorders* (3rd edn), pp. 945–66. Baltimore, MD: Williams & Wilkins, 1998.

Table 29.5 lists the movement disorders associated with other viral infections.

Bacteria

Bacterial infections can lead to movement disorders through both antibody-mediated and direct mechanisms. Classic examples of both mechanisms are discussed below.

Antibody-mediated disorders

Sydenham's disease (SD) is a consequence of infection with group A beta-haemolytic streptococcus (GABHS). Though once relatively common, SD is now encountered relatively rarely in developed countries because of the widespread use of antibiotics, which represents a key advance. SD is most common between the ages of 8 and 9, is more common in females than males, and usually appears 1–6 months after the acute pharyngitis (104). SD is characterized by chorea, which is generalized in 80% of cases, but may also present as pure hemichorea in 20% of cases (104). Other features of SD can include ballism, facial grimacing, tics, dysarthria, oculomotor abnormalities, motor impersistence, gait abnormalities, seizures, hyperactivity, obsessions, compulsions, anxiety, and even psychosis (104).

High titres of antistreptolysin are typical but non-specific as group G is associated with similarly high titres. It is not yet clear whether identification of the B-cell alloantigen D8/17, which indicates increased risk for rheumatic fever, may be useful as a diagnostic test (104). Imaging is usually normal, although some cases may show enlargement of the caudate, putamen, and globus pallidus (36). PET and SPECT studies may show reversible striatal hypermetabolism (104). Autopsy studies show widespread cell loss in the basal ganglia, frontal cortex, and temporal cortex, along with vasculitis of small vessels (104). Antineuronal antibodies (ANABs) cross-reacting with caudate and subthalamic nuclei neurons have been found in the serum of 95% of acute SD patients (105). Animal models suggest that ANABs cause autoimmune subthalamotomy, leading to disinhibition of the ventrolateral thalamus and subsequent hyperexcitability of the motor cortex (104).

In order to prevent SD, accurate diagnosis and proper antibiotic treatment of the acute pharyngitis is needed. Symptomatic treatment can be achieved with valproic acid or neuroleptics until the condition spontaneously resolves. Prednisone was also shown to be effective in a double-blind placebo-controlled study (106).

The acronym PANDAS (paediatric autoimmune neuropsychiatric disorders after streptococcal infections) was introduced in 1998. According to this theory, which was based on an initial series of 50 patients, a subset of patients with Tourette's syndrome, obsessive–compulsive disorder (OCD), and other neuropsychiatric disorders may be attributable to streptococcal infections (107). Five diagnostic criteria for PANDAS have been proposed: the presence of OCD or tic disorder, pre-pubertal onset, abrupt onset and dramatic exacerbations, temporal association with GABHS infection, and associated neurological abnormalities. These criteria are vague and have yet to be validated. Thus the PANDAS hypothesis remains controversial, and it is unclear whether PANDAS is simply a variant of SD or a separate entity (108). Over the past decade several studies have provided compelling data against any pathogenic link between PANDAS and Tourette's syndrome (109, 110).

Direct mechanisms

CNS tuberculosis can cause tremor, chorea, ballism, dystonia, myoclonus, and parkinsonism. Both tuberculous meningitis and intracranial tuberculomas can cause movement disorders. Movement disorders may occur in up to 16.6% of tuberculous meningitis cases (1). Neuroimaging may be normal or may show ischaemic or haemorrhagic infarcts in the basal ganglia (1). Alternatively, diffuse lesions at the diencephalic–mesencephalic level can occur (1). Hydrocephalus is common (1). Thirty per cent of intracranial tuberculomas are associated with movement disorders (111). Chorea and dystonia are associated with deep tuberculomas, while tremor is associated with surface lesions (111). Tremor and myoclonus can occur in spinal tuberculosis (1). Diagnosis is usually made via culture of *Mycobacterium tuberculosis* from CSF, although CSF PCR may also be useful in diagnosis. Therapy includes anti-tuberculosis drugs for a minimum of 6 months. Movement disorders generally improve within a few weeks.

Whipple's disease (WD) is a rare multisystem illness caused by *Tropheryma whipplei* infection. Classic WD is characterized by malabsorption with steatorrhoea, arthralgia and arthritis, lymphadenopathy, and rarely neurological involvement. Neurological symptoms include dementia, visual impairment, papilloedema, supranuclear ophthalmoplegia, seizures, myoclonus, ataxia, and a depressed level of consciousness. Oculomasticatory myorhythmia is a movement disorder unique to WD in which there are slow, repetitive synchronous rhythmic contractions in ocular, facial, and masticatory muscles (112). Ocular myorhythmia presents with continuous, horizontal, pendular, small-amplitude, vergence oscillations of the eyes, occurring approximately every second. Movements of the face and jaw may be somewhat quicker and resemble rhythmic myoclonus. These movements may persist in sleep. In the past, diagnosis of WD was made by jejunal biopsy, which reveals macrophages laden with periodic acid–Schiff-positive granules and bacilli within macrophages (113). Recent molecular characterization of *T. whipplei*, a key advance in the field, has enabled development of polymerase chain reaction (PCR) techniques for detection in various samples (113). Current recommended treatment is with oral administration of trimethprim–sulfamethoxazole for 1–2 years, preceded by parenteral administration of streptomycin and penicillin G or ceftriaxone for 2 weeks (113).

Movement disorders may occur in the course of bacterial meningitis caused by a variety of organisms (see Table 29.6). The pathogenesis of these movement disorders is poorly understood, and a detailed discussion of each causative agent is beyond the scope of this chapter.

Parasitic infections

Infection with *Falciparum malaria* can be complicated by movement disorders. Cerebellar involvement with opsoclonus and tremor can occur acutely or as part of a delayed neurological syndrome (114). Opsoclonus–myoclonus syndrome, chorea, dystonia, and parkinsonism have also been described (115). The pathophysiological mechanisms are uncertain. CT and MRI images are usually normal. Antimalarial treatments are essential. The opsoclonus–myoclonus syndrome has been reported to respond well to oral clonazepam (115).

Table 29.6 Agents causing bacterial meningitis and movement disorders

Mycoplasma pneumoniae
Salmonella
Legionella pneumophila
Borrelia burgdorferi
Treponema pallidum
Streptococcus viridans
Haemophilus influenzae
Streptococcus pneumoniae
Neisseria meningitides

Adapted from Janavs JL, Aminoff MJ. Dystonia and chorea in acquired systemic disorders. *J Neurol Neurosurg Psychiatry* 1998; 65: 436–45.

Neurocysticercosis (NCC) is caused by the encysted larvae of the *Taenia solium* tapeworm. Movement disorders occur in 3.5% of cases of NCC, with parkinsonism and tremor being the most common (1). Rarely, chorea, myoclonus, hemifacial spasm, and dystonia have been described (1). The presence of cysts in the basal ganglia and related structures is the presumed pathogenic mechanism. Chorea and dystonia are associated with deep lesions, while tremor is associated with surface cysts (1). Parkinsonism is associated with hydrocephalus (1). Movement disorders improve after treatment with albendazole, praziquantel, or surgery (1).

Conclusion

The variety of systemic diseases associated with movement disorders and the diverse mechanisms whereby these diseases elicit abnormal movements pose a formidable challenge for clinicians. The authors hope that the information in this chapter will serve as a guide for movement disorder clinicians in this often challenging process.

Top clinical tips

- Movement disorders may be the presenting feature of a systemic disease.
- The mechanisms by which systemic diseases lead to movement disorders are diverse, even within the context of individual diseases.
- In all cases, identification and treatment of the underlying systemic disease is essential, although symptomatic treatment of the associated movement disorders may also be required.
- Chorea, which can occur in all categories of systemic disease, is the most common symptomatic movement disorder.

References

1. Alarcon F, Gimenez-Roldan S. Systemic diseases that cause movement disorders. *Parkinsonism Relat Disord* 2005; 11: 1–18.
2. Kranick SM, Mowry EM, Colcher A, et al. Movement disorders and pregnancy: a review of the literature. *Mov Disord* 2010; 25: 665–71.
3. Grant R, Graus F. Paraneoplastic movement disorders. *Mov Disord* 2009; 24: 1715–24.

4. Bataller L, Dalmau J. Neuro-ophthalmology and paraneoplastic syndromes. *Curr Opin Neurol* 2004; 17: 3–8.
5. Shams'ili S, Grefkens J, de Leeuw B, et al. Paraneoplastic cerebellar degeneration associated with antineuronal antibodies: analysis of 50 patients. *Brain* 2003; 126: 1409–18.
6. Hammack J, Kotanides H, Rosenblum MK, et al. Paraneoplastic cerebellar degeneration. II: Clinical and immunologic findings in 21 patients with Hodgkin's disease. *Neurology* 1992; 42: 1938–43.
7. Peterson K, Rosenblum MK, Kotanides H, et al. Paraneoplastic cerebellar degeneration. I: A clinical analysis of 55 anti-Yo antibody-positive patients. *Neurology* 1992; 42: 1931–7.
8. Murinson BB, Guarnaccia JB. Stiff-person syndrome with amphiphysin antibodies: distinctive features of a rare disease. *Neurology* 2008; 71: 1955–8.
9. Butler MH, Hayashi A, Ohkoshi N, et al. Autoimmunity to gephyrin in stiff-man syndrome. *Neuron* 2000; 26: 307–12.
10. McHugh JC, Murray B, Renganathan R, et al. GAD antibody positive paraneoplastic stiff person syndrome in a patient with renal cell carcinoma. *Mov Disord* 2007; 22: 1343–6.
11. McCabe DJ, Turner NC, Chao D, et al. Paraneoplastic 'stiff person syndrome' with metastatic adenocarcinoma and anti-Ri antibodies. *Neurology* 2004; 62: 1402–4.
12. Nguyen-Huu BK, Urban PP, Schreckenberger M, et al. Antiamphiphysin-positive stiff-person syndrome associated with small cell lung cancer. *Mov Disord* 2006; 21: 1285–7.
13. Saiz A, Minguez A, Graus F, et al. Stiff-man syndrome with vacuolar degeneration of anterior horn motor neurons. *J Neurol* 1999; 246: 858–60.
14. Rudnick E, Khakoo Y, Antunes NL, et al. Opsoclonus–myoclonus–ataxia syndrome in neuroblastoma: clinical outcome and antineuronal antibodies: a report from the Children's Cancer Group Study. *Med Pediatr Oncol* 2001; 36: 612–22.
15. Pranzatelli MR, Tate ED, Wheeler A, et al. Screening for autoantibodies in children with opsoclonus–myoclonus-ataxia. *Pediatr Neurol* 2002; 27: 384–7.
16. Bataller L, Graus F, Saiz A, et al. Clinical outcome in adult onset idiopathic or paraneoplastic opsoclonus–myoclonus. *Brain* 2001; 124: 437–43.
17. Giordana MT, Soffietti R, Schiffer D. Paraneoplastic opsoclonus: a neuropathologic study of two cases. *Clin Neuropathol* 1989; 8: 295–300.
18. Mehta SH, Morgan JC, Sethi KD. Paraneoplastic movement disorders. *Curr Neurol Neurosci Rep* 2009; 9: 285–91.
19. Vernino S, Tuite P, Adler CH, et al. Paraneoplastic chorea associated with CRMP-5 neuronal antibody and lung carcinoma. *Ann Neurol* 2002; 51: 625–30.
20. Iizuka T. [Clinical features and pathogenesis of anti-NMDA receptor encephalitis.] *Rinsho Shinkeigaku* 2008; 48: 920–2.
21. Irani SR, Bera K, Waters P, et al. *N*-methyl-D-aspartate antibody encephalitis: temporal progression of clinical and paraclinical observations in a predominantly non-paraneoplastic disorder of both sexes. *Brain* 2010; 133: 1655–67.
22. Florance NR, Davis RL, Lam C, et al. Anti-*N*-methyl-D-aspartate receptor (NMDAR) encephalitis in children and adolescents. *Ann Neurol* 2009; 66: 11–18.
23. Dalmau J, Lancaster E, Martinez-Hernandez E, et al. Clinical experience and laboratory investigations in patients with anti-NMDAR encephalitis. *Lancet Neurol* 2010; 10: 63–74.
24. Camdessanche JP, Streichenberger N, Cavillon G, et al. *Brain* immunohistopathological study in a patient with anti-NMDAR encephalitis. *Eur J Neurol* 2010.
25. Baizabal-Carvallo JF, et al. The spectrum of movement disorders in children with anti-NMDA receptor encephalitis. *Movement disorders : official journal of the Movement Disorder Society* 2013; 28(4): 543–7.
26. Linke R, Schroeder M, Helmberger T, et al. Antibody-positive paraneoplastic neurologic syndromes: value of CT and PET for tumor diagnosis. *Neurology* 2004; 63: 282–6.
27. Baizabal-Carvallo JF, Jankovic J. Movement disorders in autoimmune diseases. *Movement disorders : official journal of the Movement Disorder Society* 2012; 27(8): 935–46.
28. Ha AD, Jankovic J. Parkinsonism and dystonia associated with adalimumab. *Mov Disord* 2011; 26: 1556–8.
29. Tamagno G, Celik Y, Simo R, et al. Encephalopathy associated with autoimmune thyroid disease in patients with Graves' disease: clinical manifestations, follow-up, and outcomes. *BMC Neurol* 2010; 10: 27.
30. Burk K, Bosch S, Muller CA, et al. Sporadic cerebellar ataxia associated with gluten sensitivity. *Brain* 2001; 124: 1013–19.
31. Burk K, Farecki ML, Lamprecht G, et al. Neurological symptoms in patients with biopsy proven celiac disease. *Mov Disord* 2009; 24: 2358–62.
32. Freeman HJ. Neurological disorders in adult celiac disease. *Can J Gastroenterol* 2008; 22: 909–11.
33. Mauro A, Orsi L, Mortara P, et al. Cerebellar syndrome in adult celiac disease with vitamin E deficiency. *Acta Neurol Scand* 1991; 84: 167–70.
34. Bushara KO, Goebel SU, Shill H, et al. Gluten sensitivity in sporadic and hereditary cerebellar ataxia. *Ann Neurol* 2001; 49: 540–3.
35. Burk K, Melms A, Schulz JB, et al. Effectiveness of intravenous immunoglobin therapy in cerebellar ataxia associated with gluten sensitivity. *Ann Neurol* 2001; 50: 827–8.
36. Janavs JL, Aminoff MJ. Dystonia and chorea in acquired systemic disorders. *J Neurol Neurosurg Psychiatry* 1998; 65: 436–45.
37. Baizabal-Carvallo JF, Bonnet C, Jankovic J. Movement disorders in systemic lupus erythematosus and the antiphospholipid syndrome. *Journal of neural transmission* 2013.
38. Khamashta MA, Gil A, Anciones B, et al. Chorea in systemic lupus erythematosus: association with antiphospholipid antibodies. *Ann Rheum Dis* 1988; 47: 681–3.
39. Thomas D, Byrne PD, Travers RL. Systemic lupus erythematosus presenting as post-partum chorea. *Aust NZ J Med* 1979; 9: 568–70.
40. Asherson RA, Harris NE, Gharavi AE, et al. Systemic lupus erythematosus, antiphospholipid antibodies, chorea, and oral contraceptives. *Arthritis Rheum* 1986; 29: 1535–6.
41. Donaldson IM, Espiner EA. Disseminated lupus erythematosus presenting as chorea gravidarum. *Arch Neurol* 1971; 25: 240–4.
42. Kashihara K, Nakashima S, Kohira I, et al. Hyperintense basal ganglia on T_1-weighted MR images in a patient with central nervous system lupus and chorea. *Am J Neuroradiol* 1998; 19: 284–6.
43. al Jishi F, al Kawi MZ, el Ramahi K, et al. Hemichorea in systemic lupus erythematosus: significance of MRI findings. *Lupus* 1995; 4: 321–3.
44. Jankovic J. Treatment of hyperkinetic movement disorders. *Lancet Neurol* 2009; 8: 844–56.
45. Lazurova I, Macejova Z, Benhatchi K, et al. Efficacy of intravenous immunoglobulin treatment in lupus erythematosus chorea. *Clin Rheumatol* 2007; 26: 2145–7.
46. Garcia-Moreno JM, Chacon J. Juvenile parkinsonism as a manifestation of systemic lupus erythematosus: case report and review of the literature. *Mov Disord* 2002; 17: 1329–35.
47. Orzechowski NM, Wolanskyj AP, Ahlskog JE, et al. Antiphospholipid antibody-associated chorea. *J Rheumatol* 2008; 35: 2165–70.
48. Cervera R, Piette JC, Font J, et al. Antiphospholipid syndrome: clinical and immunologic manifestations and patterns of disease expression in a cohort of 1,000 patients. *Arthritis Rheum* 2002; 46: 1019–27.
49. Walker RH, Spiera H, Brin MF, et al. Parkinsonism associated with Sjögren's syndrome: three cases and a review of the literature. *Mov Disord* 1999; 14: 262–8.
50. Lin WY, Huang CC, Chang HS, et al. Various movement disorders in a patient with Sjögren syndrome. *Mov Disord* 2009; 24: 786–8.
51. Nakazato Y, Yamamoto T, Tamura N, et al. [Primary Sjögren's syndrome presenting with choreo-athetosis.] *Rinsho Shinkeigaku* 2002; 42: 946–8.
52. Papageorgiou SG, Kontaxis T, Bonakis A, et al. Orofacial dystonia related to Sjögren's syndrome. *Clin Rheumatol* 2007; 26: 1779–81.

53. Revilla FJ, Racette BA, Perlmutter JS. Chorea and jaw-opening dystonia as a manifestation of NeuroBehçet's syndrome. *Mov Disord* 2000; 15: 741–4.
54. Bogdanova D, Milanov I, Georgiev D. Parkinsonian syndrome as a neurological manifestation of Behçet's disease. *Can J Neurol* Sci 1998; 25: 82–5.
55. Bussone G, La Mantia L, Boiardi A, et al. Chorea in Behçet's syndrome. *J Neurol* 1982; 227: 89–92.
56. Serdaroglu P. Behçet's disease and the nervous system. *J Neurol* 1998; 245: 197–205.
57. Scott TF. Neurosarcoidosis: progress and clinical aspects. *Neurology* 1993; 43: 8–12.
58. Caviness JN, Knox CA. Hemidystonia occurring in a patient with sarcoidosis. *Mov Disord* 1996; 11: 340–1.
59. Lexa FJ, Grossman RI. MR of sarcoidosis in the head and spine: spectrum of manifestations and radiographic response to steroid therapy. *Am J Neuroradiol* 1994; 15: 973–82.
60. Cunnah D, Chew S, Wass J. Cyclosporin for central nervous system sarcoidosis. *Am J Med* 1988; 85: 580–1.
61. Swanson JW, Kelly JJ, Jr, McConahey WM. Neurologic aspects of thyroid dysfunction. *Mayo Clin Proc* 1981; 56: 504–12.
62. Fischbeck KH, Layzer RB. Paroxysmal choreoathetosis associated with thyrotoxicosis. *Ann Neurol* 1979; 6: 453–4.
63. Klawans HL, Jr, Shenker DM. Observations on the dopaminergic nature of hyperthyroid chorea. *J Neural Transm* 1972; 33: 73–81.
64. Harayama H, Ohno T, Miyatake T. Quantitative analysis of stance in ataxic myxoedema. *J Neurol Neurosurg Psychiatry* 1983; 46: 579–81.
65. Athappan G, Ariyamuthu VK. Images in clinical medicine. Chvostek's sign and carpopedal spasm. *N Engl J Med* 2009; 360: e24.
66. Sachs C, Sjoberg HE, Ericson K. Basal ganglia calcifications on CT: relation to hypoparathyroidism. *Neurology* 1982; 32: 779–82.
67. Kaminski HJ, Ruff RL. Neurologic complications of endocrine diseases. *Neurol Clin* 1989; 7: 489–508.
68. Christiansen NJ, Hansen PF. Choreiform movements in hypoparathyroidism. *N Engl J Med* 1972; 287: 569–70.
69. Barabas G, Tucker SM. Idiopathic hypoparathyroidism and paroxysmal dystonic choreoathetosis. *Ann Neurol* 1988; 24: 585.
70. Newman RP, Kinkel WR. Paroxysmal choreoathetosis due to hypoglycemia. *Arch Neurol* 1984; 41: 341–2.
71. Rector WG, Jr, Herlong HF, Moses H 3rd. Nonketotic hyperglycemia appearing as choreoathetosis or ballism. *Arch Intern Med* 1982; 142: 154–5.
72. Hefter H, Mayer P, Benecke R. Persistent chorea after recurrent hypoglycemia: a case report. *Eur Neurol* 1993; 33: 244–7.
73. Ifergane G, Masalha R, Herishanu YO. Transient hemichorea/hemiballismus associated with new onset hyperglycemia. *Can J Neurol Sci* 2001; 28: 365–8.
74. Ohmori H, Hirashima K, Ishihara D, et al. Two cases of hemiballism–hemichorea with T_1-weighted MR image hyperintensities. *Intern Med* 2005; 44: 1280–5.
75. Lin JJ, Chang MK. Hemiballism–hemichorea and non-ketotic hyperglycaemia. *J Neurol Neurosurg Psychiatry* 1994; 57: 748–50.
76. Nabatame H, Nakamura K, Matsuda M, et al. Hemichorea in hyperglycemia associated with increased blood flow in the contralateral striatum and thalamus. *Intern Med* 1994; 33: 472–5.
77. Sitburana O, Ondo WG. Tetrabenazine for hyperglycemic-induced hemichorea-hemiballismus. *Mov Disord* 2006; 21: 2023–5.
78. Andermann E, Andermann F, Carpenter S, et al. Action myoclonus-renal failure syndrome: a previously unrecognized neurological disorder unmasked by advances in nephrology. *Adv Neurol* 1986; 43: 87–103.
79. Raskin NH, Fishman RA. Neurologic disorders in renal failure (second of two parts). *N Engl J Med* 1976; 294: 204–10.
80. Stark RJ. Reversible myoclonus with uraemia. *Br Med J (Clin Res Ed)* 1981; 282: 1119–20.
81. Young RR, Shahani BT. Asterixis: one type of negative myoclonus. *Adv Neurol* 1986; 43: 137–56.
82. Mucsi I, Molnar MZ, Ambrus C, et al. Restless legs syndrome, insomnia and quality of life in patients on maintenance dialysis. *Nephrol Dial Transplant* 2005; 20: 571–7.
83. Winkelmann J, Stautner A, Samtleben W, et al. Long-term course of restless legs syndrome in dialysis patients after kidney transplantation. *Mov Disord* 2002; 17: 1072–6.
84. Molnar MZ, Novak M, Ambrus C, et al. Restless legs syndrome in patients after renal transplantation. *Am J Kidney Dis* 2005; 45: 388–96.
85. Layrargues GP. Movement dysfunction and hepatic encephalopathy. *Metab Brain Dis* 2001; 16: 27–35.
86. Saporta MA, Andre C, Bahia PR, et al. Acquired hepatocerebral degeneration without overt liver disease. *Neurology* 2004; 63: 1981–2.
87. Jog MS, Lang AE. Chronic acquired hepatocerebral degeneration: case reports and new insights. *Mov Disord* 1995; 10: 714–22.
88. Victor M, Adams RD, Cole M. The acquired (non-Wilsonian) type of chronic hepatocerebral degeneration. *Medicine (Baltimore)* 1965; 44: 345–96.
89. Ferrara J, Jankovic J. Acquired hepatocerebral degeneration. *J Neurol* 2009; 256: 320–32.
90. Burkhard PR, Delavelle J, Du Pasquier R, et al. Chronic parkinsonism associated with cirrhosis: a distinct subset of acquired hepatocerebral degeneration. *Arch Neurol* 2003; 60: 521–8.
91. Aggarwal A, Vaidya S, Shah S, et al. Reversible Parkinsonism and T_1W pallidal hyperintensities in acute liver failure. *Mov Disord* 2006; 21: 1986–90.
92. Powell EE, Pender MP, Chalk JB, et al. Improvement in chronic hepatocerebral degeneration following liver transplantation. *Gastroenterology* 1990; 98: 1079–82.
93. Albers JW, Nostrant TT, Riggs JE. Neurologic manifestations of gastrointestinal disease. *Neurol Clin* 1989; 7: 525–48.
94. Mostile G, Jankovic J. Alcohol in essential tremor and other movement disorders. *Mov Disord* 2010; 25: 2274–84.
95. Brust JC. Substance abuse and movement disorders. *Mov Disord* 2010; 25: 2010–20.
96. Shandling M, Carlen PL, Lang AE. Parkinsonism in alcohol withdrawal: a follow-up study. *Mov Disord* 1990; 5: 36–9.
97. Neiman J, Lang AE, Fornazzari L, et al. Movement disorders in alcoholism: a review. *Neurology* 1990; 40: 741–6.
98. Yokota O, Tsuchiya K, Terada S, et al. Alcoholic cerebellar degeneration: a clinicopathological study of six Japanese autopsy cases and proposed potential progression pattern in the cerebellar lesion. *Neuropathology* 2007; 27: 99–113.
99. Mirsattari SM, Power C, Nath A. Parkinsonism with HIV infection. *Mov Disord* 1998; 13: 684–9.
100. Nath A, Jankovic J, Pettigrew LC. Movement disorders and AIDS. *Neurology* 1987; 37: 37–41.
101. Mirsattari SM, Berry ME, Holden JK, et al. Paroxysmal dyskinesias in patients with HIV infection. *Neurology* 1999; 52: 109–14.
102. Cornford ME, Holden JK, Boyd MC, et al. Neuropathology of the acquired immune deficiency syndrome (AIDS): report of 39 autopsies from Vancouver, British Columbia. *Can J Neurol Sci* 1992; 19: 442–52.
103. Hriso E, Kuhn T, Masdeu JC, et al. Extrapyramidal symptoms due to dopamine-blocking agents in patients with AIDS encephalopathy. *Am J Psychiatry* 1991; 148: 1558–61.
104. Cardoso F. Infectious and transmissible movement disorders. In: Jankovic J, Tolosa E (eds) *Parkinson's disease and movement disorders* (3rd edn), pp. 945–66. Baltimore, MD: Williams & Wilkins, 1998.
105. Church AJ, Cardoso F, Dale RC, et al. Anti-basal ganglia antibodies in acute and persistent Sydenham's chorea. *Neurology* 2002; 59: 227–31.
106. Paz JA, Silva CA, Marques-Dias MJ. Randomized double-blind study with prednisone in Sydenham's chorea. *Pediatr Neurol* 2006; 34: 264–9.

107. Swedo SE, Leonard HL, Garvey M, et al. Pediatric autoimmune neuropsychiatric disorders associated with streptococcal infections: clinical description of the first 50 cases. *Am J Psychiatry* 1998; 155: 264–71.
108. Kurlan R. The PANDAS hypothesis: losing its bite? *Mov Disord* 2004; 19: 371–4.
109. Singer HS, Gause C, Morris C, et al. Serial immune markers do not correlate with clinical exacerbations in pediatric autoimmune neuropsychiatric disorders associated with streptococcal infections. *Pediatrics* 2008; 121: 1198–205.
110. Schrag A, Gilbert R, Giovannoni G, et al. Streptococcal infection, Tourette syndrome, and OCD: is there a connection? *Neurology* 2009; 73: 1256–63.
111. Alarcon F, Maldonado JC, Rivera JW. Movement disorders identified in patients with intracranial tuberculomas. *Neurologia* 2011; 26: 343–50.
112. Schwartz MA, Selhorst JB, Ochs AL, et al. Oculomasticatory myorhythmia: a unique movement disorder occurring in Whipple's disease. *Ann Neurol* 1986; 20: 677–83.
113. Desnues B, Al Moussawi K, Fenollar F. New insights into Whipple's disease and *Tropheryma whipplei* infections. *Microbes Infect* 2010; 12: 1102–10.
114. Senanayake N, de Silva HJ. Delayed cerebellar ataxia complicating falciparum malaria: a clinical study of 74 patients. *J Neurol* 1994; 241: 456–9.
115. Garg RK, Karak B, Misra S. Neurological manifestations of malaria: an update. *Neurol India* 1999; 47: 85–91.

CHAPTER 30

Sleep-related Movement Disorders

Paul J. Reading

Introduction

As in many areas of sleep medicine, it is often a challenge deciding whether or not movements during sleep reflect truly abnormal nocturnal phenomenona or are simply physiological variants. Indeed, when asleep, subconscious shifts of body position occurring every 15 minutes or so are considered entirely normal, as are minor jerks of the extremities and face, particularly during periods of rapid eye movement (REM) sleep. However, if nocturnal movements are observed to be excessive, violent, or arousing, either to the subject or bed partner, they will usually indicate a defined disorder, especially if the events are stereotypic through the night. Although the second edition of the International Classification of Sleep Disorders (ICSD) was revised in 2005 (1) to include a new section dedicated to movement disorders occurring specifically during the state of sleep, diagnostic precision of such phenomena is often lacking and evidenced-based treatment protocols, when indicated, are poorly developed. Furthermore, if a sleep-related movement disorder is recognized, it can be very difficult to determine its true clinical significance for sleep quality and subsequent daytime wakefulness, especially in the elderly patient.

With the exception of rare conditions such as palatal tremor or spinal segmental myoclonus, it is a common perception that the vast majority of 'waking' movement disorders effectively disappear during sleep. This is only partly true, since parkinsonian tremor, for example, may persist into light non-REM sleep stages (2), as may dyskinesias (3), potentially contributing to impaired sleep maintenance and poor-quality nocturnal sleep. Moreover, most hyperkinetic movement disorders, such as Huntington's disease, are associated with generalized restlessness during sleep, again interfering with its quality, even at early disease stages (4). Perhaps counter-intuitively, motor tics and even vocalizations are seen throughout all stages of sleep in the majority of subjects with Tourette's syndrome (5).

However, this chapter will address those movement disorders that are intimately or exclusively related to the state of sleep or the sleep–wake transition. By convention, parasomnias causing abnormal arousals from deep non-REM sleep, such as sleepwalking or night terrors, will not be covered, although restless legs syndrome is discussed, partly because of its close association with periodic limb movements during sleep. Similarly, nocturnal epilepsy will not be addressed, and REM sleep behaviour disorder is discussed in Chapter 9.

Restless legs syndrome and periodic limb movements

Restless legs syndrome (RLS) is best conceived as a sensorimotor disorder, defined wholly by subjective symptoms and characterized predominantly by a strong urge to move the legs, particularly in the late evening (6). There is nearly always associated limb discomfort that can be difficult both to describe and to localize. A common report is that of an unpleasant 'crawling' sensation under the skin around the shins. Symptomatic but temporary relief is obtained by moving or rubbing the affected limb(s). The adverse consequences on both sleep onset and maintenance are often severe (Case 30.1) and may lead to the potentially sterile debate of whether RLS is more a movement or a sleep disorder. In any event, RLS is common and affects around 3% of Caucasian populations when screened by personal interview using validated criteria (7). Given the relatively non-specific nature of these symptom-based diagnostic criteria, self-completed questionnaires may lack diagnostic precision and have led to overestimates of RLS prevalence in the past (8). Furthermore, there is clearly an extremely wide spectrum of RLS symptom severity and frequency with approximately 20% of subjects reporting clinically significant symptoms on more than two evenings each week, potentially justifying attempts at drug therapy (9). In severe or atypical cases, leg restlessness and discomfort may extend to other body parts, particularly the arms.

RLS affects females preferentially and there is an association with increasing age up until the eighth decade (10). However, RLS also affects children and, as such, is often unrecognized in younger populations (11). A positive family history is frequently obtained, especially if symptom onset occurs before 40 years of age (12).

Many subjects with RLS will also be aware of involuntary limb movements which may occur at regular intervals during the wakeful state, usually when drowsy or at the point of sleep onset.

Case 30.1 A 57-year-old graphic designer was referred with a 10-year history of 'restless sleep' such that he was prone to 'wearing out' the bed sheets, invariably waking in a reportedly exhausted state. On direct questioning, he admitted to an unpleasant sensation of 'creeping discomfort' in both shins that always came on at 8 p.m. and was relieved by vigorous rubbing or moving around the room. He was experiencing severe somnolence at work, particularly in the mid-afternoon period. He was taking an opiate preparation for persistent shoulder pain which also improved his leg symptoms to some extent. There was no relevant family history and no markers for iron deficiency in his routine blood tests.

A polysomnogram revealed sleep onset insomnia and an extremely high number of periodic limb movements when asleep (Fig. 30.1). He rarely entered deep non-REM sleep during the night of recording, potentially explaining the unrefreshing nature of the nocturnal sleep period.

He was started on a rotigotine patch (2 mg once daily) and made an excellent response in terms of reducing his general restlessness and daytime somnolence.

Case 30.2 A 40-year-old man was referred to the sleep clinic with a 2-year history of severe excessive daytime sleepiness. A detailed sleep history failed to reveal any obvious cause for his somnolence, although he awoke after 8 hours of nocturnal sleep feeling unrefreshed. He had no bed partner, but was not known to be a snorer and was not aware of excessive leg movements during sleep. For several years, he reported mild and unobtrusive symptoms of restless legs syndrome on one or two evenings a week. All routine blood tests were normal.

His polysomnogram was abnormal and demonstrated difficulty falling asleep and several arousals from deep non-REM sleep (Fig. 30.2). Of likely significance, he exhibited numerous PLMs throughout the night which were thought to be adversely affecting his sleep quality. Video 30.1 shows a representative clip of his polysomnogram recording which demonstrates regular leg movements at 26-second intervals typical for PLMs. His left leg appears particularly involved as revealed by the EMG trace. The movements themselves appear quite subtle but are associated with micro-arousals on the EEG.

He responded well to dopamine agonist therapy, supporting the diagnosis of PLMD.

However, these periodic limb movements (PLMs) are most frequently observed or noticed by bed partners during non-REM sleep in the first third of the night and affect the vast majority of RLS subjects (Case 30.2). Most authorities consider the clinical phenomena of RLS and PLMs to share both a common underlying neurobiology and a potential for adverse health consequences (13). Phenotypically, PLMs usually resemble a slowed version of a withdrawal reflex in a lower limb, starting with great toe and then foot dorsiflexion. The slow flexor jerk may then extend to involve the knee and hip over 0.5–1 seconds, potentially leading to a more generalized movement or arousal from sleep which may mimic simple restlessness (Case 30.3). The duration of movements associated with a PLM may last up to 10 seconds, as recognized by recently modified scoring criteria (14). Automated polysomnograms using bilateral lower limb EMG monitors will usually record movements as PLMs if they recur with a precise periodicity (typically around 25 seconds) at least four times in succession. PLMs can continue in clusters for several minutes, sometimes hours. An index of the number of PLMs per hour is often calculated, with severely affected subjects exhibiting levels of 150 or more. The deeper the level of non-REM sleep, the longer the inter-movement interval tends to be (15). PLMs can also occur in REM sleep but are usually of shorter duration and less frequent.

The striking and defining periodicity of PLMs remains unexplained. Of possible relevance, as early as 1972 it was proposed there was an endogenous pacemaker to explain the apparent subtle periodicity (20–40 seconds duration) of minor changes in several physiological measures such as heart rate and blood pressure (16). This comparison has intuitive appeal given the observation that subtle EEG and ECG changes may precede the actual observed movement associated with a PLM (17). The location of any putative pacemaker needs to explain the presence of PLMs observed in patients with complete spinal transactions or significant syringomyelia (18). The similarity of PLMs to an abnormal plantar (Babinski) response has led to the suggestion that they arise due to diminished supraspinal inhibitory influences (19). Of note, an extensor plantar response can be elicited in control subjects during normal non-REM sleep, suggesting that there may be an exaggeration of this observed phenomenon in PLMs (20). Certainly, the relative lack of supraspinal inhibitory influences is supported by the observation that the spinal

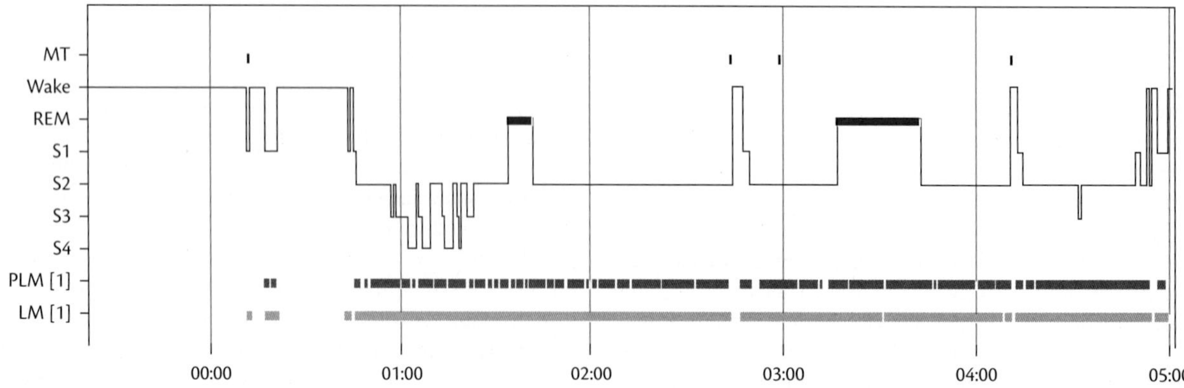

Fig. 30.1 Polysomnogram for the subject in Case 30.1. MT, movement time; S1–S4, non-REM sleep stages 1–4; PLM, periodic limb movement; LM, leg movement.

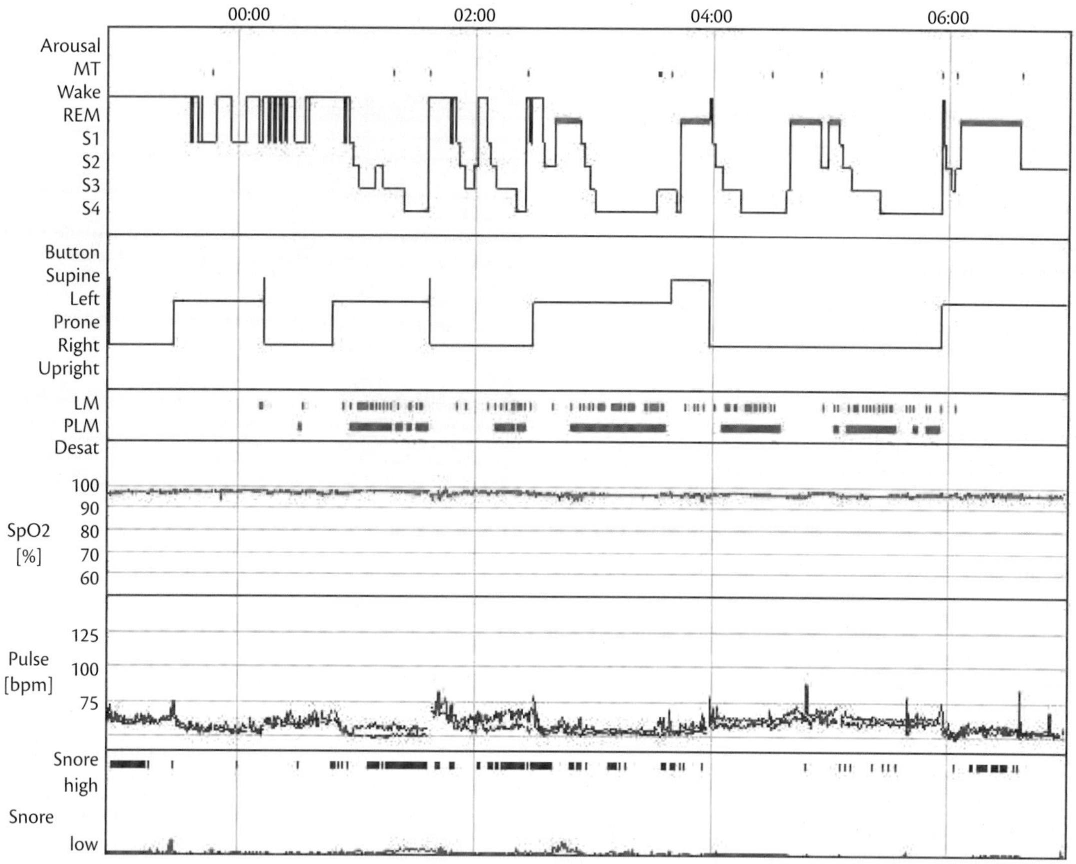

Fig. 30.2 Polysomnogram for the subject in Case 30.2. MT, movement time; S1–S4, non-REM sleep stages 1–4; PLM, periodic limb movement; LM, leg movement.

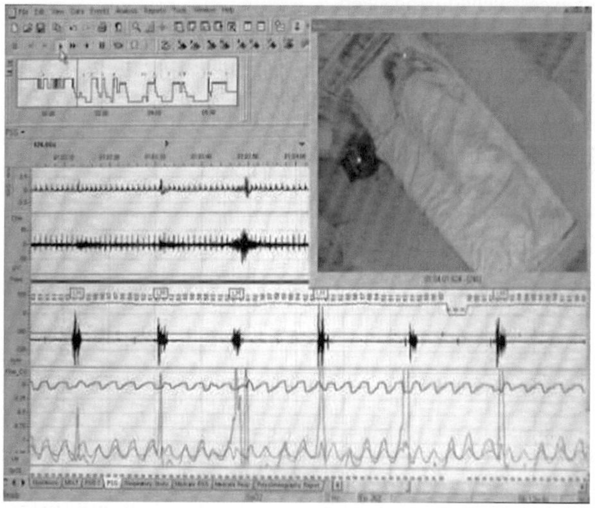

Video 30.1 A short clip showing Case 30.2 during his polysomnogram. Periodic limb movements predominantly involving the left leg are demonstrated.

flexor reflex has a lower threshold and a greater spatial spread in those with PLMs in the context of RLS (21).

PLMs during sleep can affect the sleep quality of bed partners but may well not be recognized or recalled by the subjects themselves. When monitored, transient heart rate rises often coincide with PLMs, indicating minor associated autonomic arousals in the absence of definite EEG changes. In general, up to a third of PLMs are linked to micro-arousals, defined as a return to alpha or theta EEG activity for 3–15 seconds (22). However, this remains a controversial area, largely due to issues around reliably scoring and defining these minor EEG changes (23).

PLMs during sleep may also be observed in up to 30% of normal elderly populations, but are usually at a low level and have no likely clinical significance (24). Indeed, a number of studies have failed to demonstrate a clear relation between the frequency of PLMs during the night and reports of poor sleep quality or daytime somnolence, even when the PLMs are reported to have caused micro-arousals (25).

Rarely, subjects are identified with significant and potentially arousing PLMs seen during sleep recordings in the absence of RLS, reflecting periodic limb movement disorder (PLMD). In such subjects, especially if there is no bed partner, PLMs may not be suspected from history alone even though sleep continuity is adversely affected and the deeper stages of non-REM sleep are poorly maintained (Case 30.2). As a result, it is important to recognize and treat PLMD is it may rarely cause significant daytime somnolence. Furthermore, troublesome adult sleepwalking may sometimes be triggered by sleep disorders such as PLMD when subjects are partially aroused from deep slow-wave non-REM sleep by their excessive limb movements (Case 30.4).

Pathophysiology

Despite major recent advances in unravelling the complex genetics of RLS and associated PLMs, the precise underlying neurobiological basis remains elusive and most likely has several elements. Although

Case 30.3 A 42-year-old businessman was referred with a six-month history of disturbed sleep. His wife reported virtually continuous non-specific movements throughout the sleep period involving all four limbs. He did not report waking through the night, but was unrefreshed in the morning and experiencing severe fatigue during the day. However, he was able to avoid napping. He denied symptoms suggestive of restless legs syndrome in the evening or before bed.

An overnight recording revealed that he was a heavy snorer in the absence of sleep apnoea or significant nocturnal oxygen desaturations. He spent the majority of the sleep period in light non-REM sleep and appeared to fidget continuously. The automated sleep analysis software did not report any periodicity in the leg movements.

Two representative video clips are shown (Videos 30.2 and 30.3). On the second clip, the initial movement is seen to start with great toe extension, almost certainly reflecting a form of PLM. On detailed examination of his restlessness, it was apparent that many of the movements were preceded by great toe extension before more generalized movements that lasted for 10 seconds or more.

Routine investigations revealed unexpected and severe iron-deficient anaemia (haemoglobin level was 5.2 g/L), subsequently found to be secondary to slowly bleeding haemorrhoids. Appropriate treatment of these and a prolonged course of oral iron replacement restored his haemoglobin levels and led to complete resolution of his sleep problems.

In retrospect, during sleep, he was almost certainly exhibiting atypical PLMs which were causing more generalized and prolonged movements, reflecting partial arousals. His severe iron deficiency had almost certainly triggered the PLMD.

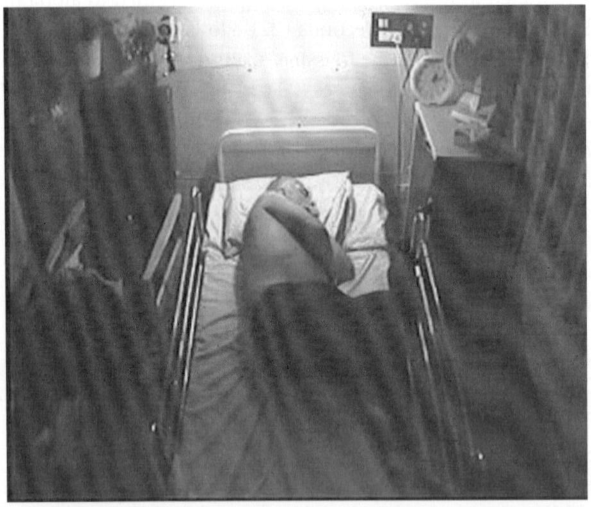

Video 30.2 A short clip early in the night of Case 30.3. He exhibits general fidgeting in light non-REM sleep.

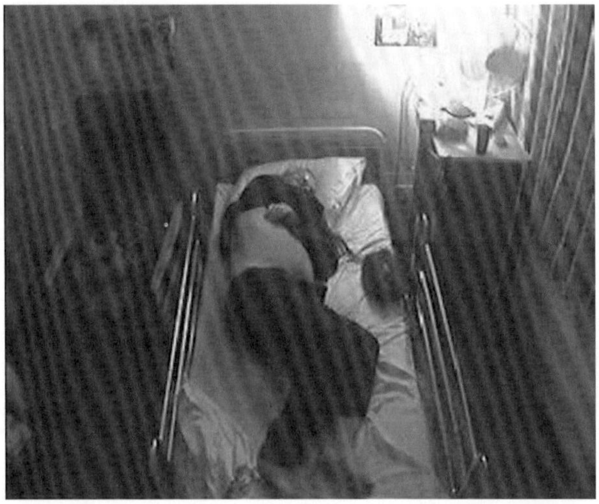

Video 30.3 A clip of Case 30.3 from later in the same night. This bout of generalized movement starts with extension of his great toe suggesting that he is exhibiting a form of extended arousal in the context of periodic limb movement disorder (see text for fuller explanation).

Case 30.4 A 26-year-old marine with a long history of benign childhood sleepwalking caused concern to his colleagues when he started to experience agitated nocturnal disturbances on active duty in Iraq. On several nights during the week, within an hour of sleep onset, he reportedly screamed and would run from the dormitory, often brandishing his army weapon. He also reported that his nocturnal sleep was generally unrefreshing, potentially fuelling a moderate degree of excessive daytime sleepiness. He denied symptoms of RLS although was aware his legs may have moved excessively during sleep.

His polysomnogram (Fig. 30.3) reveals an excess of light non-REM sleep (stage 2 occupies 71% of total sleep time) and an extremely high number of leg movements throughout the night. The vast majority of these are periodic in nature and many appear to cause micro-arousals, most likely preventing him achieving deep non-REM sleep. On the few occasions he enters deep sleep, he arouses abruptly to apparent wakefulness although appears confused. This feature reflects his propensity for non-REM sleep parasomnia activity, his main symptom of concern.

Treatment of his PLMs with a dopamine agonist before bed improved his sleep quality and reduced both his parasomnia activity and daytime somnolence.

the distinction may be somewhat artificial, RLS can be considered 'primary' or 'secondary' when it is associated with a variety of other conditions such as iron deficiency, uraemia, and pregnancy (26). RLS is also worsened by dopamine-blocking agents and antihistamines. These observations have led to two possibly related theories of RLS causation. First, supported by the fact that dopaminergic drugs are usually effective treatments, RLS may reflect dysfunction or underactivity of dopaminergic pathways, perhaps in the small but extensive descending A11 projection from the hypothalamus to the spinal cord (27). Secondly, the link to iron depletion or disorders of iron handling might suggest that there is actual or functional iron deficiency in specific parts of the brain (28). Certainly, intravenous iron infusions may be an effective treatment even in the absence of obvious systemic deficiency (29). The fact that the rate-limiting enzyme for dopamine production in the brain, tyrosine hydroxylase, requires iron as a co-factor has been proposed as a link between these two putative pathophysiological mechanisms.

Recent data from a variety of sources may have clarified some of the issues, although many unanswered questions remain. There is little evidence for direct pathology of dopaminergic systems,

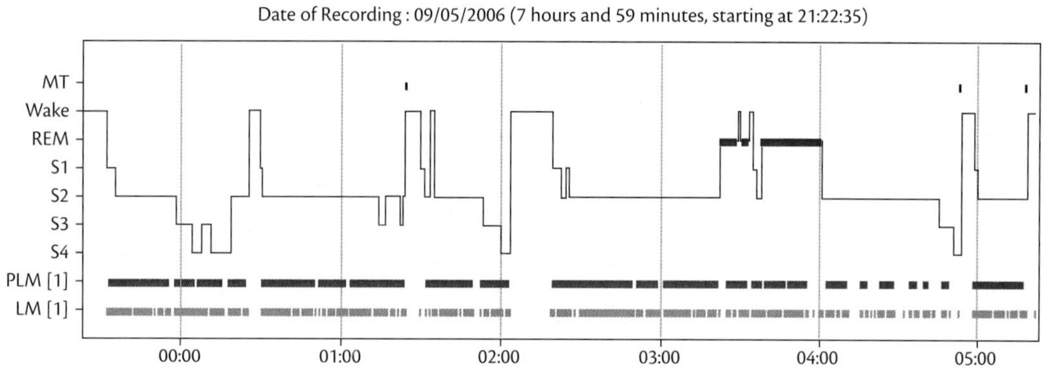

Limb Movements [1]

EMG-Tib	Total	Index	During PLM Number	During PLM Index
LM	730	139,7	689	131,9
LM with Arousal	0	-	0	-
LM following apnea	95	18,2	95	18,2
LM with no association	635	121,5	594	113,7
LM during wake	0	-	-	-
LM during sleep stage S1	46	204,4	35	155,6
LM during sleep stage S2	498	133,4	487	130,4
LM during sleep stage S3	61	149,4	56	137,1
LM during sleep stage S4	36	130,9	34	123,6
LM during REM sleep	82	146,9	74	132,5
LM during movement time	5	200	3	120

Limb Movements [1]

Number of LM 730	Mean	Shortest	Longest
Sequence duration	1,6 seconds	1 seconds	3,5 seconds

Periodic Limb Movements [1]

Number of PLM-sequences 56	Mean	Shortest	Longest
Sequence duration	4,6 minutes	0,4 minutes	18,9 minutes

Fig. 30.3 Polysomnogram for the subject in Case 30.4. MT, large body movements; S1–S4, stages 1–4 of non-REM sleep; LM, leg movement.

although some imaging studies have demonstrated reduced putaminal D2 postsynaptic receptor density (30), recently confirmed by post-mortem data (31). The latter study also implied that there were significantly higher levels of phosphorylated tyrosine hydroxylase, paradoxically suggestive of increased dopamine turnover. This counter-intuitive finding may explain the reduced levels of postsynaptic dopamine receptors as a result of 'downregulation'. Of potential relevance, rodent models of iron deficiency have shown similar dynamic changes in dopaminergic pathways (32). Furthermore, there were striking and enhanced diurnal changes in brain dopamine levels in the iron-deficient mice such that, during the active period, extracellular striatal levels were particularly high (32). In the presence of reduced postsynaptic receptor density, the relative underactivity of the dopaminergic pathways in the rest period might produce a functional dopamine deficiency and have relevance for the human condition.

Accumulating evidence appears to suggest that alterations in brain iron handling are important, even in those with primary or idiopathic RLS. For example, both imaging and limited post-mortem data imply reduced brain iron stores and lower CSF levels of ferritin than expected in seemingly idiopathic cases (31, 33, 34). Although cytosolic levels of ferritin are reduced, mitochondrial ferritin appears increased. Together with the observation that mitochondria numbers overall are significantly increased in the substantia nigra neurons of RLS subjects, it has been proposed that there is a cellular response resembling that seen in hypoxia (35). This may produce increased dopamine turnover, as seen in animal models of simple iron deficiency, and possibly a relative dopamine deficiency during the evening to explain the diurnal pattern of RLS symptoms. The ultimate reason why RLS patients may have altered brain iron handling even when peripheral stores are superficially normal remains elusive.

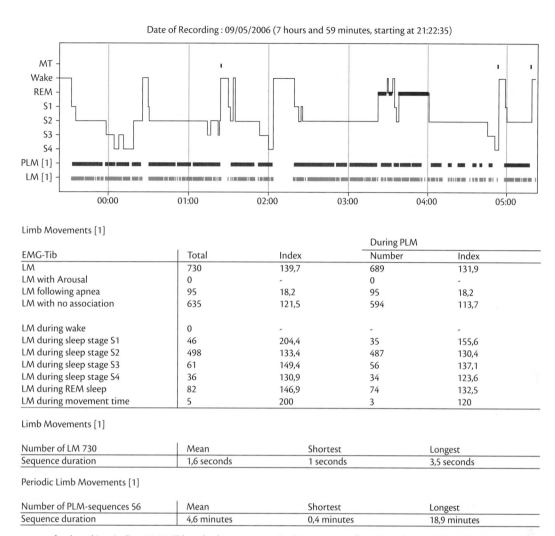

A strong association of three genetic loci with RLS and PLM prevalence was discovered through several genome-wide searches in a range of geographical populations (36). Perhaps disappointingly and contrary to expectations, none of the likely gene products appeared to have direct involvement in either iron or dopamine metabolism. In fact, the relevant single-nucleotide polymorphisms (SNPs) were intronic or intergenic, strongly suggesting a regulatory role in neural development, perhaps in the spinal cord. However, intriguingly and through an unknown mechanism, one of the loci (BTBD9) did seem to correlate directly with low levels of serum ferritin and was particularly seen in subjects with PLMs rather than isolated RLS without PLMs (37). Remarkably, at least in European populations, the population attributable risk of RLS for the BTBD9 marker was 50%. In other words, in the absence of this polymorphism, the number of clinical cases would be expected to halve.

Treatment

It is mandatory to address and possibly treat reversible conditions that may be causing or fuelling significant symptoms of RLS and PLMs. The most common is iron deficiency even in the absence of frank anaemia. By consensus, iron replacement is recommended if serum ferritin levels are less than 45 μg/L (38), although any subsequent clinical response to oral iron is usually slow. Furthermore, drugs such as neuroleptics, antihistamines, and the majority of commonly used antidepressants, namely SSRIs and tricyclics, should be discontinued if possible as they frequently exacerbate symptoms. Anecdotally, excessive caffeine or chocolate can also worsen RLS.

If there are no obvious remediable factors and clinical symptoms are deemed severe or frequent enough to warrant drug therapy, dopamine agonists are considered first-line agents (39). Although levodopa is often effective, its use is reserved for occasional or intermittent RLS symptoms, given the high risk of augmentation (39). In this phenomenon, symptoms are experienced earlier in the day than previously and are more severe, frequently with spread to other body parts such as the upper limbs. However, augmentation can also be seen with dopamine agonists, and an increasing trend is to use long-acting preparations such as the transdermal dopamine patch, rotigotine, in an attempt to minimize the problem (40). Dopamine agonist doses are typically much lower than those used in Parkinson's disease although standard side effects, including the development of impulse control disorders, need to be continually monitored (41).

In the absence of significant controlled evidence or data, second-line therapies can be used as either alternatives or supplements to dopaminergic agents (39). These include gabapentin or pregabalin at standard doses, which may be particularly helpful if the dysaesthetic component of the RLS symptomology is prominent. Some authorities recommend long-acting opiates such as methadone as an alternative, although side effects and concerns over dependency often limit this approach (42).

Extremely severe or resistant cases may become tolerant to standard therapies and pose a significant management problem. Anecdotal evidence suggests that it may be worthwhile using apomorphine infusions through the evening and overnight (43), potentially with other more conventional treatments during the afternoon or even morning, if required. Although there are potential concerns regarding severe allergic reactions that necessitate strict administration protocols, infusions of intravenous iron can also be effective in resistant RLS subjects even in the absence of obvious iron deficiency (29). It appears that the precise formulation may be important (44). In particular, iron dextran is probably the most likely to increase brain iron levels as a putative mechanism of symptom relief that may last for several months (45).

Sleep starts

The majority of people will recognize or recall infrequent mildly unsettling episodes of abrupt generalized jolts occurring just at the point of sleep onset. The sensation is often likened to briefly 'falling through space'. Phenotypically, these myoclonic jerks are not stereotyped and may produce either flexion or extension movements of trunk and limbs. The jerks superficially resemble startle reflexes (46) although, unlike these, asymmetry of limb movements is commonly observed. Generally, these wake–sleep transition phenomena are infrequent and more likely to occur in a sleep-deprived young population, potentially aggravated by caffeine excess. If events are captured during sleep investigations, brief autonomic and EEG arousals usually follow the jerks but sleep onset occurs normally thereafter and there are no adverse clinical consequences.

Rarely, sleep starts may be frequent or dramatic enough to cause significant insomnia (1), especially if they recur through the night at each sleep–wake transition. Occasionally, myoclonic seizure activity may be mistakenly suspected (47). Anxiety secondary to the sleep starts may also fuel the subject's inability to fall asleep. Furthermore, a minority of subjects experience prominent auditory or even visual phenomena, occasionally in the absence of any motor phenomena or myoclonic movements (48). Sensory descriptions of 'bangs', 'shocks', or even 'explosions', usually in the head, are typical. Understandably, these can produce concern and require reassurances that they are not due to epilepsy or cerebral vascular pathology.

Because of their benign nature, systematic studies of sleep starts are minimal and their pathophysiology is poorly understood. They usually arise from early stage I sleep and may be preceded by a vertex sharp wave or K-complex (49). There is brief generalized EMG activation which many assume reflects activation of the descending audiogenic startle reflex pathways from the brainstem. The return of an alpha rhythm on the EEG reflects cortical arousal. At a simplistic level, sleep starts probably reflect a temporary fault in the usually smooth transition from wake to sleep such that part of the brain fails to 'fall asleep' and an alerting brainstem mechanism is subsequently activated when this mismatch is detected. An interesting and somewhat bizarre probably related phenomenon, the 'blip syndrome', has been described in which subjects suddenly feel as though only part of their brain has lost consciousness when drowsy (50). This brief disconcerting phenomenon probably rarely comes to medical attention but may also reflect a partial failure of smooth transition from wake to light sleep.

Sleep starts rarely necessitate drug therapy unless there is resulting significant insomnia. In such cases, brief courses of routinely used hypnotic agents such as short-acting benzodiazepines are usually effective, although controlled trials are lacking.

Propriospinal myoclonus at sleep onset

The term 'propriospinal myoclonus' (PSM) was introduced in 1991 to describe non-rhythmic axial jerks causing symmetric flexion of the neck, trunk, and lower limbs in three index cases (51). Detailed electrophysiology implied that the movements were caused by electrical discharges arising from a spinal 'pattern' generator with spread both rostrally and caudally via relatively slow (<5 m/s) pathways presumed, from animal evidence, to be in the long propriospinal tracts. In some subjects, there are long-duration bursts (100–300 ms) of EMG activity causing repetitive jerks with a frequency of 1–7 Hz (52). Subsequent reports of the phenomenon have emphasized the important roles of body position and behavioural state. In particular, PSM was observed to be much more common when the subject was recumbent and extremely drowsy, at the point of sleep onset (53). Indeed, when the movements are confined to the wake–sleep transition, it can be considered a parasomnia, adversely affecting sleep onset and altering subsequent sleep structure. In this situation, it is commonly observed that mental activity, voluntary movements of the limbs and indeed sleep itself can all suppress the myoclonic movements. Rarely, as seen in other forms of myoclonus, PSM appears to be stimulus sensitive, triggered variously by sudden noises or external tactile stimulation to either the back or the abdomen (54).

A variety of spinal cord pathologies, including trauma, have been reported to trigger or precipitate PSM, often with considerable delay in symptom onset after the presumed primary pathology (55). Although the majority of cases have normal conventional spinal cord MRI, one recent review suggests that detailed diffusion tensor imaging may reveal subtle disorganization of white matter tracts in the majority of cases (56).

Confirming PSM by investigation can be laborious and requires significant resources as full video-polysomnography is required to demonstrate the specific association of the movements with the drowsy state (53, 57). In addition, numerous EMG electrodes situated at 2-cm intervals along the bellies of involved muscles are advocated in order to document the slow spread of EMG activation from a putative spinal source, usually in the mid-thoracic region (Fig. 30.4). The pattern of propagation, absence of a cortical pre-movement potential, and lack of involvement of cranial muscles all distinguish PSM from other disorders such as cortical and reticular reflex myoclonus.

Intensified hypnic jerks or sleep starts may mimic PSM, especially when they result in significant sleep-onset insomnia. However, they usually involve isolated body segments and do not primarily affect the abdominal musculature. Focal abnormal involuntary movements of the abdominal wall, variously described as 'moving umbilicus syndrome', 'belly dancer's dyskinesia', or 'diaphragmatic flutter', appear as different phenomena to PSM. In these, the affected muscles demonstrate irregular or writhing contractions at high rates of 30–90 per minute. PLMs, although fairly frequently seen in relaxed wakefulness, invariably start in the distal musculature and, in stark contrast to PSM, predominate during non-REM sleep. However, when PLMs are associated with restless legs syndrome they may co-exist with PSM (58).

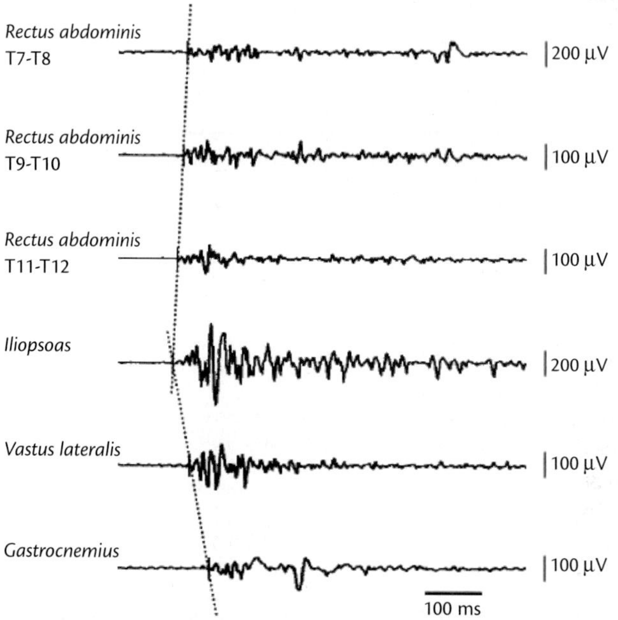

Fig. 30.4 A neurophysiological demonstration of a typical axial jerk of a subject with propriospinal myoclonus at sleep onset. Using a number of EMG electrodes spaced across several myotomes, the electrical discharge is seen to spread proximally and distally from a presumed spinal source that innervates the iliopsoas muscle. Conventional MRI of the subject's cervical and thoracic spinal cord was normal.

The surprising demonstration that the characteristic EMG pattern of muscle activation ascribed to PSM can be identically observed in healthy volunteer subjects asked to mimic the axial myoclonic movements has led some to question the organicity of PSM in otherwise typical cases (59). The disappearance of PSM with mental distraction and sleep onset might also suggest a psychological aetiology. Indeed, a striking 34 of 35 consecutive patients with possible PSM referred to a Dutch tertiary movement disorders service were ultimately diagnosed with a psychogenic movement disorder (60). Clinical clues pointing to a functional disorder were the presence of a *Bereitschaftspotential* prior to movements, regular eye blinking, sustained eye gaze, or head movements in association with axial jerks, or inconsistent polygraphic findings over prolonged recording. In addition, the fact that some subjects with PSM report a premonitory 'inner tension' or 'shock-like' sensation just prior to the movements might suggest an adult-onset tic disorder, especially if there are associated vocalizations or rebound phenomena after movement suppression (56, 61).

Not surprisingly, given the rarity of PSM, evidence for effective clinical management is very limited. Even in the absence of clinical signs of spinal cord pathology, it is probably appropriate to image cervical and thoracic regions, as benign unsuspected lesions have rarely been reported as likely precipitants (62). PSM tends not to improve spontaneously and can produce severe insomnia, warranting drug therapy. Clonazepam before bedtime has been used with variable success, and anecdotal evidence suggests that the antiepileptic agent zonisamide may occasionally help in resistant cases (59). Other agents that have been reported to be helpful are gabapentin (up to 800 mg/day), levetiracetam (up to 2000 mg/day), and carbamazepine (up to 400 mg/day) (52, 53). Transcutaneous electrical nerve stimulation (TENS) applied to an area supplied by the low-thoracic spinal level has been reported to be useful in a middle-aged man with probable PSM (63).

Rhythmical movement disorder of sleep

Sleep-related rhythmic movement disorder (RMD) is a relatively poorly researched phenomenon that is most commonly seen at the wake–sleep transition, although it can occur in drowsy wakefulness or, surprisingly given its nature, during any stage of sleep including REM sleep (64–66). Occasionally it can be seen in association with partial arousals from sleep (65). RMD is characterized by a variety of sustained stereotypic movements involving the major muscle groups. The cadence of movements is strikingly regular at a frequency of 0.5–2 Hz. Typical movements include head rolling or banging, axial rocking, and even rhythmical striking of the head with the hands. Some subjects exhibit more than one type of RMD, depending on body position during sleep (67), with vigorous head rolling most commonly seen in the prone position. Synchronous humming or moaning is not uncommon, although subsequent recollection of such activity is usually absent. It is relatively rare for RMD to be of major concern to the subjects themselves and, certainly in adults, it is the bed partner whose sleep is predominantly disturbed, especially since the movements can continue for periods of 30 minutes or so.

The prototypical RMD, namely head banging, was first described in children in 1905 independently by German and French workers who coined the terms *jactatio capitas nocturna* and *tics dans le sommeil*, respectively (see ref. 68 for a historical review). Head banging is common and may affect up to 5% of young children (69). It is seen more often in males and is more persistent if there is developmental disability, in which case similar rocking movements may also be witnessed during wakefulness. Indeed, many adult subjects may exhibit similar patterns of movement in quiet wakefulness, such as when listening to music. Secondary injuries are very rare although soft tissue damage or dermal scarring has been reported. Body rocking is even more prevalent as a rhythmic movement of sleep (around 15% of young children), but is rarely perceived as a problem and usually resolves before 5 years of age (70). In children, an association of RMD with attention deficit hyperactivity disorder has been reported, although sample sizes were small (71).

In a minority of subjects, RMD persists into adulthood, although prevalence figures are difficult to establish as it is relatively rare for the phenomenon to present to a sleep clinic. Of interest, in adults movements may be more varied and can be seen even in deep non-REM sleep, or even REM sleep when all significant movements would normally be suppressed (72). The diagnosis is usually clear simply from a video recording without the need for detailed polysomnography (Case 30.5). However, investigations may sometimes usefully demonstrate a degree of sleep disruption or an association of RMD with other sleep disorders such as periodic limb movements or apnoea-induced arousals.

The mechanisms behind RMD remain obscure although a variety of behavioural or psychological theories have been espoused, especially for childhood forms. A form of anxiety relief has been thought likely even if there is no overt psychopathology (73). Of possible relevance, RMD, like many sleep disorders, usually worsens during stressful periods. However, most authorities regard RMD as a 'tic-like' phenomenon or simply as a 'bad habit' which may be under partial voluntary control, at least in the early stages.

Case 30.5 The wife of a 35-year-old man with narcolepsy and cataplexy complained that he moved continuously for several minutes prior to sleep onset, disturbing her. This could recur through the night in association with spontaneous arousals and his attempts to return to sleep. The subject was not particularly concerned by these movements and thought that they had developed as a comforting 'reaction' to frequent unpleasant perceptions that a stranger was in the room as he entered sleep from drowsiness—so-called extra-campine hallucinations, a phenomenon occasionally reported in narcolepsy.

Video 30.4 shows him attempting to sleep, with an increasing frequency of lateral rhythmic movements involving his trunk and head occurring in the drowsy state. No treatment was thought necessary for this phenomenon which was characteristic of rhythmic movement disorder of sleep.

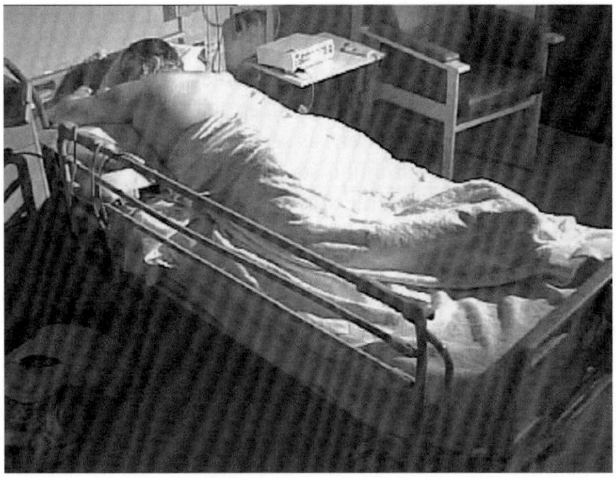

Video 30.4 A clip of Case 30.5 demonstrating an unusual form of rhythmical movement disorder of sleep in a narcoleptic patient (see text for full details).

If treatment is thought necessary, benzodiazepines such as clonazepam have been used, but only with limited success (74). Behavioural therapies including hypnosis have also been studied in small series (75). In children, some have advocated techniques such as sleep restriction and, perhaps more intriguingly, the use of a water bed (76).

Sleep-related bruxism

Sleep bruxism (SB) is probably an exaggerated form of normal masticatory movements or 'chewing automatisms' commonly witnessed during sleep, with additional tooth grinding as a potentially troublesome feature. Well over 50% of normal subjects will have episodes of rhythmic masticatory muscle activity, defined as three or more consecutive rhythmic contractions at 1 Hz frequency, once or twice an hour during sleep (77). These contractions are sustained or phasic, in which case the disturbing sounds of tooth-grinding occur. Although SB has a prevalence of around 8% in adults (78), many subjects are unaware that they grind their teeth at night and the bed partner is the main complainant. However, excessive tooth wear, dental or temporomandibular pain, and a strong association with migrainous and other headache syndromes are frequent observations. Of note, tooth grinding has been seen in over 50% of children diagnosed with tension-type headaches (79).

Secondary SB has been associated with a wide variety of medications and drugs of abuse, including most psychoactive agents and central stimulants. SSRIs and haloperidol have been most strongly implicated (80). Not surprisingly, hyperkinetic disorders, such as generalized dystonia and Huntington's disease, have also been linked to significant SB (81). Furthermore, SB tends to worsen when sleep patterns are non-specifically poor, either in the context of psychological distress or when there are frequent arousals due to obstructive sleep apnoea for example. It is rare for SB itself to trigger a full arousal from sleep, and it seems that the jaw activity is simultaneous or secondary to EEG arousals (82). In general, SB also appears to be more common in those with hypervigilant or highly motivated personalities (83).

Not infrequently, SB is picked up incidentally on polysomnographic recordings as a 1 Hz interference or movement artefact seen throughout the EEG traces. Episodes last between 0.25 and 2 seconds, occurring at intervals of 3 seconds or more. For a specific diagnosis of SB, contemporaneous audio recordings are strongly recommended, as are extra EMG electrodes in either masseter or temporalis muscles alongside the standard submental lead (14). Somewhat arbitrarily, SB can be diagnosed if there are at least four episodes per hour or at least 25 individual muscle bursts per hour of sleep (1). The EMG activity also needs to be accompanied by at least two episodes of teeth-grinding noises. Typically, subjects are symptomatic between three and five nights a week over a period of months. Masseter muscle hypertrophy may be observed in severe cases. SB is seen mostly in light non-REM sleep, although some subjects seem particularly affected at sleep stage transitions, particularly from light non-REM sleep to REM sleep (84).

If SB is deemed significant, most would advocate the use of soft or hard occlusal appliances. Mandibular advancement devices may also provide benefit and have the added advantage of improving snoring or any associated obstructive breathing-related disorder (85). Orthodontic procedures probably do not help SB specifically but can limit any potential secondary tooth damage. Various drug treatments have been studied in small randomized trials, usually with negative results. Examples include propranolol and a variety of antidepressants such as tricyclics and serotonergic agents (86). Muscle relaxants, including benzodiazepines and botulinum toxin, have not been studied systematically. Of interest, the alpha-2-agonist, clonidine, appeared to reduce SB by 60% in a small study, although early morning hypotension was seen in some subjects as a limiting side effect and REM sleep was strongly inhibited in most (87).

Fragmentary myoclonus

Infrequent small 'quivering' movements of the mouth or extremities, particularly during sleep, are physiological and of no clinical significance. However, in some individuals, the frequency of these minor movements can appear striking and the term 'excessive fragmentary myoclonus' (EFM) has been used (1). When studied systematically, it appears that the frequency of such movements during sleep is inversely related to the degree of EEG synchronization, such that stage I non-REM and REM sleep have the highest incidence. The EMG potentials are very brief (75–150 ms) and occur both asynchronously and asymmetrically, most often in the extremities. If there are more than five minor jerks per minute continuously for more than 20 minutes, it may be deemed excessive.

EFM is a controversial entity since the relationship with either sleep disruption or any consequent daytime somnolence is far from established. In a detailed study of 11 subjects, compared with a control group, an index of fragmentary myoclonus was calculated throughout the sleep cycle (88). The affected subjects had significantly increased movements throughout all sleep stages, especially early in the night, but no overall deterioration of sleep structure and no change in levels of deep slow-wave sleep. This implies that EFM, even when prominent, is not usually a serious cause of sleep maintenance insomnia.

It is very rarely considered necessary to treat EFM, but clonazepam and carbamazepine may reduce the movements clinically whereas they may be worsened by serotonergic agents (89).

Hypnagogic foot tremor

Hypnagogic foot tremor (HFT) and the related phenomenon alternating leg muscle activation (ALMA) represent further benign movement disorders commonly witnessed in subjects who are drowsy or in light sleep (1). Although often overlooked, regular dorsiflexion of either one foot or both feet in alternation with a frequency of 1–2 Hz may be seen as incidental findings in around 5% of polysomnograms, usually around the sleep–wake transition (1, 14). Rarely, these movements may disturb the bed partner, but usually they are viewed as somewhat curious or even amusing phenomena, potentially similar in nature to rhythmical movement disorders of sleep, simply requiring reassurance and no active treatment.

Key points

- Normal sleep is associated with changes in body position approximately every 15 minutes. Minor myoclonic movements of the face and extremities can also occur in any sleep stage.
- Periodic limb movements are frequently seen in the elderly, usually as incidental phenomena. They are also present in the vast majority of subjects with restless legs syndrome and appear to respond to the same drug treatment strategies. Dopaminergic agents are considered the first-line therapy if symptoms are severe and likely to be disturbing sleep continuity.
- Startling and unusual sensory phenomena may accompany sleep onset and cause insomnia, sometimes justifying short-acting hypnotic drug therapy.
- Head banging or body rocking when very drowsy and at the point of sleep onset is common in infancy and sometimes persists into adulthood, when it may occur during both non-REM and REM sleep stages. The rhythmical movements rarely disturb the subject but can adversely affect the bed partner's sleep continuity.
- Sleep bruxism is common and often overlooked. Apart from causing excessive tooth wear, it may fuel headache syndromes and disturb sleep maintenance. Dental occlusal devices are usually effective.

References

1. *International Classification of Sleep Disorders (Diagnostic and Coding Manual)* (2nd edn). Westchester, IL: American Academy of Sleep Medicine, 2005.
2. Ashkenazy JJM, Yahr MD. Parkinsonian tremor loses its alternating aspect during non-REM sleep and is inhibited by REM sleep. *J Neurol Neurosurg Psychiatry* 1990; 53: 749–53.
3. Fish DR, Sawyers D, Allen PJ, Blackie JD, Lees AJ, Marsden CD. The effect of sleep on the dyskinetic movements of Parkinson's disease, Gilles de la Tourette syndrome, Huntington's disease and torsion dystonia. *Arch Neurol* 1991; 48: 210–14.
4. Hurelbrink CB, Lewis SJ, Barker RA. The use of the Actiwatch–Neurologica system to objectively assess the involuntary movements and sleep–wake activity in patients with mild–moderate Huntington's disease. *J Neurol* 2005; 252: 642–7.
5. Glaze DG, Frost JD, Jr, Jankovic J. Sleep in Gilles de la Tourette syndrome: disorder of arousal. *Neurology* 1983; 33: 586–92.
6. Trenkwalder C, Paulus W. Restless legs syndrome: pathophysiology, clinical presentation and treatment. *Nat Rev Neurol* 2010; 6: 337–46.

7. Allen RP, Walters AS, Montplaisir J, et al. Restless legs syndrome prevalence and impact: REST general population study. *Arch Intern Med* 2005; 165: 1286–92.
8. Hening WA, Allen RP, Washburn M, Lesage SR, Earley CJ. The four diagnostic criteria for restless legs syndrome are unable to exclude confounding conditions ('mimics'). *Sleep Med* 2009; 10: 976–81.
9. Allen RP, Bharmal M, Calloway M. Prevalence and disease burden of primary restless legs syndrome: results of a general population survey in the United States. *Mov Disord* 2011; 26: 114–20.
10. Spiegelhalder K, Hornyak M. Restless legs syndrome in older adults. *Clin Geriatr Med* 2008; 24: 167–80.
11. Picchietti DL, Stevens HE. Early manifestations of restless legs syndrome in childhood and adolescence. *Sleep Med*; 9:770–81.
12. Xiong L, Montplaisir J, Desautels A, et al. Family study of restless legs syndrome in Quebec, Canada: clinical characterization of 671 familial cases. *Arch Neurol* 2010; 67: 617–22.
13. Walters AS, Rye DB. Review of the relationship of restless legs syndrome and periodic limb movements in sleep to hypertension, heart disease and stroke. *Sleep* 2009; 32: 589–97.
14. Iber C, Ancoli-Israel S, Chesson A, Quan SF, for the American Academy of Sleep Medicine. *The AASM manual for the scoring of sleep and associated events: rules, terminology and technical specifications.* Westchester, IL: American Academy of Sleep Medicine, 2007.
15. Nicolas A, Michaud M, Lavigne G, Montplaisir J. The influence of sex, age and sleep/wake state on the characteristics of periodic movements in RLS patients. *Clin Neurophysiol* 1999: 110; 1168–74.
16. Lugaresi E, Coccagna G, Mantovani M. Some periodic phenomena arising during drowsiness and sleep in man. *Electroencephalogr Clin Neurophysiol* 1972; 32: 701–5.
17. Parrino L, Boselli M, Buccino GP, Spaggiari MC, Di Giovanni G, Terzano MG. The cyclic alternating pattern plays a gate-control on periodic limb movements during non-rapid eye movement sleep. *J Clin Neurophysiol* 1996; 13: 14–23.
18. Lee MS, Choi YC, Lee SH, Lee SB. Sleep-related periodic leg movements associated with spinal cord lesions. *Mov Disord* 1996; 11: 719–22.
19. Smith RC. Relationship of periodic movements in sleep (nocturnal myoclonus) and the Babinski sign. *Sleep* 1985; 8: 239–43.
20. Fujiki A, Shimizu A, Yamada Y, Yamamoto A, Kaneko Z. The Babinski reflex during sleep and wakefulness. *Electroencephalogr Clin Neurophysiol* 1971; 31: 610–13.
21. Bara-Jiminex W, Asku M, Graham B, Sato S, Hallett M. Periodic limb movements in sleep: state-dependent excitability of the spinal flexor reflex. *Neurology* 2000; 54; 1609–16.
22. Sforza E, Nicolas A, Lavigne G, Gosselin A, Petit D, Montplaisir J. EEG and cardiac activation during periodic leg movements in sleep: support for a hierarchy of arousal responses. *Neurology* 1999; 52: 786–91.
23. Bliwise DL, Keenan S, Burnburg D, et al. Inter-rater reliability for scoring periodic limb movements in sleep. *Sleep* 1991; 14: 249–51.
24. Bliwise D, Petta D, Seidel W, Dement W. Periodic leg movements during sleep in the elderly. *Arch Gerontol Geriatr* 1985; 4: 273–81.
25. Mendelson WB. Are periodic leg movements associated with clinical sleep disturbance? *Sleep* 1996; 19: 219–23.
26. Ondo W, Jancovic J. Restless legs syndrome: clinicoetiologic correlates. *Neurology* 1996; 47: 1435–41.
27. Ondo WG, He Y, Rajasekaran S, Le WD. Clinical correlates of 6-hydroxydopamine injections into A11 dopaminergic neurons rats: a possible model for restless legs syndrome. *Mov Disord* 2000; 15: 154–8.
28. Allen RP, Earley CJ. The role of iron in restless legs syndrome. *Mov Disord* 2008; 22 (Suppl 18), S440–8.
29. Grote L, Leissner L, Hedner J, Ulfberg J. A randomized, double-blind, placebo controlled, multi-center study of intravenous iron sucrose and placebo in the treatment of restless legs syndrome. *Mov Disord* 2009; 24: 1445–52.
30. Turjanski N, Lees AJ, Brooks DJ. Striatal dopaminergic function in restless legs syndrome: ^{18}F-dopa and ^{11}C-raclopride PET studies. *Neurology* 1999; 52: 932–7.
31. Connor JR, Wang X, Patton SM, et al. Altered dopaminergic profile in the putamen and substantia nigra in restless legs syndrome. *Brain* 2009; 132: 2403–12.
32. Bianco LE, Unger EL, Earley CJ, Beard JL. Iron deficiency alters the day-night variation in monoamine levels in mice. *Chronobiol Int* 2009; 26: 447–63.
33. Earley CJ, Connor JR, Beard JL, Malecki EA, Epstein DK, Aleen RP. Abnormalities in CSF concentrations of ferritin and transferrin in restless legs syndrome. *Neurology* 2000; 54: 1698–700.
34. Mizuno S, Mihara T, Miyaoka T, Inagaki, T, Horiguchi J. CSF iron, ferritin and transferring levels in restless legs syndrome. *J Sleep Res* 2005; 14: 43–7.
35. Snyder AM, Wang X, Patton SM, et al. Mitochondrial ferritin in the substantia nigra in restless legs syndrome. *J Neuropathol Exp Neurol* 2009; 68: 1193–9.
36. Mignot E. A step forward for restless legs syndrome. *Nat Genet* 2007; 39: 938–9.
37. Stefansson H, Rye DB, Hicks A, et al. A genetic risk factor for periodic limb movements in sleep. *N Engl J Med* 2007; 357: 639–47.
38. O'Keeffe ST, Gavin K, Lavan JN. Iron status and restless legs syndrome in the elderly. *Age Ageing* 1994; 23: 200–3.
39. Trenkwalder C, Hening WA, Montagna P, et al. Treatment of restless legs syndrome: an evidence-based review and implications for clinical practice. *Mov Disord* 2008; 23: 2267–302.
40. Baldwin CB, Keating GM. Rotigotine transdermal patch: in restless legs syndrome. *CNS Drugs* 2008; 22: 797–806.
41. Cornelius JR, Tippmann-Peikert M, Slocumb NL, Frerichs CF, Silber MH. Impulse control disorders with the use of dopaminergic agents in restless legs syndrome: a case–control study. *Sleep* 2010; 33: 81–7.
42. Ondo WG. Methadone for refractory restless legs syndrome. *Mov Disord* 2005; 20: 345–8.
43. Tribl GG, Sycha T, Kotzailias N, Zeithofer J, Auff E. Apomorphine in idiopathic restless legs syndrome: an exploratory study. *J Neurol Neurosurg Psychiatry* 2005; 76: 181–5.
44. Earley CJ, Horska A, Mohamed MA, Barker PB, Beard JL, Allen RP. A randomized, double-blind, placebo-controlled trial of intravenous iron sucrose in restless legs syndrome. *Sleep Med* 2009; 10: 206–11.
45. Ondo WG. Intravenous iron dextran for severe refractory restless legs syndrome. *Sleep Med* 2010; 11: 494–6.
46. Leitner LS, Powers AS, Hoffman HS. The neural substrate of the startle response. *Physiol Behav* 1980; 25: 291–7.
47. Conigliari M, Quinto C, Masdeu J, Chokroverty S. An unusual presentation of hypnic jerks misdiagnosed as myoclonic seizure. *Neurology* 1999: 52 (Suppl 2): A80.
48. Sander HW, Geisse H, Quinto C, Sachdeo R, Chokroverty S. Sensory sleep starts. *J Neurol Neurosurg Psychiatry* 1998; 64: 690.
49. Montagna P. Physiologic body jerks and movements at sleep onset and during sleep. In: Chokroverty S, Hening W, Walters A (eds) *Sleep and movement disorders.* Boston, MA: Butterworth–Heinemann, 2003.
50. Lance JW. Transient sensations of impending loss of consciousness: the 'blip' syndrome. *J Neurol Neurosurg Psychiatry* 1996; 60: 437–8.
51. Brown P, Thompson PD, Marsden CD. Axial myoclonus of propriospinal origin. *Brain* 1991; 114: 197–214.
52. Montagna P, Provini F, Plazzi G, Liguori R, Lugaresi E. Propriospinal myoclonus upon relaxation and drowsiness: a cause of severe insomnia. *Mov Disord* 1997; 12: 66–72.
53. Vetrugno R, Provini F, Plazzi G, et al. Propriospinal myoclonus at the sleep–wake transition: a new type of parasomnia. *Sleep* 2001; 24: 835–43.
54. Schulze-Bonhage A, Knott H, Ferbert A. Pure stimulus sensitive truncal myoclonus of propriospinal origin. *Mov Disord* 1996; 11: 87–90.

55. Fouillet N, Wiart L, Arne P, Alaoui P, Petit H, Barat M. Propriospinal myoclonus in tetraplegic patients: clinical, electrophysiological and therapeutic aspects. *Paraplegia* 1995; 33: 678–81.
56. Roze E, Bounolleau P, Ducreux D, et al. Propriospinal myoclonus revisited: clinical, neurophysiologic and neuroradiologic findings. *Neurology* 2009; 72: 1301–9.
57. Vetrugno R, Provini F, Plazzi G, et al. Focal myoclonus and propriospinal propagation. *Clin Neurophysiol* 2000; 111: 2175–9.
58. Vetrugno R, Provini F, Plazzi G, Cortelli P, Montagna P. Propriospinal myoclonus: a motor phenomenon found in restless legs syndrome different from periodic limb movements during sleep. *Mov Disord* 2005; 20: 1323–9.
59. Kang SY, Sohn YH. Electromyography patterns of propriospinal myoclonus can be mimicked voluntarily. *Mov Disord* 2006; 21: 1241–4.
60. van der Salm SM, Koelman JH, Henneke S, van Rootselaar AF, Tijssen MA. Axial jerks: a clinical spectrum ranging from propriospinal to psychogenic myoclonus. *J Neurol* 2010; 257: 1349–55.
61. Davies L, King PJ, Leicester J, Morris JG. Recumbent tic. *Mov Disord* 1992; 7: 359–63.
62. Kapoor R, Brown P, Thompson PD, Miller DH. Propriospinal myoclonus in multiple sclerosis. *J Neurol Neurosurg Psychiatry* 1992; 55: 1086–8.
63. Maltête D, Verdure P, Roze E, et al. TENS for the treatment of propriospinal myoclonus. *Mov Disord* 2008; 23: 2256–7.
64. Stepanova I, Nevsimalova S, Hanosova J. Rhythmic movement disorder in sleep persisting into childhood and adulthood. *Sleep* 2005; 28: 851–7.
65. Manni R, Terzhaghi M, Sartori I, Veggiotti P, Parrino L. Rhythmic movement disorder and cyclic alternating pattern during sleep: a video-polysomnographic study in a 9-year old boy. *Mov Disord* 2004; 19: 1186–90.
66. Gagnon P, Koninck J. Repetitive head movements during REM sleep. *Biol Psychiatry* 1985; 20: 176–8.
67. Anderson KN, Smith IE, Shneerson JM. Rhythmic movement disorder (head banging) in an adult during rapid eye movement sleep. *Mov Disord* 2006; 21: 866–7.
68. Hoban TF. Sleep-related rhythmic movement disorder. In: Thorpy MJ, Plazzi G (eds) *The parasomnias and other sleep-related movement disorders*. Cambridge: Cambridge University Press, 2010.
69. Sallustro F, Atwell CW. Body rocking, head banging and head rolling in normal children. *J Paediatr* 1978; 93: 704–8.
70. Laberge L, Tremblay RE, Vitaro F, Montplaisir J. Development of parasomnias from childhood to early adolescence. *Pediatrics* 2000; 106: 67–74.
71. Simonds JF, Parraga H. Sleep behaviours and disorders in children and adolescents evaluated at psychiatric clinics. *J Dev Behav Pediatr* 1984; 5: 6–10.
72. Chisholm T, Morehouse RL. Adult headbanging: sleep studies and treatment. *Sleep* 1996; 19: 343–6.
73. Thorpy MJ, Glovinsky PB. Parasomnias. *Psychiatr Clin North Am* 1987; 10: 623–39.
74. Manni R, Tartara A. Clonazepam treatment of rhythmic movement disorder. *Sleep* 1997; 20: 812.
75. Rosenberg C. Elimination of a rhythmic movement disorder with hypnosis—a case report. *Sleep* 1995; 18: 608–9.
76. Wills L, Garcia J. Parasomnias: epidemiology and treatment. *CNS Drugs* 2002; 16: 803–10.
77. Lavigne GJ, Rompré PH, Poirier G, Huard H, Kato T, Montplaisir JY. Rhythmic masticatory muscle activity during sleep in humans. *J Dent Res* 2001; 80: 443–8.
78. Ohayon MM, Li KK, Guilleminault C. Risk factors for bruxism in the general population. *Chest* 2001; 119: 53–61.
79. Vendrame M, Kaleyias J, Valencia I, Legido A, Kothare SV. Polysomnographic findings in children with headaches. *Pediatr Neurol* 2008; 39: 6–11.
80. Winocur E, Gavish A, Voikovitch M, Emodi-Perlman A, Eli I. Drugs and bruxism: a critical review. *J Orofac Pain* 2003; 17: 99–111.
81. Louis ED, Tampone E. Bruxism in Huntington's disease. *Mov Disord* 2001; 16: 785–6.
82. Kato T, Rompre P, Montplaisir JY, Sessle BJ, Lavign GJ. Sleep bruxism: an oromotor activity secondary to micro-arousal. *J Dent Res* 2001; 80: 1940–4.
83. Restrepo CC, Vasquez LM, Alvarez M, Valencia I. Personality traits and temporomandibular disorders in a group of children with bruxing behaviour. *J Oral Rehabil* 2008; 35: 585–93.
84. Dutra KM, Pereira FJ, Jr, Rompré PH, Huynh N, Fleming N, Lavign GJ. Oro-facial activities in sleep bruxism patients and in normal patients: a controlled polysomnographic and audio–video study. *J Oral Rehabil* 2009; 36: 86–92.
85. Landry ML, Rompré PH, Manzini C, Guitard F, de Grandmont P, Lavigne GJ. Reduction of sleep bruxism using a mandibular advancement device: an experimental controlled study. *Int J Prosthodont* 2006; 19: 549–56.
86. Huynh N, Rompré PH, Montplaisir J, Lavign GJ. Comparison of various treatments for sleep bruxism using determinants of number needed to treat and effect size. *Int J Prosthodont* 2006; 19: 435–41.
87. Huynh N, Lavigne GJ, Lanfranchi P, Montplaisir J, de Champlain J. The effect of two sympatholytic medications, propranolol and clonidine, on sleep bruxism: experimental randomized controlled trials. *Sleep* 2006; 29: 295–304.
88. Lins O, Castonquay M, Dunham W, Nevsimalova S, Broughton R. Excessive fragmentary myoclonus: time of night and sleep stage distributions. *Can J Neurol Sci* 1993; 20: 142–6.
89. Jordan LM, Liu J, Hedlund PB, Akay T, Pearson KG. Descending command systems for the initiation of locomotion in mammals. *Brain Res Rev* 2008; 57: 183–91.

CHAPTER 31

Psychogenic Movement Disorders

Isabel Pareés and Mark J. Edwards

Introduction

Psychogenic movement disorders (PMDs) are one presentation of 'functional' neurological symptoms, one of the most common diagnoses made in neurological practice. Patients can present with tremor, fixed postures of the limbs, jerks, slowness, or other combinations of abnormal movements which are incongruous with movement disorders that occur in neurological disease. The terms used to describe these patients range from the general (functional, hysteria) to those that propose a psychological aetiology (psychogenic, psychosomatic, conversion disorder, somatization disorder) and those that indicate what patients do not have (non-organic, medically unexplained). This varied terminology highlights a lack of consensus and understanding of underlying mechanisms. Recently, there has been a shift away from pure psychodynamic explanations of PMD and other functional disorders towards the implementation of more neurobiological models. This chapter covers the current state of knowledge regarding diagnosis, pathophysiology, and management of these patients. Because of the widespread use of the term 'psychogenic' to describe these patients within medical literature we will use this term here, but in doing so we reject the assumption that PMD and other functional disorders are proved to be caused by underlying psychological trauma.

Epidemiology

The true prevalence of PMD is not certain as there is a lack of consensus on diagnostic criteria and different methodologies have been used to ascertain cases. The reported estimates of prevalence of PMD range from 1 to 9% of general neurological clinic referrals (1–3). The frequency in adult movement disorders clinics ranges from 2 to 4%, and is up to 20% in more specialized clinics (4).

The mean age at onset described in larger case series is between 37 and 50 years (5), and in about 70% of the cases patients present with tremor or dystonia. PMDs are more common in women, except for parkinsonism for which both sexes are equally predisposed (6, 7).

PMDs usually occur as a single neurological diagnosis, but can be associated with co-existent organic neurological disorders in 10–15% of patients (8). Children can also develop PMDs, with gait disorder and tremor the most commonly seen. In a series of children with PMDs the average age at onset was 12.3 years, with a clear female predominance (80%) (9). PMDs are only rarely reported in those aged over 65.

Diagnosis and phenomenology

As with other functional neurological disorders, there has been a shift in diagnostic practice away from considering the diagnosis of PMD as a diagnosis of exclusion, towards the use of positive diagnostic criteria. In addition, there has been a rejection amongst movement disorder specialists of the requirement for a co-existent psychological disorder or trauma to be present in order to make the diagnosis (10). Therefore, while psychiatric diagnoses such as conversion disorder require the presence of a psychological triggering event, most movement disorder neurologists state that they make the diagnosis on positive clinical signs (see below) and incongruity with movement disorders known to be due to neurological disease. One reason for this shift is that psychological disturbance is a common counterpart to organic neurological disease (and indeed is common in the general population) and therefore it is not reliable as a predictor of PMD. Secondly, epidemiological work in PMD (and in other functional neurological disorders) has shown a surprising similarity in numbers of life events and psychiatric disorder in most patients compared with control populations (11, 12).

General clues from history and examination

There are some general clues from history and examination which can help point to the presence of a PMD. It is important to note that none of these features are entirely specific for PMDs and diagnosis should not be based on these features alone. PMDs are often of sudden onset with rapid progression to maximum severity and they may have a pattern of spontaneous remissions, paroxysmal exacerbations, and relapses. Patients may experience a shift in phenomenology over time (tremor turning to abnormal posture, for example), and may have a history of previous unexplained medical symptoms.

General clues on clinical examination include the co-existence of other psychogenic signs such as 'give-way' weakness, 'false' weakness (e.g. positive Hoover's sign), or non-physiological patterns of sensory loss on clinical examination.

Psychogenic tremor

Psychogenic tremor (PT) is the most common form of PMD (3, 5). Patients typically have a combination of rest, postural, and intention tremor. Arm tremor is overwhelmingly the most common manifestation of PT, usually sparing the fingers, but isolated tremor of other body parts (legs, head, palate) can also be seen. The onset of the tremor is abrupt in a large number of patients, often following a physical injury (13).

A range of clinical tests, supplemented by tremor recordings using accelerometry and EMG, has been suggested to be helpful in distinguishing PT from organic tremor. These techniques generally rely on distracting the patient's attention away from the tremor. This usually makes organic tremor worse, but in PT tends to cause it to stop or significantly change in frequency.

A range of distraction tasks has been assessed, including cognitive distracters (serial subtraction), tapping with an unaffected limb at a different frequency to the tremor, and making a sudden ballistic movement with the other hand. With clinical assessment alone (without supplementation with tremor recordings), tapping tasks are most sensitive and specific for distinguishing essential tremor from PT. Self-paced cognitive tasks are not very effective. Using tremor recordings, tapping tasks have again been shown to be helpful in distinguishing PT from organic tremors (14). Here, patients with PT may 'entrain' to the tapping frequency, may show a shift in tremor frequency towards the tapping frequency, or may instead be inexplicably unable to perform the tapping task correctly with their normal hand. This illustrates an important point with distraction tasks which is that performance of the task must be adequate to draw attention away from the tremoring limb. This is probably why self-paced tasks (whether cognitive or motor) are not good at discriminating patients with PT from organic tremor. Ballistic movements of the non-tremoring limb cause a small pause in the tremor in patients with PT (15). Additional electrophysiological characteristics include a paradoxical worsening of the tremor with loading (which typically damps organic tremor), and co-contraction at the onset of tremor.

Recently these tests have been compared head to head in a group of patients with PT and a mixed group of patients with organic tremors (PD, dystonic tremor, essential tremor, neuropathic tremor) (16). No single test was found to be of sufficient sensitivity and specificity to distinguish PT from organic tremor, most probably reflecting different mechanisms in different patients for generating the tremor. For example, tremors generated by co-contraction were much more resistant to distraction. The authors calculated a cut-off score from a group of tests which could effectively distinguish PT from organic tremor, but this requires confirmation in a prospective study (Table 31.1).

Table 31.1 Summary score of a battery of electrophysiological tests for the diagnosis of psychogenic tremor (16)

Electrophysiological test	Points
Incorrect tapping performance at:	
◆ 1 Hz	1
◆ 3 Hz	1
◆ 5 Hz	1
Entrainment, suppression, or pathological frequency shift at:	
◆ 1 Hz	1
◆ 3 Hz	1
◆ 5 Hz	1
Pause or 50% reduction in amplitude of tremor with ballistic movements	1
Tonic activation before tremor onset	1
Coherence of bilateral tremors	1
Increase of TP (as surrogate of tremor amplitude)	1
Cut-off score for psychogenic tremor: ≥3 points	

TP, total power of the spectra between 1 and 30 Hz

Psychogenic dystonia

The concept of psychogenic dystonia classically refers to patients with fixed abnormal postures of the limb that typically are triggered by apparently minor injury. There is considerable disagreement and debate about the nature of fixed dystonia, and whether it should be classified as a PMD or a form of organic movement disorder. Almost two decades after Bhatia and colleagues concluded that 'at present it is impossible to decide whether this distressing syndrome is a true functional disorder of the CNS, or is of psychogenic origin' (17), the concept of fixed dystonia is in transition towards a more integrated view of brain dysfunction beyond the dualistic vision of this disorder (18).

Psychogenic dystonia affects predominantly the limbs, and rarely the neck–shoulder region or jaw (19). Psychogenic blepharospasm has recently been reported (20). Patients are typically female and in their twenties and thirties.

Psychogenic dystonia is typically fixed, while organic dystonia tends to produce mobile abnormal postures. Fixed postures can be seen in certain organic disorders such as corticobasal degeneration or dystonia due to basal ganglia lesions, but additional clinical signs and abnormal neuroimaging tests help to make the correct diagnosis in these cases. Less commonly, patients with psychogenic dystonia can present with non-fixed postures of the limbs, trunk, and neck.

Psychogenic dystonia usually has a clear precipitating factor (typically a peripheral injury) and an abrupt onset. Patients with fixed dystonia commonly have pain as a major feature of the disorder, overlapping with chronic regional pain syndrome type 1 (21). The role of psychological factors underlying dystonia complicating chronic regional pain syndrome remains a source of considerable controversy.

An unusual distribution of dystonia given the age of onset can be a further clue that points toward psychogenic dystonia. Primary dystonia has a very typical anatomical distribution which depends on age of onset: generalized (with classic limb onset) in individuals younger than 25 years, focal involving upper limb in individuals aged between 25 and 45 years, and focal involving the craniocervical area in individuals aged more than 45–50 years. Importantly, unusual distribution given the age of onset can also be a clue to secondary/neurodegenerative dystonia and these disorders should be ruled out. In psychogenic dystonia there is typically an absence of task/position specificity commonly seen in organic dystonia and patients often do not have sensory tricks. Some patients do develop limb contractures, demonstrating maintenance of postures even when unobserved.

It can be difficult to demonstrate distractibility of postures in fixed dystonia. This may be because, in contrast with psychogenic tremor, maintenance of postures does not require significant attentional resources, although critics of the suggestion that these patients have a psychogenic origin of dystonia could equally argue that distractibility is not seen as the condition is not psychogenic. However, in some patients rhythmic movements of another limb performed while manipulating the fixed limb can reveal some 'giving way' of the fixed posture.

It has recently been reported that some patients with fixed dystonia can respond immediately (within minutes) and dramatically to botulinum toxin injections (22). This is in contrast with the known physiological effects of botulinum toxin which usually take 36–72 hours to become apparent. Therefore the response seen in these patients is likely to be due to a placebo effect and helps to confirm that such patients are different from those with typical organic dystonia.

Psychogenic myoclonus

Up to 10% of patients with myoclonus have been reported to have a psychogenic aetiology (23, 24). Psychogenic myoclonus can be challenging to differentiate from organic myoclonus as it is difficult to convincingly demonstrate distractibility in patients with intermittent movements. Variability in the distribution of jerks from day to day, distractibility (in those with very frequent jerks), unusual triggering of jerks, excessive startle response, or response to suggestion can suggest a psychogenic origin. Electrophysiological tests can be particularly helpful in supporting the clinical diagnosis. Simple recording of the duration of the jerks can be of benefit, particularly to demonstrate variability in duration and recruitment pattern of EMG bursts, suggestive of a non-organic cause. Consistent bursts of duration less than 75 ms are unlikely to be psychogenic, as EMG bursts of this duration cannot be generated voluntarily. However, the converse is not true, as some forms of organic myoclonus (e.g. brainstem myoclonus, spinal segmental myoclonus) may have EMG burst lengths longer than 75ms. If jerks are stimulus sensitive and the latency between the stimulus and the jerk is within the range of voluntary reaction time (>150ms), this supports the diagnosis of psychogenic myoclonus. A cortical spike 20 ms before the jerk and/or the presence of a giant somatosensory evoked potential would not be expected in psychogenic myoclonus. The most definitive test to confirm the psychogenic origin of the myoclonus is detection of the readiness potential or *Bereitschaftspotential* (BP). This slowly rising EEG potential starts around 1.5 seconds before voluntary self-paced movement, and reflects activity in brain areas associated with movement preparation (25). This potential can be recorded in patients with psychogenic myoclonus, but has never been reported in patients with organic myoclonus. It requires a number of jerks to be recorded and averaged (usually at least 30), so is not suitable for those with very infrequent jerks. Those with jerks more than every 4–5 seconds are also unsuitable for recording. A recent study of the presence of BP preceding abnormal movements demonstrated that the clinical diagnosis of organic spinal myoclonus made by movement disorders experts is commonly incorrect, as many of them were preceded by a BP (26). This study and an independent study confirmed that most patients carrying a diagnosis of idiopathic spinal myoclonus or propriospinal myoclonus were best classified as psychogenic (27).

Psychogenic parkinsonism

Psychogenic parkinsonism (PP) is relatively rare, accounting for 10% of cases of PMD (28). The diagnosis is not always easy, and a detailed clinical history and physical examination looking for positive clinical signs of psychogenicity is required. All features of parkinsonism can be present. In a series of nine patients, seven had a predominant tremor form and only two had an akinetic-rigid form (29). This indicates that 'true' psychogenic parkinsonism, rather than people who have psychogenic rest tremor, is probably very rare. In such patients, rigidity may be present but feels similar to voluntary oppositional resistance against passive movements rather than true cogwheel rigidity. Movements may appear to be very effortful and slow, but true bradykinesia with decrementing amplitude with rapid repetitive movements is not seen. When patients with PP are distracted, the velocity of the movements can normalize. Postural stability testing may lead to dramatic loss of balance and falls. Speech often becomes stuttering or 'baby-like', or is produced with an unusual accent. Handwriting is laboured and irregular, but without typical micrographia (6). It is important to recognize that placebo response can be quite sizeable in patients with organic Parkinson's disease where it is associated with dopamine release (30), so caution needs to be taken in interpreting response to placebo in patients with suspected PP. Dopamine transporter (DAT) SPECT scanning is a useful test for investigating the integrity of the nigrostriatal system and discriminating PP from PD. This test will be abnormal in patients with organic PD and normal in PP. It is important to emphasize that normal DAT scans are also seen in patients with organic postsynaptic causes for parkinsonism, such as drug-induced parkinsonism. It has been suggested that some patients with PP may have underlying organic PD (28, 29, 31). Again, positive clinical signs rather than imaging studies are essential to make the correct diagnosis.

Psychogenic gait disorder

Psychogenic disorders of posture and gait are common, and are the major manifestation in 8–10% of patients with psychogenic movement disorders (32). Abnormal gait can be an isolated phenomenon in patients with PMD or mixed with other clinical manifestations. In the largest series reported (33) the proportion of pure psychogenic gait disorder was 5.7% of PMD, and this increased to 42.3% when the mixed type was included. Clinical descriptions date back to the nineteenth century. Paul Blocq was the first to use the term astasia–abasia. In this manifestation of psychogenic gait disturbance, patients veer from side to side when walking, often waving the arms at the same time. They seem continuously about to lose their balance, but tend not to. This ability to shift the centre of gravity from one side to the other without losing balance is a demonstration of good balance in contrast with the patient's subjective report of poor balance. Other features of psychogenic gait disorders include narrow base, hesitation, dramatic response to Romberg's test and tests of postural stability, 'uneconomic' postures, or excessive slowness. Because patterns of gait can be rather unusual in some organic disorders (e.g. Huntington's disease, generalized dystonia), considerable clinical experience in both psychogenic and organic disorders can be required to make a clear diagnosis.

Other PMDs: psychogenic chorea, tics, and paroxysmal movement disorders

Psychogenic chorea is extremely rare. So far, only two patients have been reported, one of them with a family history of Huntington's disease (34). Here, clues to the diagnosis were normal saccadic eye movements, absence of motor impersistence, and a marked decrease in chorea when the patient was distracted during performance of voluntary repetitive movements.

Psychogenic tics are also rarely described. Surprisingly, in a series of patients with tics reported by Mejia and Jankovic (35), 16 out of 155 (10.3%) were considered to have psychogenic tics (35). The rather high frequency of psychogenic tics in this sample was subsequently questioned. It was argued that the criteria used to give the diagnosis of psychogenicity in these patients was not specified and that typical indicators of PMD, such as abrupt onset, response to placebo or suggestion, or increase with attention and cessation with distraction, may not help to differentiate organic from psychogenic tics as organic tics may also begin abruptly and be under some voluntary control, and intensity can vary with attention. This highlighted the need for well-defined criteria to characterize psychogenic tics.

A 'paroxysmal' component to the disorder is an important clue that the disorder may be psychogenic, but 'pure' psychogenic paroxysmal disorders have rarely been mentioned in the literature (3). As organic paroxysmal disorders such as paroxysmal kinesigenic dyskinesia, paroxysmal non-kinesigenic dyskinesia, and paroxysmal exercise-induced dyskinesia, or even focal seizures, are by definition brief and reversible, the clinical diagnosis can be very difficult. However, organic counterparts have typical precipitating factors and the length of the attacks is also well defined for each type; therefore incongruous features can raise suspicion of a psychogenic basis. It is of great importance to see an attack (e.g. by getting the patient to video an episode). Often, EEG and video-recording of the attack are important in reaching the diagnosis.

Diagnostic criteria

Diagnostic criteria have been developed to operationalize diagnosis of PMDs. The most widely used criteria, developed by Fahn and Williams (36), divide PMDs into four categories of diagnostic certainty: documented, clinically established, probable, and possible. In fact, these criteria were first developed for psychogenic dystonia alone, but were later expanded to cover all PMDs. Gupta and Lang (37) have suggested revisions to these criteria (Table 31.2) which delete the 'possible' category as being not sufficiently specific for PMDs, and also seek to introduce the

Table 31.2 Diagnostic classification of psychogenic movement disorders

	Fahn and Williams (36)	Gupta and Lang (37)
Documented	Persistent relief by psychotherapy, suggestion, or placebo has been demonstrated, which may be helped by physiotherapy, or the patient was seen without the movement disorder when believing him/herself unobserved	Persistent relief by psychotherapy, suggestion, or placebo has been demonstrated, which may be helped by physiotherapy, or the patient was seen without the movement disorder when believing him/herself unobserved[1]
Clinically established	The movement disorder is incongruent/inconsistent with typical movement disorder plus at least one of the following three: ◆ other psychogenic signs ◆ multiple somatizations ◆ obvious psychiatric disturbance	Plus other features: the movement disorder is incongruent/inconsistent with typical movement disorder plus at least one of the following three*: ◆ other psychogenic signs ◆ multiple somatizations ◆ obvious psychiatric disturbance Minus other features: the movement disorder is incongruent/inconsistent with typical movement disorder without any other features*
Probable**	◆ The movement disorder is incongruent/inconsistent with typical movement disorder ◆ The movement disorder is congruent/consistent and there are psychogenic signs ◆ The movement disorder is congruent/consistent and there are multiple somatizations	
Possible***	◆ The movement disorder is congruent/consistent and there is evidence of an emotional disturbance	◆ The movement disorder is congruent/consistent and there are psychogenic signs ◆ The movement disorder is congruent/consistent and there are multiple somatizations ◆ The movement disorder is congruent/consistent and there is evidence of an emotional disturbance
Laboratory-supported definite		◆ Electrophysiological evidence proving a psychogenic movement disorder (primarily in cases of psychogenic tremor and psychogenic myoclonus)

*According to the Gupta and Lang proposal, the 'documented' and 'clinically established' 'plus or minus other features' categories can be grouped under the term 'clinically definite'.

**Gupta and Lang propose reclassifying patients in the 'probable' category according to the Fahn and Williams classification, under 'clinically established' (those with incongruent/inconsistent movement disorders) or 'possible' (those with congruent/consistent movement disorders).

***Gupta and Lang also questioned the utility of retaining the 'possible' category as this generally represents patients with organic movement disorders with additional psychiatric problems rather than a true 'possible psychogenic movement disorder'.

concept of a laboratory-supported level of certainty, for example using recordings of pre-movement potentials in psychogenic myoclonus. Shill and Gerber (38) proposed alternative criteria, but these have been criticized for relying so heavily on historical factors such as 'disease modelling' that it is possible to make a diagnosis of PMD without reference to the movement disorder phenomenology.

Recently, these criteria have been assessed with regard to inter-rater reliability, and have been found to demonstrate moderate to poor reliability for the probable and possible categories. This work suggests that new criteria, which perhaps include more specific direction as to the positive physical signs that predict PMDs rather than the unspecified 'incongruency' with organic movement disorders, might improve reliability.

Pathophysiology

We have already discussed how the movements that occur as part of PMDs are quantifiably different from those seen in organic movement disorders mainly by virtue of the fact that they resemble movements that are made voluntarily. This leads naturally to two logical possibilities. Either movements are deliberately feigned by patients, or there must be another process by which movements that appear voluntary are not experienced as such by patients.

It is generally acknowledged to be very difficult to distinguish malingering from 'true' psychogenic movement disorder, but the consensus of opinion is that malingering is likely to be rare and is not a satisfying explanation for the disorder in the majority of patients with PMDs (and indeed other functional disorders). This opinion is given some limited but important support from functional imaging studies in functional paralysis, where patterns of brain activation in patients attempting to move their apparently paralysed leg are different from those in subjects feigning paralysis (39, 40). This does not amount to proof that these patients are not malingering, but it is at least supportive evidence.

The current categorization of functional symptoms found in the Diagnostic and Statistical Manual of Mental Disorders (DSM-IV TR) reflects influential psychologically based models to explain pathophysiology of functional symptoms. It recognizes three diagnostic groups: somatoform disorders, conversion disorder, and dissociative disorder. Somatoform disorders are those where somatic complaints such as pain and fatigue are present with no clear physical cause, and encompass somatization disorder (Briquet's syndrome), where there is a history of multiple physical complaints including pain affecting at least four different parts or functions of the body, at least two gastrointestinal symptoms, at least one sexual or reproductive symptom, and at least one symptom that mimics a neurological condition. Conversion disorder is defined as occurring when patients present with one or more symptoms affecting movement or senses that cannot be explained by a physical cause and is preceded by conflicts or stressors in the patient's life. Dissociative disorders are those where there is a specific abnormality of memory, perception, or identity which cannot be explained by a physical cause.

This current tripartite classification system is underpinned by three partially overlapping theoretical approaches to functional symptoms. The category of somatoform disorders is based heavily on Briquet's original description of chronically affected polysymptomatic patients, and perhaps also Briquet's original theory that the disorder arose from a malfunction in the part of the brain receiving and interpreting sensory and affective information. More modern conceptions of somatoform disorders have tended to focus on the way in which normal physiological sensory input might be misinterpreted by an individual as pathological and signifying illness (41). Models, such as that proposed by Kirmayer and Taillefer (41), propose an interaction between somatic sensations (normal physiological experiences, those induced by emotional arousal, sensations arising from organic physical illness), pre-existing personality, previous illness experience, and societal factors that enhance the secondary gain of the sick role (disability benefits, social response of others to illness) (41). The fundamental neurobiological process that underpins this model is excessive attention that is directed towards the triggering somatic sensations which amplifies them and maintains the patient's abnormal (enhanced) perception of these sensations. These are then reported by the patient as symptoms (e.g. pain).

The category of conversion disorder is based on the concept introduced by Breuer and Freud between 1893 and 1895, and later extended by Freud alone. Here, the role of a psychological stressor is paramount. This stressor is proposed to set off a defensive reaction of suppressing (or repressing) the memory of this stressor. While this may relieve the distress associated with the stressor, Breuer and Freud proposed that the 'psychic energy' displaced from its proper place by this process is 'converted' into a somatic symptom which may bear some symbolic association with the original stressor (42). This somatic symptom is unconscious as the source of the energetic displacement is repressed and the process occurs outside awareness. Although the energy displacement mechanism proposed by Freud has been discarded, the idea that functional symptoms relate to a conversion of psychological distress retains considerable popularity.

The category of dissociative disorder is based on another nineteenth century formulation to explain functional symptoms proposed by Janet (43). Here, in individuals with a pathologically weak mental state, psychological stressors were proposed to lead to a narrowing of attentional focus and a resulting disregard of certain sensory input. This provided an explanation for hysterical sensory loss, a symptom which both Janet and Charcot proposed as being an essential clinical feature of hysteria. The attentional dysfunction proposed by this theory has continued to influence more modern models of functional symptoms. These modern theories have rejected the concept that dissociation only occurs in those with pre-existing 'mental weakness', but have instead conceptualized it as a normal phenomenon that becomes disrupted in those with functional symptoms. Thus dissociation is a normal and advantageous mode of cognitive processing that allows intentional activity to continue in an automatic non-attended fashion while attentional resources are directed elsewhere. However, in pathological states (hypnosis, functional symptoms), certain patterns of automatic activity (e.g. inhibition of limb movement) can be triggered unconsciously, and therefore are experienced by the person as outside their control.

The logical position taken by all of these theories is that patients are unaware of the way symptoms are produced (i.e. they are not feigning) as the locus of symptom production is at a low level within the nervous system. For somatoform disorders, this is the amplification of bottom-up sensory input. For conversion disorder, this is the inhibition of primary motor or sensory areas. In dissociative disorders, this is the 'automatic' activation of pre-established patterns of motor or sensory activity. In all these models, functional symptoms have a bottom-up *cause* but no top-down *purpose*, leading to symptoms that are experienced as involuntary and 'unwilled'. This contrasts directly with symptoms produced by feigning/malingering which involve top-down *purposes*, but no bottom-up *cause*, and as a result should be experienced by the individual as deliberate willed acts.

There are difficulties with all these approaches. First, the expected high rates of psychological trauma in patients with functional symptoms, including PMD, are not found in controlled studies (11). One explanation for this is that memory for such traumatic events is repressed, and therefore is not available for conscious report, but the circularity of this argument makes it difficult to test experimentally. Secondly, the characteristics of the physical symptoms in patients with functional disorders, including PMD, that differentiate them from patients with organic disorders suggest a high-level or 'top-down' process. Movement impairments disappear when attention is drawn away from them, and they often fit with beliefs about illness rather than physiological reality (e.g. patients who report tubular visual field defects which break the laws of optics). Most of the theories discussed above suggest that an 'emotional' area of the brain inhibits or disrupts a low-level motor or sensory brain region, producing a symptom which is not accessible to conscious control. Why then should such symptoms require attention to manifest and conform to high-level beliefs?

Functional imaging seems a natural method with which to approach the pathophysiology of these disorders, and recent studies in patients with PMD provide some interesting data. Voon and colleagues (44) have demonstrated abnormal connectivity between the amygdala and supplementary motor area in patients with PMD when shown emotionally arousing images, suggesting a link between emotional processing and an area involved in motor planning/preparation. The same group has also shown a relative decline in activation of the right inferior parietal lobule in patients with psychogenic tremor by comparing activation patterns while they were tremoring and when they were voluntarily producing tremor (45). This area is important in making comparisons between expected and perceived sensory data, and the authors suggest that its underactivation during psychogenic tremor would help generate a mismatch between expected and perceived sensory data, leading to a perception of lack of agency for the movement. On the same theme, Edwards and colleagues (46) have shown impairment in the normal timing of the sense of intention when making a voluntary movement in patients with PMDs compared with controls.

In a recent study, patients with psychogenic tremor and with organic tremor were given an actigraphy device to wear, similar in size to a wristwatch, capable of continuously monitoring tremor for days, and at the same time they were asked to fill out diaries indicating how much of the day they perceived they had tremor (47). Both patient groups overestimated the amount of time they had tremor as measured by actigraphy, but the psychogenic tremor group did so to a much greater extent. Indeed, this group had on average only 4% of the day with tremor measured by the actigraph, compared with diary ratings indicating that they perceived tremor to be present for 84% of the day. The subjects were all explicitly informed of the purpose of the study, and therefore these results do not support the suggestion that these patients are malingering. Instead, it suggests that an important component of belief or expectation about symptoms is driving perception of symptom severity. The interaction between expectations (or prior predictions) about sensory data and the sensory data actually received is central to modern Bayesian theories of brain function (48). These data fit within that framework, and may provide a novel direction for future pathophysiological work.

Unfortunately, this discussion of the pathophysiology of PMDs does not provide a clear answer to the origins of these perplexing symptoms, but it does highlight the deficiencies of purely psychodynamic explanations for symptoms, and the need for any theory to be implemented neurobiologically within known brain structures and mechanisms.

Treatment

PMD treatment begins with an effective communication of the diagnosis to the patient. The previous discussion regarding the absence of triggering life events in many patients may provide an explanation for the incredulity (and sometimes hostility) that patients may demonstrate when receiving a diagnostic explanation for their physical symptoms that is based on psychological factors. A more general explanation which does not ignore psychological factors, but acknowledges the physical triggering factors present in many patients, is often more successful. The benefit of simply explaining the diagnosis, at least in the early stages, has been found to lead to long-term resolution of symptoms in patients with psychogenic disorders in general (49). As the outcome for patients with PMDs worsens with delayed diagnosis and treatment, a therapeutic strategy should be planned immediately after giving the diagnosis.

Most treatments used in patients with organic movement disorders are not effective in patients with PMDs, and iatrogenic damage can occur through use of unnecessary medications and interventions. Unfortunately, there is little controlled trial data to guide treatment in PMDs, but the limited evidence that is available suggests that a multidisciplinary approach gives the best chance of benefit.

Psychological intervention can be helpful in patients who consider psychological factors to be relevant in symptom development or maintenance. In patients with clear psychological stressors but who are reluctant to engage with this strategy, explaining that cognitive techniques are commonly used in medicine to help to control physical symptoms (e.g. modern management of chronic pain) may encourage them to try this approach. Hinson and colleagues (50) conducted a single-blinded clinical trial in 10 patients with PMDs in which the patients received 12 one-hour sessions per week of psychodynamic psychotherapy. Patients also received antidepressants or anxiolytics as indicated. Means for the PMDs rating scale, function scores, Hamilton depression scores, and Beck anxiety scores all improved. A recent large controlled study assessed whether adding input from a guided self-help workbook based on cognitive–behavioural therapy (CBT) to the usual care received by patients with psychogenic disorders improved outcomes (51). Patients receiving CBT-based guided and usual care reported greater improvement in presenting symptoms and physical function than patients receiving usual care alone. In a prospective treatment trial of PMDs with antidepressants, 15 patients with PMDs were treated with citalopram or paroxetine (52). Those who did not respond after 4 weeks of taking an optimal dose were switched to venlafaxine. Significant improvements were found only in patients with 'primary conversion symptoms' and recent or current depressive or anxiety disorder, and not in those with a diagnosis of somatization disorder.

Rehabilitation with physiotherapy and occupational therapy has face validity as a technique to treat motor symptoms and is likely to be acceptable to more patients than psychotherapeutic treatments. Physical rehabilitation may improve outcome in PMD in combination with psychotherapy (19), but controlled studies are lacking. Preliminary evidence for regular low- to medium-intensity walking exercise, which is known to be effective in the treatment of depression or anxiety, has been investigated in a single-blind study of 16 patients with PMDs (53). After a 12-week programme, 62% of the enrolled patients showed a marked improvement (mean improvement of 70% in total score in the Psychogenic Movement Disorder Rating scale compared with baseline) with no adverse effects in any participant.

There is continued debate concerning the use of suggestion and placebo as a treatment strategy for PMDs. The traditional objection to its use is that it erodes patient autonomy and the doctor–patient relationship. However, an informal survey of participants at the Second International Conference on Psychogenic Movement Disorders in April 2009 found that over 50% of the experts present had witnessed the beneficial effects of suggestion in patients with PMDs (54). No long-term controlled studies with placebo have been reported to date.

Additional treatments have been suggested to be effective in PMD. For example, intrathecal baclofen was reported to be effective in fixed dystonia compared with placebo (55). However, placebo control was only used for the initial test dose of intrathecal baclofen, and it is not known whether there was systematic unblinding of the participant by systematic effects of the baclofen. Low-frequency repetitive transcranial magnetic stimulation (TMS) achieved symptom relief in 11 patients with psychogenic tremor. Thirty TMS pulses were applied over the hand area of the primary motor cortex contralateral to the affected hand (15 pulses at a rate of 0.2 Hz and intensities of 120% and 140% of the resting motor threshold, respectively). All patients experienced a significant reduction of their symptoms and four of them had lasting symptom relief (up to 12 months) (56). It is noteworthy that such stimulation parameters used in healthy subjects or in those with organic movement disorders have only small transitory effects on electrophysiological parameters and no effects on behaviour. Therefore a placebo response seems most likely.

Prognosis

Data on long-term prognosis are scarce, but most studies point to significant impact on quality of life. For example, one study comparing PMD patients and PD patients on different measures of disability and quality of life showed that patients with PMDs reported levels of disability similar to those seen in Parkinson's disease (57). In a long-term follow-up study, 90% of a group of 80 patients with a range of PMDs still had abnormal movements after a mean of 3.2 years after their initial assessment (58). In another study, a third of patients were employed at the time of follow-up, while 11.5% were on disability benefits and 1.3% were involved in litigation (59).

More optimistic studies of long-term outcome in PMD have shown that half the patients report an improvement in their symptoms at last follow-up (3–5 years after presentation) (13). Factors that predicted a favourable outcome were a short duration of illness, the patient's perception of effective treatment by the physician, and the presence of a co-morbid psychiatric diagnosis of depression or anxiety (which is therefore amenable to treatment) (58, 59). Negative outcome at long-term follow-up is associated with long-standing symptoms (more than 6 months) (3), insidious onset of movements, and a primary psychiatric disorder of hypochondriasis, factitious disorder, or malingering (52).

Conclusions

PMDs are common and disabling conditions, and as part of the spectrum of functional neurological illness represent a major source of distress and a huge financial burden to health and social care systems. Diagnosis is often challenging, and an important future line of research is to develop improved objective standardized diagnostic criteria. There has been a recent resurgence of research interest in functional disorders in general, and it is hoped that this will lead to improved biological understanding of these disorders. Even without this understanding, pragmatic treatment trials are feasible within this patient group. Patients with PMDs can recover, and research is urgently needed to find the most efficient treatments and service structures to manage their disabling symptoms.

References

1. Lempert T, Dieterich M, Huppert D, Brandt T. Psychogenic disorders in neurology: frequency and clinical spectrum. *Acta Neurol Scand* 1990; 82: 335–40.
2. Marsden CD. Hysteria—a neurologist's view. *Psychol Med* 1986; 16: 277–88.
3. Factor SA, Podskalny GD, Molho ES. Psychogenic movement disorders: frequency, clinical profile, and characteristics. *J Neurol Neurosurg Psychiatry* 1995; 59: 406–12.
4. Hallett M. Psychogenic movement disorders: a crisis for neurology. *Curr Neurol Neurosci Rep* 2006; 6: 269–71.
5. Hinson VK, Haren WB. Psychogenic movement disorders. *Lancet Neurol* 2006; 5: 695–700.
6. Jankovic J. Diagnosis and treatment of psychogenic parkinsonism. *J Neurol Neurosurg Psychiatry* 2011; 82: 1300–3.
7. Bhatia KP, Schneider SA. Psychogenic tremor and related disorders. *J Neurol* 2007; 254: 569–74.
8. Ranawaya R, Riley D, Lang A. Psychogenic dyskinesias in patients with organic movement disorders. *Mov Disord* 1990; 5: 127–33.
9. Schwingenschuh P, Pont-Sunyer C, Surtees R, Edwards MJ, Bhatia KP. Psychogenic movement disorders in children: a report of 15 cases and a review of the literature. *Mov Disord* 2008; 23: 1882–8.
10. Stone J, Carson A. Movement disorders: Psychogenic movement disorders. What do neurologists do? *Nat Rev Neurol* 2009; 5: 415–16.
11. Kranick S, Ekanayake V, Martinez V, Ameli R, Hallett M, Voon V. Psychopathology and psychogenic movement disorders. *Mov Disord* 2011; 26: 1844–50.
12. Stone J, Sharpe M, Binzer M. Motor conversion symptoms and pseudoseizures: a comparison of clinical characteristics. *Psychosomatics* 2004; 45: 492–9.
13. Jankovic J, Vuong KD, Thomas M. Psychogenic tremor: long-term outcome. *CNS Spectr* 2006; 11: 501–8.
14. O'Suilleabhain PE, Matsumoto JY. Time-frequency analysis of tremors. *Brain* 1998; 121: 2127–34.
15. Kumru H, Valls-Sole J, Valldeoriola F, Marti MJ, Sanegre MT, Tolosa E. Transient arrest of psychogenic tremor induced by contralateral ballistic movements. *Neurosci Lett* 2004; 370: 135–9.

16. Schwingenschuh P, Katschnig P, Seiler S, et al. Moving toward 'laboratory-supported' criteria for psychogenic tremor. *Mov Disord* 2011; 26: 2509–15.
17. Bhatia KP, Bhatt MH, Marsden CD. The causalgia–dystonia syndrome. *Brain* 1993; 116: 843–51.
18. Edwards MJ, Alonso-Canovas A, Schrag A, Bloem BR, Thompson PD, Bhatia K. Limb amputations in fixed dystonia: a form of body integrity identity disorder? *Mov Disord* 2011; 26: 1410–14.
19. Schrag A, Trimble M, Quinn N, Bhatia K. The syndrome of fixed dystonia: an evaluation of 103 patients. *Brain* 2004; 127: 2360–72.
20. Schwingenschuh P, Katschnig P, Edwards MJ, et al. The blink reflex recovery cycle differs between essential and presumed psychogenic blepharospasm. *Neurology* 2011; 76: 610–14.
21. van Rijn MA, Marinus J, Putter H, van Hilten JJ. Onset and progression of dystonia in complex regional pain syndrome. *Pain* 2007; 130: 287–93.
22. Edwards MJ, Bhatia KP, Cordivari C. Immediate response to botulinum toxin injections in patients with fixed dystonia. *Mov Disord* 2011; 26: 917–18.
23. Monday K, Jankovic J. Psychogenic myoclonus. *Neurology* 1993; 43: 349–52.
24. Fahn S. Psychogenic movement disorders. In: Marsden CD, Fahn S (eds) *Movement Disorders*, pp. 359–72. Oxford: Butterworth–Heinemann, 1994.
25. Shibasaki H, Hallett M. What is the Bereitschaftspotential? *Clin Neurophysiol* 2006; 117: 2341–56.
26. Esposito M, Edwards MJ, Bhatia KP, Brown P, Cordivari C. Idiopathic spinal myoclonus: a clinical and neurophysiological assessment of a movement disorder of uncertain origin. *Mov Disord* 2009; 24: 2344–9.
27. van der Salm SM, Koelman JH, Henneke S, van Rootselaar AF, Tijssen MA. Axial jerks: a clinical spectrum ranging from propriospinal to psychogenic myoclonus. *J Neurol* 2010; 257: 1349–55.
28. Hallett M. Psychogenic parkinsonism. *J Neurol Sci* 2011; 310: 163–5.
29. Benaderette S, Zanotti Fregonara P, Apartis E, et al. Psychogenic parkinsonism: a combination of clinical, electrophysiological, and [^{123}I]-FP-CIT SPECT scan explorations improves diagnostic accuracy. *Mov Disord* 2006; 21: 310–17.
30. de la Fuente-Fernandez R, Ruth TJ, Sossi V, Schulzer M, Calne DB, Stoessl AJ. Expectation and dopamine release: mechanism of the placebo effect in Parkinson's disease. *Science* 2001; 293: 1164–6.
31. Onofrj M, Bonanni L, Manzoli L, Thomas A. Cohort study on somatoform disorders in Parkinson disease and dementia with Lewy bodies. *Neurology* 2010: 74; 1598–606.
32. Sudarsky L. Psychogenic gait disorders. *Semin Neurol* 2006; 26: 351–6.
33. Baik JS, Lang AE. Gait abnormalities in psychogenic movement disorders. *Mov Disord* 2007; 22: 395–9.
34. Fekete R, Jankovic J. Psychogenic chorea associated with family history of Huntington disease. *Mov Disord* 2010; 25: 503–4.
35. Mejia NI, Jankovic J. Secondary tics and tourettism. *Rev Bras Psiquiatr* 2005; 27: 11–17.
36. Fahn S, Williams DT. Psychogenic dystonia. *Adv Neurol* 1988; 50: 431–55.
37. Gupta A, Lang AE. Psychogenic movement disorders. *Curr Opin Neurol* 2009; 22: 430–6.
38. Shill H, Gerber P. Evaluation of clinical diagnostic criteria for psychogenic movement disorders. *Mov Disord* 2006; 21: 1163–8.
39. Cojan Y, Waber L, Carruzzo A, Vuilleumier P. Motor inhibition in hysterical conversion paralysis. *NeuroImage* 2009; 47: 1026–37.
40. Stone J, Zeman A, Simonotto E, et al. FMRI in patients with motor conversion symptoms and controls with simulated weakness. *Psychosom Med* 2007; 69: 961–9.
41. Kirmayer LJ, Taillefer S. Somatoform disorders. In: Turner M, Hersen M (eds) *Adult psychopathology and diagnosis*, pp. 333–83. New York: John Wiley,1997.
42. Breuer J, Freud S. *Studies on hysteria*. Harmondsworth: Penguin, 1991.
43. Janet P. *The major symptoms of hysteria*. New York: Macmillan, 1907.
44. Voon V, Brezing C, Gallea C, Hallett M. Aberrant supplementary motor complex and limbic activity during motor preparation in motor conversion disorder. *Mov Disord* 2011; 26: 2396–403.
45. Voon V, Gallea C, Hattori N, Bruno M, Ekanayake V, Hallett M. The involuntary nature of conversion disorder. *Neurology* 2010; 74: 223–8.
46. Edwards MJ, Moretto G, Schwingenschuh P, Katschnig P, Bhatia KP, Haggard P. Abnormal sense of intention preceding voluntary movement in patients with psychogenic tremor. *Neuropsychologia* 2011; 49: 2791–3.
47. Pareés I, Saifee TA, Kassavetis P, et al. Believing is perceiving: mismatch between self-report and actigraphy in psychogenic tremor. *Brain* 2012; 135: 117–23.
48. Friston K. The free-energy principle: a unified brain theory? *Nat Rev Neurosci* 2010; 11: 127–38.
49. Hall-Patch L, Brown R, House A, et al. Acceptability and effectiveness of a strategy for the communication of the diagnosis of psychogenic nonepileptic seizures. *Epilepsia* 2010; 51: 70–8.
50. Hinson VK, Weinstein S, Bernard B, Leurgans SE, Goetz CG. Single-blind clinical trial of psychotherapy for treatment of psychogenic movement disorders. *Parkinsonism Relat Disord* 2006; 12: 177–80.
51. Sharpe M, Walker J, Williams C, et al. Guided self-help for functional (psychogenic) symptoms: a randomized controlled efficacy trial. *Neurology* 2011; 77: 564–72.
52. Voon V, Lang AE. Antidepressant treatment outcomes of psychogenic movement disorder. *J Clin Psychiatry* 2005; 66: 1529–34.
53. Dallocchio C, Arbasino C, Klersy C, Marchioni E. The effects of physical activity on psychogenic movement disorders. *Mov Disord* 2010; 25: 421–5.
54. Shamy MC. The treatment of psychogenic movement disorders with suggestion is ethically justified. *Mov Disord* 2010; 25: 260–4.
55. van Hilten BJ, van de Beek WJ, Hoff JI, Voormolen JH, Delhaas EM. Intrathecal baclofen for the treatment of dystonia in patients with reflex sympathetic dystrophy. *N Engl J Med* 2000; 343: 625–30.
56. Dafotakis M, Ameli M, Vitinius F, et al. [Transcranial magnetic stimulation for psychogenic tremor—a pilot study.] *Fortschr Neurol Psychiatr* 2011; 79: 226–33.
57. Anderson KE, Gruber-Baldini AL, Vaughan CG, et al. Impact of psychogenic movement disorders versus Parkinson's on disability, quality of life, and psychopathology. *Mov Disord* 2007; 22: 2204–9.
58. Feinstein A, Stergiopoulos V, Fine J, Lang AE. Psychiatric outcome in patients with a psychogenic movement disorder: a prospective study. *Neuropsychiatry Neuropsychol Behav Neurol* 2001; 14: 169–76.
59. Thomas M, Vuong KD, Jankovic J. Long-term prognosis of patients with psychogenic movement disorders. *Parkinsonism Relat Disord* 2006; 12: 382–7.

Index